F*CK PORTION CONTROL

A Rational Guide to Health and Happiness

NATHAN GUY HATCH

Seventh Edition, November 2025

ABOUT THIS BOOK

The concepts on human physiology and wellness put forth here are not always supported by studies, and a great part is derived only from my personal experience and unique observation of the human condition, hence the philosophical nature of this book and the recommendation that all personal medical decisions be made with a qualified and capable health professional. While broad, this work is hardly comprehensive and will change in future editions. Though there is much science it is not a book on science, and studies referenced during my hard-won quest for health are not cited because my aim is not to medically advise nor educate readers but to share my personal journey and insight.

Never in human history has information been so readily accessible, and through the efforts of fellow health-conscious advocates I was lucky to be exposed to the work of many biologists and researchers both present and deceased which helped me get well. I sincerely thank those who have uncovered the design of the natural world and the many scientists whose work underlies my own, for without their contributions I would be dead, and to those who supported my work and research as I would not have been able to accomplish this without your assistance and patronage.

To my LGBTQIA+ forefathers and advocates like Harvey Milk, Gloria Allred, Coretta Scott King, and the many tragic victims and champions of the HIV crisis who helped forge a more compassionate world—thank you. My life and this book were only possible because of you.

Content

For "family."

Nightbird

Nightbird singing on the wire outside,
Do you know that something's wrong?
Yes it seems like morning's on its way—
The city lights look like dawn.
Little Sentry keep on singing,
Not till morning cease your song.
For the restless hear your peaceful hymn
And the lonely get along.

INTRODUCTION

After a debilitating struggle with health and approaching death, unaided by doctors and abandoned by most people in my life I was forced to find my own solutions to health in order to not die. I was lucky to find such answers. But I also discovered answers to health problems which have plagued man for generations and I began excitedly sharing them with everyone on whose ear I could impose. Unfortunately I was still very sick, fat, and unhappy, and although I knew of what I was speaking not a single person listened. I watched in frustration as those around me fell into the same health traps as had complicated my own life, as the majority of people cannot see past their own nose let alone understand what the hell *nicotinamide adenine dinucleotide* is and why they should exhaust spare brainpower about it, for life these days does demand far more brainpower than it used to.

Eventually I gave up trying to help those around me, yet one day after a substantial number of requests for insight from internet strangers I was compelled to start a blog. I had previously attempted my hand at writing and was a little disheartened realizing my life was probably destined to spread boring health information rather than exciting tales of adventure and romance. After all, most people's eyes glazed over mere moments into discussing thyroid disease or the importance of coconut oil.

Soon however I found the unintended style of my personal experience and unmatched insight into human biology was relished by others suffering just as I had. The title of my book and blog, *Fuck Portion Control,* was the only title that popped into mind and it stayed there with as much persistence as the inspiration to start. These words originate from my great joy in realizing the error of everyone who ever promoted self-deprivation as a way to health and wellness which had instead led me headlong into so much misery and illness. The proper way to health and wellness it seemed was not in starvation, overexertion, and fanaticism of diet and lifestyle but from an almost hedonist approach. More and more my work continued to impress upon me the new realization that life trends not toward death and decay but to life and health, and the way there is always rooted in reason and common sense.

Part of the irreverent nature of my writing also required readers to remove preconceived entertainments which handicap not just pathways to good health but also to commonality among our fellows, which the lack thereof is a very real impediment to physical health due to stress of conflict, separation, bias, economic inequality, and misunderstanding which weighs heavily upon the endocrine system. As well, more interesting than truth to us is often what we *wish* to be true. Even when facing death, confirmation bias is far more comforting to a person than healing. Given a choice to survive cancer or an ideology which contributes to its development most people will choose the ideology and die, which just so happens to be the reason a cure has not yet been achieved as scientists and medical researchers charge down boulevards of discovery in every direction but the correct, as biases of yesterday turn the compass point of research today. Take for instance the great hormone serotonin. Considered for decades to be the so-called *'happiness hormone'* it has spurred countless studies, drugs, and reshaped the course of medical history, yet depression, anxiety, and other such diseases persist unchecked. Influenced by the bias that serotonin is "good," authors of new studies on the hormone take for granted that those assumed characteristics might not in fact be correct. What if serotonin isn't as has been described? It would mean that *all* studies on serotonin which assume its characteristics to be of a healing nature are flawed. This would certainly account for some of the failure of this particular arc of research to cure depression. Serotonin, as it turns out and as some studies are finally revealing, is not at all involved in happiness but is in fact a hormone of torpor (to slow things down). The mistaken characterization of it came from the apparent calming effect it had during experiments on the severely ill, who prior to treatment were excitable and erratic. By lowering the metabolic rate serotonin caused an *appearance* of therapy, which seemed to validate what was still entirely hypothetical. To the dismay of both patients and practitioners serotonin based medications often failed to heal these debilitating diseases in spite of much promise, and worsened things for countless others with side effects of such drugs as suicide and other mental deterioration. How could the hormone of happiness possibly carry a risk of suicide?

Our instinct to comply with authority and the status quo is so strong we often willingly sacrifice our own wellbeing, even our lives, rather than question it. Several years ago a young woman with advanced breast cancer was referred to me by someone else I helped. I gave her this book and told her to read the chapter on cancer right away, then the rest after, and to keep me updated on her progress. I had helped another person with stage-four breast cancer which had moved into her bones get an NED diagnosis (no evidence of disease), but about six months after giving this other woman my book she wrote and asked if I would post her crowdsource cancer fundraiser on my social media. I was confused and asked what she had been doing from my book, and she replied that she hadn't read any of it, not even the chapter on cancer, which only takes about thirty minutes to read. She still didn't read it after that, and sadly died a few months later.

I suffered from suicidal depression since the age of twelve, and after trying to commit suicide at twenty-one slowly drank myself to death for another fourteen years. Having discovered the cure for depression I would often try to help others, but nineteen in twenty will tell me to go fuck myself and that only doctors and pharmaceutical companies which have kept them chronically medicated have the authority to understand disease, which is not at all how knowledge works. One of my friends tragically took his life after refusing even to hear what I had to say about it. Had I known he was suicidal I would have been more forceful, but the reason that antidepressants don't cure depression is *because they don't fucking cure depression.* It is also well known that hair loss medications come with debilitating side effects including depression, loss of sex drive, and even more hair loss! But people continue taking and promoting them even while continuing to lose hair or suffering other harmful side effects. Most medications are in fact quite harmful and medications for things like depression, hair loss, thyroid dysfunction, diabetes, etc., which don't cure illness outright don't actually cure those conditions because it is more profitable to keep people chronically medicated. We then stay on our meds because we're told to. We exercise and diet because we're told to. We go to church because we're told to. We get chemo injected into our spine as a last resort during cancer and die an excruciating death worse than what would have occurred naturally because we're told to. We refuse to question authority, even in the face of irrefutable evidence that it harms us, and what we're NOT told to do is to treat ourselves with compassion, nor what nutrients and resources we need to care for the body and resist disease, nor how to get them and how to use them because that would be empowering, and if we're empowered we won't then have to buy what they are selling.

Ironically even the very studies used to support incorrect theories about health and medicine do contain valuable information, if you know how to look for it. I found answers and solutions to my own health problems from these studies, among others, because I learned how to read the information and find the evidence I was searching for. Thankfully there seems to be a growing motivation, in part from the backlash against the medical professions for failing to protect the health of the public, but also from increased awareness through social media and community organization to more willingly revisit accepted practices.

What *I* want to be true is that I am young and healthy again and have no problems whatsoever. Unfortunately there are and will always be limits to mortality that we must submit, but recognizing the bias of wanting something to be true helped me arrive at such accomplishments as what is in these pages, which stem from a new and comprehensive understanding of *why* diseases happen to the body and how to fix such conditions.

After being failed by institutions and finding some success through my own work I sought to discover the answers to so many health challenges and the practical and accessible ways in which healing could be accomplished so that barriers to good health might be more easily overcome. It is a good idea when reading this book to keep a notepad and paper handy to write down specific things which may be relevant to you.

This book is *not* professionally edited, so you must excuse my mistakes. tDo not make the mistake of thinking that because you don't identify with some of the chapters that you can afford not to read them—you, your friends, parents, siblings, and children are all human and subject to the same environmental factors which cause *all* disorders, and if you skip, say, the chapter on alcoholism you will miss very important information about the human body which can serve you in other capacities. Generally this book should be read from beginning to end, not skipping around at will as information is generally built upon and reliant on earlier chapters. And again, a paper and pencil are going to be your best tools in reading this book because you will not remember particular things due to the vast amount of information and will need to write down what you must do to improve your own condition.

Remember, like any worthwhile activity in life being healthy is not a destination, it is a practice. It is almost never too late to improve health, and you will be surprised how much healing the body is capable, if you only give it the chance.

Good luck.

CHAPTER 1
THE STAFF OF LIFE

A small town in northern Utah encircles a United States Air Force base, once maudlin farmland spattered by a few small cloned tract-home developments now as dense as a Los Angeles suburb, with as many or more shopping malls and certainly more malcontent, middle-class religionists. When I was eight the town had yet to reach its adolescence, and the only destinations of note was a small gas station at the entrance to our dirty little hillside neighborhood, the first place I ever ventured without the watchful eye of a parent, or the immense trash incinerator complex next door where in its scattered cooling ponds I and my brother and our friends would collect tadpoles into empty paint buckets and sentence them to an unintended yet ignominious death by asphyxiation in the bare-ribbed garage of our unfinished suburban-American rambler. As I was only eight, a dearth of amenities was not so high on my list of concerns, but that this void of a place where rocket-powered fighter planes shook our house with frightening regularity was the most idyllic place my parents could find to raise their burgeoning young family was perplexing even at that age because previous to this one-traffic-light seed of urban sprawl we had lived a few peaceful and joyous years on the island of Oahu, where the air is a weighted blanket scented with flowers and saltwater, playing under the burning sun and eating fresh road-side fruit after a long day of boogie-boarding in the kiddie surf, where I and my siblings possessed all the glee of naive, young island children and enjoyed the company of a diverse set of friends.

Before Hawaii too we lived in Newport Beach, California, though our time there well preceded the invasion of the rich obtuse, a small aluminum washing bin for our pool was more enchanting than any fancy, olympic-sized luxury, minutes from the ocean and secure in the swaddling arms of the Southern Californian economy. Yet as well my birth, which had transpired a year previous to Newport occurred just outside of Phoenix, Arizona where my architect father and beauty-queen mother had begun their union after finding Los Angeles a little too hot-blooded for their conservative sentiments, where after winning the title of Miss Arizona in 1972 and achieving tenth most beautiful in the Miss America pageant my mother effortlessly segued into Hollywood as one of the original *Barker's Beauties* on *The Price is Right*, a scene in the television show *CHiPs*, and a contract as an Orange Crush Soda spokesmodel till my suave, red-meat-and-potatoes and cream-on-his-cereal working class father seduced her away from a wealthy surgeon and the glitzy lights of fame and fortune with promises of a quiet life of six children, financial uncertainty, and forty years traipsing across the western half of the United States. I don't blame her—If I met a man like my father, even knowing what my future held, I would make the exact same decision. But moderately cosmopolitain couple they were, living in such a small town did prove suffocating, so trips to Europe or Mexico were frequent, my siblings and I distracted from our regular abandonment by the lavishing of small prizes won from adventures far and exotic. Asked later why they carted us off from an island paradise my parents said they had grown tired of constantly good weather. In reality my dad had been offered a lucrative involvement in a real estate development scheme, which unfortunately never materialized. My father *did* love skiing though, at a level resembling religious devotion, and as Oahu has no ski resorts I can see how the call of the Rocky Mountains might also have won out.

So rather than basking in the heat of Phoenix, partying on the shores Orange County, or surfing the tranquil tides of Oahu it was in this dreary, sullen Northern Utah town I one day found myself at eight-years of age dancing in my underwear atop spare carpet squares in an unfinished concrete basement to Whitney Houston's '*I Want to Dance With Somebody.' Yes!* I thought with all the naivety of an eight-year-old, *how great that would be to dance with somebody. That's all I need to be happy.* The song was full of pining joy, an uninhibited lust for life, and no less than a very angel of heaven was confirming that the hopes and wishes being instilled within me as a child would bear out unfettered through a life of inclusion and togetherness, and that my deepest wish fulfilled merely required its utterance. In such a crowded house, as all five of my siblings had now been born, it was indeed a rare moment to be alone. As the soaring vocals punched through the cold basement air my limbs bounced and twirled with all the delight a child like me could summon. At the height of this party for one, in the midst of a blissfully ignorant celebration of life the strange and unexpected thought occurred that I was perhaps enjoying this song a lot more than might other boys. The horror that they would outright despise it was a thought to be banished! For a moment I felt embarrassed, but also perplexed as to why my lovely time was so suddenly spoiled with what I would later come to know as shame. In a moment I knew for the first time that I was different, though not a soul had yet to tell me so. Perhaps I simply knew by instinct that dancing to Whitney Houston in his underwear was not something my very male father would do, the man I so much wanted to be like. A satisfying resolution to my dilemma was not forthcoming, so I did not stop dancing, but there was a little less enthusiasm, a little less innocence. My childhood naivety had sprung its first leak.

In that dry, empty cul-de-sac there were three other boys my age. Sean, who lived in the house to our left was missing one hand and forearm, retaining only a few inches of limb past his elbow which ended in a blunt but perfectly smooth stump save for a button of skin at the end tied like the knot of a balloon. Sean was kind and fun and anticipated that others might consider his lost arm and immediately offered an explanation for the absence of it the first time I met him (he was born that way). Cody, who lived to my right was a specimen of a young man—brazen, hot-headed, and handsome as the devil. I could never quite decide if I loved or feared Cody, trying my best to keep up with his feverish athleticism and determination I more often found myself stymied by an inability to match the inexhaustible energy and aggressiveness, which only served to inflame my obsession which of course I had no understanding of, as I was only eight. Brian, who lived far up the hill, was a different story. Less complex, I found ease in relating to him. Brian and I played together constantly. We seemed to be the same kind of boy, finding refuge with each other from those unspecified characteristics possessed of other boys. That he had a brother the same age as my own made us four a common sight roaming the dusty hilltop neighborhood.

One bright spring day I bounded up to Brian's house and knocked on the door. His mother answered, as she always did, and directed me to the basement to join my friends. Like our house the Smith's basement was also unfinished, but where our stairs were carpeted and walls painted theirs was entirely a bare skeleton of construction lumber and makeshift storage. Stepping into the dim, muted light was like descending into the abandoned lair of a mad scientist—perfect for a handful of small-town American boys. While it wasn't unusual for us to lack some clothing in the hot, dry summers, all of my friends were in various stages of total undress. The air was quiet, stiff with an unfamiliar expectation.

"What are you doing?" I asked, immediately infected by the energy which seemed to jump from one boy to another. "Playing," said Brian.

"Guess what?" said our friend Jeff.

"What?"

"Michael can do the naked boogie dance."

The what?" I replied, giggling at the word naked, my curiosity immediately piqued since I had never heard of such a dance. Michael smiled nervously, but unhesitatingly removed his underwear, buck naked on the bare concrete in all his glory and began to swing his wiener around and around in what we grown men later learn is properly called a *helicopter.* "HA!" I shouted, suddenly feeling nervous but also excited. I had never seen another person be so free with their own body. I was *not* supposed to get naked with other people, my mother had said. Well, specifically she had warned us against *touching* privates, not so much being naked, so technically I was not yet in violation of her rigid expectations. The other boys laughed too, no doubt confused by similarly strange new feelings which began to tumble around inside my stomach. I was smart enough to know this would not pass muster, and keen to obey my parents, but it really did not seem like a dangerous situation, and I loved my friends and had many questions roaming my mind about the human body which had yet to be addressed by anyone. The thought of twirling my own wiener in such a manner seemed like something that really would be quite fun, and harmless.

Our neighbor friend and Brian's brother joined in too, little boy wieners twirling everywhere though I could not muster the courage to remove my own clothes, as the conflict between what I wanted to do and what I had been told had not yet come to a consensus. "Want to play a game?" said Brian, segueing into a new idea as if twirling our penises was the most normal thing in the world, which for boys our age actually is if they don't grow up in body-shaming, abusive communities. I didn't reply, as my mouth had sealed up from anticipation. "It's called mommy-cow, baby-cow," he explained before gathering together two old barstools in the corner of the room. He placed them methodically about a foot apart, and laid across both to let his wiener hang down between them. My excitement fully shifted to panic as Michael got on his knees beneath Brian and put his mouth where I never expected a mouth could be put.

I would not see the remainder of this scenario since I was suddenly outside and running breathless down the hill toward home. Halfway I immediately knew I regretted this decision, being both brave and a coward in the same moment, and that somehow I would regret it for the rest of my life. I almost turned around to go back, but then I would have felt embarrassed for running away. I was missing out on something important, something that would bring me closer to my friends but which I didn't have the perspective to fully understand. The fear of my parents was stronger than my desire to belong, already knowing I was different, a doubling of my efforts to conform would be needed in order to survive. So I continued home, missing out on the first of many coming of age experiences.

Boys have been playing with each other since the dawn of man (and for that matter boys and girls, and girls and girls). A very thoughtful perspective from author Jane Ward considers that straight males engage in sexual contact with each other as children and young adults to confirm their heterosexuality. By experiencing intimacy with other men their attraction to women, which is many degrees greater, is made more obvious by comparison and thus cements their sexual identity. This is devastating to us homosexual boys who fall in love with them at these intersections of growing up only to find those boys veer off toward women when they begin adolescence, something we do not comprehend. Indeed the many gay men I know who had sexual contact with peers now partnered with women shows how men as boys find out that they are attracted to one sex or the other by comparing the degree of response to interactions with each (not all sexual) but which contact also brings inclusion and acceptance and love with their fellows as well. For young gay boys such as I these encounters are our first foray into the sexual contact of our different orientation (although I would not even kiss another person until I was nineteen), and we enter into adulthood and find contact with our own sex the overwhelming satisfaction. This lack of inhibition in children toward one another is in fact one of the reasons why sexual abuse by adults is so traumatic to them, because the adult who is by definition not a peer and by exploiting this vulnerability in children is not an appropriate object of the child's psychological curiosity, and so their actions destroy this part of development in their victims. That fateful day as an eight-year-old boy where I chose to obey my parents at the price of my own wellbeing may be described by those with a prudish attitude as a moment in which I turned away from temptation. But sexual abuse can occur without physical contact whatsoever, when cultures expose children to excessive and inappropriate discussions about sex and private parts, especially when accompanied by shame, which may even be motivated from an adult's own experience of abuse but which is actually disruptive to a child's normal development. My friends might have even got the idea for their games from the constant obsession with sex and its characterization by the conservative, religious community in which we were raised, which usually begins before we were even old enough to comprehend it. What actually occurred that day in my friends basement was a severance of my ability to relate to others, regardless of gender, in order to comply with perceived expectations, to act on fear rather than courage because of inappropriate conditioning, and was the beginning of a life sentenced to psychological and emotional isolation, never learning the talent of drawing close to others, a debility which would compound the long, harsh decline of of my physical and mental health over the next thirty years and which would eventually nearly cost me my life not once, but twice.

A few weeks later my dad came home one day with bikes for us four older children, all of which except mine had training wheels. "Don't I need training wheels?" I asked as he steadied the little blue *Husky* brand bike while I fiddled with the black, velcro strapped pad wrapped round the crossbar between the handles. "I'm pretty sure I need training wheels."

"You don't need training wheels," chided my father. "Riding a bike is easy." "But dad—" I protested. I knew I needed to be tough, like Cody, especially since he might well be watching from his front windows and might only be interested in being friends with someone who was tough like he was, or so I thought. I also knew I didn't know how to ride a bike, and training wheels were supposed to help one learn. "I think I should start with training wheels."

"Training wheels are for wimps," my dad continued. "I'll keep it steady." His assurance was nothing of the sort, but having accepted responsibility for my well-being and seeing that he was my father after all and I was supposed to trust him, climbed on the bike. It wobbled under my weight but his strong hands, dwarfing the handlebars, kept it upright. "Alright," he said, and began to slowly advance me down the driveway toward my siblings, who joyfully and naively careened around the cul-de-sac, training wheels scraping loudly on the hot asphalt, as I envied their immediate, naive indulgence. "Start pedaling," he said. "I'll give you a push."

"What?" I shouted. "Don't let go!" "You'll do fine—" the reply was curt, unconcerned at an unacceptable level. He began to push harder. "No, dad!" I started to protest, but he was so big the bike kept moving forward. "You'll be fine" he repeated, pushing faster. "NO!" I yelled louder, my shoulders shoved up under my ears, hands welded to the plastic handles from which blue plastic streamers fluttered gaily in the summer breeze, taunting me. The fixed-gear pedals moved my feet, not the other way around as the bike moved faster and faster across the open cul-de-sac, whizzing past the asphalt ground as I cut through the group of my siblings.

"Pedal!" shouted my dad, whose voice was now far behind me. I was alone. *He had let go.* But the bike was inexplicably upright, held by some ghostly and unreliable mechanism, yet the curb on the other side was fast approaching like a tsunami of concrete, and dried tumble weeds in the empty lot beyond portended a swift and painful death. "Turn!" he then shouted, "turn the handlebars!" His voice was distant, mocking, but I could not turn. No one had taught me. The information was not in my brain and would not be by the time death arrived. If I moved the handle bars the bike would surely plant me into the asphalt, which on account of things was definitely worse than the relatively softer, dry brush. It did not matter anyway since it seemed I had lost control of my body entirely. The volume at which he shouted did nothing to help my little brain scramble for instructions to save myself. How could he not see all of this? *Stop shouting!*

The bike's front tire smashed into the end of the street and I let out what was surely neither a brave nor manly scream as I went over the front of the bike. As I watched the weeds pass beneath my soaring body the fear of dying was immediately supplanted by a hatred for my father. I had put my trust with him, my very life into his hands, and over my own intelligent protests had condemned me to an embarrassing end to a very short and uneventful life. If I lived beyond this moment, which I surely would not, I would never trust him again. The ground hit me hard, tumbleweeds ripping my face, arms, and ears. I suddenly found myself staring into the sky as the bike fell into the dirt next to me, a moment later flooded by a delayed onset of pain that was really more psychological that physical. Even so, I could not subdue my tears, especially not as my father wrested me from the ground and began to roughly smack the dust from my clothes. I did not want to cry but I could not stop it. My dad laughed a nervous, ungainly laugh which is laughed by men who have failed at the only job that truly matters but who are too proud to say they are sorry. Being the age I was only heard laughing, and through a torrent of furious sobs swore that I would never get on that bike again until it had training wheels, and ran into the house.

Later that night my mother made us grilled cheese sandwiches for dinner, because if my childhood had a theme that theme is wheat and melted cheese, as it was these two ingredients which formed the foundation of almost all our nutrition. No doubt I was smiling and happy again by dinnertime, presented with the sight of gooey, drippy grilled cheese sandwiches or macaroni swimming in cheese sauce accompanied by slices of hot-dog, or perhaps what my mother called *cheese crisps*, which were large flour tortillas topped with cheddar cheese and broiled under the broiler until blistering and crispy, dripping with delicious cheese-oil and served with tomato soup. Even meals already composed of wheat like macaroni or other pasta had bread and butter as a regular actor, although butter at this time was not actually butter but that obscene imposter, margarine. Not quite the behemoth I would become I nonetheless resented the size of the macaroni box, which when distributed evenly among six children and two adults hardly served to satisfy the hedonist portions of which all macaroni and cheese should be enjoyed. Like most middle-class suburban families during the closing years of the twentieth century, variety was not a priority because it was also not an option. We were, however, lucky to be indulged by my father's culinary talents on weekends and holidays, when dinners consisted of roasts, chicken fettuccini, or even Kalua Pig which had come with us from our time on Oahu as a cherished family tradition, all of which came with bread and margarine because this was the eighties when food conglomerates tried to convince people their cheap, disgusting butter substitutes were healthy. Other variations on bread were of course delicious peanut butter and jelly or honey sandwiches, that blessed smell which wafts from a freshly opened lunchbox at noon of crystallized honey and the melding of bread and peanuts still invades my memory on quiet days.

One night when my father was away my infant sister would not stop crying. I had never been truly scared before and seeing the look of fear in my mother's face terrified me to my core. The pain was so severe my little sister passed out, though by that time I had thankfully gone to bed. I can't imagine my own mother's pain at experiencing something like that. Eventually she made it to the emergency room and it was discovered that my sister had a severe ear infection (and also that it is not uncommon for children to cry so hard they actually pass out). The doctor made her well with antibiotics, but infections plagued her for years until the age of four when she underwent an uncomfortable operation to install plastic tubes in her ear canal to keep them open but which also prevented her from swimming most of her childhood because the tubes made water entry into the ear dangerous, and the whole experience was rather traumatic for her.

It turns out this condition, and many like it such as that I would soon suffer, is actually caused by wheat. Though wheat has traditionally been a cornerstone of Western civilization, enshrined even in scripture, it was adulterated around 1960 when a well-meaning man named Norman Borlaug worked to make breeds of wheat more robust and hearty and could survive in more climates around the world and feed more hungry people (which it did). Novel artificial fertilizers which made it possible to grow crops in arid, poor quality soil also made wheat grow too tall and thin, and a strong wind would come along and easily destroy an entire year's crop. So he hybridized a stouter and sturdier version of wheat, and in so doing helped stabilize food resources in many parts of the world and helped to spare countless people from hunger. His intentions were noble, and he rightly received a Nobel Prize for his work, but the resulting wheat which makes up most wheat and wheat products available today is also much harder to digest, the same characteristics that make it resistant to wind and climate also make it more resistant to digestion, although some were already more difficult anyway through previous agricultural hybridization.

Wheat flour is also often mandated by law to have added iron which is a valuable nutrient required by pathogenic opportunistic microbes to infect us and cause disease. Normally iron in food is bound to the food matrix and is safer for us to ingest, but iron fortification of food is nothing more than added metal shavings which freely supports opportunistic microbes to then more easily cause disease such as what was suffered by my sister. Over the intervening decades more and more people have become aware of the difficulty of digesting common wheat, which is what has led to the increase in gluten allergies and gluten free trends but which is a very real impediment to not only digestive health but that of the body as a whole. Proteins and peptides (which are fragments of protein) have signaling effects within the human body and undigested gluten acts like an over-excited kid in a high-rise elevator, pressing all sorts of unhelpful buttons. It creates massive inflammation and discomfort in the gut and the body, causing or contributing to everything from migraines to shutting down the immune system and even promoting cancer. Fortifying food with iron is then like adding gasoline to a fire, with gluten suppressing the immune response and iron fueling the growth of disease causing organisms. The gut is rich in nutrients and a major target for literally thousands of different microorganisms (discussed more thoroughly in the upcoming chapter on gut health), but because of the hardiness of youthful digestive systems, which enviously seem to get away with murder, adults take many years before they are forced to accept the limited ability of our system to dismantle certain foods. By then it often seems a mystery as to what exactly has caused the accursed wretchedness which becomes the eventual state of the human gut.

Contrary to long held belief, not a single thing in in all of creation aside from fruit and milk are intended as food for humans. Potatoes, oats, lettuce, broccoli, chicken, beef, and fish all do not want to be eaten, and nature has done its damnedest not only to dissuade consumption of these organisms but in some cases developed methods for actually surviving or impairing digestion. Most plants contain astringent, bitter traits not to build character but because they are chemical deterrents to being eaten, or to protect their own nutritional resources which our tongue senses knowing these anti-nutritive chemicals are a warning not that this unpalatable thing will make us lean and healthy but that it has something in it which disagrees with our physiology, because the role of the tongue is to do just this—prompt us to what is good and what is not. Many grains, legumes, and tough leaves also contain enzyme inhibitors and cannot be digested at all without cooking (try chewing on some raw wheat berries sometime and no matter how long it is chewed it will not break down). Some of these properties of plants are truly toxic, such as the solanine toxins in the family of nightshades, although the varieties we consume as food have been skillfully bred by our ancestors to reduce their potency, which also addresses the little known fact that almost none of the plants we consume from the grocery store appear as they did in nature but have been coaxed and prodded by generations of farmers to become what they are now. Gluten is not a part of wheat so that bread will rise—it is there to enable the wheat plant to grow robustly from the seed, to survive harsh conditions until it germinates, and to help store energy and nutrients. Indeed it is the tougher gluten which allows wheat to grow in the harsh conditions of different climates under the influence of artificial fertilizers, but which then makes it less digestible to the very creatures who created it. Cynical voices deride gluten-free 'trends,' but people don't often do things just for the hell of it—that takes too much time, energy, and inconvenience, and there has simply been a growing recognition that the long gastrointestinal suffering of many millions of people is rooted in wheat.

Another characteristic of all grains, as well as legumes and most plants, is the presence of a compound called *phytic acid*, which is a molecule designed by nature to prevent leaching of nutrients out of the plant when wet. If the plant did not have phytic acid water would then leach precious calcium, magnesium, zinc, sulfur, and other nutrients and thus rob it of the ability to survive and grow. Unfortunately in the last few decades it has become commonly thought that eating whole and unrefined grains is healthier, because our parents and grandparents were apparently lazy and indulgent with all their peeling and threshing and refining and all that. Nothing could be further from the truth, and our parents prepared food the way they did not because refined flour is more palatable (although it is, remember that the tongue's job is to detect what is edible) but because our ancestors intuitively discovered that preparing food in such a way *improved* health and outcomes of mortality. They recognized the apparent skill of the tongue as an organ and used its guidance to find out what things we could eat and which we cannot (although there was some trial and error too). Peeling a plant food such as potatoes or carrots removes the part which contains what is generally referred to as anti-nutrients, not for the plant, but for us, and can be anything from a rather benign compound to ones which are outright toxic. Solanine in nightshades such as the potato is contained mostly in the skin (but also in any green parts), so failing to remove the skin puts a potent toxin into food. The role of solanine and related glycoalkaloids is to protect plants like potatoes, tomatoes, eggplant, and peppers from nematodes. The toxin functions by overstimulating their parasympathetic nervous cells and the nematodes are killed by their own nervous system. Because we are so large the small amounts of solanine aren't obviously harmful to us, but with repeated exposure it still can and does cause neurological damage which results in agitation, restlessness, insomnia, and even diseases like alcoholism and drug addiction as discussed in that upcoming chapter. It is no coincidence that when my family decided to stop peeling potatoes because we had heard it was "healthy" we also experienced some of our most emotionally turbulent years. Similarly, phytic acid is contained mostly in skins or the outer coverings in many vegetables, nuts, seeds, and whole grains, which is why the unrefined grain tastes less pleasant to us than the refined portion, because the tongue senses the presence of phytic acid, and is why our ancestors intuitively evolved technology to refine, peel, process, remove, or separate those parts which are undesirable and other methods of treating food for our safe consumption such as the sprouting, soaking, and fermenting of grains, seeds, and nuts which thusly inactivates phytic acid. If not properly treated by soaking or fermenting, whole grain diets can actually cause catastrophic tooth loss, insomnia, and bone disorders because of the inhibitory effect of phytic acid on calcium (especially if the diet is low in calcium). My generation was the first to be subjugated to the hastily borne craze of whole wheat bread and grain products, to say nothing of the toxic and allergenic additives that are in commercial bread, and it was no coincidence that my sister began developing ear problems at the same time my mother began feeding her the first tastes of solid foods which, as most parents know, includes soft pieces of bread but if made from common wheat and fortified with added iron is like the opposite of antibiotics and a potent promoter of pathogenic microbes.

Historically, bread has been healthy when it was made of pre-hybridized grain, especially because fermentation by yeasts not only helps break down phytate but also generate B vitamins and other nutrients which make them more digestible, but the inclusion of modern, common wheat in industrial food systems and the addition of toxic iron and other additives strongly promote opportunistic micro-organisms which then colonize the gut and body to produce outsized amounts of toxic metabolic byproducts which then overwhelm our body's detoxification organs. Over time (or immediately in those more sensitive) this causes tissues to swell, and the swelling causes a loss of robust metabolic function in what is generally referred to as inflammation, further causing or contributing to degenerative illnesses. For my young sister it meant her body could not fight nor repair the bacterial infection in the ear canal, nor prevent the swelling which shrank them, and so a chronic condition developed which would have cleared naturally if the offending food been simply identified and removed and the diet anchored in more healthful fruits and vegetables. But even parents who know their children's conditions are exacerbated by gluten still feed it to their children, too comfortable with their routine to bother making the healthy choice which would not only spare their children, but themselves as well, persisting even with debilitating stomachaches and other metabolic diseases directly related to consumption of common wheat because of how we attempt to control our lives and those within it in response to our own experiences of trauma. Common wheat has rightly been implicated as a contributing factor to the symptoms in those with autism, and it is not as common as it should be for families to notice this and to rethink their diets. But this does not mean that only gluten allergic types have issues with wheat as every human has difficulty digesting the hardier gluten strains. It is only that some bodies are healthy enough to overcome the consequences more easily than others. Every time a heavy meal of pasta, pizza, or a sandwich results in fatigue, stomachaches, or indigestion it is evidence that gluten or similarly incompatible foods are tearing apart your gut and thus your metabolic health. Less obviously, connections of sleep troubles, difficulty staying lean, building muscle, and even problems like erectile dysfunction or depression are all also related to such inflammatory dietary factors, and surprisingly resolved quickly when the offending food is simply replaced with better options. One day when discussing her children's health issues I recommended to another sister that she serve fruit and cheese for lunches instead of sandwiches, to alleviate the stressful mood swings exhibited by her high-strung young ones. She retorted that making sandwiches was easier, and would not change. In a way she is right, change is difficult. But putting a pile of cheese and apple slices on a plate is demonstrably a less demanding task than preparing sandwiches. If you also factor the relief which comes from calmer, less ill children the benefit would add up even more. But mentally it is easier to cling to our traditions, to do what we know, even if it is harmful, and so our problems compound themselves from an unwillingness to change.

At twenty-six, still spreading my wings in the great city of Los Angeles, I one day realized I hadn't been able to breathe through both nostrils simultaneously for some time. My health had improved somewhat since moving to the balmy climate of Southern California, but I now frustratingly struggled to clear my sinuses at any moment of the day and tried to use nasal sprays, antihistamines, or more exercise to clear the passages, but was soon driven mad by constant blockage and nothing seemed to work. Even after trying prescription decongestant the condition soon worsened into a full-blown sinus infection which required a visit to an emergency room for antibiotics. The infection cleared but my sinuses continued to tango with each other, and before a month was over I got *another* sinus infection after which another round of antibiotics also failed to permanently clear the passageways, and before I knew it was going on a year bouncing from one sinus infection to the next about once a month. It was the first serious physical health complication that I would endure and my doctor suggested I have surgery, but I didn't understand why surgery would fix a problem obviously caused by germs and was not as eager to go under the knife as other people. I had also developed sleep issues, though not as severe as they would become, and problems with my emotional health had accompanied me for so long I was now taking them as the condition of my life. I also had frequent and debilitating stomachaches, almost daily, sometimes so severe I would have to call in sick to work, but because my father and so many other adults were also plagued with chronic stomach problems I assumed that gut-tearing pain was a normal condition of adulthood and accepted my miserable fate as something to be endured rather than cured until one day on a lunch date with a handsome nurse when I mentioned my sinus and gut issues. "You're probably allergic to gluten." "What's gluten?" I asked. Actually, I knew what gluten was. I'd been cooking for some time and liked to even make my own breads occasionally, especially as pizza. I had also tried going without meat or dairy for months in an attempt to cure myself, and been consuming meat-free alternatives which are often made from gluten. He explained how gluten can cause allergic reactions, that most aren't aware of it because it takes up to a full day or more for food to transit to the lower intestine which is where the allergic reaction takes place, and many people erroneously identify other foods as the source of their complaint. True to this misidentification I had assumed dairy might be the problem, even though long-term abstinence did nothing to improve my condition, nor had a vegetarian diet. Desperate for some relief I immediately tried avoiding all sources of gluten—wheat, barley, even oats, as well as fake meat made from gluten and not one week later both of my sinuses suddenly opened at once for the first time in more than a year, an epiphany heralded by the triumphant return of fresh air flowing freely through my head. I didn't need any more convincing that wheat was causing my health problems, but the disappearance of those debilitating stomachaches and a notable increase in my energy levels two weeks later seemed to show that wheat had been a lot more of a liability than I ever could have imagined, and I would never again be bothered by even small stomachaches except on occasions when the temptation for a pizza or doughnut rudely reminded me just how real were the problems with common wheat.

Excited by my discovery I right away told my parents, who had experienced similar although less debilitating symptoms over the years. "But wheat is the staff of life," said my mother. She said it not so much in rebuttal but I think in coming to terms with new, contradicting information to what she had always believed. It took more than ten years to get them to even cut back on wheat, even with the obviousness of its burden to their own health, and still do not entirely avoid and willingly persisting with the same health problems they have endured for decades while I have been entirely relieved of those health problems. Our dietary traditions are sometimes so entrenched in emotion and family sentiment we are unable to step back and objectively analyze the situation for what it is. The resistance comes in the fear of change, of newness, of letting go of control, but the results from improving diet can mean less stress and suffering over the long term and resolution of health problems, not only of a metabolic nature but also those which are aesthetic. If my parents had known the myriad of physical challenges suffered by their children were rooted in diet, those terrifying nights with my little sister, and my life-long health issues which were all rooted in the presence of this undigestible allergen would never have happened. Sadly what was meant to help the world has instead contributed to disease and discomfort. Many of us are no longer dying from hunger, but we *are* still dying. Initially my experience with gluten was one of necessary total abstinence, because I did not yet know the intricacies of food chemistry. Even after years without having even a single bit of wheat a slip-up would send my health crashing. But bread and other grain products can still have a place in the diet, if they are made of safe grains and properly prepared as discussed in the upcoming chapter *Good Bread*. The thought of giving up pizza and pasta is rightly a depressing one and isn't even necessary if care and effort are taken to make them healthy, and my journey has been nothing if not one to confirm the joys of living. Importantly, eating the way which promotes health is not one of deprivation nor of limitation, but rather *replacement*, and exchanging allergic and problematic foods for those which are equally satisfying and indulgent rather than just avoiding them is the best approach to achieving success, otherwise the pain of deprivation prevents compliance and makes us miserable. Instead of making pancakes from conventional flour I enjoy spelt, yeast-risen pancakes every weekend, slathered in heaping amounts of delicious, organic grass-fed butter and indulgent maple syrup, or occasionally sprouted oats cooked in grass-fed milk. Where there were almost a daily occurrence I have now had only about three or four stomachaches over the last ten years of my life, and not only are these foods not hurting my health, they are actually healing and often more tasty than the options which are harmful to begin with.

Replacing foods which contribute to illness is not an arduous, joyless process. Quite the opposite the diet becomes one which is more satisfying and indulgent, and only requires a little knowledge and some careful planning. When visiting my late grandparents shortly after my gluten discovery I mentioned to my Nana that I had given up bread and found great relief, thinking I might enlighten her since her own children seemed to suffer the same condition. "Oh yes," she replied. "I haven't had a piece of bread since 1974. It gave me stomachaches."

Thanks Nana.

CHAPTER 2
THE TRUTH ABOUT FAT

By the age of twelve we had relocated to Salt Lake City. The move had been difficult but I was finally developing into a young man, already around six feet in height, and the crowds of people and things to do in a real city made life much more exciting than that drab little town in Northern Utah. One bright summer day I bounded up the brand new polished oak staircase of the second-floor addition to our new home my father had spent the last six months building. With no open land in the city on which to develop homes my father had taken to restoring old and dilapidated properties, usually while we lived in them. My whole family was gathered on my parents huge master bed, laughing and chatting and playing games. The sight of my loving family gathered in such joy and harmony filled me with a sense of peace and serenity. "You're getting fat," said my dad as I stood at the top of the staircase. *What?* I thought, my smile instantly replaced by a red-hot flush of shame. Instinctively I sucked in my gut, peering down at my torso in shame, less to inspect my own figure than to escape their gaze. My shirt was tucked into my jeans which made it impossible to hide the gut spilling over them. Suddenly I was an outcast, an awkward teenager, stuck between adolescence and the shelter of childhood enjoyed even at that moment by my ignorant siblings, unable to escape the temperamental whims of those two adults who ran this house but who kept me continually at arms length. "You need to go on a diet," mom agreed. "You should workout," said my dad. "Yes," agreed my mom as she pet my dad's chest. "Women like big chest muscles." Both of them smiled as if they had imparted valuable insight for which I should be grateful. But I turned around and fled downstairs before the tears could give me away. In the bathroom, tears streaming down my face, I looked at my stomach in the mirror. *Was I really fat?* My gut did seem to extend outward a little. I sucked it in again, and it disappeared entirely, an acceptable fix for now but what was *a diet?* What was working out? I had never done any of these things. Even if I had known what diet to do, my parents were the food providers for the family. I wasn't the one shopping or preparing food, nor could I even if I wanted to. At the time neither of my parents exercised, and I had never been to a gym or even knew that people ran on treadmills or lifted weights in order to be thin and fit. I spent every day that summer and the following school year sucking in my gut, terrified of being perceived as fat, but my parents never mentioned the words diet or workout to me again.

In reality my twelve-year-old body was perfect. Most children gain weight at the onset of puberty as the body prepares for a demanding growth process to come, because fats are required for the massive increase in hormones required of puberty, and indeed I grew a great deal shortly after, reaching nearly six-foot seven-inches tall by the time I turned nineteen. While all children should eat a healthy diet, no child should ever *go on a diet*, and too many people are terrorized by inappropriate conceptions of fat, health, and diet, shamed by misguided and manipulative people and incorrect ideas of physical wellness. For instance, the word *gluttony* does not actually mean that someone eats too much and gets fat—gluttony means to eat in excess *while others go hungry*. It is a Santa Claus type guilt-trip meant to address food inequality, to enlighten the well-off of their ignorance, selfishness, and neglect of those who suffer, to encourage them to help their fellow man, but its meaning has been corrupted to avail those with wealth and abundance and relieve them of the responsibility of sharing, to absolve their selfishness and instead shift shame to those who have difficulty with weight as if weight is amoral but not the refusal to help those in need.

And yet many still go hungry while those more fortunate choose to give up food voluntarily, not to help others mind you but in attempts to achieve self-centered satisfaction of vanity. If you really believe calorie deprivation makes good aesthetics, switch socioeconomic classes—You'll never have enough to eat. But poor people are often overweight, even when they go hungry. I once heard some asshole claim that poor minorities with obesity drank too much orange juice. As if they could afford it. But fat as macronutrient is the densest source of calories we can eat. At 5% cow milk has about the same saturated fat content as human milk, though store bought whole cow milk has less fat than human milk, having some cream removed to sell separately and to make butter. Removal of fat from milk for other products is why there is also for sale things like 2%, 1%, and skim milk which are marketed to ignorant consumers as a health product and not, in fact, actually an opportunistic industry trying to sell waste products to consumer in order to increase their profit margins.

Fats also come in three different chemical types—saturated, monounsaturated, and polyunsaturated. The term *saturation* is a reference to the frequency of chemical bonds on a fatty acid molecule. Fully saturated fats have no shared bonds, monounsaturated have one shared bond (*mono* means one), and polyunsaturated have two or more shared bonds (*poly* means many). Saturated fats which occur in high percentages in foods like butter, cream, and milk, is claimed to be the root of much disease and obesity, which is why more than three quarters of all infants are considered obese.

Are you paying attention to what you're reading? Babies aren't considered obese, yet they feed exclusively on full-fat, highly saturated-fat milk. If saturated fat causes obesity, why are babies not obese? Why aren't they dying of heart disease at alarming rates, since it is the highly saturated fat of milk on which they feed entirely? If it was the case that saturated fats cause human illness then babies should be the prime reflection of those illnesses. They are pretty slovenly after all.

They can't even wipe themselves. Harp seals whose milk-fat is almost 50% are even more lazy, sunning on ice floes all day, hardly spending much time in the freezing saltwater to hunt. If fat is bad then why is it in the food made by nature for our precious and fragile babies? Why do young people go through states of life where fat is a necessary part of development? Why don't baby harp seals have a heart attack the instant they drink mother's half-fat milk?

Fat is not an unfortunate defect of life, but a reason for it. It saves the body from death. This is why the baby harp seal needs to be fat. Fat is what saves it from a harsh environment. Human baby fat saves them from death by cold as well, even though they don't sit on ice flows. Fat insulates from heat loss while also generating some heat from its metabolism. If you don't think fat saves a human adult from death by cold you don't understand thermodynamics, which is that heat constantly moves toward cold, from inside our bodies to out. The entire reason we have metabolism is to generate energy and heat, and it is this very heat which allows our life to function, enabling the generation of energy and the movement of biological pathways. Without heat we would not be mammals, nor alive, since mammals require high body temperatures in order for their metabolism to function, and the inside of our bodies is indeed *very* hot. Ninety-four degree weather (thirty-four celsius) can make anyone wilt, but if your internal body temperature ever dropped below that you would go into a coma and die. Normally the human body is as hot as one-hundred degrees, and fat helps maintain these required internal temperatures by preventing its loss to the environment. Fat is a safety measure to spare heat, both by insulation and by generation, but before the body resorts to fat storage of the type we usually dislike it also amps up stress hormones like *cortisol* and *adrenaline* which help maintain energy and heat production and can keep a person lean but which creates an illusion of good health or fast metabolism and after enough stress or factors like pathogenic colonization the body will then increase its storage of fat to help protect and maintain health.

Because the primary role of fat storage is thermoregulation, calorie storage is a secondary purpose (or even less), metabolically expensive, unnecessary for well fed adults, and inferior to carbohydrate oxidation. But people often realize they have an insatiable appetite at the same time they struggle with their waistlines which clues us into believing there is an association between the two, which there is but it is exactly the opposite of what most people think. When the body begins to store fat due to stress it is using a great deal of eaten calories to store as fat, so not only does the body then need to have calories to synthesize and store fat but it must also have enough calories to feed the rest of the body at the same time. When the metabolic rate declines the body is also forced into backup modes of energy generation which are also less efficient. For instance, oxidation of carbohydrate in the *mitochondria* of cells can produce up to 36 molecules of our primary energy molecule, *adenosine triphosphate* (abbreviated as ATP), per 1 molecule of glucose. When this pathway is disturbed such as occurs from metabolic disease, dieting behaviors, or other metabolic stress we lose the ability to oxidize carbohydrate for energy and instead only produce 2 molecules of ATP per molecule of glucose through fermentation. While this latter reaction happens up to one-hundred times faster than oxidation of carbohydrate in mitochondria it is also up to 18 times less production of energy from the exact same quantity of calories, thus causing significantly inefficient energy production thus stimulating far greater caloric requirements to achieve the same levels of energy required for life and why those who talk about calories, fat, and sugar as problems for weight loss have no fucking idea what they are actually talking about. Fat molecules produce 129-147 molecules of ATP depending on the type of fat when metabolized for energy, which is why fat also functions as a source of energy in many animals, but this process is very, very slow compared to carbohydrate oxidation, far less efficient, and in humans also results in peroxidation stress which can and does contribute to systemic metabolic disease and why our body preferentially oxidizes carbohydrate as its primary strategy for producing energy.

Fats are also required to produce cholesterol, and most people associate cholesterol with disease due to mischaracterization and misinformation but cholesterol is the precursor to both vitamin D and most hormones and steroids in the body such as pregnenolone, testosterone, progesterone, estrogen, and the all-important corticosteroids which help our body manage electrolytes and water metabolism. Going to the emergency room for medical care often results in the administration of synthetic corticoids which in our own body are naturally synthesized from cholesterol which in turn is synthesized from fat, so guess what happens when we engage in dieting behaviors which restrict dietary fat intake? So, yes, dieting behaviors result in metabolic disease directly caused by nutritional deficiencies which then later require medical intervention to synthetically replace what is otherwise freely available in our diet. In response to metabolic stress and disease our body also increases the rate of cholesterol synthesis, in order to support greater steroid production, so while elevated cholesterol is associated with disease it is often treated as causal instead of correlated, and treatment to lower cholesterol, triglycerides, and other disorders of lipid (fat) metabolism usually exacerbates disease by further impairing the body's ability to produce steroids. Many people with high cholesterol are put on medications like statins which reduce and impair cholesterol production, but studies show that statins also disrupt microbial production of their cholesterol equivalent, ergosterol, and what benefits statins may show is not in fact from reducing production of cholesterol but from marginal inhibition of opportunistic microbes.

Most metabolic disease instead involves the presence of opportunistic pathogenic microbes including bacteria, parasites, fungi, and viruses which instead interrupt metabolic pathways like fat metabolism, and consume calories and nutrients meant for our own bodies, so in response to colonization by pathogens our appetite increases and becomes nearly insatiable since the body needs more calories for storage, to burn as fuel, and to compensate for calories and nutrients stolen by these opportunistic microbes. One major intervention caused by fungi and parasites is the *saponification* of dietary fats as discussed in upcoming chapters, which is the conversion of fatty acids to biosoaps that act as surfactants which dissolve protective mucosal barrier lining of the gut and other mucosal organs and disrupt populations of healthy commensal microbes. Those pathogens then use those nutrients like dietary fats to produce their own forms of sterols, so dieting can and does cut off nutrient supply to pathogens and which provides some relief and further convinces people that dieting is productive, but since we also require fat for our own cholesterol, vitamin D, and steroids the practice of dieting also always stresses and damages our own body too. But this practice does not eliminate those pathogens, and returning from a diet a body frantically packs on even more pounds to help protect against further deprivation stress while stimulating an even greater appetite and lower metabolic rate in order to adequately prepare for what it perceives to be intermittent famine and a losing battle with highly virulent microbes.

Many vitamins like carotene and vitamins A, K, and E are also fat-soluble and directly required for growth and differentiation of body tissues, and without dietary fat and fat-soluble vitamins the body fails to develop properly (dentition malformation and neurological dysregulation are particular casualties), and cholesterol and fats also serves a structural role within cells as part of the membrane, scaffolding, and internal machinery such as phospholipids which are even more important than thermoregulation (the brain is actually the most fat-dense organ in the body). One primary reason saturated fats such as what occur in butter, nuts, cocoa butter, coconut oil, or made within our own bodies are better for our health is that they are more stable in the high heat, high oxygen environment of human physiology. Animals like fish live in a veritable refrigerator and are not subjected to the same oxidative stresses and high-heat environments, and their fat composition is reflective of such, because if fish were made out of the same saturated fats we are they would turn into a solid stick of fish-butter in the cold temperatures of their environment just as butter and coconut oil do when they are refrigerated (fish oil actually originates from algae in the food-chain), and the fish would be unable even to move, let alone transport fats freely in and out of their cells. Degree of saturation affects the melting temperature of fats, so the more polyunsaturated a fat the more liquid it is in colder temperatures. But shared bonds are also weaker and therefore more susceptible to oxidation, so fish oil and other highly unsaturated fats like vegetable oil, canola oil, or soy oil oxidize rapidly when exposed to air and heat since very little energy is required to oxidize their shared bonds, and this same deterioration occurs in our bodies since, as mammals, we also have a high rate of oxygen saturation and heat required for oxidation of carbohydrate as our primary energy production strategy. Saturated and monounsaturated fats are biologically designed to be more stable in volatile bioenergetic processes high in heat and oxygen, so when we are deficient in saturated fats our cells break down more easily and function poorly like a car with old motor oil.

When the ratio of fat types shifts due to diet or metabolic stress our body purposefully lowers its metabolic rate to reduce oxidative stress in response to the increase in reactive oxygen species and inflammation which occurs from the oxidation of polyunsaturated fats, specifically factors like prostaglandins, to prevent further oxidation of tissues. Because fat deposition is primarily for thermoregulation, this then promotes and increase in fat retention to insulate against further heat loss during a low metabolic state which produces less heat. Visible adult fat accumulation is thus entirely a reflection of health stress, as an adult in good health will have little extra body fat. But this does not also mean that being skinny or lean is a reflection of good health, and there is much evidence that adults who don't gain fat during stress are more likely to die suddenly because fat is a protective response to heat loss required for our metabolic pathways to operate, and those who are lean who come under such stress are much more likely to have a severe and sudden health episode than those who have some extra weight, especially since fat can and does also function as a storage site for nutrients like of the fat-soluble vitamins. Fat retention is a reflection of other biological developments and *is not itself a disease OR the cause of health problems*, but is a response to disease. Fat is our friend, and though you may have issues with self-worth and acceptance related to fatness its presence is in fact evidence that your body is actually protecting your health and taking care of you as it is designed by nature to do.

So if fat is protective for the body, how can we prevent its accumulation in a healthy way? Do we even want to? The short answer is to improve overall health. If we have unwanted body fat, even a little, it means our body is experiencing some metabolic stress—nearly always microbiological in origin—which reduces the efficiency of cellular respiration or subject to stressors which are stimulating its deposition such as pathogenic colonization. The biggest factors which cause this are things like calorie deprivation and nutrients stress since these inherently lower the rate of metabolism and impair our immune system. But consumption of inappropriate foods, excessive physical exercise, emotional and environmental stress, some types of prescription drugs, or deficient exposure to sunlight (yes, light is a resource for our biology, or what did you think the point was in going outside to play?) are other major factors as addressed in upcoming chapters. Too little body fat should also be more alarming to people than too much, and I have personally witnessed a handful of friends suffer incidents, even death, due to insufficient body fat because though lean and fit in appearance their body was under tremendous metabolic stress, nutritional or otherwise, and the absence of fat resulted in catastrophic failure of the heart or promotion of cancer because there is no fat reserves from which the body can acquire needed nutrition or retain necessary body heat. As discussed in upcoming chapters, impaired fat absorption and saponification of dietary fats by opportunistic microbes which cause fat accumulation also cause fat-deficiency symptoms like dry skin and chronic skin fungal infections (dry biscuit heels are a major early symptom), and it is very important to address pathogenic colonization and consume regular amounts of good fats such as found in butter, ice cream, coconut oil, chocolate, nuts such as almonds and hazelnut, olive oil, etc., as well as generous amounts of carbohydrates. It is understandable to have insecurities about self-worth and acceptance based on our physical appearance such as being overweight, but these are psychological traumas which are *never* resolved by being fit and healthy but instead must be addressed through trauma therapy as discussed in my other book on psychology, *The Perfect Child*, or the chapter on spirituality later in this book, because no matter how fit or healthy we might be it does not directly address problems of insecurity or poor conceptions of self-worth which are the root of such fears and worldview.

Because simple problems with weight gain can often be resolved, superficially, by a little dieting and exercise the temptation is to believe that things like fasting or low-carbohydrate diets are healthy solutions since this weight loss can easily be achieved when young and healthy from stress behaviors like dieting and excessive exercise, because of the misguided belief that leanness equals healthy. But the metabolic rate is not a function of leanness—it is a function of the efficiency of our metabolic respiration pathways, and high fat catabolism is often a reflection of low-metabolic rate in which more fat is consumed due to a shift away from efficient carbohydrate metabolism. While stress methods to weight loss can produce results it will always, eventually, promote a declining metabolic rate and loss of youthful features of the physical body and greater susceptibility to pathogenic colonization simply due to the deficiency of cholesterol, steroids, and fat soluble vitamins which will always also make future weight loss and fitness efforts much more difficult. Eating a good diet, sustaining blood sugar, getting daily sun exposure, going sober for a short time, and eating enough dietary fat should make it entirely possible to remain at a normal, healthy weight without *any* diet or exercise. If there is a significant struggle for weight loss or weight gain accompanies even indulgent eating habits this is always a reflection of microbial pathogenic stress because the presence of pathogens disrupt normal metabolic pathways and the body responds by depositing more body fat in order to extend our lifespan since, in the context of human evolution, infection with virulent microorganisms portended the eventual death of an organism. Before the advent of medicine and sanitation technology, gum and tooth decay for instance caused loss of teeth and thus the inability to chew food, so our body has evolved knowing that infection with such pathogens means the eventual inability to eat, and packing on fat in response to their presence is a measure meant to prolong life as much as possible, and why dieting cannot fix those problems.

During disease the human body also increases its synthesis of the most stable saturated fats from carbohydrate, which has been used erroneously as evidence for saturated fats being harmful rather than the adaptive response to disease this actually is. It makes more sense that our body would do this on purpose consid- ering our body is designed to answer stress with effective coping strategies rather than just give up and submit to them, and the benefit of saturated fats can also be seen even in other natural examples such as queen bees who live more than twice as long as their other family members, where queens are exclusively fed royal jelly which has very high saturated fatty acid content. This is the same kinds of fat made by the bodies of mammalian mothers when nursing their young because it is the most compatible with our biology, resistant to oxidation and functional in high heat. Studies done on rats and other animals showing harms caused by high-fat diets also show those harms to be alleviated by the addition of sugar to those diets, where the harm is not actually the high fat but instead the unnatural, unbalanced composition of experimental diets supplying an excess of one nutrient or another, and it is the lack of other nutrients, not excess of one, which is the true cause of such negative results shown in such studies along with poor understanding of the natural world and complexities of microorganisms.

The first person to tell me about the health benefits of butter was a female personal trainer who had abs like I never will. She said she ate half a stick of butter a day. I liked the sound of that, but I hesitated to eat much of it as I still clung to old ideas of fat and negative concepts of body image. Thankfully saturated fat is finally being recognized again as a health food due to efforts of health conscious and forward-thinking researchers revisiting of problematic studies and ideas on nutrition, health, and the human body, yet people still shrink from butter while eating copious amounts of inferior fats, mostly in pre-made and restaurant food as if there are no consequences to that behavior or that restaurant food quality is often the worst of all available options. The fat profile of the diet is the number one way to guarantee health, or to doom it. Good fat is what makes us young and robust. Greatly increasing saturated fat in our diet can help restore youth, shrink waistlines, and heal metabolic diseases like insomnia, hair loss, fatigue, etc., or prevent any of it in the first place, so long as that colonization by opportunistic microbes is also addressed as discussed in upcoming chapters, because it is the most compatible fat for our physiology and is the sole source of healthy cholesterol required for the production of steroids without which our body loses the ability to run the metabolism, maintain electrolytes, metabolize water, and defend against opportunistic pathogenic organisms.

Some foods like nuts contain appreciable amounts of polyunsaturated fats but are still fine and healthy to consume, especially those like almonds, hazelnuts, macadamias, and pistachios which contain higher quantities of saturated fats, where the primary problem with high polyunsaturated fat are refined, processed, and concentrated fats such as occurs in products like canola oil, vegetable oil, margarine, fish oil, and soy oil because in the refining process they are exposed to air, light, and heat which oxidize the fats and thus deliver high concentration of oxidized polyunsaturated fats directly into the body (many of those products are actually 'deodorized' to remove the offending malodor that would otherwise indicate the oxidative damage to our sense of smell). Whole foods like nuts, if not extremely high in polyunsaturated fats content, contain important nutrients we need for our health which balances their polyunsaturated fats content such as vitamin E, zinc, selenium, manganese, and other nutrients, and being in whole food form are less likely to be oxidized. The entire purpose of vitamin E in nature is actually to inhibit oxidation of polyunsaturated fat, and because foods like nuts contain their oils inside and are not exposed to oxygen, light, etc., their fats are unoxidized and vitamin E intact, thus greatly reducing their negative effect on our physiology. Seeds and nuts which are extremely high in their ratio of polyunsaturated fats to saturated and monounsaturated are likely best avoided.

Dairy is the only source of animal fat high enough in good fats to be absolutely reliable because ruminants (beef, sheep, goats, etc.) possess intestinal bacteria which convert polyunsaturated fats into good saturated, which is why their milk and fat is high in saturated fats even when their diet is not. One of the first improvements I found from once again eating butter was the disappearance of dry biscuit heels which had begun to crack painfully, and were replaced by far softer skin since skin can be a storage site of good fats. It was also crucial in restoring my thyroid function for reasons discussed in that upcoming chapter. Other healthy sources of saturated fat like almonds, hazelnuts, macadamias, and olive oil can also be very useful and convenient, while cheap, high polyunsaturated oils like common cooking oils and fish oil are absolutely not compatible with human health, as evidenced by a recent study which found consumption of fish oil to be associated with an increase risk of sudden death, because of the profound increase in lipid peroxidation they cause, and directly contribute to problems like allergies, asthma, and premature aging as discussed in the upcoming chapter on immunity due to their higher propensity to oxidize. Coconut oil is almost entirely saturated, and there is much advice in this book on using coconut oil therapeutically (although it is low in oleic acid and should be complimented by olive oil, dairy fat, and nuts). My favorite example of the health benefits of saturated fats is the frequency by which centenarians cite chocolate as a reason for longevity. Good chocolate is almost entirely saturated fat, and cocoa butter is one of the most stable fats found in nature. Jeanne Louise Calment, who lived to be 122 years in age, is one of those who regularly cited chocolate and consumed it frequently.

Fat is our friend, most especially the types appropriate for our biology. Rather than fighting biology there is great empowerment from working with it, and doing so is delicious and satisfying anyway. Poor concepts of body image and equating metabolic health with self-worth which results from negative experiences of rejection and fear underlie our attitudes about fat, food, and motivate the behaviors which both cause and prevent resolution of health problems which in turn cause weight gain in the first place and can be resolved by addressing experiences of trauma and pain of past experiences. Fat is evidence your body loves and cares for you, and that it's working as it should. Be grateful for the body that promotes life, and the fat that protects us.

CHAPTER 3
THE TRUTH ABOUT SUGAR

Thirty-two and struggling with my weight, though I was not yet fat, I began a strict low-carb diet in a misguided attempt at weight loss. But instead of the health and fitness it promised I triggered the worst insomnia, physical discomfort, and weight gain of my life which eventually led to full-blown thyroid cancer and metabolic disease which would prove impossible to escape for several years.

Many people malign sugar also as the source of their fat deposition or health problems, and spend great effort in its avoidance. The conflict between fat-promotes-fat and sugar-promotes-fat should clue people into the inconsistencies and subjective nature of dietary moralizing. It is true that our body can and does use carbohydrates to synthesize fat but it is not true that sugar becomes fat simply because we eat it. The body stores fat when it is under metabolic stress, so if the body is free of metabolic stress it does not store sugar as fat either.

But who actually eats that much sugar anyway? Most people who whine about sugar addiction actually avoid sugar on a pathological basis. Obese people tend only to drink *diet* sodas, and none of them regularly consume fruit. Because of the shame associated with weight gain and indulgence surrounding my upbringing I avoided sugar as a general rule my entire adult life and took pride in my ability to resist desserts, candy, and soda even as I watched friends and romantic partners with better health consistently indulge in them and would instead order water or iced tea. In the recovery community many members regard sugar with the same negativity as heroin, cocaine, and alcohol yet I don't know of anyone who wrecked their car while under the influence of regular cola, suffocated during their sleep from caramel abuse, or committed murder during an ice-cream deal gone wrong. Do you?

One night early in my recovery I had an extreme craving for watermelon. I couldn't explain it. I just *needed* watermelon. Though it was one in the morning I put on my clothes and braved the night cold to head to a grocery store in downtown Los Angeles where I got the most satisfying watermelon of my life. I don't know what it was about the watermelon that I was craving. Well, my conscious mind didn't know, but my tongue did. I had plenty of sugary foods in the house—apples, oranges, cane sugar, ice cream—but just like pregnancy cravings I *had* to have watermelon. When I started eating it my brain confirmed that *yes, this was exactly what I neeeeeeded.*

The tongue's job is to decide if what we are putting into our body is good for us or not, and here is the trap that most people fall into—sugar tastes good, so it makes us feel good, so we put more into our body, but we feel guilty for feeling good, try harder not to eat it, then we feel bad again, and sugar's siren song calls once more. We know *if we eat sugar we will feel so good*, and the more we abstain the stronger the craving, so we eat it again, and again we feel good. Do you see what's going on here? The trap is not that sugar is bad for us. We have a problem with feeling good. The trap is the misinterpretation of rational biological functions and shame surrounding pleasure and satisfaction. Either the body—the tongue—is bad at its job and should be mistrusted and outsmarted and our body does in fact want to trick us into doing things which are bad for it, which doesn't make any fucking sense, or it's doing exactly what it's supposed to because it is in fact good for us and the deficiency is instead with our intellect.

Some studies claim that sugar activates the same centers of the brain as controlled substances. Of course it does! People who abuse drugs and alcohol are attempting to alleviate very serious suffering as explained in my upcoming chapter on alcohol and addiction, and sugar relieves suffering very well too but does so without the behavioral and social consequences of drugs and alcohol abuse because sugar is not only neither intoxicating nor disruptive of normal physio-logical processes, but actively improves our wellbeing. Because of the diabetes epidemic people have come to the observational but erroneous conclusion that abnormally elevated blood sugar equals high sugar diet (which also equals fat). If this were the case we'd be right to avoid sugar. I had often experienced fluctua-tions in my waist size relative to my observed sugar intake, so I used to believe this too, or at least wasn't sure of an alternative explanation. Also nothing good comes without sacrifice, or so said every self-righteous person I've met/dated/was born to, and there is no greater sacrifice than giving up a creamy mocha Frappuccino on a hot summer day. Herein lies the problem, that *every cell in the human body runs on sugar*. Some cells like parts of the brain only run on sugar. To be clear, when I refer to sugar I am not glibly referring to cakes, cookies, and candy which are so asinine-ly referred to colloquially as "sugar." Sugar is a technical term for a chemical form of energy storage, and dietary forms of sugar are things like glucose, fructose, sucrose, lactose, maltose, mannose, etc. Bread, whole grain, and pasta, contrary to what you have heard, are entirely made of sugar. The kind of sugar which they are composed is called starch and it consists of many, many molecules of glucose strung together. Once bread is digested it provides the same kind of sugar as pure corn syrup—chemically they are the same substance, and it's why eating starchy foods feels so good and comforting because starch provides our bodies with a great deal of sugar, and because sugar provides energy cells use it for fuel, and extra fuel means a well running metabolism, lower stress hormones, etc.

Going on low-carb diets is also quite misleading because the body can and does also mobilize sugar from tissues during deficient intake of carbohydrates, and even synthesizes sugars from non-sugar substrate in a process called gluco-neogenesis, because total sugar deprivation would in fact be lethal. This is why low-carbohydrate diets and starvation is so difficult to accomplish because the body is trying to tell you *to stop the fuck what you're doing and eat some goddamned carbs.* Since we as humans have a tendency to ignore and distrust our bodies and misunderstand nature I will tell you *why* sugar is not only necessary only for life and health but more importantly our outward youth and good looks. And no, I did not just get those priorities mixed up since people will gleefully spend thousands and thousands of dollars on beauty treatments, cosmetics, and surgery but tell them they can look and feel ten years younger simply by giving up gluten suddenly you're forbidden from ever again going near their children.

The tongue is no deceiver. In fact, it can taste things we aren't aware of it tasting, which is why I had that inexplicable craving for watermelon which is uncommonly high in nutrients like *molybdenum* and *citrulline* not easily gotten from other food sources. Consciously we can recognize sweet, savory, salty, umami, but the tongue can and does also help us identify minerals and vitamins we need too, in addition to calorie sources. We experience this as craving for certain foods which our body intuitively understands will contain whatever we are at that moment deficient. Because I listened to my body that night I was provided with relief and an increase in health and wellbeing. Cravings for "unhealthy" foods like carbohydrate rich pastas, sandwiches, or sugary candy or desserts comes simply because a person does not eat enough carbohydrates or calories in the first place, or cannot store enough *glycogen* in the body from years of nutritional abuse, neglect, or pathogenic colonization and metabolic disease. Glycogen is the mammalian equivalent of starch in plants, where adipose tissue is our primary storage site for fats glycogen is our primary storage site for carbohydrate, in the form of glucose. As blood sugar falls glucose is released from liver glycogen through low amounts of *adrenaline* to help maintain consistent and steady level of blood sugar. Liver glycogen is designed to be released in this manner between meals but when it becomes depleted and blood sugar drops to the point of crisis this triggers greater and greater release of adrenaline as the body attempts to squeeze every last drop of glycogen, and because the body will die if carbohydrate deficiency continues further deprivation then releases *cortisol* which serves to catabolize lean muscle tissue to release its glycogen content into circulation to sustain the internal organs, as muscle glycogen is not designed to be released. This high catabolic hormone expression due to dieting or other low-carbohydrate stress is what causes us to feel poorly, anxious, and depressed, and why starchy and sugar foods are so therapeutic to reversing this stress response. It is also why those who chronically diet and starve themselves lose muscle mass because the body cannot sustain both muscles and internal organs if there is not sufficient dietary carbohydrate. Glycogen is also hydrated and requires potassium for synthesis, and dieting and fasting causes fluctuating weight not because of fat loss but because water, potassium, muscle, and glycogen are lost from the body during glycogen depletion. Fat is ironically one of the last things to go during dieting because fat is essential for maintaining our internal body temperature. Even skin and hair are destroyed by chronically low blood sugar as the body eats itself to supply missing nutrients to keep us alive, so the tongue jumps for joy when greeted with sweet, sweet sugar and tasty starch because it knows this is going to help the body function better, and these signals are meant to reinforce those behaviors which sustain life and reduce stress. Whining children don't want sugar because they are brats—they are hurting, most likely because you yell too much or haven't fed them properly, and they instinctively understand that sugar will relieve them of that stress.

How well our body utilizes sugar and whether it stores carbohydrates as glycogen or instead coverts it to fat storage is also a barometer for health as a whole.

When sugar is converted into fat instead of glycogen (meaning there is significant weight gain from eating sugar) it is a sign our health and ability to oxidize sugar needs improvement, likely caused by the presence of infectious pathogens as discussed throughout this book, and not that sugar should be avoided which will only end up exacerbating the problem since carbohydrate deficiency decreases the body's ability to resist stress and increases the severity of the effects of stress upon the organs, muscles, connective tissue, and metabolic pathways. It is the ability to metabolize sugar, not the nature of sugar itself, which is responsible for sugar-related health problems. Non-diabetics often do a pseudo-diabetic dance, avoiding sugar/carbs but then indulging once the cravings become too strong to ignore and is very dangerous behavior because it elicits chronic and repeated exposure to high stress hormones unnecessarily which over time begin to destroy the body's ability to store and oxidize sugar in preference of fat which then shifts the metabolism primarily to one based on fat which then promotes more fat storage and less glycogen, eventually causing a host of more serious health conditions which result from a depressed metabolic rate since carbohydrate is the most effective and efficient way for our bodies to produce energy.

This is exactly what happened to me in the development of my own health problems, convinced that sugar was the cause avoided it religiously, even though I still continued to develop health problems when doing so. I was so happy when I learned that it was the metabolism of sugar and not sugar itself which was contributing to my health problems and began to consume sugar in ever increasing amounts and for the first time in my life actually began to get well. The more sugar I had the better I felt, the more energy I had, and also the more weight I lost. In addition to all the other whole meals, chocolate, fruit, candy, and desserts I was already eating I at one point was consuming *four pounds* of high-quality, organic sugar a week (mostly in smoothies made with fruit and added protein) and for the first time in my adult life not only lost weight without exercising but experienced improvement in my health rather than decline. Now that I have gotten better and my health is more stable I no longer need to sustain my blood sugar quite so vigorously, and consume about one to two pounds of unrefined sugar a week, though I also partake of generous amounts of fruit, desserts, maple syrup, potatoes, breads, pastries, and other carbohydrate rich foods while enjoying a nearly effortless ability to stay lean and retain muscle. Mentioning my nightly sugar consumption to friends or family who suffered insomnia they often replied, «*doesn't it keep you awake?*» From people with insomnia, who don't eat sugar, to someone who eats sugar, who does not have insomnia. They asked that. Seriously. I mean, is the discrepancy not blatantly obvious? Am I the only one who sees it?

We go to great lengths to feed our pets and animals the diets that are appropriate for their biology—No one would feed bird-seed to a cat and expect the cat to live, let alone thrive, or likewise meat to a horse. But when it comes to ourselves we often don't consider that there is a proper human diet. It seems like a limitation on our potential and most people don't want to believe we have those, but when it comes to diet we *do* have specific metabolic functions which require specific metabolic substrates, and when we eat the way we are meant as human animals we experience a thriving of health and metabolism, when we do the opposite we experience the reverse. Many foods on which we evolved as humans and as such dependent for our nutritional needs are full of sugar, including fruits, honey, and also lesser known options such as sedges, like the tiger nut on which our ancestors subsisted generously which is so high in sugar it tastes like a commercial breakfast cereal. Saying we are addicted to sugar is like saying we are addicted to air, or water. Our body *can. not. run. without. sugar.* Without sugar our pancreas, lungs, and brain will shut down and we die, as a friend of mine once found out the hard way during an alarming health crisis after a prolonged version of a popular, low-carb, commercial diet when he one day found himself unable to breathe and during the resulting and expensive emergency room trip was told he only needed to eat a piece of bread.

It is impossible to be addicted to sugar. We cannot be addicted to things we naturally need for health and wellness, and what is usually defined as addiction is in reality the body trying to motivate the resolution of nutritional deficiency. Of course, since sugar also relieves suffering it can feel good to eat it because it enables the body's ability to overcome stress, so people who believe it is addictive think this is true because it makes them feel good, and because of our negative opinions of life and the human condition we are suspicious of cravings and feeling well rather than sympathetic and grateful. The craving for sugar is a sign of metabolic insufficiency and requires satisfaction and attention to consistent blood sugar maintenance. If proper glycogen storage and sugar metabolism is occurring sugar and carbs are not craved as long as a person eats regularly and keeps their blood sugar steady. Liver glycogen is designed to slowly release glucose into the bloodstream between meals to sustain blood sugar but glycogen is also a mechanism to prevent the full quantity of glucose from any meal being delivered all at once and overwhelming cells, and in metabolically compromised people the ability to store glycogen is greatly diminished so carbohydrate is instead shuttled to fat for storage so that no calories are wasted. In people with deranged sugar metabolism other health problems are also usually present such as weight gain, insomnia, anxiety or emotional problems, gut dysfunction, and thyroid disease because the proper pathways for sugar metabolism have been upset, especially in severe cases such as hypothyroidism, diabetes, and cancer.

Often pathogenic microbes make it seem like sugar is causing weight gain, but like I mentioned in the previous chapter the presence of these microbes is what actually interrupts our metabolic health through their own opportunistic biological mechanisms. Inferior fats like the kind in canola, soy, or fish oil are also some primary causes of problems with sugar metabolism because the more unsaturated a fat the more susceptible it is to peroxidation which will in turn cause systemic oxidative damage to cellular organelles such as mitochondria, and chronic loss of mitochondria impairs our ability to oxidize carbohydrate which then triggers backup processes like production of lactate or fatty acid oxidation to which the body responds by reducing the metabolic rate. Vitamin deficiencies such as of riboflavin or thiamine also interrupt normal carbohydrate metabolism as they are used in enzymes which store glycogen and process carbohydrate. Disruption to the gut microbiome also purposefully redirects sugar from oxidation to fat storage and fatty acid metabolism to promote long term survival during colonization by opportunistic microbiological pathogens, to which the body also responds by decreasing its metabolic rate. Drug and alcohol use (including prescription drugs) can also interfere with hormonal and chemical pathways which regulate sugar metabolism. Some foods like yogurts or sauerkraut, because they contain lactic acid which directly impairs proper sugar metabolism, can also contribute to the derangement of the metabolic rate by inhibiting normal sugar metabolism. There are so many factors which interrupt normal and healthy sugar metabolism that have nothing to do with the nature of sugar the fact that anyone thinks sugar is bad for us shows just how misguided its vilification has been and how ignorant are gatekeepers of health and wellness research and treatment.

The primary reason our bodies crave the kinds of sugar used in desserts, candy, and beverages which is either usually *sucrose* (which is made of glucose and fructose) or *high fructose corn syrup* is because, unlike glucose, fructose does not require insulin for use in cellular pathways and directly raises metabolic respiration and mitochondrial oxidation of carbohydrate. Fructose gets its name for being the predominant sugar in ripened fruit, not because it's part of high-fructose corn syrup, and fruit was (and still should be) a primary food source for humans because we are primates and require fructose in many metabolic pathways not only limited to the production of energy. Fruit also provides many of the other nutrients we require as human beings, and part of the reason we don't synthesize vitamin C, which most animals can do, is because our evolutionary diet consisted of high-vitamin C foods like fruit, leaves, and roots which became a regulatory source of vitamin C. Because vitamin C stimulates the metabolic rate animals which produce their own vitamin C do not as easily survive famine and nutrient deprivation, and since we instead rely on its availability in the environment our metabolic rate only rises during times when the environment also contains an abundance of food such as from fruit and falls during times of scarcity like winter when vitamin C and other nutrition is unavailable, to slow the metabolic rate and thus the expenditure of spare nutrients. Unfortunately this ability to better resist nutritional deprivation which promoted our evolutionary survival also makes it possible for us as humans to endure significant starvation and dietary stress which makes their destructive effects on our physiology less obvious, thereby helping people who engage in dieting behaviors delude themselves about its actual effects on our wellbeing. The metabolic requirement for fructose and it's strong promotion of our metabolism is why fruit and other sources of sugar are so satisfying to our senses but why many animals like dogs or cats which evolutionary are more dependent on meat usually don't give a damn about fruit.

I once saw a study by actual scientists which discussed with much novelty the fact that fructose absorption rises after consuming a source of fructose. Imagine. Unknown even to most researchers is that the great majority of all glucose which enters cells *is actually converted directly into fructose* in complete opposition to general, misguided nutritional advice on the nature of fructose in human health. More peculiar, the body nearly always first converts other sugars like glucose or mannose into fructose even when it converts it back to their original form, a seemingly unnecessary or wasteful step, but this probably occurs to help maintain fructose pools which are required in so many necessary pathways, and all glucose which is taken up for use in carbohydrate oxidation is converted to fructose before entering the pathways in which it is consumed. For this reason is it not only pleasurable to consume fructose but much the way a cat suffers ill-health on a protein deficient diet so do humans suffer one which is fructose deficient. Before the medical community discovered insulin therapy to treat diabetes sucrose was actually a standard treatment because fructose assists the body in using glucose since it does not require insulin. Fructose is also the primary reason why fruitarians (a diet dangerously low in protein and fats) have such a high metabolic rate, which in fruitarians is actually too high due to the constant intake of fructose which more quickly exhausts their insufficient protein intake. Our cravings for sugar and fructose do not thus occur because the body is a trickster that wants us to suffer and fail but because fructose is a primary driver of our metabolic health, involved in all sorts of necessary metabolic processes. If fructose caused metabolic disease then fruitarians would be fat and diabetic, but they are overly lean and not diabetic. Not only can we use fructose to feel good, we can use it to help restore health, but in case you are

one of those enterprising individuals who thinks they will rush out and buy purified fructose, please be reminded that body hacking is dangerous and imbalances
interdependent pathways, and all health decisions should be based primarily in food
and health can never be achieved by doing anything in excess. Fructose is also not
absorbed into the body without the simultaneous presence of glucose, which is most
likely a regulatory mechanism meant precisely to prevent overdriving metabolism
and exhausting nutrients and glucose stores. Even sodas with high-fructose corn
syrup still contain generous amounts of glucose, and high-fructose corn syrup and
commercial beverages are unhealthy for all sorts of reasons that have nothing to do
with their sugar content. Whole food such as fruit and unrefined cane sugar (or less
refined such as occurs in organic products) also contain countless vitamins, minerals, and other biologically active components which benefit health as well which
cannot be replicated by supplements, and certainly not by reducing foods into their
mere constituent parts.

When children protest certain foods like broccoli and brussels sprouts it is
not because they are undisciplined and willful but because some foods contain
anti-nutritive compounds like phytic acid or oxalic acid which in excess can
interfere with digestion and absorption of nutrients, because children's digestive
systems are not fully developed. Children are also super-attuned by nature to
bitter flavors of food to prevent them from accidentally ingesting harmful poisons,
because many plants in nature contain poisons which can actually kill or sicken
us. If LEGOS tasted like raw broccoli no child would ever accidentally swallow
them again. For this same reason children also respond to sweet foods because
those foods are the safest and most easily digested and most compatible with
their physiology. Parents who let their children have plenty of healthy desserts,
ice cream, and high-quality sweets along with a focus on fruit consumption have
children who sleep through the night, are generally happier and easy going, and
are rarely ill. Parents who feel a moral obligation to withhold sugar from their children and instead feed them grain-based foods, raw or underprepared vegetables,
dilute their juice, or make children go hungry when upset and tired have children
who wake frequently during the night, get sick often and easily, and are quick to
fall apart emotionally, who will also develop early and severe metabolic disease as
adults (or even earlier). As much as many people would like it to be true the body
does not live on morals, discipline, or conjecture. It lives on sugar, protein, and
fat. Jeanne Calment was also reported to have a dessert with every meal, and it
was only after generously reintroducing sugar and improving my body's ability to
metabolize sugar that I was finally able to experience a restoration of my general
health. Sometimes I don't follow my own advice, and when I regained some weight
during my recovery I had stopped my usual sugar consumption. My liver could now
store enough glycogen to keep me going without constant refueling so I got lazy in
taking in enough and began to see again sugar-deficiency related stress hormones
like high cortisol, expanding waist, and return of some health problems which were
all resolved by again resuming generous consumption of sugary foods.

When we eat sugar we feel happy. Want to feel happy all day long? Go ahead.
Eat sugar. Obviously we need vitamins and minerals to properly utilize sugar, so
the use of less refined and organic sugar and whole food sources such as fruit can
increase happiness, energy, and healing. I really can't think of any good reasons to
avoid that.

Undiscerning people often refer to baked goods like cake and cookies as sugar
but these are often made with common wheat, bad fats, preservatives, iron fortification, and other unhealthy additives, all things that are not good for us which are

not actually sugar. If a food manufacturer can't make their product with healthy ingredients for you, you shouldn't be eating it and they don't deserve your money. Almost none of the candy or desserts in famous stores like Trader Joe's are made without things like potentially allergenic gums, binders, or toxic preservatives. Even most chocolate brands at Whole Foods use soy in their products—since when did soy become an ingredient in chocolate? If you buy something pre-made, you *must* read the label to avoid these potentially harmful food additives which have absolutely nothing to do with sugar.

It has also escaped the attention of researchers that most of the hydrogen atoms which make up stomach acid come from carbohydrate, so there is no better way to induce metabolic disease and gut problems by avoiding carbohydrates which then impairs the digestion of food and facilitates ingress of opportunistic microbes into the gut. Because fructose is so necessary in so many pathways it can also be used as a natural medication, because it is necessary for specific enzymes which run our most robust metabolic pathways, and studies show that sugar is an effective analgesic (pain reducer) and should be used proactively for rehabilitation from metabolic disease. Obviously those with diabetes are an exception to the use of sugar, discussed in the upcoming chapter on metabolic disease. Whenever anyone asks me about remedies to fall asleep I always tell them to put some sugar in warm milk and unless their insomnia is extremely severe they fall asleep immediately.

Fructose can also be an aid for anyone who does not feel sufficient hunger impulses, who might find themselves under-eating, as fructose stimulates the overall metabolic rate which in turn will stimulate hunger impulses, and starting each day with vitamin C and sugar can turn on the metabolic rate and start the daily process of metabolic healing. On consumption of fructose-containing sugar some immediate effects will be an increase in heart-rate, body temperature, a depressurizing of sinus and ear canals if there is chronic inflammation, mood will increase, posture will improve, and tension will subside. These are all signs that it is doing good for us. Keep it up. Over the long term it can help support the repair and rebuilding of tissues and systems which are suffering such as the thyroid, adrenals, gonads, fixing erectile dysfunction, age-related cognitive decline, hair restoration, and more. Should any increase in sugar or carbohydrate be accompanied by weight gain, bloating, or digestive or metabolic symptoms it is a definitive sign of invasive pathogenic microorganisms as discussed in upcoming chapters.

Fat is supposed to be on our body. It is part of what defines us as humans and makes us aesthetically the way we are, and sugar is what our body wants in order to thrive, and if we put in the right kind of fuel we get the right kind of benefits. If we gain weight it is not a sign that we need to stop eating but that our body is under metabolic stress. Besides, you know you want sugar. Consider this your permission. Just don't keep stuffing your face with cheap restaurant chips or processed food and blame sugar when you get fat. Your body is simply protecting you from yourself. Only when you begin to treat it right will it do what you want.

CHAPTER 4
MISLEADING SCIENCE

My alarm blared in the early morning darkness. It was 5:30 a.m. and, remembering why the alarm was set this early in the first place, was overcome with more than the usual Monday morning dread. "Good luck today," said my sleepy mother as she dropped me in front of Mountain Ridge Junior High a short while later in total darkness. "Thanks," I smiled weakly, fear growing inside me to the point I began to shake as she drove away.

Our school had been built only a few years before, so the huge gymnasium floor was shiny and free of wear, the bleachers new and nice, and the walls clean and white except for a large, vibrant Husky Dog logo. I hesitantly joined the other boys already stretching and warming on the court for ninth-grade basketball tryouts. They were numerous, but varied widely in height, build, and skill. Among us were those obvious choices for the team who would get a spot simply because they showed up, boys the rest of us secretly envied who already sported uncanny, incredible pectorals and washboard abs who could dribble without looking or run for hours without tiring as if they actually possessed a set of wings. Most of them were my friends, but I took great pains to hide my lust for the few I desired by keeping a set of less attractive, safe friends who presented no such conflict of interest. One of these friends was nearly my height, and for the last few months had been sizing me up in the hallways during school. "I'm taller than you," he would insist. In no mood this morning to entertain his competitive obsession I pushed passed him, but he stepped closer, pushing me out of my stance with his weight and raising himself on his toes to exaggerate his height. "I'm taller." He repeated. "You're cheating," I replied.

"Alright! Gather around!" shouted our coach, Mr. Hansen, a revered figure at the school, older but healthy and fit and unlike stereotypical gym teachers was kind, supportive, and inspiring. I could feel his eyes on me, the tallest kid for twenty miles, a guaranteed secret weapon in spite of my wanting skill and passive demeanor. Tryouts started with drills and though I had the longest legs in school I was not the fastest runner, but now that things had started I was feeling more relaxed and confident and surprised at how well I was actually doing. The truth was I hated basketball. Ever since my father realized I was going to be tall he had thrust me forcefully into the sport without my consent, but all the long, unpleasant work with him over the summer, playing in a club league, and his constant berating to be 'more aggressive' finally seemed to be paying off. I made shot after shot, and started to feel like I might actually justify a place on the team apart from my uncommon height. For a brief moment I fantasized about maybe become one of the jocks of the school and, though unlikely, a possible reprieve from my dad's constant criticism and lack of enthusiasm for his favorite sport.

Near the end of tryouts we were separated into teams of three to play some scrimmage. My friend happened to be on the opposing team from me and while we were handily beating them decided to use his weight advantage once more and rammed unexpectedly into me as he went up for a shot, which he missed, the force of his charge knocked me over. As I fell his legs trapped my feet and the first thing to hit the floor was my right kneecap.

The pain was sharp for a moment, stars briefly flashing in my vision, immediately followed by a dull, seeping feeling of shock which began to spread from my knee and slowly wash over my whole body. My first thought after how painful it was feeling my kneecap snap off was followed by the strangely comforting realization that I would never have to play basketball again. "Are you okay?" asked my friend as he helped me up. I avoided his gaze, afraid I might go off and unleash all my frustration at everything on him. But he clearly regretted it, so I forgave him immediately. "No," I muttered, trying to hold back tears. They helped me to the bench but with each step my knee responded with pain that felt like someone sticking in a hot needle. The coach, worried, approached me.

"I think I tore something," I said. He helped me to his office and I dialed home. "Hello?", answered my dad.

"dad," I said, trying to sound brave, "I got hurt at tryouts."

"That's too bad," he replied.

"I need you to come get me."

There was a moment of silence. "Walk it off, you're fine."

"dad, it's serious. I think I—"

"Toughen up and walk it off."

I began to feel ashamed, my face flushing in frustration. Perhaps if I could entreat him to understand the seriousness of the injury, which even now only a few minutes after had swelled noticeably. "No, dad," I said, "I think tore something—"

"I'm not coming to get you," he said angrily. Tears forced themselves out, my throat choking with sadness and anger. Not only had I failed tryouts, I was now having to convince my own father to take care of me, in front of my coach, and publicly reveal the misery which I had to deal on a daily basis. "Put mom on the phone!" I demanded.

A few hours later I was at a clinic having my now melon-sized knee drained of blood and fluid. The doctor suggested I wait a few weeks to check up on it, but my mother was not happy and instead found a renowned local surgeon known to some relatives to inspect me with an MRI. A few days later I went into to surgery to repair a torn medial patellofemoral ligament and remove a large piece of bone which had chipped off the back of my patella. It was a nice surprise as I recovered at home to find out I made first cuts for the varsity team, while my assailant did not, but it was going to be many long months until I could walk again, let alone run, and with that my basketball career was officially over as fast as it had begun.

It was the first crossroads of my young life, freed from the suffocating expectations of my parents I realized I could now choose what I wanted to do, or to even do anything at all (aside from running of course). When summer came I found myself healed enough to be active again, and swimming had always been fun. The added bonus of being nearly naked while competing if I were to join a team was an alluring perk, a fantasy kept closely guarded from my conservative family, and toward the end of the summer I finally got the courage to suggest, with pretended indifference, that in light of the fact that I could no longer run swimming might be a good option. My parents didn't object and a few days later I walked onto the deck of the pool at the American Fork Recreation Center, the sun blinding as it glanced off the choppy water full of raucous, joyful teenagers, and extended my hand to the coach. "Hi," I said, swallowing my nerves. "You're the swimming coach?" "Mr. Harris," he replied. He appeared to be in his thirties, a great big smile plastered across his face, a whistle hung around his neck and a clipboard in hand. He did not look like a swimmer, dressed in a full shirt and shorts, his skin pale, with extra weight spilling over his shorts. "I'm Nathan," I said.

"Good to meet you." He replied, looking me up and down. "Boy you're tall."

"Yeah, I get that a lot," I smiled. "I was thinking about joining the team."

"We'd love to have you. Have you swum before?"

"I used to play basketball, but I hurt my knee trying out for the team last year. I've been taking a few lessons but I've never been on a team."

There was an easy, joyful inspiration about Mr. Harris that I never saw in coaches of other sports. In spite of my nerves it seemed this was going to be fun for many reasons. I looked around at the handsome, barely clad guys my age and felt a thrill of excitement at the possibility of being one of them. Mr. Harris explained that I would need a suit, goggles, and a cap if I wanted but which wasn't necessary. It was the least amount of equipment for any sport I'd ever played.

The next day my mom reluctantly took me to a sporting goods store in a larger nearby town. "Can't you wear a normal swimsuit?" She asked, disgusted as she picked a speedo off the rack with only two fingers as if holding a dirty diaper. "No—" I said sharply, imagining the horror of walking onto the pool deck as the only one in board shorts. "Do you want me to look stupid? I'd be the only one on the team *not* wearing a speedo. It's the equipment for the sport." She grimaced but dropped her protest, much to my relief. I strolled up and down the aisle of speedos, doubling my efforts to disguise my gawking at the photos of beautiful grown men which graced the cover of each package, each promising the achievement of manhood simply through its purchase. Some speedos were clearly too sexy to get away with, like one which had barely an inch of material at the sides and was a bright fuchsia color. I settled on a plain racing suit and another with a creative green pattern across the top which still had a bit of style but was also masculine enough to buy in the presence of my mother, and suppressed my impatience as the cashier rang up the long line of customers. Arriving home I immediately went to the bathroom to try on my new equipment. Standing in front of the mirror I was suddenly no longer a boy, my head nearly passing out of view ever since I had grown taller than all the mirrors in our house. Of course I was quite skinny, but the speedo was a symbol of passing beyond the divide which separated my childhood and blind trust in parents from the oncoming autonomy of adulthood, filled with the excitement of finally getting to do something I had decided for myself.

On the first day of practice an older, insecure boy made fun of my first dive from the blocks. But the other members, the real athletes of the team, told me not to pay him any mind and so I didn't. I had never been so integrated into a group of peers. They showed me how to turn, how to have proper hand position, even how to defog my goggles. They also showed me how to laugh and joke but also how to work hard and to support each other. I had finally found my place.

The idea that there might be other boys in the world just like me never entered my mind. Certainly they were not on my swimming team, racing up and down the lanes right next to me, or standing nearby in the warm water of the locker room showers, longing for me as I did for them, and the ones passing by the showers who stared were certainly just comparing sizes, I thought. Since I was so tall I was never subject to harassment, which I learned later was frequent for the other gay boys on the team. I was unlucky to pass the entirety of High School without ever having an impetus to confront my sexual orientation such as an encounter with another boy, or learning anyone else harbored the same kinds of feelings for me, never looked at with longing, averting my eyes in the locker room for fear of getting caught, for disrespecting other boys which might not appreciate it, and so I spent the entirety of my early swimming career in constant fear.

I did catch on to swimming like a fish, however. By the end of the first year I had put on fifty-pounds of muscle and was on the relay team with older boys who had been swimming all their life. I was destined not only to be a swimmer, it seemed, but a good one, and the excitement that infected our team at the completion of our State Finals when my relay team placed fourth overall seemed to promise my life was actually going to turn out alright.

But something changed the following summer. Our coach became unhinged, as if some monster from a classic horror film had taken possession of his body. "Nobody talks to the football coach like that!" he screamed one day at a boy who had ditched practice and ran from the pool deck crying, and followed it up with, "you're off the team!" Swimming became exhausting. Emboldened by our new potential our coach added morning practice in addition to those in the afternoon, and instead of swimming during the allotted school hour we lifted weights in the school gym *and then* went to the pool for another workout afterward. On slow days we were training for two and a half hours, a total of four on the hard days. I had never pushed myself like this and my body rebelled quickly. One day during swimming practice when hooked up to long lengths of surgical tubing that prevented us from reaching the other side as a drill to improve our strength, throwing my newly massive arms forward in butterfly stroke my muscles suddenly felt as if they popped. It was a strange feeling, one I had never had before. Something was wrong, but I wrote it off as simple fatigue from that workout. I sank in the water, letting the rubber bands haul me back to the other end, floating on my back as I stared at the white bubble dome erected every winter which blocked all sunlight and sequestered chlorine gas in the air. The rest of the practice I pretended to work hard, too exhausted to push myself any more.

The next morning I missed practice. Coach was angry, but being one of his star swimmers he muted his frustration. Little did the break help my situation. My times began to plateau. One young swimmer who used to idolize me suddenly beat me in a race that was usually mine and rubbed it in my face. Normally it would have been fun camaraderie but the feeling that I was fighting something serious made me all the more worried. I tried to put more effort into training, more determination, pulling harder and turning faster and tighter. My times would not budge. I felt exhausted, and because they always responded to problems with blame it never even crossed my mind to ask my parents for help. Worse, I began to feel even more depressed than usual, and my mind ruminated continually on my sexual orientation, stolen glances at the boys in school on which I crushed but followed by guilt and shame and hatred for who I was. I redoubled efforts to suppress my fantasies, a desire to be loved, which merely fueled the desires more until they became too overpowering to resist. My newfound love for swimming had suddenly rotted away into fear and anxiety, that old thrill before each practice and the prickling anticipation of the water sliding over my dry skin replaced by fear and dread of more failure. *I would take a break*, I thought one day. *That's all I need. Just don't let anyone know you're weak.*

I made an excuse for needing to miss a length of practices and a meet, but my coach was furious. He ran into the locker room after me and screamed in front of all the other swimmers that I attend or get off the team. I didn't know what to do. If I kept it up I felt like I was going to die. "We're proud of you," said my parents on telling them of my decision to quit. I veiled my shame of my assumed weakness in pretended apathy and boredom for the sport, since I could not ask them for help with any of the kinds of problems I was having. They could have stopped there and things would have been great, but my mother added, "We didn't think you were going stick with it as long as you did anyway." That made a lot more sense.

The long needed rest which came brought life back to my soul. My attention returned to school and other friends, and my mind and body began to heal. My grades improved as did my social life. I made some different friends and began to do normal things like go to the movies, skip class for the first time, attend school plays, football games, and dances. But when the next summer came I found myself missing the pool, my teammates, the rush of water past my body, the thrill of winning, and felt I had regained the strength to try again. It was my Senior year, after all, and my last chance. I gathered my courage, swallowed my pride and asked the coach if I could rejoin the team. He seemed to bury his excitement in a reprimanding scowl, and agreed.

There was still some summer weather remaining, and the winter bubble had yet to be installed over the pool. Lap after lap seemed to welcome me back to my true home, the rotisserie of swimming under the summer sun once more gave my skin that impeccably even swimmer tan. I put on even more muscle than the year before. During a family lake trip as I lay spread across the seats of our ski boat a girl who had graduated the previous year said I "had a good body," the first time anyone had ever complimented it. I went skinny dipping for the first time and realized that men could be near each other and not be afraid of intimacy. The season began on a high note. I was elected co-captain. I walked the school halls for the first time in my life not feeling small and insignificant, but my true height, for the first time a confident, proud, and capable boy fast becoming a man.

But soon the bubble went back on the pool and shortly after my fatigue returned, and this time not only did my speed plateau, it plummeted. I also finally told the first person about my secret desires for other boys. It was not my mother or father, not even a close friend. I told our bishop, the man to whom everyone in our religious congregation was expected to confess what their religion defined as sin. I had never kissed another person, never engaged in any sexual activity. I had seen pornography for the first time that year, and was both frightened and thrilled by the feelings which an aroused, naked man holding a jock strap in his mouth evoked within me. I told the bishop I knew I was gay. But instead of reassuring me that others existed who were just like me, that God loved me and I should do the same, he counseled me that being around other boys in speedos was not good for my spiritual health, and that I needed to stop masturbating and quit the swimming team.

How could I do that? Swimming was going to get me a scholarship. It was how I was going to attend college and propel the rest of my life. It was my identity. At the beginning of the year I had been one of the fastest in the state. The humiliation of having revealed my desires was too much. I could feel the exhaustion infecting me again. It was too much to bear. So once more I failed, leaving behind the sport and people I loved, and there were no more chances.

A few years after I moved to Los Angeles, and with few friends to show for the years I had been in that enormous city I missed the scent and feel of the pool and the camaraderie of a team. Insufferably insecure I had avoided joining the gay team because I had gone on a date with one of the swimmers which had not gone well and feared seeing him again. It was ridiculous, I realized. I put in some time jogging away a few extra pounds and once more gathered my courage to strap on a speedo and joined the team. It was terrifying wearing a speedo among other gay men, who are often more cruel to each other than straight people are to us on account of growing up constantly fearing for our safety. But once I got in the pool I felt at home, like a teenager again, speeding through the water, the feel of my own strength and power recharging my bare-level confidence. Within a few weeks my strength and skill as a swimmer quickly found me leading the lanes with the other fastest swimmers and won me the adoration of my teammates, my figure quickly becoming once more fit and tight, acquiring that even coat of tan so easily got by Southern California swimmers who never have to swim in a bubble.

But my depression did not lift, and once more I began to find myself sullen and anxious outside of the pool. Worse, I began to have increasing insomnia which had fluctuated in severity over the years. I had long been interested in discovering the root of my physical and emotional adversities and now the pain was too severe to put off any longer. I began to investigate but this time instead of a psychologist I went to a psychiatrist. I got on an antidepressant, but dismay set in immediately when, although altering my mental state it failed not only to relieve my depression and anxiety but robbed me of clarity of thought and the ability to orgasm. A coach on my new team also became sexually aggressive and crossed boundaries, and being timid and once more overwhelmed I stopped showing up to practice.

Around that time I met a wonderful boy with whom I promptly fell in love and hid away from the world for a year, but toward the end found myself wearing size thirty-eight jeans instead of thirty-six and my new love avoiding my kisses. I resolved to leave him and change my heavy drinking and hapless eating habits. I would return to swimming and get my life back on track. I confronted the problem coach and asked him not to talk about my body or touch me when I returned to practice. Even though I spilled out of my racing suit and received some underhanded ridicule by some of the assholes on the team I was overjoyed to be back in the pool. I changed therapists and quit the antidepressant, tired of the castration it made me feel, and began to look for natural means of relief. Articles I found were usually from news sources or self-help books. Most of the consensus supported by 'exciting studies' were about things I'd never heard like St. John's Wort, 5-HTP, and resveratrol. I ordered them and immediately felt a change, less dramatic and specific than the prescription had been but definitely a difference. I dropped weight faster than I ever had in my whole life, and for the first time saw the clear outlines of abdominals and hip bones (which was not actually a good thing). Then one day during practice my heart skipped a beat. Not metaphorically for any of my handsome teammates. It literally skipped a beat, and my lungs terrifyingly emptied of air. I had to stop mid practice and stand up in the middle of the lane in order not to drown, trying not to appear as panicked as I was, like I was having a heart attack, which I thought I was. The episode abated quickly, but my muscles felt weak and tired. I left early, thinking some rest and food would help me recover, yet again unable to ask for help for the deafening voice of shame within me. Consequent practices continued to render me fatigued and terrified, as heart palpitations set in with regularity. Though the supplements helped give me the leanest physique of my life I stopped them altogether, worried they were doing things to my body which might be very bad. My heart returned to normal within a week, and I began to take practices with a little more leisure.

Two years later I met someone new and fell in love once again. I idolized him. He was ballsy and tough and funny and we had similar backgrounds from oppressively conservative and abusive childhoods. He was the first man to whom I ever committed sharing closet space. Later we decided to move to Palm Springs, a wonderful resort town in California for a change of pace and a chance to focus on saving money, artistic pursuits, and getting our own home with our limited financ-es, he a writer and me in search of a mentor trailing him like a puppy dog. It would also be a chance to get my health under control. Since my partner did not drink, I could also drink less too, I thought. Living in a resort town near a grocery store I could cook healthy meals and exercise under the sun to my heart's content without worrying about crowded gyms and judgmental glares.

But in spite of my efforts to remain fit and living in a resort community and plenty of time to workout and eat healthy my waist began to expand. Having gotten down to thirty-four-waist jeans I once again found myself at thirty-six and rising. In addition to a gym we joined a cross-fit group, and I went occasionally to the public pool to swim alone, and did some jogging through the neighborhoods once or twice a week. My insomnia had worsened over the last year but had now become debilitating, and I was too exhausted to workout with any resemblance of my former athletic self. Swimming also now seemed to make me irritated, like someone plugged me into a high-powered electric socket and flipped on the switch. In spite of hitting the gym and a cross-fit group and jogging and swim-ming my waist went up to thirty-eight. My partner began to withdraw, and make comments about my appearance. "Yeah," he said one day during a conversation about what I don't remember, "because you don't want to get any fatter." I was floored, not that he would say something like that since he had long shown himself capable of real cruelty but because I was an athlete. Fat wasn't who I was as a person. That was other people. *I could not get fat.* But of course I could. And I did. Growing more frustrated by this free-fall into fatigue and frumpiness I began to search for other answers, reading papers, news articles, and books and blogs by doctors, weight-loss experts, and nutritionists. Among the samplings I read during that time was a book on liver health. I followed its protocol. It failed as well. Other leading doctors and nutritionists, personalities with sprawling websites peppered with advertisements for every kind of health product outlined tips for weight loss and improving health with general sweeping statements such as "sugar is bad," and "leptin resistance causes weight gain," hocking supplements which I bought and diet manipulations that sounded scientific yet lacked any positive effects on my quality of life.

Despite all this nothing changed, my energy slowly draining like water from a partly clogged sink. One day while walking my dogs I ran into a neighbor and mentioned that losing weight was proving unsuccessful and frustrating. She was a nurse practitioner, she said, and worked for a successful and expensive weight loss clinic. "I have a program for you," she said. "Men lose weight *so fast* on it."

"Really?" I asked, feeling hope once again. As she described the program I could see the sense behind it, although the rigor and deprivation gave me some pause as it seemed to simply be calorie deprivation and portion control which had so far only ever served to add suffering, not weight-loss, to my weight-loss efforts. But the difficulty paid off. By the third day I had lost eight pounds! Not only would I be lean again, my boyfriend would probably stop dropping backhanded compliments about my appearance. In retrospect I actually still looked hot. There is a video of me from this time standing out in the rain by the pool, with huge muscles and a bright smile on my face. But my health was already like a commuter bus in the Peruvian Andes—much too close to the edge. Contrary to my hope of hopes I did not keep losing eight pounds every few days. Instead, the weight loss stalled at ten pounds, though I was nearly starving myself. Two weeks of this hell resulted in no more weight loss, and my insomnia suddenly worsened from the usual one or two in the morning to three or four, and now with a new irritating sensation not unlike what I felt after swimming, but more like someone was scraping my spine with a fork.

I abandoned the diet, much to the dismay of my disdainful partner, and resigned to investigate other options. Meanwhile, the stress of my relationship and life was proving more than I was able to handle and, unaware of it at the time, began to drink more. Unable to extract myself from ill-health and loneliness my physical health began to decline now at a steady pace until one day I finally found myself so ill I could not walk around the block with my dogs without my extremities swelling, literally gasping for air as if oxygen itself was being sucked from the earth.

I don't remember exactly how I came upon the writings of the biologist whose work would change my life, but suddenly I found myself on the website of a Dr. Raymond Peat whose articles and papers discussed hormones and women's health and included a vast and thorough understanding of cellular biology based on that of other scientific greats like Albert Szent-Györgyi, Gilbert Ling, and Otto Warburg. His writing was detailed, and though meandering I was suddenly reading information that fit not only exactly with the science I already knew but also my lived experiences which all the other books and articles had not. For the first time in my search for answers I was reading work which correctly characterized the nature of molecules and cellular processes in the context of diet, and fit exactly in line with causes, factors, and consequences of my own personal experience. Dr. Peat even talked about how nutritional deficiencies, stress, and excess physical exercise could wrought harmful effects on the body, about chlorine and it's antagonism to thyroid health (OMG I've been swimming in chlorine for most of my adulthood!) and how hypothyroid disease contributes to weight gain and depression. He mentioned 5-HT, St. John's Wort, and resveratrol as substances which promote stress and torpor to cause problems like heart disease. His insight into energy and nutrition and how both contribute to specific outcomes and metabolic conditions such as insomnia correlated *exactly* with what I had experienced in my descent into ill-health. Things I had tried which resulted in failure were described exactly as they had occurred, like some psychic retelling of my past, but on a metabolic, biological, scientific context.

I began to implement some of the things his articles talked about, but they were also filtered through forums and amateur health advocates who didn't entirely understand, as well as the complications of bias from my own life, and Dr. Peat's writing was better at pointing out problems and less effective in presenting solutions. The most effective tool I learned from him was a method of monitoring temperature and pulse as an indicator of metabolic health (which I discuss in the chapter on self therapy). I was alarmed to find my body temperature *far* below what it should be, but it was a revelation because it was the first time I could see the state of my health reflected in a measurable, objective way and not just how I felt or what I looked like in the mirror that day. Beginning some of the concepts advocated by his papers I found brief relief, but not knowing enough yet I made some mistakes, but which still continued to improve my health because they were choices better informed than I had been previously. At this same time I finally found a competent doctor, after having visited many who insisted there was nothing wrong with me though my tests had for the last four or five years consistently returned a high white blood cell count. She had the insight to image my thyroid gland, and found it was enlarged and infected with five nodes, two of which were tumor size and likely cancerous.

But already my health began to improve, though my partner couldn't see it and he left. I lost my health coverage and could not pursue cancer treatment. Abandoned to my own devices, my keenness for science finally allowed me to connect the dots of cause and consequence in my own health. I saw the flaws in the books, articles, and medical studies which had led me to adopt devastating dietary behaviors like starvation, fasting, and carbohydrate deprivation, or taking supplements like 5-HTP and resveratrol which had harmed my health. It soon became apparent that most of the health information I had heard through all my life was utter bullshit. I began to see the body for what it truly is—not a decrepit, weak vessel for the soul which must be shaped and molded in the forge of self discipline but a competent, amazing, logical construct of nature which does not trend toward death, but to life and health. I also saw the vast majority of health advice for what it was—tent poles to prop up the canopy of wishful thinking, the lengths great indeed to which we go to convince ourselves of things we most want to be true— that we are safe, that we are wanted, that there is nothing wrong with us even when life demonstrates the contrary. Most medical and nutritional information is exactly this, with biases infecting studies, research, and practice to tell us what we want to hear, what makes us feel safe and in control, to the point of leading astray even those who are intelligent and open minded, and especially those who are not.

I once saw a study on dialysis patients which charted their sodium levels in relation to the rate of death during dialysis. Those with the lowest sodium levels lived longer on dialysis than those with the most sodium, and the conclusion of the authors was that high sodium caused early death while on dialysis, because like many others they have long believed sodium to be antagonistic to good health. But if one is being truly objective and scientific there is an equal, opposite conclusion in that very same study which is that those with high sodium *were more likely to die from dialysis*. This is the more logical conclusion from such data, given that the dialysis process removes sodium from the body and thus kills those with an apparent need for extra sodium as reflected by the action of their own physiology. Similarly, research into resveratrol has made it appear to be a healthy supplement but in reality resveratrol raises cortisol by blocking carbohydrate metabolism, which is why I slimmed down so fast but also why I could not sleep and nearly lost my mind from insanity, as in excess cortisol is highly destructive to the body. 5-HTP too is converted to serotonin which is regarded as the happiness hormone, but serotonin is actually a hormone of torpor and in excess slows the metabolism of the heart. St. John's Wort does similar things, as do most antidepressants such as the one I was one previously. In studies and medical research the failure to ask *'is this a good thing?'* often goes unaddressed, and 'first, do no harm' is more of a suggestion, and bias rather than understanding is the prevalent motivation. Some studies show increases in testosterone from calorie deprivation and excessive exercise but fail to consider if that rise in testosterone is a stress response, to protect the body against the damage which is being done, which would eventually lead to a failure of testosterone production, or worse, and is immediately characterized as a positive effect leading to many people starving themselves.

Studies like one which supposedly found an association between prostate cancer and and barbecued food due to a known carcinogen called *acrylamide* caused a worldwide panic and brouhaha to avoid charred and barbecued food. Before the 1900's food was always cooked with open flame, fired by wood or charcoal. In fact we have been eating barbecue since man first discovered fire, and the fact that we cook food *is the reason* we are so advanced as a species, because heat breaks down chemical substances into elemental parts, destroying inedible barriers to nutrition and allowing easier and greater absorption of a higher quantity of nutrients, proteins, and calories. Tremendous energy is otherwise required to separate the chemical bonds that hold food together, and it takes our bodies (or microbes) the same amount of energy to do the work that can be done for us by fire. Our tongue also identifies beneficial molecular properties of food as delicious (or not), and charring food tastes amazing because it breaks it down into its most basic elements, which also allows them to be absorbed without much effort. Since we have survived for millions of years as a species while consuming charred food (*Homo erectus* first discovered how to make fire about two million years ago) I was not inclined to accept the conclusions of the study, and even less so after reading it. Even our chin is an evolutionary result of our ability to cook, specifically because our ancestors used to have enormous, protruding jaws and huge teeth for grinding plants but after our discovery of fire we no longer needed such strong teeth and jaws to chew food and our dentition rapidly shrank inward to facilitate chewing softer, cooked foods while the bone which makes up our chin did not retreat as fast (people also claim that Neanderthals did not have chins, but they clearly have chins, only ones which are flatter and less pronounced).

This study in particular was also a survey, a kind of study which is notoriously unreliable for determining cause and effect and is supposed to only be used as an investigative or jumping off point for further scientific inquiry, not to be published and distributed as proven science. It was authored by young scientists conducting phone interviews with a random assortment of people, asking them pointed questions about food habits and following up later with another phone call to inquire if they had contracted cancer. The authors then "adjusted" for variables, which means they altered the data, and arrived at this conclusion without so much as drawing a single drop of blood or running one slide of cell culture on their subjects. Not once did they confirm by observation or in clinical settings that these people actually ate burnt food, how much of it they did or didn't eat, if there was acrylamide confirmed in the foods, or exactly how burnt each meal was. There is absolutely no evidence from this or any study that charred food actually has *any* causative association with *any* type of cancer, whatsoever. In fact, it should also be argued from the results of their study that if there really was an association of prostate cancer with charred food, which there is not because if there was an association nearly every single male in the Untied States would have prostate cancer, it is equally possible that people who develop prostate cancer might naturally *crave* charred food for some yet unknown therapeutic action, which is a more probable reality since we as a species intuitively crave foods which alleviate suffering and illness.

This study is tantamount to fraud, as are most studies where people draw erroneous conclusions from sets of data they have manufactured themselves, and people consume the information from these studies as legitimate advice or insight because most people think authors of such work are motivated by a desire to help, cure disease, and advance scientific discovery. In reality the majority of scientific research is motivated by profit, prestige, and professional advancement, and most people never contemplating that a scientist's aim in performing a study may be to land a good job at some well-paying research institute, secure funding for their programs, or justify selling a medical product that may or may not actually work. Studies and articles which use subjects unfamiliar and frightening to the general public such as acrylamide sound legitimate because we often don't know what they're talking about and assume the scientists do. But many studies and scientists are outright racist or eugenic, which are primary traits of narcissism and stupidity, and discuss differences in human health as if a significant role is played by race or family genetics, which also effectively supports racism since it blames disease on heritage, rather than more causal factors like systemic economic inequality, food insecurity, lifestyle, geopolitical conflict, access to medical care, dietary traditions, pathogenic microbes, etc. One absurd study claimed that appendicitis runs in families and therefore is caused by genetic susceptibility without any supporting study to cite that claim, because there are none, because appendicitis is caused by infectious fucking microorganisms which are easily spread among close relations such as family groups and supported or inhibited by dietary behaviors or lifestyle factors which are also a product of familial conditioning. These problems are so rampant in science that studies will even outright attribute race as a factor when we know, scientifically, *THAT THERE IS NO SUCH FUCKING THING AS RACE*, and that the genetic differences between me and someone on the other side of the world to whom I have not been related for millions of generations is at most no more than 0.1%. All sorts of bias infect the scientific community which affect conclusions drawn by authors and readers alike, and bias has direct and devastating consequences for our real physical health as evidenced by the currently unchecked, undeniable, rampant rates of metabolic disease which keep getting worse in spite of advances in many other areas of science and technology. There are literally more dangerous chemicals on the grocery store receipt you handle every time you go shopping than are in charred food from barbecue, and the authors and promoters of the barbecue study failed, conveniently, to mention that acrylamide *is entirely destroyed by stomach acid*, a fact that should have rendered irrelevant the study and anyone who talks about acrylamide as a danger of barbecue.

If we are going to get cancer or diabetes it's not the fault of a delicious grilled dinner or the consumption of ice cream and other sugary foods, but instead factors like chronic pathogenic infection, exposure to environmental contaminants and stressors, and behavioral and dietary patterns which compromise the ability of cells to produce energy and cause stress to the body. Poorly done studies are exactly the reason *why* we have epidemics of metabolic disease like diabetes and cancer, because even in the age of particle accelerators and quantum computers the medical and scientific professions do not understand these diseases, else these studies would have lead to their cure, which they have not. The kind of medical and scientific malfeasance which leads to misinformation and even dangerous health consequences is also a lesson in how unscrupulous people misuse or misinterpret evidence which can influence your health and quality of life, and why it's important for the general population to understand the context of a study when using them to make important health decisions. Simply reading study titles or their abstract is not at all sufficient to glean useful information, especially since the bias of authors can obscure scientific realities, even on accident and certainly with intent. In my own experience my health was further destroyed by blindly heeding supposedly "scientific" advice, especially if backed by a study or seeming irrefutable evidence, never understanding that "science" as it exists is just as easily and commonly adulterated by incompetence, malfeasance, deceit, cheating, conflicts of interest, outright racism, and ulterior motives as any other profession. Adding to the confusion is the motivation of media and other businesses to use outrageous, exciting, novel, or emotionally exploitative sources for click-bait it begins to seem clear how little reliance should be placed on this system of dissemination. This is nothing new, of course, as humans have always used deceit and information for personal gain. Benjamin Franklin for instance concocted outright lies to increase the popularity of his newspaper. He once wrote an entirely fabricated article about caches of human scalps belonging to white Americans taken by indigenous Americans aligned with King George, because he was a revolutionary and wanted to make King George look poorly. Of course there was no cache of scalps and European colonists were in contrast responsible for the genocide of an entire continent of people. The lie enflamed prejudice against indigenous populations and contributed unnecessarily to fear and the emotional unrest of consumers of that information. Such disinformation happens to us when we listen to exploitative, misguided, and opportunistic sources of information rather than personally vetting sources for honesty and authenticity and exercising some critical thought. For me, it nearly cost my life.

The fact that countless studies also torture animals in such cruel and inhumane ways appears that scientists are often just looking for an excuse to commit heinous and immoral acts on helpless animals, and many studies being done on living animals do not even extrapolate well to human beings, often performed just to keep grant money flowing and to justify the profession, when more intelligent and productive studies using tissue cultures, computer modeling, and simply better comprehension of biochemistry would actually produce results without wasting innocent lives of helpless animals. While some of the information used in this book did come from studies on animals the most productive, accurate, and useful ones come from simple tissue cultures or ethical human studies by scientists who actually know how biology and chemistry works and don't require the barbaric torture and slaughter of dogs, monkeys, rabbits, rats, and other animals to brute force their stupidity into scientific journals. Once I learned how to find reliable information from reliable sources it became plainly obvious how to get it, and the broad strokes of truth can even be seen in every day life—The effectiveness of low-carb diets are invalidated by everyone who stays fat after dieting. Those taking prescription medications which act opposite their claimed benefits means those medications do not work. When portion control is cited as necessary for fitness it is invalidated by all those with abs who eat like porkers. Our food history has a rich tradition of good dishes made well while enjoying the benefits of youth and wellness. It is not necessary to resort to exotic solutions or extreme behaviors. It only requires a little knowledge and care and compassion for your own body. When ingesting dietary advice it behooves a consumer to ask whether it is rational, logical, and likely. If it is not those things, best to disregard. Your very life may be at stake.

CHAPTER 5
A PROPER HUMAN DIET

One day at the age of nine I came home from Cub Scouts to find my family already fed. "Warm up your dinner honey," said my mom while putting a diaper on the newest and last of my younger siblings, "it's in the fridge." I had never eaten a dinner alone at this point in my life, and while initially struck by the loneliness of eating on my own it also seemed to foreshadow my growing up, of having some autonomy, and I felt a wonderful sense of practicing some independence. I opened the fridge and found a large platter of leftover mashed potatoes, chicken, and sautéed vegetables. The portions were much too large for my age, but I wasn't about to complain. The plate was an oblong platter with an undulating edge and a fine floral motif about the rim, one of a large collection my parents had lovingly purchased for their restaurant down the street. I pulled the plastic wrap off the food then set the plate on the stove and turned on the burner.

I was nine. No one had ever taught me to cook. Or to ask for help when I needed it. I'm sure we had a microwave, but I had also never used that, and I had always seen my mom and dad prepare food on the stove or in the oven. I went to join my family in the living room while the food heated up, and a few moments later as we all watched television a loud *bang!* rang through the house followed by the sound of shattering ceramic and sizzling juices followed by my mom rushing into the kitchen.

I would learn many life lessons in a similarly hard way. Such as that hard-boiled eggs cannot be made in the microwave—they explode and cover everything, including unexpecting little sisters, in hot scrambled egg. Frozen candy bars shoot violent electric arcs of Sith-Lord style lightning bolts when thawed in the microwave if the inner wrapper is metallic (and it can ruin your microwave). Consuming an entire box of Butterfinger candy bars in a week, even if they were a birthday present and you loved them, will make you hate them for the rest of your life.

Drunk cooking will either produce a masterpiece or a disaster, there is no inbetween.

But for all the cooking my mother and father did, when finally on my own I found myself perplexingly lost when it came to food. What to cook and how to cook it, and how to manage my physical health and nutrition were as much an intellectual desert as taxes, sexually transmitted diseases, and making and maintaining friendships. For the first few years on my own I made lots of easy pastas which really means I was making boxed macaroni five nights a week, and some chicken, all of which grew boring very quickly. I began to eat fast food for lunches and sometimes for dinner. But soon I got a copy of *The Joy of Cooking,* and found some recipes on the internet which, like me, was also coming into its maturity. Later when I moved to Los Angeles I met people infected by the gastronomical glee that makes life in California so enchanting, and day trips to cooking stores and farmers markets faded into nights crafting wild boar, pairing cheese with wine, and finishing with toasty espressos. For the first time I had artichokes, chestnuts, and escargot and was smitten with food-love and became a believer in the celebration of eating not as a means to banish hunger but rather something to be respected, worshiped, and relished with gratitude and good friends (which were unfortunately in short supply). I fell in love with Ina Garten and began learning better cooking skills by watching her show, such as how to properly hold a knife, smash garlic, or get more out of chicken than I ever knew was possible. Food also became something to appreciate for its inherent qualities rather than smothering under complicated preparations. I had the best meal of my life at *Chez Panisse* in San Francisco, restaurant of famed chef Alice Waters who helped restore the concept of eating seasonally. One day at a social event at their restaurant *Ciudad* in downtown L.A. I won a copy of Mary Sue Milliken and Susan Feniger's *Cooking with Too Hot Tamales.* I had never seen food take such a place of esteem. Food was a religion.

Of course food should be revered. Food is what we are made of. But even in the midst of this cultural awakening my diet continued to suffer from the burden of nutritional hearsay and body dysmorphia—friends with killer physiques whined about their dinners of boneless, skinless chicken breast and steamed spinach. News outlets decried dairy and barbecue. Social media shamed anyone who ate sugar. I began to listen to all this nonsense and deprive myself, cutting out this food or that depending on whatever trend I became aware of. It seemed as if there was nothing really good left to eat that would not kill me or make me fat, matters made worse by a gut which for years now was constantly mangled and inflamed, a problem which grew so bad it began to interfere with my daily life, having to call in sick to work or skip social functions from crippling stomach pain and an unpredictable bowel. The first time a serious episode of digestive problems hit me was during a date at a restaurant where I became trapped on a toilet for an hour and he had to come and enquire about me. Growing up, at almost every meal my father consumed Pepto Bismol like it was a beverage, so I naturally assumed that stomachaches were a condition of adulthood and I was expected to soldier through it. Eventually I realized my health was being affected by what I ate, though I could not exactly find good answers. First I tried cutting dairy. That seemed to work, but then it didn't. I cut out red meat and found a little relief. That seemed to implicate meat, so I converted to vegetarianism and accidentally healed my acne, but which convinced me that vegetarianism was a legitimate way to go, and then I began to suffer those chronic sinus infections and for a year of my life could never breathe through both nostrils at once. Later, the calories-in-calories-out philosophy of fitness eventually gave me a glut of metabolic illnesses, including cancer, made worse by harmful medications and inferior foods which made up my diet but which I thought were healthy due to the hurricane of misinformation which swirls around us, and my appetite became increasingly insatiable precisely because of the stress I was putting on my body.

Those who laud the asinine idea of a beneficial calorie deficit are usually young, male, or eternally fit, and continue to promote calorie deprivation long after such diets have left them as beautiful as dried roadkill, as if any organism on this planet thrives on food shortage. Most women, and men who've struggled with weight problems come to intuitively understand the fallacy of calorie deficit through experience, even if we refuse to acknowledge it, because when we try it we get exactly the opposite of what is promised, with the addition of new and previously unimagined health problems.

In defense of calorie deficit proponents it does appear to work. For them anyway. They see a decrease in body fat (while ignoring muscle loss and other side effects like depression, fatigue, low libido, insomnia, etc.). Naturally, they promote what worked for them. But the way calorie deficit diets work is through the utilization of stress, and young and healthy bodies respond to stress differently than everyone else. Having not yet succumbed to the consequences of chronic stress, young bodies tend to shed fat more easily and recover more quickly, making it appear as a legitimate way of living. It eventually fails for everyone, though, even if for some it takes until they are much older. I was absolutely perplexed when the calorie deficit backfired at the age of thirty. It had worked before, and was certainly the proper way to do things. But once the method failed for me, no matter what I did I continued to retain fat, and even began to gain more in spite of my tireless and exhaustive assertion, which makes it sound like I was dieting 24/7 but in reality I could barely go a few days before the pain was too severe to resist. One day I had the thought that whomever was responsible for Chris Hemsworth surely knew the secret to health and beauty. So I looked up the work of a "nutritionist to the stars" and found a diet which prescribed eating vegetables before meat because tigers have a short digestive tract but we, who are not tigers, do have a very long intestinal tract (but not so long as gorillas) and tigers eat meat but we are not tigers with short intestinal tracts so meat rots in our non-tiger intestinal tract—It also did not work.

As far as dietary trends go the paleo and primal camps have probably come closest to understanding an optimal human diet, although none have gone so far as to suggest eating bugs which were in all likelihood a regular staple of the human diet and which many billions of people on the planet still consume, not out of necessity as assumed by xenophobic weirdos but because they have never lost the tradition of the natural dietary use for insects. While the idea of eating bugs does admittedly gross me out our past evolutionary history using insects as a food source accounts for our affinity for crunchy foods such as potato chips, which mimic the texture of the insect exoskeleton. In fact, a prominent theory of human evolution which I consider accurate is that we evolved on a coast of Africa or on the shore of an ancient African lake, as more recent research is revealing, such as ancient Lake Mega Chad, foraging and hunting not only in the forests and grasslands but a great part in the shallows near the shores because we discovered mollusks and crustaceans could be an easy food source. This observation, put forth by marine biologist Alister Hardy and further developed by anthropologist Elaine Morgan is supported by the fact that we have no body hair, and display more subcutaneous fat than our primate relatives, not to mention our great affinity for water, because our regular immersion in water searching for shellfish and other easily hunted seafoods stimulated the loss of body hair in exchange for an increase in subcutaneous fat which better protects from heat loss in water, which has also occurred in many other species including cetaceans, manatee, and even elephants which, yes, also had a marine ancestor. Proponents of the Savanah and heat or distance hunter hypotheses of hairlessness forget that insulation does not only work in one direction, and also keeps animals cool which is why wild dogs, lions, and other active animals all have fur. Fur and hair also protects against UV exposure, which is why we still retain hair on the top of our head as it serves to block sun during the most direct rays when the sun is immediately overhead. All apes are also capable of walking on just two legs but, as pointed out by Dr. Hardy, our primate relatives only do so consistently when walking through water, not in pursuit of food, prey, or during conflict, hence our later commitment to bipedal locomotion and elongation of legs which did not occur so we could see over tall grass but to better ambulate through water, and these primal man diets also make some of the classic mistakes that infect every other diet trend because they focus on the supposed flaws of our human condition rather than our strengths as an adaptable and marvelous creation.

Substantively all dieting is based on the same desecration of the human body that has plagued humanity for the last two-thousand years or more, one which views the mortal frame as intended for the grave, weak unless strengthened in the forge of discipline and deprivation, annexing responsibility for biology instead of submitting to it, which is why primal man diets are so appealing to so many who desire to view the human animal as a dominant subjugator of nature. But such ideas are a defiling of the human form, ignorance of the resiliency of life and the power of creation, and the versatility of metabolic biochemistry which fail to properly honor our actual evolutionary past. Coming near the brink of death I have seen the folly in the characterization of the human condition which is instead a magnificent organism, as are all the creatures which have survived on earth for so long, persisting in spite of our efforts to poison, starve, and abuse ourselves and our species, surviving sabotage, social and nutritional stress, and exhaustion and over-exertion we continue to live, even thrive, because contrary to the bemoaning and ill-tidings characterization of the human form the body trends not toward death, but to life, a machine of cunning construction able to outwit even our own minds in order to ensure success. Our physiological processes have backups for backups of backups, able to create energy and recycle nutrients even during extreme starvation, exhaustion, disease, and environmental poisoning. It was once believed that cells were more or less stagnant, that once damage occurred it stayed because cells did not recover or replace themselves, not because anyone ever confirmed that stupid theory but because men who considered themselves intelligent said it was so and the rest of us nodded in agreement. It is the bald-faced anthropomorphizing of biology, which to this day continues to handicap real understanding of the actual designs which makes us work, even by men and women of notable intellect and investigative resources, but whom desire not to converse with the transient nature of fate see permanence where it does not exist, misled by their search for confirmation rather than enlightenment, fertilized by the common man who seeks the same.

For instance, did you know there are no such thing as *receptors*? Not as they are described, anyway. The idea of receptors was proposed to explain the reaction of cells to molecules and in response to the concept of *signaling*, because it was difficult to comprehend how certain materials enter and exit cells, move about the body, and cause cellular functions. The idea of receptors and signaling became accepted as fact because it does not strongly contradict cellular functions, and the theory stays put because biology continues to work regardless if anyone understands precisely how it is accomplished and the speculation it actually is. In reality only one major flaw in this design is enough to refute it, though there are others, which is a physical impossibility for the surface area of a cell to support the sheer number and variety of every necessary receptor, transporter, pump, etc., required for the full function of cellular metabolism. Neither can the energy requirements for all receptor systems, pumps, transporters, etc., be satisfied by that which is actually produced in a cell. In addition, the impossible probability of molecules meeting by chance with their coordinate receptor around the limited surface area of an object which is proportionally in size to those molecules as a human to the Sun is too ridiculous to be probable.

Signaling concepts in cells and molecules was a frustrating barrier to solving many health problems because it's also not really a thing, but many, many studies and researchers emphasize in their research the supposed signaling effects of elements and molecules in cellular function so their inherent and actual function is usually entirely missing from research. What researchers mistake as signaling is instead the actual, physical effect that elements and molecules have on their surroundings inherent to their presence and atomic properties like electrochemical charge, size, weight, etc., and containing their own chemical energy potential which, upon entering a cell or interacting with other atoms and molecules, catalyze actual functions due to their own inherent nature without the need for receptors and signaling systems. For instance, *nitric oxide* is considered a gaseous signaling molecule and when received by a cell the cell receptor system then recognizes and responds according to its specific DNA programming by having received it. In reality it is the electrochemical properties of a nitric oxide molecule which directly cause those effects when it enters a cell, not the receptor system, to which the cell is changed because of the particular molecular architecture of the cell which has been constructed by our DNA so that when nitric oxide enters it will have this particular effect. This seems like a trivial difference between the accepted concept and what actually occurs but many elements and molecules are never properly understood beyond insufficient 'signaling' functions so researchers then do not understand the real atomic nature of elements or molecules which then leads to insufficient understanding of how they actually work to construct biology and thence larger biological functions like disease which then results in millions of people suffering from unchecked and untreated metabolic illness. The concept of signaling is like characterizing a piece of wood as burning itself in response to fire rather than fire being the thing that burns the wood. Concepts of signaling and reception also overcomplicate far simpler biology because systems of signals and receptors must in turn be supported by other systems since they don't on their own completely solve those functions. Those supporting systems don't exist anyway so research remains stymied in a closed loop of self imposed ignorance. It is instead simply that elements and molecules possess their own inherent properties which, upon entering cells, organelles, or interacting with other elements and molecules directly cause those observed effects.

Such concepts are also entirely unnecessary for us to understand that starvation and calorie deprivation ruin metabolic health, and I have found that the more studies or concepts invoke such lingo as receptors and the deeper it descends into biological minutiae the less actual information it contains. Ideas such as receptors are mere intellectual trivialities, where cause and effect are the real issue when it comes to getting well. It can help to understand cellular processes only inasmuch as it enables positive, effective, actionable understanding. The proliferation of minutiae in discussion and research of receptor, membrane, and signaling concepts has done squat to improve the health of the general public, as you can see by simply looking at the population of industrialized cultures who suffer from more systemic disease than at any time in history (and no, not only because we live longer). A few years ago in a meditation class I met a woman suffering from a painful and serious edematous condition of her leg and ankle. She was by no means overweight or unhealthy by other appearances, yet her foot and calf were swollen to a grotesque and misshapen two or three times their normal size. She took care to hide it with her clothing but when we were alone I was compelled to ask as the condition looked quite alarming and I knew how to treat it. She confessed her doctors were unable to help, and been suffering with it for more than a year and tried all kinds of medications. Further inquiry revealed a severe bias against sodium on account of her mother dying from heart attack many years ago, and she claimed to not have added *any* salt to her own nor her family's diet in twenty years, and now she was walking around (if you can call that walking), with a life-threatening condition which is directly caused by sodium deficiency. Her son was also currently dying of a pancreatic disease though only in his mid twenties, and on more than a few occasions I have heard from friends and acquaintances who are also black that have been told to avoid sodium *because* they are black (and some other quack, racist medical advice). Our body uses sodium and chloride to manage and balance water, and when these electrolytes become imbalanced the body can no longer control water which in turn invades tissues, suffocates them, and contributes to and causes many severe metabolic diseases. The higher rate of these kinds of diseases in minority populations is a function of economic racism and policies such as red-lining which prohibited economic development in communities composed largely of minority groups and impaired access to products, services, healthy food, and opportunity and is not in any way a function of biology except that the human body cannot thrive without sufficient quality and quantity of nutrition, and I told this woman about the biological roles of sodium and how she needed to get salt into her diet immediately (though I never went to that mediation class again and don't know if she did or not).

Because we have become the most intelligent creatures on the planet (arguably), we have the luxury of skirting consequences, or at least delaying them for a time. Because the body is so adept at adapting to diet and nutritional deficiencies we are not always confronted by the incompatibility of our actions with our existence, though it will always catch up to us. But even when stricken with cancer it is not too late to wake up and pay attention, and to work with our biology rather than in opposition. Not only is a proper human diet supportive of health and vitality, it is also indulgent and satiating. There is not a single organism on the planet which thrives on starvation, and ideas of dietary deprivation originate from society's residual obsession with discipline, of a sacrificial requirement for gain, and the religious contamination of spirituality and biology. The body does not care about whether we believe in God, or personal discipline, or whether you are resisting that urge to scarf down a tub of cookie-dough ice cream. If we run out of carbohydrate the body releases hormones to catabolize our internal tissues, regardless of your ideological beliefs, to make its own carbohydrate at the expense of lean muscle. These same hormones stimulate hunger, not to challenge your willpower but to alarm you to the damage you are doing to your body.

The first tenet of a proper human diet is to be well-fed. It does not make sense that a well-fed animal should become lethargic and diseased by an excess of nutritive quantity, and in fact the first sign of metabolic stress is an increase in appetite, because the body needs fuel and nutrients in order to resist stress whether it's caused by that insensitive boyfriend, a demanding job, too much exercise, or fallout from a radiological disaster. An organism which simply grows overweight from an excess of nutritional resources would destine the creature, and thus the entire species, to predation and death. There is no biological mechanism for the impairment of locomotion, metabolism, or social success while also increasing susceptibility to disease as a result of too much fat, sugar, or protein in the diet. Athletes and those with eating disorders subject to calorie and nutritive deficits who meet unfortunate cardiovascular crises are evidence of the fallacy of calorie deprivation, that fantasy that the body can somehow run on air, without fuel or nutrients. Often, the physical consequences of calorie and nutritional deficits present long before the unignorable episodes—thinning skin, declining energy, hair loss, changes in vision, problems sleeping, and changes to erectile function or libido are some of a cacophony of signs that the body is under nutritional stress and that such strategies are incompatible with human physiology. These are usually ignored, though, from a desire to achieve certain goals and force life to do what we desire. Always athletic, lean, and energetic, my father constantly reprimanded our family on discipline and self-deprivation, yet he has never in his entire life abstained from ice cream, sodas, or indulgent food nor embarked on a calorie, carbohydrate, or fat deprivation diet. Conversely, and like many women, my long-suffering mother spent more years in a continual battle with food than otherwise, yet found it impossible to keep lean. To my father it appears that his his lean physique was evidence of his ideals rather than his diet which did not actually reflect his ideals, and to my mother whose diet reflected her ideals never achieved a body which did. Being fed is a requirement for a healthy body, it is why your body, which decides the fate of your health, tells you to eat something before you fucking starve to death.

The therapeutic effects of foods are much greater than I ever imagined, even after I had experienced such profound healing, because my diet was for so long based on concepts of deprivation I had never had occasion to actually witness the obvious benefits which come from a repletion of nutrients and calories, and the more research and success I found the less and less supplements even played a role in my wellness and recovery, though my disease was some of the most severe any person can have. Supplements often have an obvious effect simply because they fill the deficits of a limited diet, and can be used to exaggerate pathways dependent on specific nutrients, but they are *never* a replacement for food, and the same effect can often be had from whole foods if the diet is simply replete in nutrients and calories and grounded on principles discussed throughout this book.

Several years ago when I was active in online forums trying to help people an insane lady yelled at me when I talked about how the amino acid tryptophan in milk converts in the human body either to niacin or serotonin, depending on certain metabolic conditions, where niacin promotes metabolic activity and serotonin alternatively slows down the metabolism, both regulatory branches which help to run human biology. She was insistent that milk was a perfect food and there was not only nothing wrong with it but that a person could live indefinitely on milk alone. It is these very kinds of ideological conceptions of food and human biology which seek to subvert and control nature and fate that we have not yet cured a great many diseases. Nature and food have no concern for our opinions, beliefs, tastes, desires, wants, faith, or needs, even be they great, and our desire to control life and bend fate and nature to our will is never anything but an illusion constructed by our human psyche to help us cope with the difficulty that life can be. Desiring foods to be miraculously incredible in their nutritional profile is completely delusional. There is no such thing as a perfect food, not even superfoods, which are nothing more than direct effects of marketing and advertising campaigns meant only to get you to buy shit or click on articles and not even a tiny bit meant to help you.

Milk can be very nutritious, but much of its nutrition also depends on the state of your health and not the other way around, having the ability to properly metabolize its amino acids and handle its very large phosphate content. Milk can be great for kids and while it has lots of other nutrients it is so deficient in vitamins K, E, D, and iodine, copper, iron, zinc, selenium, molybdenum, manganese, and oleic acid that it is not at all an ideal food for adults, and has too high of growth-associated animo acids and less of those which are inhibitory if it is used without complimentary foods like fruit and vegetables. Most fruit and vegetables too have been systematically bred and cultivated over centuries by our ancestors into forms which make them more palatable but even foods which are highly nutritious and helpful for our wellbeing are still based on their own original purpose, which is to perpetuate and support their own propagation, not ours, and as such are not designed to be "superfoods" for humans and usually lack sufficient nutrition for any one food to perform such a role.

One of my favorite nature facts is the trick oak trees play on squirrels in order to promote their own survival. Trees and other plants produce flowers, pollen, fruit, nuts, and seeds in part because other creatures will participate in their reproductive strategies, and as enticement will make those things tasty and nutritious in exchange. But if animals and insects consume an excess of them it would also eliminate those plant species, and having evolved to avoid this very problem oak trees normally only produce enough acorns to support a moderate quantity of squirrel population but every few years will suddenly produce an incredible bumper crop of acorns purposefully to overwhelm and confuse squirrels and by so doing increase the chances of seedling germination since the relatively small population of squirrels cannot possibly eat them all, but only do this occasionally so as not to promote squirrel overpopulation which would decimate the oak's own chances at propagation. This demonstrates how everything in nature is concerned first and foremost with its own survival, and why there is no such thing as a superfood, and while foods like milk can be extremely nutritive no food is a superfood because not one single food on this planet contains even most of the nutrients we require as a human species, as well that our nutritional needs as a human being are also not only dependent on food, for instance requiring sunlight as a nutrient as well, and many health problems which occur during our lifetime can be caused by sunlight deficiency. This is not only relevant for our levels of vitamin D but also regulatory pathways which respond to sunlight, because of our evolutionary past in which any state of sunlight deprivation is a signal to the body of wintertime and insufficient nutritive resources, and as such artificial states of winter such as excessive sequestration indoors actually alters our metabolic function even more strongly than diet which no food on this earth can change regardless of its nutritional profile.

Many things that people eat are also not natural at all and the food industry is contaminated with preservatives, emulsifiers, anti-caking agents, adulterants, food coloring, bleaches, etc., which, even when natural, can still sometimes be extremely toxic. Food colorings in cheap candies, meats, processed baked goods, drinks, and mass produced dairy products can often be very harmful to the body and when eaten by children disturb endocrinological or neurological pathways to produce or contribute to behavioral disorders, asthma, immune dysfunction, or gut health. Consuming whole foods as much as possible and avoiding those which have chemical additives in the ingredients label is extremely important to avoid significant health problems.

Our own native gut microbiome also produces many nutrients that are not even available in food, nutrients like the short chain fatty acids or vitamin K2 (there is some K2 in cheese, on account of the microbes, and vinegar contains one short chain fatty acid, but they are not replacements for a healthy gut). These microbes can also be extinguished by exposure to toxic agricultural chemicals, which is why eating organic can be very helpful, but they can also die from vitamin D deficiency as well since, like the oak to the squirrel, we share vitamin D with our microbes in order to cultivate them for our own purposes. The reason we have such a broad, omnivorous diet as a species is precisely because no one food is even close to sufficient to provide for the demanding nutritional needs of such a biologically complex animal. To be who we are biologically requires a much greater scope of micro and macro nutrients than any few foods can provide. Indeed, we evolved into the species we are in the first place because our ancestors developed physical traits which enabled the acquisition of nutrients from a wide variety of sources. When it comes to human nutrition a broader, not limited diet is the true superfood, one which gets for us the broad range of nutrients required in so many metabolic pathways that no one can provide on its own.

Because we are primates, and mammals, we are designed by nature to subsist primarily from carbohydrates, especially those which are within fruit and root vegetables. Our little, flat nails evolved to better open and peel the skins of fruit, to dismantle the skin away from flesh and seeds, so that our fingers could be more tactile from the absence of claws to better handle delicate fruit and succeed in our type of foraging. Fructose is the reason for the seeming paradox for that person you know who regularly consumes regular Coke but stays thin and energetic while you struggle to lose weight drinking diet, because the fructose in normal drinks, though artificially derived, actually provides ample amounts of this necessary biological intermediate for the proper functioning of their metabolism while diet products and your lack of fruit consumption does not. Fructose is also why we crave something sweet like dessert after dinner even when that dinner was high in carbohydrates and calories because fructose is also needed to properly metabolize many other macros including glucose and protein, and our body instinctively sends those biological signals to our brain to make us search out the needed nutrient when it is in short supply, not because your body wants to sabotage your diet plan but because you have already sabotaged the way the body is supposed to work and our protective instincts are kicking in trying to deal with those problems trying to save you from yourself.

Those who adhere to an idea of a paleo diet while condemning sugar do not understand what role sugar plays in biochemistry nor that *all carbs are sugar!* While it is true that refined sucrose is devoid of most other vitamins and minerals nobody ever eats plain sugar, and there is plenty of less refined or unrefined sugar available which also tastes better than fully refined sugar due to the presence of other nutrients and a more complex flavor profile, and sugar is usually combined with other ingredients which do contain vitamins and minerals that support the function of sugar in our biology. In animals such as us which are designed to run on carbohydrates, the robust metabolism that defines mammals like us characterized by leanness, high heat, high-energy personalities cannot happen during a deficit of sugar (that is to say all carbohydrate), and so our metabolic rate descends and reverts to backup forms of other energy production which cannot sustain good health, wellness, and function. For instance, carbohydrate deficiency activates catabolism of the amnio acid proline in our tissues which is largely incorporated into cartilage and extracellular matrix because proline is an efficient source of energy during glucose deprivation, and one of the age-promoting stresses of dieting and low-carbohydrate intake is the depletion of proline otherwise required to keep and maintain healthy skin, joints, and enzymatic function. Even in the case of diabetics the solution is not to deprive the body of sugar and carbohydrates but to restore the ability to metabolize it. Any diet that does not include fruit as a regular staple is incomplete, but dessert has come to take the place of fruit in our natural diet and is not a problem except for other factors in the dessert such as harmful types of grain, bad fats, or additives which are incompatible with our physiology. Sugar as it occurs naturally is fuel, a very proper and necessary one. Candy, desserts, and junk food which are asininely and collectively referred as "sugar" are not bad for your health because of sugar but for their quality of manufacture. Are they made with vitamin deficient products? Do they contain industrial additives? Is it actually food? Chocolate made with inferior additives like soy lecithin is not the same as good chocolate made properly with good ingredients. Properly made chocolate does not need lecithin added to it. The additive is a cheat and a shortcut used by the manufacturer which also renders chocolate so molecularly smooth in my opinion as to prevent tasting it properly anyway. A cheap candy bar with a list of unfamiliar chemicals is not going to hurt your health because it has sugar, but for all the other shit which is in it. Because it contains an abundance of nutrition in addition to sugar there is no more important human food than fruit, which should be consumed daily, in generous quantities, especially with breakfast which helps to wake up the metabolism and promote energy and happiness.

Dietary fat is similarly important to metabolic health, but many people often deprive themselves of fat as if calories are a liability rather than the every energy which keeps us living. Most people do not know that most hormones in our body, including sex hormones and the mineralocorticoids which are vital for maintaining electrolyte balance, are made from fats, so low fat diets impair libido, reproduction, and cause the body to lose electrolytes more rapidly. The greatest gains I achieved in my health came simply from switching the types of my dietary fat intake, and eating more of it (from unsaturated to saturated, conversely the greatest decline in my health came from consumption of the most unsaturated fats such as from fish oil and vegetable oil), while also eating a low-fat diet. As the chapter on fat elucidates, saturated and monounsaturated fatty acids are more stable in high heat, high oxygen environments such as occurs within our own body and best promote health because they easily resist the stresses of oxidation, and includes fats like butter, coconut oil, cocoa butter, shea butter, olive oil, almonds and their oil and butter, hazelnuts, or high-oleic sunflower oil (but not regular sunflower oil). Those products highest in polyunsaturated fats like canola, corn, soy, and vegetable oil would quickly turn rancid and smelly if you had pressed them yourself, but manufacturers deodorize and treat those oils to obscure the olfactory and visual cues which would otherwise clue the consumer to their rancid state, and consuming such products is akin to poisoning the mitochondria and lowering the metabolic rate, and the prevalence of such oils in the food industry is the sole reason for such pandemic levels of obesity across industrialized nations because the peroxidation stress caused by high intake of polyunsaturated fat so strongly destroys metabolic health. Unfortunately, most olive oil is counterfeit and cut with cheaper, harmful oils, and should be expensive, fruity, and taste very strongly of olives otherwise it is most likely cut with cheaper oils.

Though perceived as healthy, low-fat diets usually contain mostly bad fats and without good fats to help protect the metabolism they have a disproportional effect on health, weighing down the metabolic rate and is one of the reasons why diets backfire. It is much better to eat a diet which includes butter and low in all other fats than it is to do a low-fat diet. A good example of this phenomenon is the classic low-fat meal for muscle builders of a skinless chicken breast and steamed vegetables. While high in protein the chicken breast has enough bad fat to cause metabolic problems because of the absence of better fats, and some of the obvious outward effects of this type of diet are the decline in skin quality and hair loss in body builders and athletes because bad fats are so easily prone to destructive oxidation and contribute to the production of lipid peroxides and other reactive oxygen species which harm the body and lower the metabolic rate. A low fat diet also makes it difficult to obtain the necessary fat-soluble vitamins A, K, and E from the diet, as they are only absorbed when eaten in the presence of fat and deficiencies of those will lead to weight gain and immune dysfunction anyway.

Some sources of harmful fats enter our diets in sneaky ways. For instance because chickens and pigs are not ruminants and cannot convert harmful fats into good fats the way that cows, sheep, and goats can do, much of that fat on their body is the same as what is in their diet, and industrialized food systems which feed animals mostly soy and corn means their fats also strongly reflect that composition and eating chicken, eggs, and pigs fed poor diets can thus contribute to metabolic illness. Coconut oil survives unchanged in the cupboard for years at a time because it is so stable, and fats which are supportive of the human metabolic rate not only improve and sustain energy levels and health but prolong the youthful characteristics of our physiology since fat also participates in the structural components of every cell's construction. The French are famous for having a high fat diet but low occurrence of metabolic diseases. Ignoramuses in the United States characterize this as a paradox, as if everyone else would not experience the same results if you were not French, which is like the most stupid thing I've ever heard. The French have this benefit precisely because of the types of fats they consume and the quality of their food supply. For this reason French foods are very often compatible with good health. Thai food with its ubiquitous use of coconut milk and coconut oil is also more commonly healthful. Real olive oil is very high in the healthy monounsaturated fats and some saturated, so Mediterranean food in general is usually very healthy. At the very least the ubiquitous use of good quality butter and olive oil should replace inferior vegetable oils and substitutes. That these are also delicious is not only a plus, it is an indication the body knows what is good for our health.

Because of the pervasively negative conception of the human body, vegetables which are bitter and flavorless tend to take up an inappropriately greater portion of our contemporary diets, and more masochistic types consider the displeasure of eating these raw a sign of self control and health promotion, which has absolutely no foundation in reality. Green leaves like kale often contain phytotoxic substances (*phyto* means plant-based) that can interrupt our physiological pathways and should *always* be cooked. These toxins are why such plants taste so horrible. The tongue is an intelligent and capable organ and the signals it receives from tasting is meant to warn us of potentially harmful substances or conversely to promote those which benefit health. Putting something in your mouth which is alarmingly acrid such as raw kale is tantamount to long and slow suicide, because those same things which taste bad are either poisonous or prevent proper digestion which in turn prevent assimilation of the very vitamins and minerals which are the reason you're eating the kale in the first place. Phytic acid binds minerals in the digestive tract and can entirely rob you of calcium, magnesium, and even zinc, iron, or sulfur among others which in turn can cause tooth decay, bone loss, and insomnia due to subsequent mineral deficiencies. Cooking can often diminish or destroy these toxins which is one of the reasons why long-cooking methods are traditionally associated with healing foods such as soups and stews and why we have a long history of cooking, the action of which improves the bioavailability of most nutrients and why raw diets, while well-meaning, are completely misguided. Plants do not want to be food, so they have developed means of protecting their nutrients by dissuading would-be grazers from feasting. The reason our ancestors processed and cooked all their food was not because they were slovenly hedonists who paid no attention to nutrition but because they already knew what we are having to relearn, which is that these anti-nutrients can actually harm our health and wellbeing.

Root vegetables are also an important cornerstone in human primate health because they directly support gastroinestinal bacteria on which we depend for nutrients not available in the diet like many B vitamins and the short chain fatty acids such as acetic acid, butyric acid, propionic acid, etc., which have direct effects on cellular function and gut health. Our ancestors ate a great deal of different varieties of root vegetables but unfortunately grain has overtaken root vegetables as the most common source of dietary starch where grain is often less nutritious. We have also never evolved to efficiently digest grains that are not properly prepared, and they often come with deleterious health consequences when eaten before preparing properly or if they entirely replace root vegetables as a foundation for the diet. French fries are not bad for us because they are cooked in copious amounts of oil, they are bad for us when made in cheap, crappy vege-table oil as they are in most restaurants in order to make more profit from them, as even when potatoes are fried they contain lots of useful starch to promote our wellbeing, promote the microbiome, and contain enough vitamin C to supply our needs. French fries made at home in coconut oil become a health-promoting indulgence rather than a liability since coconut oil helps promote healthy hormone and metabolic function. Often it is not a question of which foods but what exactly they are made of that makes the difference. Roots also don't contain the amount of bad fats which occur in grains. In those with robust digestive systems our bacteria can produce helpful metabolic products from other foods like fruits, meat, and grains, and even things that aren't really food, but when the digestive tract is at all compromised (which often occurs *because* of excessive consumption of grains like corn and common wheat) the gut will require the best substrates such as fruit and root vegetables like sweet potato, yam, potato, yuca (also known as cassava and not to be confused with yucca), taro, carrots, etc. As a general rule, fruit yields acetic acid and roots yield butyric acid, although the variation is wide and dependent on other factors. Butyrate has the additional benefit of reducing insatiable appetite, because butyrate directs sugars directly into oxidation as fuel while a deficiency shifts the metabolism to fat storage. Incidentally, butyrate is shown to improve diabetes and other sugar-related metabolic disorders. Roots are not only filling but full of nutrients, and promote others which are manufactured in our gut.

Sedges are a long forgotten type of root vegetable which used to be a staple of the human diet, replaced by the advent of agriculture and more novel and attrac-tive vegetables, grains, and other commodities but which are in fact part of our obligatory, native nutritional requirements and required to resolve gut problems and directly combat gastrointestinal infection. Related to grasses the starchy tubers of sedges are eaten by a great many animals in the world and evidence of their consumption also appears in the ancient, anthropological record with sites of human ancestors containing remains of sedge tubers and other wild plants. Ancient Egypt cultivated the sedges we call *chufa, tiger nuts,* or *yellow nutsedge* which is widely cultivated around the Mediterranean region (Chinese water chestnuts are another common and delicious sedge). Horchata is a popular drink originally made from chufa (tiger nuts) which originated in North Africa before its popularity spread to Spain, and other forms of horchata are now made with other things like rice which are not tiger nuts, where tiger nuts are highly nutritious, delicious, and synergize better with human digestive and microbiome. Although they can be tough to chew if eaten dried it is a good workout for lazy jaw muscles, and chufa can be prepared in a variety of ways, including delicious horchata but also used as flour added to other foods, smoothies, or baked goods. The fatty acid profile of tiger nuts is also even better than olive oil and contains other useful dietary compounds like tannin and polyphenols which have further benefits to health and wellness. Tiger nuts are one of the most filling foods I've ever sampled, because they so strongly promote the commensal microbiome and thus synthesis of other nutrients made by our microbiome, and snacking on tiger nuts or making real horchata is a great strategy to start changing the diet.

Stomach acid required to digest food in the first place is regulated most strongly by *potassium,* which is exchanged with hydrogen atoms across the parietal cells barrier of the stomach, and potassium is also required for the pancreas to produce digestive enzymes and insulin and for the digestive tract to synthesize the mucin barrier, but grains and animal products are typically very low in potassium and general potassium deficiency due to insufficient consumption of fruit and root vegetables is a significant catalyst for metabolic illness since stomach acid is not only required to digest food but also acts as one of the first barriers against pathogenic ingress into the human body. For example our potassium requirements are about 5,000 mg a day (5 grams), depending on size, but a cup of wheat flour only contains about 134 mg total, and a cup of rice even less at 55 mg. A hamburger patty has about 250 mg, a cup of milk can have about 360 mg, corn 400 mg, and a cup of apricots 427 mg. One cup of potato has 630 mg, one cup of sorghum 696 mg, sunflower seeds 900 mg, hazelnuts 920 mg, and yam an amazing 1,224 mg. Especially when compared to the amounts our ancient ancestors used to consume which some researchers estimate to be around 10 grams a day (in my experience 5-6 grams is plenty), it is clear how contemporary diets easily promote potassium deficiency to catalyze a great many metabolic diseases due to its effect on gastrointestinal function. Potassium inhibition is actually how proton pump inhibitors are used to treat conditions like acid reflux, because interfering with potassium stops the secretion of hydrogen into the gut, but stomach acid is how we digest food and any impairments to this system, including the use of medications but especially from dietary potassium deficiency can collapse the system of digestion (acid reflux is discussed in upcoming chapters). Because potassium is extremely water soluble, boiling and draining plant foods as is common practice can cause loss of 50-70% of potassium, making it very easy to acquire potassium deficiency even when eating foods high in potassium, and foods high in potassium are best steamed, baked, or fried rather than boiled. Many people with poor digestion try supplements like betaine HCL which supposedly helps increase stomach acid, but in my experience such supplements almost never work and when digestion problems first begin to develop the first step should always be to increase dietary potassium through the daily consumption of high potassium foods.

It is easier than it has ever been to acquire enough protein for our needs and protein is a requirement for a well-functioning metabolic system, but some people can still develop a protein deficiency, especially during fasting or dieting when protein and other nutrient intakes are diminished. Protein deficiencies can result in ruining the detoxification organs like the liver and kidneys or prevent the formation of lean muscle and the maintenance of cardiovascular integrity. Protein is in lots of foods, most obviously meat, but also occurs in milk, cheese, nuts, seeds, grains, and even in smaller quantities in fruits and vegetables. Though it is less abundant than other sources the quality of protein in fruits and vegetables is actually higher than high protein foods, and our health gut microbiome can and does also produce protein required for our wellbeing and regulation of the gut, immunity, and other body systems. Protein is made up of amino acids, which are the building blocks of life and, much like fat, protein has more roles than is known by its common stereotype and not only makes up structures like muscles but forms important enzymes, hormones, neurotransmitters, detoxification, and other dynamic metabolic processes. Even asteroids which exist in the dead of space have been found to contain amino acids, and for established life such as our own the purpose of obtaining protein through diet is to acquire the particular amino acids in the proper ratios by which are needed to run our biology. Some important amino acids like glycine and proline can also be made within our body from other amino acids but this function is often impaired in disease states and addressing disease as discussed in upcoming chapters can restore these processes to repair damage and regenerate the body.

Protein excess is also a problem, however, especially as we age, because pathogens exploit protein for their own purposes and use it to produce toxic byproducts like ammonia and hydrogen sulfide which destroy the gut microbiome and inhibit the immune system as discussed in upcoming chapters. The body actually requires carbohydrate to metabolize protein, so every time we eat protein the body also consumes large amounts of carbohydrate in order to metabolize that protein, and should protein exceed dietary carbohydrate this causes the body to exhaust glycogen stores, and when glycogen stores are depleted this in turn stimulates the production of those stress hormones which catabolize lean tissues to release more sugar, which can complicate a host of metabolic problems such as insomnia or cancer, so carbohydrate intake should always greatly exceed protein consumption, and cravings for more carbohydrate after a meal indicates too low a ratio of carbohydrate to protein, which is usually caused because people think foods like bread or pasta are only carbohydrate when in fact they also contain substantial quantities of protein.

Some foods like potatoes, though low in actual protein, have compounds called keto acids which are easily converted into protein in the body, all plants contain amino acids which are the building blocks of protein. I love a good hamburger but many meat and hunting advocates believe we ate meat for much of our history and try to justify consuming large amounts of meat or killing wild animals who have difficult lives as if it's good for our health, which it is not, simply due to the fact that excess protein causes harmful side effects such as by excess ammonia and promotion of opportunistic pathogens. Exploiting big, slow game is what allowed our species to colonize the planet, but it also shortened our lifespan, and our ancestors are the reason why amazing Pleistocene megafauna like the mammoth, Irish elk, giant sloth, or woolly rhino no longer exist (mostly because we also hunted their babies which were easy to catch and large enough to feed entire villages...which also killed off the predators like dire wolves and short-faced bears which preyed on those animals). But we still do this as humans, and more recently caused extinctions of the aurochs, the enormous flocks of passenger pigeons that used to darken the skies in the Americas, or the loss of the only parrot native to the United States because vain consumers wanted to stick feathers in their fucking hats.

In reality our evolutionary protein sources as humans came from consumption of insects, mollusks like snails and clams, and nuts and seeds, and our physiology is designed more around plant foods, not meat. The problem is that we require a healthy microbiome to break down plant foods, and when those microbes are deficient instead have greater cravings for easily digested food like animal products and refined foods, even though they are less healthy for us, because they can be digested easily. We certainly have never as a species eaten raw meat except for insects, shellfish, and probably some fish and did not begin hunting as a species until after we discovered fire, probably from foraging on natural barbecue after wildfires swept a landscape, otherwise raw meat would taste as delicious to us as a peach.

Most people are unaware that our gut microbiome actually produces protein (amino acids), and when the gut is health a significant amount of important amino acids like lysine, tryptophan, alanine, etc., are produced by microbes from healthy foods like fruit and other plants, and plant foods can also help spare dietary protein from interception by opportunistic pathogens, making dietary protein more effective.

Indulging in hedonistic and satisfying food can actually be therapy for the body if they are made of high quality ingredients which are full of nutrients and appropriately compatible with our physiology, and rather than simply avoiding foods which are incompatible with human physiology, *replacing* them with generous amounts of healthy options is the key to success. Having ample choices is also useful, and when I was early in recovery I found it necessary to carry with me a large thermos full of a sweet, frozen-fruit smoothie (with a little added protein) to sustain my blood sugar between meals, which had the advantage of keeping me satiated and never bored or distracted from want of food. I lost more than sixty pounds of unwanted body fat consuming more than four pounds of unrefined sugar in fruit smoothies per week in addition to all the other food and calories I was consuming during regular meals and snacking. It was all indulgent, sugary, healthy, and most importantly, satiating but also for the first time in my life I got the kind of results I had always wanted all while participating in very little physical activity and entirely hedonistic eating behaviors.

Food boredom is often a problem for those of us trying to be healthy, but it is actually a biological instinct when the diet lacks required nutritive quality which, when resolved, does not occur even when we eat the same things day in and day out. Whole meals which incorporate cooking best leverage the nutritional potential of food, supported by sources of carbohydrate-rich snacks from human-appropriate sources like fruit to sustain blood sugar inbetween meals. Adjusting the diet to avoid lapses in hunger, including a wide array of easily digested and satiating, stable foods not only improves health but rescues the eating ritual to become once more something which is both satisfying, satiating, and restorative.

One of the worst problems with food and nutrition is the hybridization and breeding of plants to yield greater quantity which has the unfortunate effect of diluting nutrient density of fruits and vegetables which can have as much as half the amount of vitamins and minerals as their more heritage parent plants. Because farming is usually controlled by larger agriculture conglomerates that produce very poor quality food it's best to obtain food from locally grown, independent farmers growing heritage plants in regenerative agricultural practices which end up producing far higher quality products. Even if they are more expensive you're paying for greater quantities of important nutrients like calcium, magnesium, potassium, vitamin C, etc. The state of our food supply really is abysmal, and only those who don't pay attention think it's not getting worse. There are some options for well-to-do consumers to purchase organic and healthy foods, but unless more people become involved in consumer awareness, run for office, and engage in the active policymaking which surrounds the governance of how our food is made and distributed it is likely to become a situation where more people must be sickened and die in order for the rest of us to be forcefully woken from our ignorance. Even organic food can be deficient in nutrients because soil microbiology is easily destroyed in most farming practices and it is the soil biology which feeds the plant which in turn feeds us. Industry and government would have you believe that toxic chemicals like the pesticides poured over our agriculture have no consequences to our health, and egoist doctors with no experience in biochemistry claim that organic eating is fruitless. Listening to these people are exactly why systemic metabolic disease runs rampant through Western civilization. Most of the treatments in this book will absolutely not work if you are exposed to certain agricultural chemicals and pesticides which are far more destructive than any healthy eating can compensate. If you don't want the fate of yourself and your family and loved ones to be worse than it already is, get involved. Many people are leaving the empty promises of industry and finding purpose again in growing and producing for themselves and their communities. Farming is part of who we are as humans, and needn't destroy the Earth when using responsible, regenerative practices. Even if you're not able to grow healthy things you can still be part of the solution by supporting people who do, and you will benefit along with everyone else. Vote. Speak out. Get active. Create change. Advocate for farmers, quality food, and food workers. Support regenerative agriculture. Buy only high-quality, honest products. Eat locally. Help us once more make great food.

CHAPTER 6
FOOD SUPPLY, NOT GENETICS, DETERMINES HEALTH AND SEX APPEAL

There is a photograph of my father at eighteen in Mexico with two of his High School friends on a last big hurrah road trip. All three are wearing midriff, sleeveless cutoff shirts and jean shorts and wide brimmed sun hats. It was the seventies and America was not yet the great prude it has become, and both my father and his friends were unabashedly showing off their six-packs, well built for their age. The stories from his road trip were always entertaining for us growing up, and inspired within me ideas of doing the same when I came of age.

But my father's easy six-pack and freewheeling athleticism never came to me. My efforts to excel in physical development were strenuous and taxing. Even while I was a competitive swimmer I sported a layer of extra fat about my waist, which obviously was not a problem except that it was accompanied by a chronic deficit of vital energy and body dysmorphia enflamed by my shame-based upbringing. There was a year when my muscles grew and my body increased in thickness, and I was still handsome, but the devastating physique and unstoppable vitality that came so effortlessly to my parents and most other young people never materialized for myself, even though I was made from their very genes. Most of my friends too never morphed into the roaming bands of washboard abs and pectorals that deceptively populate Instagram these days. In reality most of the Untied States and other developed nations are in the same or worse condition in which I found myself. The effortless leanness of the generations of the twentieth century is something lost to history, where people used to eat normally and regularly without engaging in any form of dieting or exercise yet found their physical appearance not often something to worry about. Now we find it impossible to eat without suffering the consequences of a contaminated and insufficient food supply which destroys our health and ruins our appearance, all while exerting strenuous effort to shape and form our bodies and minds for what sadly seems a futile effort.

I once met a young man from New Jersey who was almost as tall as I am and he and his brothers were all clad in effortless muscle though he had never touched a weight in his life (his brothers who had were humongous) and had as much of a physique as I did now after years of hard work, though I had been a competitive swimmer and athlete for years and was still pushing my body with weight lifting, running, and yoga. On the face of it no one would accuse New Jersey of having healthy diets and yet they consistently turn out young men who turn the heads of the country so fast it gets whiplash. Brazilians too are often some of the most beautiful people in the whole world even though their heritage comes directly from a mix of societies which do not maintain a similar reputation, and after a visit to the Polynesian Cultural Center in Hawaii when I was eighteen was forever haunted afterward by dreams of a particular boy wearing only a sarong, and Kānaka Maoli in my opinion are the most beautiful people to live on this Earth though many now suffer serious metabolic diseases which did not exist prior to the introduction of white Europeans and the eventual advent of the processed food industry. Some Africans like the Senegalese have an abundance of incredibly fit and striking people because of the absence of western industrialized food systems, and thankfully the United States suffers from an invasion of gorgeous, kind, and talented Canadians who, though descended from the very same gene pool as their fat, angry American cousins do not suffer the same because of better attitudes and policies concerning food.

Beauty, though, is more than aesthetics. The well-formed features of youth are hallmarks of wellness which is why we instinctively recognize it and why many of us try desperately to cheat it, because as hallmarks of wellness they often determine our perceived social fate and ability to act effectively in life. But this also turns many of us into social cannibals, destroying relationships, fostering discontent and derision of others to cover up our own fears of growing old, sick, or dying. As someone who both benefited from the shallow profits of heightened aesthetics and suffered from the social consequences of physical decline and illness I have great sympathy for the fears which motivate the feats of sophomoric social engineering and pretended youth, those vast swathes of restless malcontents who feed on victims of aging and metabolic disease but whom are or will also become them eventually because no one can avert the laws of nature. While these side effects of beauty and sexual attraction are a benefit, the real value of such a state is the absence of disease and suffering within the body. Real health promotes energy, vitality, contentedness, and heightens personality and betters the life not only of the healthy person but all those around them.

All societies which churn out beautiful progeny do not share genetics, but diet. Specific cuisines are not so important but rather the composition of macros and nutrients and absence of anti-nutrients or harmful chemicals which occur in food. One staple in New Jersey is a meat product produced with sugar, and because the body needs sugar to process proteins, providing both simultaneously has far greater benefit to protein assimilation than eating protein alone. Brazilians eat lots of meats accompanied by high-carbohydrate foods like plantains and manioc which also have compounds that help protect the gut and immune system from the consequences of a high protein diet. Hawaiians traditionally dined on meats with fruits and taro for similar effects, and the French have a storied culinary history high in fat and calories and famously suffer less metabolic illness than other industrialized societies. Americans and other developed cultures plagued by an increase in obesity and metabolic diseases who suffer a dearth of beautiful people and abundance of hatred and anger eat industrial food products made of bad fats and harmful chemicals and additives made worse by misinformation about foods like sugar and lack of culinary skills which would afford them a broader, more healthful diet. This is not a superficial concern but one which is alarming because youth and beauty are a reflection of the interior metabolic processes, and having lost our culinary and dietary traditions which previously guarded against metabolic decline and fed by an industrial food system which does not pay attention to the quality of its products our diet has been made vulnerable to contamination with foods which are not appropriate for the human body and has thus destroyed the physical integrity, wellness, and outward appearance of its population. This does not mean there cannot be an industrial food system, only that it has mistaken what is acceptable for consumption. Even more specific, maternal and paternal diet also directly affects the biological integrity of offspring, and dietary quality can affect progeny as far as a handful of generations into the future. In fact, science has found that dietary behavior in parents might contribute to diseases which occur in their children later in life like schizophrenia and autism. Thankfully this does not always mean that progeny are doomed to suffer because of what their parents ate, as a good diet can and does also fix health issues even if they started during gestation, but usually children inherit their parents dietary traditions as well as their microbiome which is sustained and determined by diet and environment, not only during gestation for but for the entirety of their development and even into adulthood, which can perpetuate nutritionally related metabolic diseases, and because diet has such profound effect on our biology even problems which appear to be genetic are in fact most often rooted in diet.

Darwin, the father of evolutionary science, begins his book *On the Origins of Species* by quoting Aristotle—"The rain does not fall in order to make the corn grow," he said, pointing to the plain observation that life was not appointed to earth but evolved to exploit natural resources through competition and evolution. During the intervening years from his profound discovery man has gradually shifted the bulk of our survival exploration from appeasing the supernatural to exposing the nuance of biological function, and while this has resulted in many wonderful and important changes in the way we live like running water and penicillin it has also supported terror and exploitation like the sterilization of people against their knowledge in the United States during the nineteen-hundreds, not because any of these atrocities were based in actual science or logic but because specious scientific theories and observations were paraded as science to support the bigoted goals of terrible people. Were such programs based on actual science rather than bigotry and bias they would still present an incredible ignorance of genetics because by their very existence genes which are still around are by definition superior since they have passed the long evolutionary test which weeds out ineffective genes. Genetics continue to be a *Hail Mary* in health and wellness because genetics are so abstract and so difficult to understand it is easier to cite genes and be done with an argument than confront errors in human judgment or the fallibility of human nature and culpability, the seeming complexity of life and mystery of biology an empty hat from which arguments can be pulled and which no one can question because it is something larger than our ability to comprehend. But inconsistencies are rampant and simple. It is often remarked in awe how much of our genetics are shared with our cousins the chimpanzees, with a genetic similarity of 95%. Even with mice we share 80% similar genetics. Imagine how little the variation is between you and someone who lives all the way on the other side of the world. At most it is 0.1 %, no matter the difference in height, weight, eye color, gender, orientation, or skin color.

A high-profile health advocate who suffered a heart-attack at a relatively young age blamed the episode, without evidence, on an inherited "weakness" passed down from his parents who also suffered heart attacks. Many people feel shame in being mortal, and the accepted tradition of inherited weakness is a contributing factor, but this conclusion was probably an effort to shift blame from the diet and excessive physical exercise he so publicly espoused to uncontrollable genetics and thus more socially acceptable than making a mistake. True, it would be heartbreaking to admit your life's work was in error, and I don't blame him for reaching for something beyond his control. No doubt things in this book will and have been proven errant and I must also confront and accept my own fallibility. But considering how much more evidence is accumulating that genes are *also altered* by diet and behavior and no longer accepted to be the stagnant, cemented destiny they once were it becomes clearer how misguided the emphasis on heredity has been and how destructive to the betterment of mankind. There is no heart-attack gene. No weak-heart gene. That the heart pumps at all is evidence of good genetics. The idea that genes can predispose a person to some unfortunate and random accident years after their birth originates from the anthropomorphized sadism of two thousand years of religionist desecration of the human condition and total disregard for the influence of food, tradition, and the environment on our biological destiny. There are literally billions of human hearts all around the world working just fine. We survive starvation, poisoning, infection, stress, and literal injurious trauma and hearts keep beating even in the bodies of people who have lived more than a century. But because of nihilistic conceptions of death and the mortal body we put our hope in dead, lifeless technology more than our own living cells which are literally designed by nature to spontaneously regenerate and pump blood reliably day in and day out. A heart can literally perform self repair, something it has done for millions of years, which no machine or medicine can yet actually achieve, and the purpose of genes is to form a heart, not to handicap it during later years of life. Genetics are by their very nature intended not for us to suffer and die, but to *thrive*. Genes determine that we have two eyes, a mouth, or stand up on two feet. They do not determine that we contract cancer or heart disease any more than we might lose our legs in war, or that our heart gives out after decades of being overworked and underfed, except in the sense that we do not have the genes to be supermen.

Charles Darwin's all-important work on the origin of species discovered how biology changes in response to the environment, and showed that traits which are not effective in the quest for resources fall by the wayside and disappear from the gene pool. His work did not, however, establish how the biochemistry of food intertwines with that genetic development, since science was not advanced enough to investigate the nuances of vitamins, molecules, and minerals and their effect on biology, nor by the actual mechanisms which cause the determinant genes to achieve success or disappear from a lineage, only that they do. But even then it is clear that if the goal of genetics is to enable the competition for resources, then those resources are inexorably valuable to our biology. Physical observations such as the lengths of beaks, the speed of predators, or the height of a man are on the face of it something that seems like a genetically determined characteristic until we consider that height is actually a function of calcium and protein supply, then it becomes more clear how the quality of the food supply actually supports and determines the quality of the organism rather than the other way around. Speed and beak size would not have any effect on the biotin content of food nor how much sun exposure and thus vitamin D an organism obtains, and a deficiency of biotin or vitamin D can lead to problems in growth, reproduction, and even death. As such, most characteristics of human development are determined by nutrition, not genetics. Populations with low-calcium diets result in shorter stature, not that there is anything advantageous to being tall (trust me, I'd much rather fit into clothes, cars, airplanes, and not hit my head all the time), only that diet is the determinant factor. The fact that calcium can also be stolen or inhibited by certain dietary compounds and pathogens contributes another link in the complicated cause-and-consequence nature of biology, which is more than the sum of its parts and certainly not limited by the genetic makeup of an individual. The work of the famous scientist Weston A. Price catalogued how modern industrial diets damaged physical features in just one generation, where native peoples all around the world eating traditional diets (which yes sometimes even included lots of dairy and sugary foods) typically had perfectly straight teeth and properly formed facial structures even without any dental health services and institutions while those with access to modern industrial foods (foods created through efficient, cheap, industrial production) showed highly deranged dental growth and severely underdeveloped facial bones. Genes control that an organism can absorb calcium and make use of it, but it does not extend the atomic nature of calcium nor replicate the ion and cannot compensate for dietary deficiency or other exogenous (outside) sources of interruption. Without enough calcium, vitamin D, healthy microbiota, or proper hormone balance an individual will suffer calcium deficiency and thus fail to thrive regardless of their genetic makeup. Considering that many environmental factors like pesticides, microbes, and radiation can and do also alter genes and their expression it becomes even more apparent how environment and food exert an even greater control over biology than do genetics. In fact, there is much evidence that DNA is a dynamic and ever-changing element of biology and *entirely* reflective of the state of life rather than determining it. At the point of conception an offspring will obviously inherit the DNA of parents, but that does not mean that parents' or children's DNA is unchanging.

Not even gender is determined by genetics, as there are no genes which directly determine gender but is rather a process which occurs in the environment of the womb during gestation in response to population demographics surrounding the mother. It is often suggested that male sperm determines the sex and gender of a fetus but this is entirely untrue, and while male sperm carries options for genetic traits and gender the sperm which carry gender options are chosen instead by the environment of the body of the mother, probably as a function of temperature or other mechanism similar in other animals in response to their environment, with certain genetic gender characteristics then becoming more or less prominent during gestation where each of us is based on a gender-neutral foundation which develops in either direction of gender-variable traits, or combinations of them which is why there also results in various other gender types including those whom are born homosexual, bisexual, intersex, or transgender, but which is not at all a random process since the balance of gender ratios holds constant across all populations except in cases of purposeful human intervention such as has occurred in places like India and China. As a gay man I often wondered why I existed, especially since my existence seemed so painful because of the rejection and persecution by others including my own bigoted friends and family indoctrination by religion. Differently gendered behavior has been documented in over 1,500 animal species, especially mammals, and after all my work discovering the purpose and function of human biology I realized one day that we who are differently gendered offspring are an evolutionary survival adaptation meant by nature to improve rates of childhood mortality by increasing the ratio of caretakers to offspring. Wolves display a more obvious and similar strategy in which only the dominant male and female of each pack are permitted to mate, so there are more caretakers to young and thus an increase in young survival, and those who are born lesbian, gay, transgender, bisexual, intersex, etc., are the result of a process specifically designed by nature to increase supervision, care, protection, instruction, and mentoring of offspring in species like humans, other primates, lions, horses, swans, sheep, etc., to distribute the responsibilities of rearing offspring and thus increase their chance of survival to adulthood. If all adults in such social species all reproduced the adults could and can be easily overwhelmed by the number of offspring and, like my own parents and others with large families living emotionally isolated from others thus become unable to care effectively for and protect them all. Industrialized, suburban human societies where most couples live entirely apart from other family members, parenting entirely on their own and separated from opportunity by car dependent infrastructure devoid of third spaces in which to find social connection and chosen family, or burdened by bigoted, hateful consideration of their differently gendered family members who are otherwise born literally to assist with the raising of children, quickly become depressed, abusive, and neglectful to then produce traumatized, ineffectual offspring prone to addiction, antisocial behavior, and perpetuation of intergenerational abuse and societal dysfunction.

Families also not only pass down genetics but food culture, which includes eating habits like frequency, amount, and prioritization of certain food stuffs (or not), as well as ideas about what even constitutes food and how much of it to eat (or not). All across the southern United States a candy bar made mostly of industrial chemicals dipped in flour and fried in bad oil is considered "food," whereas I would never let something so horrific pass my lips. Just because something can go in our mouths doesn't mean it should. But this unhealthy "food" is not bad because it's a fried candy bar, only because of its ingredients. The very same dessert could be made from a nutritious candy bar made from real, whole food ingredients, battered in safe flour, and fried in coconut oil which would actually *promote* health rather than destroy it. Like many Americans my own family inherited the toxic attitude of food deprivation as a means to achieve leanness, mistaking leanness for self worth which then brought devastating effects to our physical and emotional health. Ideas of what to eat and when to eat it have almost nothing to do with genetics, certainly not the way we think it does, and long traditions of consuming foods that are actually quite inedible persist in large populations as if they have no bearing on health, as if we are not made from the very food we eat, which is the entire point of food and our biological traits evolved to acquire it. Darwin's work showed the ability of an organism to compete for food supply. If the food supply itself is not sufficient for the organism it doesn't matter what the genetics are. Genetics cannot bridge the requirement for calories and nutrients. Even my own intelligence, which has enabled me to uncover broad solutions to many health challenges eluding man for millennia is not rooted in genetics but comes from my access to education, learning to read at an early age, environmental stimuli such as video games, and ironically health problems to which the body responds by accelerating cognition (which is explained in the upcoming chapters on autism and hair loss).

Obesity, aging, and disease sadly are severe impediments to romantic and social engagement, although it may seem so these are not actually cultural constructs but find their roots in our biology and instinctual fears of death, disease, and rejection where mechanisms have evolved in our species to facilitate the most successful replication of the species possible, even at the expense of the individual. The instinct to reject those who suffer physically is partly determined by genetics and the fear response, because disease can actually compromise the quality of genetic inheritance from parent to offspring and survival of the individual, especially since most metabolic disease is caused by opportunistic and infectious microorganisms which can and are easily communicated by close contact such as occurs during sex, but this too is also influenced by the very same poor dietary and environmental standards which cause those outward manifestation of disease and poor health where those who are slave to baser natures who shame and reject our outwardly suffering brothers and sisters also suffer from within, an imbalance of metabolic function which instead of a fat waistline promotes an increase in fear, hatred, anger, shame, shallowness, stupidity, and other undesirable qualities through deranged endocrine and neurological function, resulting in low intelligence and deficient emotional and mental cognition. When stricken with cancer and weight problems I was not only left by my fiancé but shunned and condescended to by a host of family and friends as well, even doctors, all of whom presented also with some manifestation of outward or inward metabolic and mental stress themselves. Those in the medical profession often treat patients poorly because many people who enter medicine do so from a desire not to help people but to control the disease and death we fear, and sick patients are a direct refutation of our desire for control. Unfortunately, the physical cues to disease result in too much emotional suffering for those already stricken with health problems and not only are these people sentenced to grueling, devastating health challenges but social ones as well. People who reject others on physical appearance are unenlightened to and complicit with an animalistic, compassionless nature of self preservation, brought about in part also by imbalance in their own metabolic health which will, at some point, be their undoing too.

Since food quality affects genetics it is the quality of an individual's food supply and not genetics which determine growth, sexual attraction, and general overall health. Individuals with access to generous amounts of high-quality food sources exhibit the best physical attributes, and the opposite occurs in restricted access to lesser quality food sources. The reason lust overtakes us at the sight of a well-muscled, vibrant man with a great jaw line and thick, beautiful hair is not because our brain is unconsciously concerned with obtaining his genetic DNA but rather that we instinctively know he has access to superior nutritional resources and we and our offspring will benefit from proximity to those resources through association. His body shows that he has access to the things which enable his DNA to function its best, but not the DNA itself. It is also why this attraction impulse occurs between non-sexual interactions as well, such as in social groups or in business and politics, and also why it is relative to the accounting of options where the most attractive or resourceful person in the room becomes the nexus of attention among those enslaved to their baser instincts, not because the most attractive person has the best DNA but because the most attractive person has access to the best food supply and behaviors and attitudes toward food (at least to this point in their life). This is why attraction also can sometimes feel so intense, as if our life actually depends on it, especially for those who are mentally or metabolically ill our instincts drive us to associate with those who are healthier and thus perhaps a chance to benefit from their resources and behavior, and is not sexual attraction although when that is also a factor it is easily confused for the former.

Our desire to associate with those who are healthier than ourselves so that we may by extension benefit extends even to the most absurd and even heinous of human behaviors such as those who support obvious predators and the endless line of harmful junk and misinformation they peddle, or to the support of violent and hateful politicians which always comes with both a financial and moral reckoning, no matter how many times history repeats this difficult lesson, and human beings who are sick, stressed, and angry will willingly hand over their money, integrity, and humanity for nothing more than even the feeling of access. Since food supply can be manipulated much more easily than genetics this means that regardless of genetics it is in fact possible for anyone to achieve physical health, including sexual attractiveness, which is merely a reflection of internal health and overall state of wellbeing and vitality of life. I will offer even an extreme example of those affected by autism who, on the part of their parents, often continue to eat foods which inflame the condition even though it is now common knowledge that foods such as wheat gluten make symptoms worse, and that abstaining from such foods will dramatically improve their physical, emotional, and mental wellbeing. Those with Downs Syndrome, which is certainly related to chromosomes, often spend too much time indoors because of the attitudes of their families and caretakers and so do not get enough vitamin D which not only accounts for weight gain but can also causes emotional and cognitive problems and has nothing to do with their genetics. Even such seemingly unrelated conditions to diet as misaligned teeth or being knock-kneed (which I was) are defined by diet, not genetics, because certain foods or lack of others, by lowering the metabolic rate and promoting colonization by opportunistic and pathogenic microbes, do not have sufficient nutrition to support biological integrity to stand up to the stressors of gravity, chewing, entropy, and life, and so structural integrity wanes, teeth slip apart, bones fall out of alignment, skin sags, etc. During the worst of my health issues my front teeth began overlapping, and my knees, skin, and hair quality got considerably worse as my health and metabolic rate declined. After my metabolic rate was restored both my teeth and my knees returned to their usual position and my appearance improved, all the while possessed of the same genetics with which I was born.

The attraction response is triggered by an observation that a person has been well fed and thus able to achieve their best genetic potential not only through access to good nutritional resources but also usually good dietary behavioral skills, and is not simply an observation of genetics. Not only this, but the state of overall health is determined by quality of the food supply, so all aspects of life from the physical to the emotional and spiritual reflect the overall quality of nutrition. Ensuring a diet which is appropriate for humans, absent industrial contaminants, and generous in nutrients and calories will thus allow anyone to achieve the pinnacle of every part of the human condition, regardless of genetic composition.

Pair of Hearts

I traded my eyes
For a pair of hearts
But found myself holding ashes.
So I traded my heart
For a pair of eyes
And found myself holding diamonds.

CHAPTER 7
HOW TO PERFORM SELF-THERAPY

A home video of me at the age of eight is marred with scan lines and poor sound quality. Standing expectantly in place I sway slowly from side to side with the impatience of a little kid told to stand still. My dad's voice calls from behind the camera, "Hi Nathan," he says. "Hi," I reply excitedly, a large smile plastered over my young face, arms dangling and bouncing freely and restless. He has already interviewed all of my five younger siblings on a range of topics not particularly important to children but which are easy to capture on film. "How old are you?" he continues.

"Eight," I reply.

"And where do you live?"

"Layton, Utah."

"What do you want to be when you grow up?"

My face lights up too quickly to have done much thinking on the matter, clearly I have long known the answer and with a twinkle in my eye, a lisp more obvious than a house on fire, and a wrist so limp any father, no matter how open-minded, would question which sex his child will be fantasizing about when he finally learns to masturbate replied, "A clo-th-ing de-th-igner." But without even skipping a beat my very male, very working-class father segued effortlessly into the next question, and for all their shortcomings I am grateful my parents did not attempt to dissuade my effervescent personality anymore than they did, nor my interest in doing things usually considered the realm of girls like playing barbies or dress-up for if they had, as is the result for so many different-gendered children subjected to harsher, pitiless parenting I would not have become any more heterosexual but sunk even deeper into the morass of despair and isolation to which I was already doomed, being raised in a culture of shame and fear as we were.

If we are at all aware of our surroundings young gay men are already confused as children, realizing intuitively that though we may share the same outward appearance of gender as our beloved and revered fathers we do not exactly operate as them. My dad once called me a homophobic slur when when we were all playing in the living room, not out of anger or shame but simply in the moment of teasing and I think it slipped out with his other teasing jabs. I had no idea what the word meant and only remember it happening because of the look of surprise on his own face, knowing from his expression he knew something about it I did not. Mostly, my parents let me run around in my mother's high heels with a towel on my head pretending to as beautiful as she, or showed patience and kindness when my obvious lisp took longer to disappear, or when I screamed at the top of my lungs during my third or fourth Christmas when they tried to take away the large, plush, blue and purple-haired *My Little Pony* which had in fact been meant for my little sister.

Which makes their reaction a decade later to the confirmation of my being gay more than a little puzzling. As a late-teen my father employed us as janitorial staff at his commercial buildings and I frequently found myself alone at night. Not having internet access at home first discovered the intoxicating erotica of naked men in the silent darkness. The very first image of a beautiful, nude, erotically posed man I ever saw was on his knees with a jock strap in his mouth is as clear in my mind today as when I was seventeen. It was only the advent of the internet and the image took so long to download I finished before the picture even fully loaded.

Though there was thereafter no doubt in my mind I was gay these incidents only happened on a handful of occasions, but one day I walked into my dad's office ready for work to find him scowling at his desk. He motioned to the computer screen, shame dripping off his tongue like a thick beverage. "Nathan," he said, "have you been looking at—at *images*?" The question was incomplete but his tone made every other unutterable detail very clear. *Are you looking at images of naked MEN* was what he meant to say. I hung my head, not out of shame but because at that moment I knew I should appear embarrassed but was surprised and over-whelmed at a sudden and totally unexpected urge to smile, or even laugh. *I was finally found out!* I thought. No more would I have to hide who I was and endure the suffocating weight of my isolation. "Yes," I said. His scowl was searing, so I continued to avoid his gaze. "My secretary found those websites," he said, angrily. Apparently I did not yet known about browsing history. "She thought I was visiting them." He then paused, no doubt waiting for me to explain the mysteries of fate which had handed him such a disappointment for a son. Being just a teenager, I could not give such an answer.

"Are you gay?" he finally said, angrily, as if such a thing were *my* fault. I paused, unsure what I was. I mean yes, any fucking idiot of a man would know I was gay, most certainly the stupid fucking people who raised me. But I had nothing to compare this to, no point of reference. I was only a kid, I had never been straight and had no life experience to provide the answers desired by this frightened, bigoted, grown ass adult.

But I also had no wise and perceptive counsel from older, experienced role models for what being gay meant because those who could have been were either also in hiding for their safety because of the very people like my parents or died during the HIV epidemic.

There was also the supposed possibility in our family's religion that I was not gay, but simply confused, and could be changed with enough faith and pleading which logically implied that no, homosexuality didn't really exist and therefore the theocratical answer to his question was no, I just have a problem with enjoying the beauty of men. But years of prayer and pleading with God to change me had yielded no satisfactory answer to their demands.

Though confounded by the impossible contradiction of my predicament I still knew I was overpowered by an inexplicable and uncontrollable attraction to other boys, but confusion was the best word to describe my current state of mind and I finally grumbled a noncommittal, "I don't know," still working hard to suppress my urge to smile but also navigate the apparent danger sitting before me. My dad's rage grew more intense, seething under carefully chosen words and rigid posture and suddenly my relief turned to resentment for this man who was supposed to love me, to protect me, to show me how to live and to thrive and protect me from dangers such as he instead himself presented. That he could even look at me that way, as if I was some kind of adversary, not his son, destroyed the last of what little respect for him remained. "I have to tell your mom," he said.

"Please don't," I begged. "Let me do it." He said nothing more and we remained silent the remainder of the night, until at home when he called me into their bedroom and announced that I had something to tell my mother. I recalled the earlier events in censored detail, something along the lines of *dad caught me looking at porn and I think I like guys*. I will never forget the way she looked at me either, as I stood there alone and frightened at the end of their bed, their son who used to put a towel around his head and run around the house in her clothes and heels, who cared for his younger siblings with every ounce of his being, who strove for good grades and to excel in everything he did, who always obeyed everything that was asked of him even at great cost to his own individuality—none of it saved me from that look.

The remaining year at home was one of constant anger, shouting, and pent up frustration between my parents and I and between themselves. I began to resent them for their failure to accept me, their failure to assuage those fears which haunted my life and assure that yes, they unequivocally loved me for who I was. I was a stranger in my own home before even moving out, and shortly thereafter came the day came they told me to leave.

A few years later during an infrequent visit to my family, having been on my own long enough to discuss my sexuality with more objectivity I asked my mother why she had been so surprised that I was gay, considering how effeminate I was as a child. "Oh, I thought you were kind of fruity as a kid," she said. "But I didn't say anything because I didn't want to hurt your feelings." It answered so many questions, just not the one I asked.

All humanity's problems stem from one single malady—personal dishonesty. To put the onus of her behavior on me instead of answering the question directly is a perfect illustration of why we descend into physical and mental illness, choosing to avoid reality rather than accept it for lacking the tools which would otherwise empower us. Sometimes it is not deliberate as many of us lack the skills which are required in living, but it is always nonetheless consequential. Though it took me two decades (and more) to discover real answers to my health problems my ability to accept most of my reality is what helped me solve not only a good part of my own problems but also many of which have been plaguing humanity since the ascent of the modern age, during a time when even unfathomable amounts of investment capital into the healthcare industry didn't. When tackling personal health issues whether they are nutritional, metabolic, or emotional the very best skill to adopt is a self-honest attitude. Some of the most deluded of us are we who exclaim our body to respond differently than others, that tired trope of different things working for different people, thus exempt from the laws of physics and biochemistry and the consequences of diet, environment, and fate. Such an attitude serves to not protect our health nor enable success against challenges but only to reinforce already established beliefs and behaviors regardless of their effectiveness or benefit and condemn us to persist in cycles of self destruction. These special cases aside, it is advantageous to anyone seeking healing to accept the reality of our physical bodies and of life in general, mostly that we have very little control over anything except our choices and behavior, as resisting only brings further pain and suffering and often leads away from the path back to good health. This is not a macabre evaluation of any one person's fallibility but instead a tool through which we can be productive and effective rather than sabotage our own best interests. When it comes to health most of us fail because we are beset by perceptions about life and food which are not useful and get in the way of the reality of biochemistry. We cling to our perceptions. They are the measure by which we navigate life and without them a visceral fear rises of being unable to live which then prevent us from changing those things which, in fact, must change. My best function as a biologist, researcher, and philosopher is not really to enlighten people to information or truths but instead to the biases and fears we retain which subvert our intended goals. This was surprisingly productive when I began helping people who approached me for counseling because although they would resist suggestions their motivation was not to insist they were right but instead eager for satisfactory replacements for their existing prejudices, which they usually already suspect of hurting their health, even if they aren't able to admit it quite yet. Deep down we usually recognize when things aren't working but we hesitate for the absence of a convincing alternative.

Some, it is true, do not actually want relief even though they insist, such as one woman who asked for help with her emaciated form and absence of a menstrual cycle promptly retracted from my assistance when I directly addressed her painfully obvious eating disorder. I suppose she expected me, like everyone else in her life, to also pretend it didn't exist and was probably embarrassed by it. Life is hard, we are subject to mortality, and nobody should be ashamed at having problems, no matter what they are, which is a primary reason I discuss my life in this book, to demonstrate the principle that there is value in all our experiences, including our weaknesses. Similarly, many people want to retain ideas of calorie deprivation and other abuses to their body as if they have any benefit to their health, even after years of evidence to the contrary with deteriorating health and energy. Long before I ever got diagnosed with anything I began to notice changes in my body. I began feel cold frequently, and sweat easily even when I was not engaged in physical activity. My hair began to thin, to grey prematurely. My eyes were easily blood shot and my vision became less sharp. But because nothing catastrophic had yet occurred no doctor would help me, and I was not so motivated to actively search for solutions because it was easier to sit in ignorance and hope things just didn't get worse. The consequence was to suffer much more later on.

There are no such thing as cleanses or protocols that can be used to address any health problems. Organs like the liver, kidney, and intestines are either healthy or unhealthy, which is dependent on factors like pathogenic microbes and attitudes about food, diet, and the body, and metabolic health is a direct function of our body's ability to produce *energy*. Specifically, the consumption of food and related metabolic pathways culminate in the production our primary metabolic molecule adenosine triphosphate (ATP), and how much ATP we are able to produce and use directly correlates with metabolic wellness, a function which is not restored or promoted by cleanses, products, or protocols but by consistent, daily practice of healthy dietary and self-care habits, because cells cannot function properly if they are deprived of energy, and if the entire body lacks sufficient ATP it means tissues and organs cannot perform to their optimal purpose. Dr. Peat described this concept as "energy begets structure" which means that cells are only able to organize themselves properly as designed by our genetics and function accordingly if they are also able to produce and use sufficient ATP. This is exactly the reason why stress and dieting promotes metabolic decline, because stress and starvation most strongly interferes with both ATP production and utilization (pathogens can also be a major problem), and accomplishing the opposite can instead restore the body as cells are supplied with plenty of energy to accomplish their proper function.

A major impediment to getting well is the absence of any consequential way to measure or perceive health. If there could be a tangible measure of the state of the metabolism besides looking at oneself in the mirror or standing on a scale, such as a *Star Trek* tricorder, it would be quite easy to assess and address health concerns. It just so happens that there is an entirely easy and accessible way to measure and diagnose one's own metabolic health, at home, without a doctor, and it's just as effective as a tricorder. Using this while also under the care of a medical professional during illness can provide self-empowerment and help anyone track their own progress from illness back to health in a way that is objective and helpful, and it can even be used to monitor good health and head off potential downturns in metabolic integrity. When sick we have a tendency, though, to focus on everything that is wrong. This is a natural instinct to recognize when we are having problems as anyone with serious metabolic diseases will remember the first moments when they suspected something to be off. But as we really get desperate for understanding what is going on or become used to a continuous downward spiral we can miss obvious but small signs of improvement and tend to focus on the symptoms rather than data, thus contributing unintentionally to prolonging the problem. Psychological trauma surrounding body image, mortality, death, illness, and control can also complicate efforts to get well and even undermine them as we strive desperately to control the things we are afraid of. One person I coached continued to communicate to me every little, unpleasant development in their symptoms even though we had only just begun a new diet and though they also refused to integrate every part of my advice. More than a few times I had to council them to stop focusing on the symptoms and fears and instead to chart improvements described in this chapter. Finally, it turned out that they were in fact seeing progress and with that revelation they finally felt empowered to effectively care for their own wellness.

I learned about these diagnostic tools from the work of Dr. Peat, and they are an absolutely useful tool for improving health regardless of your personal medical condition, especially in medical systems that are uninterested in the wellbeing of patients except for what profit can be extracted. When attempting to get well we can use evidence from our body to recognize if things are working or not. The first marker of the metabolic state is the fingertips and toes. At various times of day the color of the fingertips changes. When blood flow is slowest such as in the morning or under metabolic stress the fingertips, toes, and the nail bed will be more pale than when the metabolic rate is high during which which they appear flushed with blood and thus more red. In sufferers of metabolic disease the fingers stay pale even far into the day and this is an indication of slow metabolic activity. Reynaud's disease, where the fingers turn completely white for long periods of time and is accompanied by severe discomfort due to the lack of blood flow is an extreme manifestation of this phenomenon which usually develops in aged individuals and is dismissed by medical professionals as 'usual' even though it causes pain and disquiet and does not occur in healthy individuals. Even sufferers of Reynaud's can avoid the attacks using the tools in this book. This problem of blood flow to the extremities occurs because during stress the body redirects blood flow to the core and away from less important extremities like the fingers and toes but which then causes discomfort and other issues as well as the reduction in visual circulation. Reduction of blood flow to the periphery such as this, no matter the severity, indicates high stress hormones and will result in other problems like hair loss, erectile dysfunction, depression, and even cancer since high stress also impairs healthy metabolic pathways. So, using blood flow to the fingertips and toes is very useful in ascertaining the metabolic rate.

Factors contributing to the stress response which redirects circulation is anything that raises stress hormones like adrenaline and cortisol such as gluten from common wheat, bad fats, going without food for a given period of time, or engaging in chronic strenuous physical activity. Even volatile emotional experiences and chronic sunlight deficiency can induce strong stress responses and raise stress hormones. Such occurrences will directly lower the color of the toes and fingertips in those who are metabolically ill as the body responds to the elicitation of stress hormones by redirecting blood flow. Because stress and stressful dieting behaviors interfere with the body's ability to produce energy it adapts metabolic function and lowers the metabolic rate in order to preserve spare ATP so we don't die. The opposite occurs with generous consumption of calories, carbohydrates, B vitamins, good fats, consistent blood sugar, reduction of stress, daily exposure to sunlight, and avoiding volatile emotional experiences which allows the body to produce sufficient energy which in turn allows blood to redistribute across the entirety of the body, thus raising the temperature and color of the fingertips and other extremities. Elevation of metabolism also enables systems in the body which facilitate healing because it is reflective of the body's ability to make and use energy and energy is required for regenerative pathways. The first time I began using thyroid medication I remember seeing my fingers turn pink, only then realizing how pale they had really become over the intervening years. Paying attention to the color of our fingers and how it correlates with symptoms and behaviors can help diagnostically and functions as a quick shortcut to establishing the current state of the metabolism—pale means it needs to be raised, flush with blood means things are generally going well. If the fingers do not appear flush it can be an indicator to eat, or to utilize therapies which are better at improving metabolic function. Sustaining blood flow to the fingers and toes with a consistent and high-quality diet and good self-care behaviors is an indication that deeper metabolic processes are also recovering and that stress hormones are low, because the fingers cannot be their normal, fleshy warm color in the presence of metabolic stress and high stress hormones.

The second diagnostic tools and which should be written down when first embarking on health restoration is to monitor *heart rate* and *body temperature* such as is done during every doctor's visit. Because heart rate and temperature are directly dependent on energy production (ATP) they are diagnostic data which correlate directly with ATP and metabolism and thus are empirical, not subjective, and thus useful for evaluating metabolic status.

First, pulse is measured by placing two fingers on the neck over the *carotid artery*, which runs between the neck muscles on either side of the neck immediately beneath the hinge of the jaw, and counting beats for an entire minute. Do not only count for thirty-seconds and multiply by two or other strategies because this can provide inaccurate results. Maybe it's difficult to feel a pulse but you have one because you are alive. But a body with robust health and metabolic rate will have a strong *resting* heartbeat which presses back firmly against the fingers at a fairly rapid pace depending on the time since your last meal as calories (especially carbo-hydrate) will always increase the heart rate. Heart rate elevated by exercise, stress, confrontation, or other physical exertion is not useful for this purpose because that elevation in heart rate is achieved by the release of adrenaline and other stress hormones which instead must be at rest when the heart is unstimulated. The function of the heart is also sorely misunderstood and is not strengthened or exer-cised as a muscle in the way that as arms, legs, or pectorals, and instead functions directly in relation to available nutrients and beating rises or slows depending on available glucose, sodium, potassium, calcium, ATP, and other important dietary nutrients.

Pulse and Temperature Diagnostic

	Waking	After Breakfast	After Lunch	After Dinner	Bedtime
Temperature					
Pulse (BPM)					

The heart is also directly regulated by hormones of torpor like serotonin and during periods of stress and high stress hormone expression the heart may increase or decrease in speed and strength depending on the various composi-tion of stress hormones and degree of stress and disease. It is assumed that a low resting heart rate indicates a healthy heart but this conception of cardiovascu-lar health is justified only by the idolization of athletes and is not supported by science or biology. Many athletes, especially endurance and distance runners, experience sudden cardiovascular events because the stress of chronic exercise chronically depletes ATP and required nutrients to then stop the heart. I mean seriously what do you think the heart is running on? Willpower? The heart requires carbohydrate and nutrients to run and because it is constantly running it also requires a constant supply of nutrients, otherwise It. Will. Fail. In order to protect the heart from failure during chronic nutritional stress and energy deficit the body will release hormones of torpor to slow the heart rate to prevent the overconsump-tion of spare nutrients, so the low resting heart rate of athletes is an adaptation to chronic cardiovascular stress, not a benefit.

A slow pulse that pushes back weakly against the fingers or a fast pulse that pushes back weakly are both signs of stress because the heart is not able to fully relax and fill with sufficient volume of blood to deliver a strong heartbeat, and so must beat more shallowly to effectively move blood. A slow, weak heartbeat is a sign of high hormones of torpor which slow the metabolic rate entirely, and a fast, weak heartbeat is a sign of high fight-or-flight stress hormones which temporar-ily raise the metabolic ability of cells but which compromise long-term health stability by depleting nutrients like carbohydrate. A healthy heart also follows a stair-stepping pattern where it beats harder as it beats faster, a function which increases the delivery of blood and nutrients but which becomes disturbed as the heart and body become stressed and depleted of nutrients required to achieve this state. The third state of the pulse we are thus looking for which is desirable is a good heartbeat which pumps with vigor, both quick and with appreciable force which pushes back firmly against the fingertips. This is because a heart able to relax fully also fills fully with blood between each beat to push more blood with every pump, and plenty of nutrients and energy, not discipline and stress, allow the heart to work at the full force at which it works best.

Sometimes a slow beat but strong pushback occurs briefly when transitioning from poor health but this rarely lasts longer than a few minutes and can sometimes even occur with arrhythmia. On occasion when I was first getting better I experienced a skipped heartbeat which resulted in a strange deflating of my lungs and was slightly alarming but never lasted more than thirty seconds and was not accompanied by any pain. This can happen when the body is not entirely used to the increase in CO_2 produced during an elevated metabolism which can then cause a harmless skip of heartbeat by displacing some oxygen. Usually this occurs because we are unconsciously holding our breath in response to a low metabolic rate to retain more CO_2, so if this does occur during recovery deep, steady breaths (not fast) will vent excess CO_2 and the problem will stop.

Once you are well practiced with this diagnostic, checking the pulse with two fingers on the carotid is a great way to spot-check the metabolic rate—if it is fast and weak or slow and weak it means that nutrition is required to keep it sustained in order to keep the body in a state of recovery. During my recovery I would check my pulse many times throughout the day when first recovering and could evaluate my metabolic state all day long. Writing down the pulse according to the chart shown in this chapter showed me at what times of day I was most vulnerable to metabolic insufficiency, such as the morning, and could take measures to boost and support my metabolic rate at those times by eating more and better food or getting sunshine earlier in the day. It also showed me which foods were more successful in raising the metabolic rate and which were not.

Like the pulse rate, *body temperature* is a direct reflection of the overall metabolic state because a body with normal metabolism will produce more heat than one which is burdened by excessive stress or unable to maintain a healthy metabolic rate. Where stress of the heart is primarily mediated by adrenaline body temperature is primarily maintained during stress by cortisol, and when we are unhealthy the pulse and temperature will not move together as they normally should, with separately elevated heart rate indicating excess adrenaline and low heart rate but high temperature showing excess cortisol. Oral thermometers are most relevant for taking temperature, as skin is always several degrees colder than the interior of the body, especially when blood flow is cut off to the periphery by stress, and underarm or forehead monitors are not actually useful for these purposes. Blood in the back of the throat rising in the carotid comes immediately out of the heart and as such better reflects the core temperature of the body so long as no food or drink has been taken within 30 minutes at the time of measure. It is important to remember that eating or drinking anything will naturally change oral temperature readings and care should be taken to take these factors into consideration, using readings as an overall pattern and not fixating on any one single measurement.

It is most helpful to take measurements at certain times of day—on waking, after breakfast, after lunch, after dinner, and immediately before bed. If a person is healthy it will be noticed that numbers are low in the morning and usually rise, together, after eating, especially if the food is good for the person's health, and then steadily throughout the day to peak in the afternoon or early evening before falling once more as the body prepares for sleep. Often those who are ill or diet will present with abnormal patterns such as high morning pulse that falls after breakfast. This specifically indicates high nightly adrenaline which can be resolved by eating more before bed and fixing glycogen storage. Medications and supplements can strongly affect these numbers as well, for instance if thyroid medication is taken before bed it can keep the metabolic rate on too high during the night, causing the body burn rapidly through carbohydrate stores which will then result in very high morning heart rate numbers.

A healthy pulse should meet or exceed 85 beats per minute after eating, especially later in the day, even sometimes easily passing 100 (higher would be abnormal). A diet and lifestyle which enables a resting heart rate to rise in excess of 85 beats per minute without stimulation by stress hormones and accompanied by good body temperature is reflective of effective nutrient delivery to the heart and low stress hormones, and these same pathways also facilitate the healing processes as other parts of the body benefit from the same repletion of nutrients and mitigation of stress, so measuring the pulse along with temperature can precisely establish the state of the metabolism and thus the overall health, or potential for health, and so becomes an indispensable tool in recovering from metabolic diseases of any sort. The goal to achieve for healthy body temperature will be a daily peak once a day of 99° Fahrenheit or greater (37.2° C) which typically occurs in the afternoon or early evening. When I was sickest my morning temperatures were regularly 95.1 and the highest only ever barely passed 97 if I took great strains to get there. I was in quite dire straits indeed, but it didn't take very long to normalize these numbers. If you are metabolically ill it does not help at all to focus on low numbers, only the high ones, because when the high numbers reach their peak this means means the metabolism and body are healing, and the low numbers will come up automatically, while it is the inability to reach the peaks which indicates chronic stresses that will always impair progress.

For those desiring to heal *any* kind of metabolic condition, whether it be cancer, hypothyroidism, diabetes, stalling or reversing the aging process, or simply just losing weight or regrowing hair the ultimate goal and singular focus should be to elevate the general temperature and pulse through food and nutritional based therapies, to achieve through the coaxing of metabolic pathways as described in this book the eventual and consistent rise in all temperature and pulse to that which is stable and characteristic of a youthful and healthy metabolism. In doing this diseases will heal because the same pathways which raise these indicators also facilitate healing of the body through the production of energy. There may be other specific points to pay attention to when it comes to certain conditions, but aside from those it should be priority to monitor and elevate these numbers no matter what. It is a good practice to spend two weeks measuring pulse and temperature each day, writing it down in the chart, then after use periodic testing as you improve to monitor your progress (or lack of it) and through this tool it becomes extremely easy to monitor the state of your health and your progress back to wellness and to understand exactly what is going on with the body.

Taking thyroid medication or progesterone along with good food immediately raised both my temperature and pulse, along with a relief from a great many of my symptoms, but things like aspirin, coffee, pregnenolone, niacinamide, coconut oil, butter, ice cream, fruit, sugar, vitamin C, and sunlight are all tools be used as discussed in upcoming chapters to improve markers of the metabolic rate, in addition to a generous and nutritive diet and the resolution of pathogenic factors. Some people have trouble healing metabolic illness, depression, and even alcoholism and addiction because of eating disorders like *anorexia* which itself is a problem of high torporific hormones and can be treated with a daily, low-dose of *niacinamide* (vitamin B3) which will help raise the appetite to facilitate sufficient eating to keep the metabolic rate up. The torporific state catalyzed by undereating forces the body's metabolism down in order to spare nutrients, so metabolic healing can never occur without consuming sufficient and regular calories, especially carbohydrate, fruit, and other nutritive food, and addressing trauma such as is discussed in the upcoming chapter on spirituality or my other book can help resolve psychological stress which motivates behaviors of dieting, undereating, excessive exercise, and other negative conceptions of the human body which prevent recovery from illness. A *magnesium* supplement such as magnesium bicarbonate, magnesium citrate, or magnesium glycinate can also be very useful for raising the metabolic rate for reasons which will be come clear in later chapters. The three *strongest* promoters of metabolic activation are sunlight, sugar, and vitamin C, and getting all three of these first first thing in the morning with breakfast is the absolute best way to get the metabolism started (while sugar can come from any source fruit is most useful). The longer the metabolism is turned on each day, supported by a constant supply of food, the more rapid the metabolism will regenerate, so eating first thing on waking is best. While coffee can help raise the metabolism it will absolutely raise stress hormones if taken before food, as it strongly stimulates the metabolic rate, and should never be used on an empty stomach.

The last diagnostic, which doesn't need to be written down, which is helpful and fairly obvious is *mood*. Mood is a very strong indicator of metabolic health. Happy, calm, and productive feelings are generally signs that health is good and metabolic rate is high due to adequate blood sugar and production of energy and will not occur in those with a compromised metabolic rate. Irritability, anxiety, lack of motivation, fatigue, restlessness, inexplicable or excessive anger, depression, etc., are all signs of high stress hormones, low blood sugar, and often pathogenic colonization and that the diet and environment is wanting for improvement as discussed in upcoming chapters. Emotions are in fact hormones, and hormones also directly effect the metabolic rate, so paying close attention to mood within the context of our diet and metabolic rate is extremely helpful in managing our health, where the pulse and temperature can support that with empirical data, and the onset of unpleasant moods is one of the first indicators that you probably need to eat, get sunshine, or that perhaps you ate something which does not agree with our physiology.

Eating can be annoying, and most of us would starve to death if we did not feel discomfort by going hungry, but this can be alleviated by choosing delicious and indulgent foods and cultivating culinary culture and skills, to learn cooking if you do not know how, to enjoy food if you do not know how, and eating a wide variety of food options to avoid food boredom which is an indication of missing dietary nutrients. Sweetened whole milk warmed with added sugar is ideal for demonstrating the effect of the diet on pulse and temperature and works best at the time of day when the metabolism is typically at its peak, after measures like sugar and vitamin c to start the metabolism many hours before. Warm a cup or two of milk, add a generous amount of sugar (1/4 cup?), and drink after it is all dissolved. Pay attention to resulting changes in pulse, temperature, and finger color over the next thirty minutes to an hour after consuming. The character of this heartbeat is the ideal state to achieve with diet overall, and this milk tonic can be used any time it is difficult to get the temperature and pulse to their peak numbers (mindful of the principles of dietary calcium as discussed in upcoming chapters).

Another easy and effective tool for raising the metabolic rate is what I call the *coconut oil swish* which consists of using a small spoonful of coconut oil much like a mouth wash, holding it in the mouth and swishing it around slowly for five to ten minutes until salivary enzymes break down the fatty triglycerides into their individual fatty acids, then swallowing once it is very liquid. Practicing this daily works because most people with metabolic issues have trouble digesting fats so using salivary enzymes to break down a healthy fat like in coconut oil guarantees the release of helpful fatty acids which will in turn rapidly help heat up the metabolic rate. Coconut oil is specifically useful because it is high in *lauric acid* which promotes the endogenous (inside) synthesis of the master hormone of the body, pregnenolone, which in turn promotes other hormones like thyroid, testosterone, progesterone, etc., which help increase metabolic rate and will strongly compliment the use of carbohydrates and other rehabilitating factors. This method is also the concept known as 'oil pulling,' but oil doesn't pull anything and the benefit which comes to oral health from using oil as a mouthwash is from the liberation of fatty acids by saliva as they absorb into tissues of the oral cavity. Spitting it out is also a waste of those fatty acids which would do the same in circulation for the rest of the body once swallowed (gargling also with this fluid once it becomes watery, not just melted, is also strongly effective in treating conditions like sore throats as discussed in the upcoming chapter on infectious illnesses).

Sometimes people use the temperature and pulse diagnostic but don't get good numbers and run in place expecting change without actually doing anything to change them. This is a tool, a source of information from which to then make informed decisions. If numbers aren't moving there is something wrong or missing which needs to be discovered, and that can only occur by changing dietary habits, your environment, and trying new strategies. Other metabolic issues that might prevent elevation in pulse and temperature are covered in the remainder of the book, especially those of a pathogenic nature. With practice, taking the pulse and temperature to monitor the state of health will become second nature, simplify the healing process, and aid in exploration to understand what is effective for restoring health.

Like my experience with resveratrol and 5-HTP we can in our desperation to get well cause more disease by using products and supplements marketed and sold as healthful, but not even things which are natural are necessarily safe or useful for our wellbeing. Most supplements are actually harmful to our health, and if something is not explicitly recommended in this book it is probably *not* useful and should be avoided (and be wary of fraudsters and cheats using my name and work to sell products as I never endorse anything or sell through other parties).

Many people have metabolisms that are entirely sustained through stress hormones which is evident by higher morning numbers and lower peak numbers, or temperature and pulse which does not rise and fall together, and embarking on this type of eating and lifestyle which reduces stress may at first actually cause your numbers to fall, especially the restoration of carbohydrate and sodium since those most strongly lower stress hormones. The function of stress hormones is to bridge the distance between what our body can do without them, but the removal of stimulus for stress hormones will actually cause some numbers to decline if they are irregular to begin with, and will rise later as stress hormones are consistently suppressed through diet and healthy practices. It is important to remember that if your body has been running on stress you will mistake the lowering of stress hormones as being tired, and will probably be tempted to continue chasing your conception of "energy" through the use of stimulants and behaviors which continue to raise adrenaline. This is a consequence of being so depleted of nutrition due to long term, chronic stress hormones but will in turn allow the restoration of a healthy metabolic state and return of healthy energy and vitality.

Similarly, the experience of waking very early in the morning anxious to start the day is a typical symptom of high adrenaline due to exhausted glycogen stores, and restoration of glycogen, sodium, sunlight, and will result in feeling sleepy in the morning and afternoon due to the restoration of our natural circadian rhythm cycle otherwise inhibited by stress hormones, so don't confuse sleepiness as a negative development because of obsessions with productivity and materialism. Being sleepy is good, it means low stress and more healing and direct sunlight exposure is the best way to wake up and being alert (and coffee or tea can help too), and you must have some compassion for your physical body during this time and recognize the requirement for rest and rejuvenation for our overall health, and other chapters, therapies, and increased healing will soon bring your energy levels back up to normal through sustainable metabolic health. Improvements should also always be constant and obvious—there are no walls or plateaus in metabolic health and if ever you feel stuck or stagnant it means you are simply missing something and should reevaluate if you are accomplishing all the requirements mentioned throughout this book, and because symptoms and hope are not a diagnostic tool always use the temperature and pulse diagnostic as your reliable guide to wellness.

CHAPTER 8
A HEALTHY GUT

Though my parents always produced a mountain of food to keep us well fed, there was always a rush at dinnertime. The first to finish got seconds, and all of us wanted seconds. As an athlete my caloric needs were astronomical, but even during periods of relative inactivity I had an overwhelming need to eat and eat. I got tired of this drive to eat or felt insecure about my body and would skip meals only to later find myself shoveling mac and cheese or mashed potatoes like I'd recently been rescued from a desert island. My dad used to call me a "human garbage disposal," which as an adult I realize sounds like more of an insult than it was probably meant. Actually, maybe it was. Not surprisingly, I always struggled with my weight and appearance and like most people heard and believed that weight gain and health were a product of discipline, not biology. This dangerous mindset led me to starve and abuse my body until it finally rebelled and brought me almost to death. It turns out that health—including weight and outward appearance—have nothing to do with morals or willpower and everything to do with the state of our gut.

The expression "no man is an island" is never truer than in our reliance on microbes for our overall health, and it seems strange to realize that significant parts of us on which we are wholly dependent aren't even the same species. The large intestine, confusingly also called the lower intestine or colon, is actually an incubator or farm wherein each of us carries around our very own bacterial agriculture, producing many nutrients like vitamin K2, the B vitamins, and short-chain fatty acids but which even synthesizes amino acids and protects us from pathogens. Food is first digested in the stomach and small (or upper) intestine where we absorb as much nutrient potential as possible to prevent competition with bacterial species further down, which consume the same nutrients as we do, and the remainder which we cannot metabolize is carried on to the farm in the lower intestine, which actually at one point sits higher than the upper intestine, rising up into the abdominal cavity before descending back down to the exit as the terms 'upper' and 'lower' refer to the progression along the intestinal tract from the stomach and not its physical location in the body. This becomes important because of the many faces of digestive stress because misidentification of the part of the intestines in which pain, gas, bloating, or discomfort appear usually leads to incorrect self-diagnoses. For instance, gas in the lower intestine can occur in the part where the lower intestine rises higher inside the body than the upper intestine, making it seem like the problem is with the stomach or upper intestine when in fact it is not. Gut problems which occur from the consumption of common wheat (due to its iron fortification and hybridized gluten) do not appear until that food is pushed into the lower intestine by the eating of later meals where it is then exploited by opportunistic microbes which can then lead people to be believe what they ate last gave them the discomfort rather than from several meals prior.

One of the first correlations perceived with metabolic problems is eating speed. Without evidence, the general consensus between chew-speed and weight gain is considered a consequence of calorie intake, wolfing down excess calories which are then packed on as fat. But the calorie model of weight loss is total bullshit, as is evident by the many millions of failed and frustrated dieters whose even dedicated and consistent efforts do nothing to relieve their metabolic problems. There is actually a direct relationship between weight gain and eating speed but it has nothing to do with willpower or calories, and many lean people can eat huge amounts of calories and do not gain weight, and self-righteous egoists will tell you their body burns more calories and thus they are lean, as if they themselves are actually responsible for their biology, as if they are not walking contradictions to their own philosophy demonstrating that weight gain is in fact *not* a function of calories and willpower, but of biochemistry.

Yet most healthy people who are lean do tend to chew more slowly and eat less calories, so what is going on? Most people assume that anything we eat is dissolved by stomach acid and absorbed into the body but this sometimes isn't true at all since pathogens like *H. pylori* and parasites can entirely disrupt stomach acid production, and when food passes out of the stomach and enters the intestinal system it is acted on by bacteria and other microbes which reside there, and any failure of the body to produce sufficient stomach acid or effective digestive enzymes secreted by the pancreas during digestion results in food entering undigested into the intestines which makes nutrients available to microbes in our gut which produces an explosion in microbial overgrowth and deprives us of valuable nutrition. This microbial burden then causes bloating, fatigue, lethargy, metabolic disease, thyroid problems, and eventually even cancer, and the presence of harmful microbes is why fast eaters are hungrier, eat more food, and gain more weight because we eat not only to feed ourselves but also to compete with opportunistic microbes also consuming our food and the harm this directly causes to our body, which is why the normal amount of food for a healthy person does not produce satiation for those who are ill. Because sick people even produce less ATP from the exact same amount of calories as a healthy person it becomes impossible to benefit from the same amount and type of calories, and thus those who have the impulse to panic eat and to eat in excess suffer not from caloric excess but from microbial dysbiosis.

Our human ancestors only experienced metabolic stress during times of real danger such as famine, disease, and competition, but our modern, cramped and self-centered societies polluted with social inequality, poor food quality,

environmental toxins, antagonistic politics, car-dependent lifestyles, toxic pharmacological products, childhood abuse, unresolved psychological trauma, and lack
of sunlight exposure causes constant and unceasing metabolic stress, and those of
us who experience such stress in turn respond to our biological programming to
panic eat because our evolutionary biology is concerned about our literal survival,
not being skinny. But it then appears to the ignorant and asinine that fast eaters
eat more calories and so gain more weight, but the natural world does not operate
the way undisciplined observers can see with their eyes, especially not the dimwit-
ted, and the cause of weight gain is not caloric intake because fat deposition is a
biochemical process, not one of statistics, morality, or beliefs. Groups of people
who feel socially ostracized or economically vulnerable will also naturally express
higher levels of stress hormones which in turn promote panic eating, as a safe-
guard against compromised food security as isolated animals. Such populations
also tend to have limited access to nutritive food, or are exposed to more to toxic
chemicals which interrupt the gut and endocrine system anyway.

Because pathogens do cause disease many people try using antibiotics to
reverse gastrointestinal and metabolic illness and while they can sometimes have
beneficial effects they primarily risk eliminating our commensal microbes on
which we rely for nutrients and protection from pathogens. Our body does possess
strategies to manage pathogens such as with a salivary enzyme called *lysozyme*
in the saliva which kills bacteria by dissolving their outer cell wall. But one study
showed that stress decreases the expression of lysozyme and that participants
experienced an *increase* of salivary lysozyme if they first watched a funny video.
So, cute kitten videos are part of this cure but it also demonstrates how the body
manages the microbiome in response to stress, during times of calm and joy is less
concerned with acquiring microbes but increases acquisition of microbes during
stress to purposefully accomplish things like increased caloric absorption and
retention to better promote long term survival during stress. Healthy, self-care
skills such as having a fulfilling food culture in the cooking of meals for ourselves
and sharing food with our friends and loved ones instead of just eating to satiate
hunger can lower stress and thus increase lysozyme and reverse metabolic decline,
where the lack of self-care skills, culinary skills, a good food supply, and fulfilling
interpersonal relationships and lifestyles actively increases stress and thus the
ingress of opportunistic microbes. Interestingly, humans produce many times more
lysozyme in breast milk compared to other mammals which seems to be related to
our consumption of milk as a food staple and thus increased exposure to milk-as-
sociated microbes.

Though they may seem virulent, microbes are only opportunistic and, contrary
to what many people believe, cannot just move in and cause infection without
conditions being favorable to their survival, much like a seed cannot grow in the
wrong kind of soil. It's why bacteria don't feed on your phone or computer—they
are not able to invade environments that do not support their growth. The same
thing is no less true when it comes to biology and the body is normally very good
at controlling which microbes are allowed to live in and on our bodies simply by
maintaining an environment inhospitable to opportunistic species but favorable
to commensals. One of the first lines of defense against opportunistic colonization
of the gut is stomach acid, which creates an impassible barrier to many types of
harmful microbes while also neutralizing some potentially harmful factors. After
stomach acid, we are then primarily protected by our commensal, native microbiome. When we are born the gut is more or less sterile of microbial growth but
this begins to change as soon as the baby is born and the systems which select for

healthy microbes begin to screen for helpful species to populate the gut and oral cavity to establish a viable commensal microbiome. Breast milk also contains a special prebiotic fiber called *human milk oligosaccharides* which selectively feed only those species of bacteria which are most helpful to our physiology, and these beneficial bacteria then use those oligosaccharides to produce helpful *short chain fatty acids* like acetic acid, butyric acid, propionic acid, formic acid, etc., which fuel cells of the gastrointestinal system and consume free oxygen to promote a *hypoxic* (low oxygen) environment which then naturally prevents the ingress of fast-growing, opportunistic, aerobic microorganisms.

The infant gut is also almost entirely devoid of *iron* unless they consume any iron-fortified products like common bread or iron-fortified infant formula such as what occurred to my sister with her ear infections, because pathogens require iron to cause disease, and a baby's liver stores a large quantity of iron during gestation to provide their iron needs until they begin consuming solid food. Iron fortification to formula is the likely cause of *sudden infant death syndrome* as iron is an extremely inappropriate nutrient to feed a newborn, and one poorly written study which claimed no association with bottle feeding actually showed just 17 of 98 babies which died were exclusively breast fed, which is an extremely high association with bottle feeding opposite to the author's conclusions, where they considered a mix of breast and bottle as 'not bottle fed' which is another example of bad studies presenting misinformation confused as science, where there is not specifically a problem with bottle feeding except for potential contamination of product by pathogens, chemicals, or formulated incorrectly for the real needs of a human infant as most milk formula is formulated for the profit of corporations, not the health of your child. Iron fortification is also the primary reason for debilitating stomachaches which often follow consumption of foods such as breads, pastas, pizza, burgers, and other baked goods because iron fortification is nothing more than added iron shavings, and the ingredient labels on these products will use the words 'iron,' 'ferric,' or 'ferrous' in various combinations. It really is fucking insane to be adding iron to foods, especially those marketed for children like cereal or infant formula, since iron is one of the primary targets for pathogenic, disease causing microorganisms, and is comparable to putting gasoline in a fire extinguisher. Because of the changes in my diet reflected in the pages of this book I have had less stomachaches in the last ten years than I can count on one hand, where before they were a near daily occurrence and often so debilitating and frequent as to interrupt my personal and professional obligations. That it was so easy for someone as ill as myself to entirely resolve stomachaches simply by avoiding wheat and iron fortification (since rice and other grains are also now fortified with iron) shows just how dangerous and destructive it really is.

Mammalian milk even contains molecules like *lactoferrin* which actively bind free iron to prevent its acquisition by pathogenic species, and iron in whole foods such as from spinach or meat is always bound up in the food matrix such as with phytochemicals or proteins which makes it far safer for consumption, but iron-fortified foods introduce an abundance of unbound iron into an environment teeming with microbes in opposition to everything nature is trying to do to protect us from the effects of iron excess and it is absolutely impossible to heal the gut while consuming any foods with added iron or using iron containing supplements. Even meat, which is extremely high in the most bioavailable form of iron (heme), is shown in studies to be associated with contracting diabetes when eating in excess because the pancreas becomes oversaturated with excess iron which then allows microbes to colonize the pancreas and disrupt its function (the pancreas produces insulin). As mentioned earlier, the B vitamin *riboflavin* (vitamin B2) is normally produced by commensal microbes and used in their own immune and defensive functions and has a strong affinity for iron and can be used as a supplement to mop up free iron in the gut to help reverse iron excess problems and arrest many of the pathogens which cause acute intestinal distress for more rapid resolution of acute gut problems like stomachaches, IBS, Crohn's, etc. Pathogens which produce the riboflavin analog roseoflavin inhibit commensal riboflavin producers, so symptoms like stomachaches are also symptoms of colonization by roseoflavin producing opportunists which causes other symptoms and disease sine riboflavin pathways are extremely important to our metabolic health. While riboflavin supplementation will not reverse gut dysbiosis in the long term anyone with frequent stomachaches should make use of a riboflavin supplement until stomach pain fully resolves without requiring it. Not much is needed (a dose of 10 mg should be plenty) but riboflavin is highly water soluble and very safe to take in any dose and can be taken with meals to prevent adverse reactions until the healthy microbiome is restored.

Specifically, overgrowth of bacteria in the gut which promotes bloating, poor digestion, weight gain, and other metabolic problems is called *small intestine bacterial overgrowth (SIBO)* because large populations of bacteria begin to grow in the small intestine where normally they are contained only to the large intestine. The small intestine is the site of absorption for most of our dietary nutrients—starch, sugar, proteins, fats, and vitamins and minerals, which is why microbes are usually contained to the large intestine so they do not compete with us for these nutrients. So when bacteria access the small intestine they in turn have greater access to all these nutrients and thus grow unchecked on the abundance of nutrition, competing with us and stealing our nutrition but also producing gas and bloating, slowing digestion and producing digestive stress, and opportunistic and pathogenic organisms take advantage of this state to further contribute to metabolic illness by producing enzymes, proteins, and toxins which interfere with our biology. Normally the intestinal system has a built-in regulation response meant to prevent SIBO called the *migrating motor complex* which is a sustained wave of peristalsis (contraction of gut muscles) which manually moves food and bacteria out of the small intestine and down to the large intestine. Aside from the immune system and mucosal tissue this is the body's primary way of guarding against bacterial overgrowth and pathogenic colonization by literally pushing bacteria away from undigested food so those nutrients can be properly absorbed before passing the remnants we cannot digest onto our bacterial farm and then out of the body.

Humans, other primates, pigs, guinea pigs, and many other mammals also have only one stomach and accomplish our necessary microbial fermentation after the stomach and we are referred to as "hindgut fermenters" to distinguish us from other mammals like ruminants which are cows, sheep, bison, etc., whom have multiple stomachs whose bacterial farm occurs in the foregut and are thus "foregut fermenters." This fascinating difference in evolutionary strategies means that animals like ruminants benefit directly from bacterial nutrient production where those who are hindgut fermenters benefit indirectly, but foregut fermenters must also share their nutrients with microbes, and cows, for instance, only run on about 30% of the carbohydrates they consume while humans not suffering SIBO can use most digestible carbohydrate we eat for our own nutritive purposes which allows us to have a higher metabolic rate. Even though we are a hindgut fermenter our microbiome is still a primary source of many nutrients, and the most important factor in the maintenance of a healthy microbiome is *cobalamin* (vitamin B12) which is not only important for our survival, without which we would die, but also that of our commensal microbiome without which they also die. Microbes have the same negative electromagnetic charge as the indigestible substrate they consume in our gut and, like two of the same ends of battery or magnet, are electromagnetically repelled from food substrate if they are not able to neutralize that charge such as with highly positively charged B12. Plants (and other life including humans) use principles of electromagnetic *polarity* to defend against microbial adhesion and for this reason plant foods are very difficult to break down without a properly working microbiome supplied with B12, so deficiency of B12 then prevents liberation of nutrients from plant cells by microbes as well as the nutrients produce by our microbes such as other B vitamins, short chain fatty acids, and even the production of amino acids like lysine and GABA since commensal microbes must first adhere to substrate to metabolize it.

This principle of polarity and the function of B12 is why some foods like peas and corn can pass through the gut entirely undigested, as while plants possess other anti-digestive factors like enzyme inhibitors polarity is the most effective defense mechanism. Our own tissues like the epithelial lining of mucosal tissue also uses this same principle to protect ourselves first and foremost from colonization by pathogens. While much of our B12 comes from consumption of meat, shellfish, and insects only microbes can actually produce B12. Researchers wrongly believe the liver can store up to three years of B12, which is an absurd proposition, and cobalamin deficiency is instead one of the catalysts which triggers SIBO because the body adapts to deficiency by stopping the migrating motor complex to purposefully *allow* microbes to ascend into the small intestine where B12 can be absorbed to prevent fatal deficiency since we would literally die without B12. Gut distension often mistaken for a fat gut is characteristic of this shift from hindgut fermentation to SIBO because the overgrowth of gastrointestinal microbes and presence of parasites like *Giardia* literally increases the size of the intestinal system and we start to look more like our gorilla cousins as our body adapts to nutritional deficiency and pathogenic ingress. Evolutionarily we obtained dietary B12 mostly from insects and easily forgeable shellfish from the shallows of ancient Lake Mega Chad (or the Mediterranean or other body of water) where we evolved our most defining human characteristics as mollusks are also very high in B12, but if our supply of B12 only came from the diet as is commonly believed we would perish from meat deficiency, which we don't, and considering that B12 production occurs right here in our gut it is ridiculous to think B12 repletion comes only from the diet.

Without cobalamin not only do our commensal microbes fail and die off but competitive microbes such as *methanogens* (methane producers) take over and instead consume food substrate which leads to the production of *methane* gas instead of healthful B vitamins and short chain fatty acids. This means that gas and flatulence is a primary symptom of poor B12 status, and one study found that the microbiome composition of adults who experienced sudden death were dominated either by methanogens or hydrogen sulfide producers. This does not mean that having B12 available to microbes is nice but that its absence actively impairs our commensal microbes and thus also our health, so restoration of local B12 production is required to be healthy and to recover from any metabolic disease. During my research there was no science which identified commensal microbial cobalamin producers, but the most prolific cobalamin producers in the world, which also happen to live on and in the human body, are not actually bacteria but an *archaea* called *Thaumarchaeota* (archaea are single-celled organisms). Most people don't know that methanogens are also archaea, specifically *Methanobrevibacter*, and *Thaumarchaeota* are some of the most abundant microbes on the planet and occupy nearly every environmental niche from ocean water to human bodies, with *Thaumarchaeota* representing about 20-40% of the ocean's plankton as well as being found on nearly every surface of the human body, including mucosal tissue. There are very few bacterial B12 producers and though it has not yet been confirmed by studies it is obvious our body proactively cultivates *Thaumarchaeota* on mucosal tissues, including the gut, to supply needed B12 to our other commensal microbes which then helps them properly metabolize food substrate and makes it appear as if the liver can store large quantities due to its constant local production.

Thaumarchaeota consume ammonia as an energy source and feed on the probiotic glycoproteins produced by mucosal tissue which cultivate commensal microbes. But *Thaumarchaeota* effluence is also found to contain vitamin D, implying vitamin D dependence and it has long been known that vitamin D actively supports and promotes the gut microbiome, although how this occurs has also eluded science, but since *Thaumarchaeota* are dependent on vitamin D and are a primary cobalamin producer in the environment even in and on the human body it is clear that *Thaumarchaeota* are the primary beneficiaries of our vitamin D which stimulates their production of B12 to support the healthful microbiome. Because glycans which compose glycoprotein are made of sugar the body also cannot produce glycans without both dietary protein and sugar, and another mechanism by which dieting contributes to disease is by impairing the production of glycans and glycoprotein which, among other functions, help cultivate healthy mucosal populations. Human milk oligosaccharides are glycans, and children born to mothers who engage in harmful dieting behaviors or whom suffer conditions like diabetes which impair metabolism of sugar risk not only their own health but also that of nursing children due to glycoprotein deficient milk to perpetuate developmental problems like autism or childhood diabetes. Dietary sugars used to produce glycans are mostly converted into the sugar *mannose* for this pathway which, if you or anyone you know have ever dealt with urinary tract infections might have heard, cranberry is widely recommended because of its high mannose content which helps by quickly restoring glycan production to then directly promote commensal microbes which outcompete pathogens that cause infection of mucosal tissues such as what line the genitourinary organs. But mannose is primarily synthesized in the body from glucose and fructose and the need to use cranberry or presence of genitourinary infections are instead a consequence of dieting or diabetes.

While this mechanism for gut dysbiosis is highly technical it is very easy to understand and diagnose since its primary symptom is farting excessively, since methanogens take over when commensal microbes suffer deficiency of B12, and any excessive gas and flatulence is an easy way to diagnose it. Most people simply require adequate carbs, protein, and getting daily sunshine exposure (and no, sun on your face and hands for fifteen minutes is not sufficient), but vitamin D metabolism is highly complex and if daily sunshine exposure and daily consumption of fruit, sugar, and carbohydrate does not result in resolution of gas, flatulence, and gut dysbiosis the steps in the upcoming chapter on vitamin D will need to be addressed in order to restore vitamin D production and function (and sorry no a supplement of vitamin D usually does not solve this problem). But another very reliable symptom to diagnose this problem is also whether or not there are cravings for leafy greens. Being impossible to break down without commensal microbes supplied with B12 the absence of B12 prevents cravings for hard to digest food like vegetables and instead shifts cravings to easily digestible foods like meat and starches, so absence of cravings for leafy greens is always an indicator of poor microbial B12 status and thus also that of vitamin D and *Thaumarchaeota* activity. Especially during the summertime there should be strong, daily cravings for fresh, healthy vegetables, especially leafy greens, which indicates the presence of flourishing commensal microbes and an ability to break down tough foods and release of their nutrients for our benefit, while the absence of such cravings is a symptom of deficiency of vitamin D and B12.

While it cannot replace local production of B12 this problem can be temporarily addressed by adding a low-dose supplement of B12 to foods daily, but must be mixed into food and not just taken along with it, which will help provide B12 for our commensal microbes to break down plant foods (which can also be done during wintertime to prevent gut dysbiosis). Once daily is usually sufficient, such as in breakfast or a large salad mixed into the dressing (no more than about 1-5 mg per dose is required). I prefer to avoid *methylcobalamin* since this can potentially add excessive methylation to the body, but other types like *cyanocobalamin* are great. Supplemental cobalamin has also been thought to be absorbed under the tongue, sublingually, which is why many B12 supplements are flavored, but this is not true and saliva actually contains a protein called *haptocorrin* (confusingly also called R-factor) which binds B12 during chewing to help protect it from stomach acid during digestion. In the stomach B12 then bound by *intrinsic factor* and haptocorrin is cleaved from B12 by the proteolytic enzyme *trypsin* to promote absorption into the body (not all will be absorbed). Some bacterial species like those used to make Swiss cheese, called *Propionibacterium*, are also prolific producers of cobalamin and a little Swiss cheese or *Propionibacterium* culture can also be used to increase B12 in the diet when added to things like bread dough (as discussed in the upcoming chapter on bread) or other ferments like kimchi, kombucha, pickles, etc., to get more dietary B12 directly into foods for these purposes (B12 bread is especially delicious), and I initially discovered this therapy and function through the strategic use of *Propionibacterium* cultures, although simply crushing up a B12 supplement and adding it to foods is much easier while long term, permanent resolution of this problem will be entirely dependent on restoration of vitamin D as discussed in that upcoming chapter.

The gastrointestinal system is also fundamentally dependent on the chemical elements themselves such as sodium, potassium, magnesium, manganese, chloride, zinc, copper, lithium, and calcium. Proper balance of elements both within and without the gut regulates pH, water, mucus secretion, acid production, bile production, neutralization of acid in the intestines, and the ability (or not) of the migrating motor complex to contract. Calcification of tissues disturbs gut homeostasis as opportunistic microbes exploit calcium to colonize the gut and chelate zinc to inhibit our immune defenses, and when conditions such as constipation, gut dysbiosis, SIBO, etc., occur the tissues which contract to engage peristalsis have lost their normal elemental and electrolyte balance to cause inflammation which reduces electrical conductivity of cells which thus inhibits contractile stimulus. Inflammation is water, and restoring elements such as with a dose of salt or magnesium dissolved in water can often stimulate a bowel movement because the increase in electrical charge draws water from the surrounding tissues into the gut thus reducing inflammation and producing a laxative effect, restoring electrical conductance of cells which then reengages peristalsis and the migrating motor complex while also making feces more watery, reversing constipation. Because ammonia produced by parasites and other pathogens impairs the normal uptake of electrolytes failure to inhibit ammonia prevents the elements from permanently reversing these problems which then sustains inflammation, constipation, and gut dysbiosis but using those tools constantly in the diet can and will help reverse this imbalance and restore normal metabolism of water, peristalsis, and the microbiome from dietary and supplemental salts and other electrolytes.

One particularly nefarious source of mineral depletion which strongly interferes with our electrolyte balance required for normal gut function is the popular use of water softeners, reverse osmosis systems, or distilled water and other excessive filtration systems because purified water strongly and catastrophically dilutes electrolyte concentration in cells and tissues. This problem also cannot be reversed by adding minerals back into filtered water because excessive filtration also removes *carbonic acid* from water, which is dissolved carbon required to balance water pH and to dissolve other elements into aqueous suspension which more strongly neutralizes the chemical potential of water than minerals alone. Contrary to popular belief water is not inert at all, which is instead a function of its other dissolved elements, and in the right experiments water can actually be made to explode as it is, after all, nothing but hydrogen and oxygen, two of the most combustible elements in existence, and by removing other dissolved elements drinking excessively filtered water strongly dilutes electrolytes, carbonic acid, and bicarbonate which then destabilizes the body's ability to manage water in the first place which then causes intestinal tissues to swell dramatically to promote profound water retention, turning our bodies into a sponge, which is extremely dangerous because it also dilutes electrical conductivity and electrochemical functions of cells. I suspect distilled, reverse osmosis, or other excessively filtered drinking water to be a probable factor in *Ehlers-Danlos Syndrome* (the stretchy joints condition) because purified water so strongly dilutes the halides chloride and bromide which are required for healthy collagen synthesis, though this could also be caused by other factors that interfere with halides, and during all metabolic disease it is requisite to avoid highly filtered water while also increasing the consumption of electrolytes (seaweed is a good supplement for those with Ehlers-Danlos). Because elements are also needed to form urine in order to remove excess water, drinking water can thus be either harmful or helpful depending on its dissolved mineral content and should never, ever come from excessively filtered sources like distillation or reverse osmosis. Gentle carbon filters, tap water, or genuine spring or mineral water are best and should be drunk only according to thirst and not any stupid advice about number of glasses per day or any of that bullshit, and adding a small amount of salt to beverages like juice or tea can help reverse electrolyte dysfunction which contributes to gut dysbiosis which will compliment efforts to suppress ammonia producers and resolve parasitism and pathogenesis.

Similarly, consumption of iced beverages is highly detrimental to gut health when trying to recover from metabolic illness because the function of most digestive enzymes is dependent on body temperature and thus reduced by cold foods and beverages. In a body which is healthy and produces an abundance of heat this isn't usually a problem, and consumption of cold drinks or ice cream can also result in greater heat production due to their caloric content in those who are even moderately healthy. But in those who are metabolically ill most calories have to be put toward production of energy, not heat, which is why the body temperature drops and fat retention occurs, and drinking cold beverages lowers gut temperature for long periods of time which then further prevents digestion and leaves food intact for more opportunistic microbes to consume instead. Digestive enzymes lose about half their function for about every ten degrees (Fahrenheit) of temperature drop, so cold beverages or foods can in those who are very ill entirely stop digestion altogether, while warm beverages and food like tea can oppositely help promote their function. Often people with metabolic disease use cold foods because it helps stop sweating but sweating is mediated by calcium and stress hormones so resolving excessive calcification of tissues which also promotes parasitism and pathogenicity will also help resolve problems with excess and spontaneous sweat.

While it is not a major cause of gut dysbiosis, exogenous sources of oxygen also strongly fuel aerobic bacteria and directly contribute to and exacerbate SIBO problems. One such source is the kitchen sink because most water faucets, dispensers, or filters contain aeration grills which aerates water as it is dispensed which is why it turns white and foamy. This basically adds supplemental oxygen directly to the gut which in turn promotes aerobic pathogenic microbes and oxidative damage. Normally this oxygen is consumed by the epithelial layer of the gut lining using short chain fatty acids but in those who are ill there is too little production of short chain fatty acids by microbes to fulfill this function which then results in promotion of aerobic, opportunistic microbes to worsen disease. Around the age of forty I suddenly and inexplicably stopped being able to enjoy coffee (which often happens to people as they age) and like most people initially supposed this was an effect of the caffeine. We do not in fact drink coffee for its caffeine, although that is nice, but because coffee is in fact a source of potent *prebiotic* polyphenols which strongly promote the growth of commensal microbes (if they are functioning properly) which results in an increase in B vitamins and short chain fatty acids, but the new apartment to which I had moved had very high water pressure and the aeration grille in the sink faucet caused the water used to brew coffee to become highly oxygenated, then because coffee is extremely high in prebiotics the combination of oxygen and prebiotics caused massive overgrowth of aerobic gut microbes to then cause discomfort rather than joy from consuming coffee. Because the filter was not removable, running the water slowly enough to avoid aeration (no fizziness or bubbles) completely resolved this issue. Likewise, smoothies blended at high speed with a deep, swirling vortex thoroughly oxygenates the entire solution, while blending on slow and low to avoid a deep vortex helps reduce oxygenation. Homogenized milk is an unfortunate source of oxygen entry to the gut with food because the homogenization process forces milk at high pressure through a nozzle against a hard surface which also fully aerates the milk, causing the liquid to absorb high amounts of oxygen and studies even show that homogenized milk does not last as long on the shelf as non-homogenized milk, and this is an entirely unnecessary and harmful process (pasteurization is fine, though). Oxygen supplementation to the gut accounts for a great deal of the increased symptoms like bloating or discomfort which accompany conditions like SIBO, and avoiding these sources of additional oxygen is required for their resolution and maintenance of a healthy gut.

Because pathogens use iron to make reactive oxygen species and cause blood and cellular leakage on purpose to feed on our tissues dietary *vitamin K* (phylloquinone) is also very important for preventing and resolving gut dysbiosis through the process of *coagulation*. This effect of vitamin K can be illustrated by what happened when I had a young puppy named Charlie who woke me one night because he was very sick and vomited and defecated blood. It was very scary and on getting to the vet it was discovered that he had eaten a tube of antibiotic cream I left on the coffee table. The antibiotic ointment killed all but the most virulent and resistant strains of gut microbes which then caused severe gastrointestinal bleeding. The vet cured him by injecting a high dose of vitamin K and he improved rapidly and without any lingering complications. For this same reason, regular intake of foods high in vitamin K is absolutely necessary to prevent gut dysbiosis by preventing the introduction of blood and iron products like hemoglobin and oxygen into the digestive tract.

But, just like vitamin B12, our commensal microbes also require vitamin K for their own metabolism too and use vitamin K in their respiratory pathways, and the regular consumption of dietary sources of vitamin K is especially effective supporting commensal microbes which protect the gut and produce other nutrients we require. Beneficial microbes also produce derivatives of vitamin K called *vitamin K2* (also known as menaquinone) which are even more healthful for us than normal vitamin K1, and there are at least thirteen different types of vitamin K2 and we do not fully understand them all and which absolutely cannot be replaced by a supplement but must instead come from the microbiome. Normally the body can also recycle vitamin K many thousands of times and some people can get away with having vitamin K only rarely, but in those who are ill this ability to recycle vitamin K is severely impaired or even nonexistent so it can often be required to consume vitamin K every single day. Foods high in vitamin K are typically green, leafy vegetables like spinach, basil, kale, parsley, broccoli, etc., but because commensal microbes require B12 to adhere to these foods their ability to metabolize vegetables and access vitamin K to produce vitamin K is also entirely dependent on B12, so the ability to effectively benefit from dietary vitamin K is also entirely dependent on the aforementioned pathways which result in local microbial B12 production or the use of supplemental B12—mixed into and not just lazily taken alongside it as that does not guarantee effective distribution. Many cultures around the world still consume foods high in vitamin K even for breakfast, and vitamin K is one of those fat soluble nutrients lacking from industrial food systems as shown in Weston A. Price's 1922 survey of pre-industrial cultures which affects human development such as dentition since vitamin K is required to manage calcium, and vitamin K is especially important for the proper formation and positioning of teeth alignment, bone structure, prevention of tooth decay, and a healthy nervous system which is highly dependent on calcium.

Leafy greens are also usually high in calcium which also makes them an ideal source for nutrients which directly support tooth, bone, and neurological health, and because cobalamin deficiency impairs commensal microbial adhesion to these foods any excess gas means also deficiency of vitamin K even when consuming vitamin K foods which requires first reversing B12 deficiency. Many also people try to overcompensate for a lack of leafy greens by embarking on dogmatic and excessive consumption of the most unpleasant preparations of high vitamin K foods such raw kale or adding spinach to a smoothie, but being miserable does nothing to promote the health benefits of vitamin K and in some cases can even prevent benefit. Very tough plants like kale contain enzyme inhibitors which prevent digestion and so are best cooked (baby greens are usually fine raw), and the long-term success of sustaining a healthy diet requires that meals be delicious, satisfying, even hedonistic, otherwise we get sick of such foods and fail to eat them consistently, which is far more important than large doses of unpalatable foods based in dogmatic and unreasonable ideas of health and nutrition (one of my favorite ways to have spinach is simply pre-boiled briefly, drained, then sautéed in a LOT of salted butter). This fundamental problem of doing things in excess is rooted in hatred of the body and mistrust of biology, when in fact our body is just as interested in being alive and healthy as we are, and it must be treated with the same kind of compassion and care that we desire for ourselves which includes serving good and delicious meals and taking the time to learn how if you don't. Even a little bit of intense heat can destroy enzyme inhibitors in less than a few minutes so instead of choking down a disgusting green smoothie make creamed spinach with garlic and mushrooms, collard greens with bacon, or an incredible salad full of different selections like baby spinach, arugula, basil, cucumber, bell peppers, olives, artichoke, asparagus, radishes, raisins, tomatoes, cheese, seasoned with salt and pepper tossed in a high quality vinaigrette with added B12. Even adding parsley, cilantro, or basil which are all very high in vitamin K to meals or having pesto regularly can supply much needed vitamin K for the commensal microbiome to thrive, and if access to greens is difficult basil, parsley, and even spinach can be grown in pots under a windowsill or on a porch and harvest into meals regularly.

When it comes to gut health a primary focus is *probiotics* which are commercial products containing supposedly healthy microbes, especially *lactic acid* producing bacteria and products like yogurt as lactic acid is often advertised as being effective against pathogenic bacteria, which it is, but lactic acid is *also* effective against our own beneficial bacteria, and bacterial lactic acid actually has very little nutritive benefit to our physiology. An old study attempting to discover a good milk replacement for infants actually showed an increase in infant mortality (meaning they died) from lactic acid added to cow milk, but a decrease in mortality from cow milk containing the short chain fatty acid, *acetic acid*. The reason lactic acid is not actually very helpful for our own health is that lactic acid is an inhibitor of cellular respiration and directly lowers the metabolic rate, because its production in our tissues is a result of insufficient carbohydrate metabolism so this downregulates the metabolic rate as an adaptive response, so consuming foods like yogurt which contain high quantities not only of lactic acid but also prolific lactic acid producers causes significant deterioration of both gastrointestinal tissue, the composition of gut microflora, and the body's general metabolism by directly lowering metabolic respiration. When I was in my early twenties struggling with my weight, insomnia, and suicidal depression I was consuming a pint of yogurt daily because I had been told it was good for me. Lactic acid is so powerful that yogurt can measurably lower body temperature, and while there's nothing wrong with healthy people consuming small amounts of raita or sour cream occasionally the fermentation of dairy should never be a dietary staple, and avoided entirely in those who are struggling with their health. In severely diseased persons such as I was lactic acid production in the body is already extremely high so adding yogurt on top of it is like committing suicide, and especially if developing cancer this effect can lead to inexplicable fatigue from the most mundane activities such as walking the dogs around the block let alone going to boot camp four days a week *I'm trying my hardest don't you think I would work out more if I could? FUCK.*

I'm okay, I'm okay.

One strain of lactic acid producing bacteria was found to actually change good fats into toxic trans-fatty-acids which downregulate the metabolism, destroy the immune system, and which are more susceptible to peroxidation and contribute to conditions such as diabetes, cancer, hypothyroidism, hypogonadism, and mental health disorders, which is why it seems impossible sometimes to get better even when changing the diet since unhelpful microbes can even make bad things out of good. Most of my struggle back to good health in truth was entirely a struggle against such microbes, but add to this the barrage of other environmental, chemical, and nutritional stressors which destroy our health and it's a wonder any of us are alive at all, let alone *billions,* and nowhere in my journey back to health has lactic acid ever played a beneficial role. Probiotic products like yogurt are *not* formulated because they are part of our innate microbial gut populations nor particularly beneficial to human health but because they are easily manufactured and distributed while having enough scientific studies to justify their sale. Most people do not realize that *all* health products for purchase are not intended to get you well but to make a profit for the manufacturer, whom are often actively disinterested in your wellbeing because their entire business model literally depends on your continued illness. It is assumed by most consumers that the probiotics in yogurt are naturally associated with dairy, or even with our native gut microbiome, but this is actually a lie meant to increase profit margins and is not true at all and the primary strain of bacteria used in the manufacture of yogurt, *Lactobacillus delbrueckii,* cannot be found in any natural milk of any species outside of starter cultures, nor does it colonize the human gut as we are led to believe. Studies on the use of lactic acid bacteria for diabetes show reductions in blood sugar but this mechanism is achieved because lactic acid directly impairs absorption of sugar into the body due to its effect on gastrointestinal pH, so disturbances in pH such as from highly acidic lactic acid or highly alkaline ammonia directly impairs sugar absorption. Diabetics always present with excessive lactic acid in feces compared to healthy controls anyway, so using lactic acid in studies trying to treat diabetes just represents complete stupidity. The entire function of the *citric acid cycle* which is the beginning of energy production is entirely dependent on sugar, and because so many systems in the body from stomach acid to glycoproteins to the immune system are dependent directly or indirectly on the consumption of sugar, dominance of the gut by lactic acid producers is always found in those with metabolic diseases like diabetes and obesity which, if lactic acid was so great, should instead be the most healthy, but they aren't because it isn't, and if diabetes is caused by sugar then lactic acid foods should cure diabetes, but they don't, and it doesn't, and actually makes it worse.

Many *Lactobacillus* are also excessive producers of histamine, which can trigger inflammation and cause chronic excess mucus production and irritate the nervous system. While there are a few species of *Lactobacillus* that are beneficial, microorganisms which are truly beneficial to the human gut such as *Clostridium, Faecalibacterium, Akkermansia, Roseburia, Prevotella, Blautia*, etc., are harder to package and distribute, which is why you've also never heard of them, and so are not typically available for purchase. This does not mean however that helpful bacterial strains cannot be easily gotten. Commensal microbes which populate the human gut originate from all around us and even in us already but are simply not abundant or may be suppressed by bad microbes or bad dietary habits. Normal human interaction is the best way to acquire beneficial microbes, which occurs as easily as contracting those which cause disease like strep throat, flu, and food poisoning, and the seeming difficulty in restoring gut health has nothing to do with actually buying probiotic supplements which almost never help anybody but everything to do with restoring a gut environment which is every bit as hospitable to healthy microbes as it should be inhospitable to those which are harmful. While humans can also carry disease causing microbes healthy humans harbor healthy commensal microbes which protect us from pathogens, and cohabitating or other close contact with other humans through friendship, touching, and especially sex can transmit commensals also, and if our diet and dietary behaviors support their populations then we will benefit from exposure. Some people get fecal microbiome transplants for this very reason and while this can help they also don't last very long (several months to a year) because the problem *is not lacking exposure* to these microbes but the diet and gut environment. Even animals can be a source of probiotics and studies show that having a pet prolongs human lifespan, this is wrongfully attributed to the stress relief caused by their presence, which is nice, but animals like healthy dogs and cats harbor other helpful microorganisms and lick their fur and our faces and being around them exposes us to their microbes (adopt shelter animals and fucking spay and neuter your pets people). Gardening and interacting with healthy soils and freshly harvested plant foods not sprayed with chemicals also exposes us to many, many types of beneficial soil microbes which help not only to break down foods but also protect our bodies from pathogens and opportunists. The environment truly is a far more prolific resource for beneficial microbes than any product which can be purchased.

Some of the most important microbes to human health are from the *Bifidobacterium* genus which are found to be dominant in the gut of infants which are acquired from parents and the environment by gleefully trying to shove everything and everything into their mouths, even and especially dirt which is actually safer for children to do than grown humans due to their absence of sex hormones, low iron content (if not fed iron fortified food), and overproduction of saliva which helps select for commensals like *Bifidobacterium*. Many *bifido* species such as *B. bifidium*, *B. longum*, *B. lactis*, or *B. breve* also degrade histamine, and unlike most *Lactobacillus* strains *Bifidobacteria* also produce vitamin B6 which is used in our enzyme *diamine oxidase* which also degrades histamine, not only destroying excess histamine themselves but also providing us the tools to do so too. Additionally, all *bifido* species also produce the same type of lactic acid as our own body rather than the more harmful D-lactic acid that is more common to other microbes, but more importantly they also preferentially produce short chain fatty acids from most carbohydrate substrates and far less lactic acid anyway. Many *Bifidobacterium* also produce folate (vitamin B9), which is so necessary for our growth and wellness and to prevent severe birth defects. The need for bifido bacteria in the gut is so important, in fact, the term *bifidogenic* is used to describe anything which increases their population. *Propionibacterium* bacteria used in the manufacture of Swiss cheeses are themselves bifidogenic as they are also dependent on *Bifidobacterium* for their own growth. *P. freudenreichii* is one such variety but it is very susceptible to pesticides and herbicides and is easily eradicated from the gut from exposure to toxic agrochemicals like *glyphosate*, so reinoculation would not occur unless a person actually avoids contaminated food and then consumes products like Swiss cheese or exposed from the environment. Consumption of *P. freudenreichii* has an immediate effect on the gut microbiome through the promotion of B12 and short chain fatty acids (which are what give Swiss cheese its nutty flavor), and is particularly effective in reducing water retention around the gastrointestinal system. So Swiss-type cheese is an effective and cost-efficient way to promote helpful *bifido* species, especially when actual *bifido* supplements can be prohibitively expensive.

Justification for lactic acid probiotics is usually explained as its severely low pH, but acetate is a whole degree less acidic than lactic acid yet its bactericidal effect against pathogenic bacteria strains is a number of times *more* potent than lactic acid, for instance killing the species which cause tuberculosis at tiny concentrations in solution compared to lactic acid, so the idea that lactic acid is beneficial simply for its pH value is a complete misunderstanding of how biology works. Acetic acid is also used by our friendly gut flora and most species of butyric acid bacteria actually use acetic acid to make butyric acid, and if yogurt was actually made with acetic or butyric acid producing bacteria and contained little lactic acid it would instead become a healthy food. One of the reasons the fermented drink *kombucha* can be healthful is because kombucha is traditionally made with acetic acid bacteria (much like apple cider vinegar), although due to overzealous, conservative government overreach now often requires kombucha to have lactic acid bacteria added to control its alcohol content which entirely negates its benefit. Studies also show that regulation of tryptophan catabolism by commensals or opportunistic bacteria is regulated by the availability of indigestible carbohydrate, especially that of *pectin* which is abundant in fruits and vegetables. Unlike other carbohydrates, pectin cannot be metabolized to lactic acid, and fruit, pectin, and other indigestible carbohydrate are supposed to be our primary dietary source for acetic acid via commensal microbes which, when available, advantages them over lactic acid producers and proteolytic (protein consuming) opportunists. Acetic acid is also the primary constituent of vinegar, and while some vinegar in salad dressings or diluted supplementally in smoothies or juice can be very helpful it can never fully replace the function and benefit of local production from dietary pectin by the microbiome, which our commensal microbes absolutely love, and because children can also be affected by pathogens but greatly dislike the taste of vinegar the use of fruit is far more helpful.

Apples are especially high in pectin, which is why apples are used to make apple cider vinegar, but it also accounts for the genesis of that age-old adage '*an apple a day keeps the doctor away*' as people intuitively recognized the unique benefit of apples on health. But in order to access the pectin in plant foods our gut microbiome also requires access to B12 which thus means that periods of vitamin D deficiency, which is required by commensal *Thaumarchaeota* to produce B12, also prevents our microbiome from breaking down plant foods and releasing their pectin content so that opportunistic microbes instead use their methane, hydrogen sulfide, or ammonia to break down food and harm our health in the process. Not only then does the use of B12 with plant foods like fruit help those with chronic gut problems but the cooking of fruits to break down their plant matrix and liberate pectin or the use of supplemental pectin with meals can help circumvent this problem and restore gut health and a commensal gut microbiome by feeing commensal microbes directly and protecting tryptophan from catabolism by opportunists. Products like apple sauce, apple butter (which is especially delicious), and marmalade and common, high-pectin fruit products which can be used, but pectin itself is also widely available for culinary use which can and should also be used as a supplement preceding or accompanying meals in anyone requiring gut rehabilitation, and can rapidly help restore gut function and increase gut transit time (do not use excess, though, as that can turn the gut into a vinegar factory, and no more than about 1/2-1 tsp, depending on size, mixed into water or juice, or daily consumption of apple butter or apple sauce should be required).

Acetic acid is in fact more vital to our health than anyone has ever realized, and is actually a base for most fundamental and indispensable metabolic pathways including the synthesis of cholesterol, steroids, bile, fatty acids, and acetyl-CoA which is a cofactor in many metabolic pathways, so when the gut fails to produce acetic acid due to B12 deficiency or deficiency of vitamin D and pectin our metabolic health in turn plummets from resultant deficiencies of things like hormones and respiration pathways. In many studies acetic acid is shown to inhibit things like obesity and diabetes, as well as stimulating the storage of glycogen when taken with food. One popular but completely misunderstood theory for poor health in humans is the MTHFR debate and the concept of 'over-methylators' and 'under-methylators.' While it is based on some facts *methylation* is essentially how the body turns off genes and pathways while *acetylation* with acetic acid turns them on, and the real problem underlying disturbed methylation processes is actually deficiency of acetylation due to poor production of acetic acid in the gut. Acetate also helps acidify nutrients like chloride, calcium, silicon, sodium, etc., which helps promote their absorption. Supplemental acetic acid can be highly effective in supporting recovery from metabolic disease and gut dysbiosis, but straight vinegar can be very caustic and unpleasant and frequent use can actually erode the enamel on teeth as unreacted acid reacts with tooth enamel or burns the sensitive tissues of the mouth and throat. If supplementing straight apple cider vinegar had any health benefits I didn't notice them because of my overwhelming desire to never again put that shit in my mouth, which is another reason the use of pectin and high pectin fruits is so useful because they are pleasant to consume and promote acetogens in the gut, thus eliminating any need to supplement vinegar. Many candies are even made from pectin (and they are very good) which can be a good choice especially for children since this will also directly support healthy gut microbes and better digestion of food in those with metabolic illness like diabetes, autism, cystic fibrosis, etc.A medicinal form of acetic acid I found useful for treating many illnesses is *sodium acetate*. Because acetic acid in sodium acetate is reacted with sodium the acid is no longer as caustic to the mouth, teeth, and digestive tract such as from plain vinegar, and can be supplemented more effectively with better uptake of acetate to directly help support acetic acid dependent functions which underly many basic cellular pathways including bile, steroids, neurological function, and cellular respiration. Sodium acetate is generally recognized as safe and is used in food products like salt and vinegar chips or as a preservative in cheeses, and can be used to dose acetic acid therapeutically to immediately treat gut dysfunction and related conditions, and sodium acetate is indispensable for the treatment of alcoholism and addiction as discussed later in this book. Sodium acetate is also the byproduct of your childhood science fair volcano, mixing baking soda and vinegar together, and doctors use sodium acetate in hospital settings to treat acute lactic acidosis and metabolic acidosis as a replacement or backup for bicarbonate, with studies remarking how patients receiving sodium acetate recover faster and with fewer side effects than those receiving sodium bicarbonate, even though the mechanism of action for sodium acetate is actually to raise endogenous bicarbonate and does so more effectively than actual bicarbonate, which is likely due to activation of pathways by acetylation. One study showed that sodium acetate also reduces the amount of CO_2 ventilated from the lungs, meaning more is retained which translates into higher metabolic rate and lower lactic acid production. Some studies show acetate supplementation alleviating diseases like Polycystic Ovary Syndrome (PCOS), which makes sense since acetate is also the foundation for hormones which are dysregulated in PCOS and endometriosis, or diabetes-like conditions since all of these diseases originate from parasitic disruption of the microbiome and resultant deficiencies in short chain fatty acids made by a healthy gut microbiome. Fruit is plenty sufficient when taken frequently (daily) for healthy people, those who are moderately ill may benefit from simply using fruit and supplemental pectin, and those who are very ill will require use of sodium acetate, and a recipe can be found at the end of this chapter, taken once a day can strongly help treat many of the conditions discussed throughout this book.

It is also important when recovering from gut dysbiosis to consume generous amounts of healthful food. Stomach acid secretion is entirely dependent on potassium, and low potassium diets like those low in fruits and vegetables rapidly promote ingress of opportunistic microbes into the gut simply due to hypochlorhydria (low stomach acid), and there is no faster way to restore a healthy microbiome than with carbohydrates and sugar, especially from fruit which are high in potassium, and oppositely no faster way to kill off the microbiome than with dieting, especially low-carb eating and the avoidance of sugar and fruit. People also often have a glucose or calorie deficiency and though they take all the right supplements and eat foods which are "safe" do not see improvements due to the stress of caloric and carbohydrate deficiency, blaming supplements rather than poor, dissatisfying diets and limited culinary skills. Eating disorders like anorexia can also be an impediment to getting well, since plenty of food and carbs are required to restore a healthy microbiome. Anorexia is caused by high torporific hormones and can be easily treated by using a daily, low-dose supplement of *niacin* or *niacinamide* to stimulate a higher metabolic rate and hunger impulses, and resolution of trauma as discussed in the upcoming chapter on God and spirituality or my book on psychology, *The Perfect Child*, which more deeply explores childhood trauma and its effective resolution as misconceptions of our self worth are some of the most significant impediments to getting well because they motivate self-destructive behaviors like dieting. If you do not enjoy eating and cooking you are focusing too much on what you can't eat rather than finding *replacements*, because there are far more options to eat than otherwise (some often say too many after reading this book), and watching cooking-centric media such as Michael Pollan's *"Cooked"* or *"The Great British Baking Show"* or other good and inspiring cooking shows and social media channels can help inspire appreciation for food and a desire to care for your body through cooking. Stop relying on other people to feed you and learn to do what your ancestors have done for literally millions of years.

Additionally, many people with gut dysbiosis also suffer from chronic lower back pain because such injuries are *not* the result of physical injury or sitting, even in the case of conditions like herniated disks. For years as a young man I suffered intense lower back pain and my job as a motion graphics artist kept me at a desk for ten to twelve hours every day and was so painful I often had to call in sick to let my back rest. I tried all sorts of therapies for back pain short of surgery, which is unfortunately common, even buying special chairs which promised relief and good posture which in reality did shit. While herniated discs can cause some back pain this problem is in fact caused stiffening *psoas muscles* which transit directly through the gut and are thus directly affected by the state of the gut and production of toxic metabolites like ammonia, hydrogen sulfide, and lactic acid by pathogens and opportunistic microbes. The psoas connect the legs with the spine and their atrophy and stiffening due to poor gut health makes them more prone to injury and very slow to heal. I have not had any back pain at all now for almost a decade even though I am forty-four, still six-foot seven-inches and two-hundred sixty pounds, sitting in cheap chairs with no back support for up to ten hours a day, because the restoration of a healthy gut microbiome frees the psoas to regenerate and once again become strong, flexible, and resilient. Specifically, a microbe which gave me such debilitating back pain I had to lift myself out of the seating position like old man was *Bacillus subtilis* which is a common probiotic and used in the preparation of some foods like natto, and should be avoided entirely and eliminated from the supplement market as bacillus species are *not* probiotics but are potential proteolytic pathogens. If back pain is a problem the principles in this chapter can rapidly and effectively help treat chronic low back pain but will likely also require the use of *iodine* as instructed in the upcoming chapter on immunity to fully resolve.

All metabolic disorders have their origins in the gut. Restoring and promoting stomach acid is the primary protective mechanism for a healthy gut, and supporting and nurturing our commensal microbiome, not taking probiotics, is the best way to fix problems with digestion which lead to illness. Considering how effective sodium acetate is at reducing lactic acidosis I'm surprised it isn't standard treatment for metabolic diseases like cancer considering lactic acid is one of the most devastating byproducts of metabolic illness. As an effective and "generally recognized as safe" distinction from the FDA it should have a larger role in our medical arsenal and available as a common and easily accessible medication or supplement. The upcoming chapters, especially that on immunity, will be required to achieve a full recovery from gut dysbiosis and related metabolic conditions.

If you are annoyed by a limited availability and increased cost of eating organic, the food supply situation is only the way it is because people like you do nothing to demand and implement better standards. In the late eighteen-hundreds in the United States 90% of honey sold was just corn syrup bottled by deceitful manufacturers. The food production industry is not meant to produce food, but profit, and we only ever have the food supply we demand if people like you follow the example of indomitable chemist Dr. Harvey Wiley and stand up for what is right and demand better. Stop eating at restaurants that serve only toxic, pesticide-laden food or buying from grocery stores that stock inferior, poorly produced products. Plant fruit and nut yielding trees and bushes on your property and in your community. Get involved in civics and elect officials who support clean and quality food supplies, reduce pollution, and promote higher culinary standards and regulations, or run for office and do it yourself. Boycott companies, products, and politicians who do not actively protect our nutritional and environmental health and a safe agricultural system. Or grow your own food or start a community garden using the principles of regenerative agriculture which will give you and your family the most nutrient dense and healthy food possible.

SODIUM ACETATE

*never mix in a sealed container—reaction is volatile and will burst
1 tsp baking soda
3 tablespoons vinegar (plus more if needed)
Place baking soda in an open cup or bowl, slowly adding vinegar until foaming stops (agitate solution to react all bicarbonate). Dilute this solution with water or juice, or milk. Divide into two doses the first time, separated by at least an hour. The benefit of this comes from consistency, not excess, which can be unhelpful or cause sodium overdose.

CHAPTER 9
PATHOGENS AND METABOLIC DISEASE

If someone wished to become a great ballet dancer they would never become so by studying bad ballet. A good ballet dancer becomes good by spending their time and energy understanding and studying good dancers, and learning the definition and requirements for what makes good dance. A student who worked to achieve excellence by studying bad dancing could possibly improve upon the definitions of bad dancing but they would most likely not become the best dancer themselves, never having seen for themselves what it means to be a good dancer.

So much fixation on what constitutes disease has likewise failed to define what constitutes *not disease*, and this has lead to misguided observations about human biology which impair progress and prevent the discovery of cures for common diseases like cancer, diabetes, erectile dysfunction, Alzheimer's, or depression even though we can magically speak face to face to people on the entire other side of the planet in real time or smash together subatomic particles at near the speed of light.

What's worse is that while people assume the goals of medical research industries is to find cures for illness their actual goal is to find products to sell to ill people, which is not at all the same thing, and thusly treats disease as commodities for profit, to thus actively undermine research and understanding of human biology and medicine.

All illnesses in fact are not really conditions of separate diseases but are the varying symptoms of a single state of non-health, a failure of the fully integrated biological system to perform as intended at differing intersections, and the consequences of misdirected research and medical discovery are such things as calorie deprivation, prohibition of sugar, or excessive physical exercise which destroys the cardiovascular system. For instance the proper course of discovery in treating diabetes should have been how to restore normal sugar metabolism such as occurs in a healthy state, because healthy people have no problems metabolizing sugar, but instead has been treated by trying to cut sugar from the diet, using a supplement of insulin (which healthy people do not have to do), or to block the body from absorbing sugar, which has been catastrophic as sugar is fundamentally required for our health and wellbeing, which is why those with diabetes, who cannot metabolize sugar properly, become diseased and die, which should have been obvious, but originated from spending too much time observing disease rather than health, and a good dose of religious contamination of the human experience exploiting anything that makes us feel good as a mechanism for control.

Such doctrines have not only failed to cure diabetes but have also endangered many millions of other lives which depend on healthy intakes of carbohydrate and sugar to thrive, and countless people starve themselves or destroy their microbiomes, misinformed to the reality of their biology because of a failure to understand what really constitutes health. But this also causes people to seek out healthful diets and lifestyles only when their heath fails, such as the idea that zinc or vitamin C are only useful during a cold rather than understanding that such nutrients are *always* required for good health and wellbeing, not only when sick. Just as an aspiring dancer strives to acquire the necessary definition of a good dancer, the focus on repairing disease should be not *what is wrong* but instead *what is not right*?

One summer when I was sixteen, prior to the development of full-blown body dysmorphia (which is an unrealistic conception of and unhealthy preoccupation with ones own body), I was in the basement playing *Warcraft II*. We had just returned from a trip to Lake Powell where I had spent an entire week in the sun to the point of becoming so tanned as to not require any more sunblock even when in the sun for five hours a day. "You look so thin when you have a tan," said my mother as she paused on the staircase, looking down on me at the computer. I was wearing a white tank top which clung tightly to my torso and no doubt accentuated my taught, teenage waist. The tan had little to do with my current physique as I had in fact leaned up even more than usual because of a long summer vacation away from training as a competitive swimmer that allowed my body to relax and reduce the stress hormones which, also due to insufficient dietary habits, had been ravaging my body. It was the most lean I ever was during the entirety of my teenage years as even though I would train harder as I got older always found it impossible to replicate because of the compounding stress of under eating, excessive exercise, depression, and metabolic illness of which I was ignorant.

Any teenager is by definition beautiful no matter their appearance, because there exists in young people the innate embodiment of youth and potential of a life newly beginning. Even us teenagers who struggle with health and wellness are by wide margins more attractive than aged people who still maintain a lean or muscular figure, not only for the physical attributes but the blessed naivety and newness we who are older lost long ago, and the comment my mother made about my figure was not something a teenager should hear from a parent and only worsened my already severe feelings of insecurity and body dysmorphia. I think she said this out of envy, and not meant to harm, as she was also abused in this manner by her parents in her youth, entered in beauty pageants and no doubt encouraged to diet and starve herself and base personal worth on transient aspects of existence such as physical appearance, as we pass to our children the attitudes we adopt about life in response to its traumas. Though I was a competitive swimmer, and young, pushing my body with intense training twice a day for three to four hours, six days a week I usually found it difficult to be Though my first year of swimming netted me an increase of fifty pounds of muscle, spreading my shoulders and bulking my arms and chest it changed me from a child into a young man. But even with all this training my waist otherwise stayed comfortably padded and my muscles never grew to quite the size or cut of the other champion swimmers. Of course I was fit by *any* standard, and concern about my lack of shredding was a symptom of serious body dysmorphia and self-hatred, learning from my parents harmful attitudes about the body and self worth, and my declining endocrine system stressed by excessive strenuous physical activity, a poor diet, undiagnosed metabolic illness, exposure to pharmaceuticals like Accutane, incessant exposure to chlorine through my training, and an emotional abuse from family and our religious group which led to an emotional state more susceptible to psychological struggles that no one should have to endure, let alone children.

There is nothing wrong with wanting to be fit, but when we feel bad about ourself because we are not fulfilling any ideal of physical appearance that is dysmorphia which is rooted in poor conceptions of self worth (and addressed by resolving trauma as achieved by inventory therapy). Stress compromises the metabolic rate, whether it's nutritional, environmental, or emotional, and the body protects us from this problem by then retaining fat, without which we would simply die, so I was never able to achieve the physical state of my peers, and in fact I have known many swimmers over the years who in spite of daily, vigorous workouts remain not only overweight but even obese because of the role of fat in mediating thermoregulation which is even more difficult to maintain when submerged regularly in water since water conducts heat much more efficiently than air.

When I first became very ill in my early thirties and struggled even to walk my dogs around the block without gasping for air and was tormented by unrelenting fits of coughing a delusional doctor dismissed my white tongue and hairy leukoplakia as inconsequential as if it was normal for a man in his early thirties to have a thick, gross coating on the top and sides of their tongue. But none of the half dozen other doctors I asked for help did anything to diagnose me, let alone treat the metabolic illness rapidly taking my life. It turns out that hairy leukoplakia is a common symptom of *leukemia* which, along with diabetes, often accompanies cystic fibrosis which was the reason for my constant coughing that I would not discover to be the root cause of my major health issues until I was forty-years old. The average lifespan of someone with cystic fibrosis is only a tragic thirty years which is why my health completely collapsed in my early thirties. A nurse at the same clinic said my blood sugar levels suggested pre-diabetes (a diagnostic the doctor denied), and it made a lot of sense considering the symptoms I was suffering and later helped direct my research, inquiry, and eventual recovery.

One of the most infuriating things about the medical industry is an absence of consideration for gestational stages of conditions like diabetes, autism, cancer, Alzheimers, cystic fibrosis, etc., which would help to prevent their most devastating stages, as if we either have them or we don't and they appear suddenly and magically out of nowhere rather than gradually over years and years with more than ample time to identify and prevent them. If any of the doctors I went to while developing diabetes and cancer were competent I might have been screened for cystic fibrosis because it is not normal for a thirty-one-year-old white male (because of economic status and access to goods and services not available to minority groups because of institutionalized racism) to present with persistent cough, fatigue, insomnia, libido issues, excessive sweating, and immune dysfunction which are obvious and common symptoms of cystic fibrosis. While the naming of diseases helps to remove stereotypes and prejudice and raise awareness in the general public the problem of ineffective treatment in medicine is a consequence of the egoism which motivates the discovery, cataloguing, and institutional management of disease for the accolades and profit of researchers, doctors, scientists, and corporations which exploit disease for their personal gain, because if the condition of these diseases are not separate, disparate, spectrum of one single, interrelated state of non-health there are no separate diseases and thus no names, no products to sell, and no heroes to worship. After learning how to restore erectile function I once shared that information on a social media group of gay men, many of whom I knew personally to also suffer erectile dysfunction as it has become shockingly common for young men these days to suffer premature problems with declining libido, but I was roundly shouted down by a doctor who used his credentials, not evidence or science, not only to discredit me but also to incite harassment from the other members.

While I have now enjoyed normal erectile function for many years now, even better than my teenage years since cystic fibrosis affected it even then, I can only assume many from that group of twenty and thirty-year-olds continue to suffer erectile dysfunction along with many, many other young men due to ignorance of biology, diet, and systemic metabolic disease which the medical profession does absolutely nothing to address except prescribe useless and harmful pharmaceuticals which exploit chronic disease for profit. No doubt many people will skip this chapter because they think they don't have diabetes, or autism, or cystic fibrosis since stereotypes even more strongly inform individual behavior, when the simple fact of our shared biology makes every single person on the planet a potential victim of every single disease that can and does affect human beings, and like myself can have illnesses and conditions we don't even consider, even from the time of our birth. All diseases do have a gestational stage which the medical industry is not even interested in addressing as evident also from the absence any cures for these diseases in spite of epidemic levels of malady but centuries of scientific progress in other areas like technology and physics, because curing or preventing disease does not generate the same profits as long-term management of chronic illness.

Pathogenic fungi like *Candida* are commonly associated with metabolic conditions like diabetes, and nearly all diabetics have white tongue conditions because white tongue is a colony of opportunistic microbes including *Candida* which cause and benefit from the metabolic dysregulation of sugar metabolism that presents as diabetic conditions. *Candida* is shown to be associated with zinc deficiency and actively chelates zinc from its environment, and also causes vaginal yeast infections. Pathogenic fungi produce damaging oxidized lipids like *oxylipin* to strongly dysregulates normal sugar metabolism and immune function, which is normally inhibited by the fat-soluble antioxidant *vitamin E,* but industrialized diets are often highly deficient in vitamin E. But because *Candida* can be found in the bodies of healthy individuals there has been some contention on whether *Candida* is truly harmful or not, which is absurd because healthy people do not have thick coatings of microbial colonies on their body parts. *Candida* is in fact quite harmful, and obvious signs of *Candida* is a thick white or yellow coating on the tongue, yeast infections, thrush, angular cheilitis (cracks at the sides of the lips), dry mouth, dry eyes, chronic post-nasal drip, or leukoplakia. Advice from health professionals and laymen alike also claim that *Candida* is caused by dietary sugar or that a low-carb, low-sugar diet can be part of the solution to curing *Candida,* but dietary carbohydrate (especially sugar) is the primary substrate for the *citric acid cycle* from which energy (ATP) is produced from carbohydrate which also results in important metabolites like citric acid, CO2, and bicarbonate, so while dieting can temporarily address chronic microbial colonization it also causes long term, catastrophic metabolic stress to our own bodies and increases susceptibility to infection by impairing our ability to make the energy which keeps us alive and runs pathways like the immune system and other defensive biological systems.

Candida is also an ancient pathogen which evolved over *millions* of years to infect us and other animals long before modern dietary habits ever included refined sugar, and *Candida* is better at surviving than you are and you are more likely to kill yourself first through carbohydrate deprivation than a *Candida* infection. What is actually occurring in conditions like white tongue and other chronic microbial colonization is that our ability to metabolize *calcium* becomes deranged, by dietary or environmental stress since for instance the body requires vitamin D, vitamin E, and vitamin K to properly metabolize calcium, and opportunistic pathogens like *Candida* then harvest that calcium and use it to colonize our tissue and buffer themselves against our immune factors such as *histatin* which are specific anti-microbial proteins in our saliva. For this reason if you have white tongue you might have also noticed that eating any food high in calcium makes it temporarily thicker. Thrush is a severe condition of white tongue that can even cause death in those who are very aged, young, or immunocompromised, although its milder form is common in nursing children and breastfeeding mothers since hormones like prolactin cause greater calcium mobilization from bones to supply milk production, and since milk is the primary nutrient source for neonates there is an abundance of calcium available for colonizing pathogens, but thrush can also be caused in adults both by taking calcium excess or losing the ability to properly metabolize calcium such as occurs in milk-alkali syndrome, and any white tongue symptoms are also that of disturbed calcium homeostasis. Most people with diabetes also get "dirt" beneath the fingernails even when not ever touching any dirt because this is in fact not dirt but mold growing on sugar leaking from nails and nail beds and is also an excellent way to diagnose diabetes and metabolic disease if the nails are not extremely short. Getting fingers wet such as from showering or washing dishes will kill mold since it is an obligate aerobe (requires a constant supply of oxygen) but it will grow back within a few hours after any meal high in carbohydrate if there is diabetes.

The pathogenic bacterium *Heliobacter pylori* also infects the oral cavity and stomach where it makes toxic *ammonia* from our *urea*. Like calcium, ammonia is highly alkaline and is used by pathogens like *H. pylori* to neutralize stomach acid, but *H. pylori* also directly inhibits the hydrogen-potassium exchange channels by which stomach acid is expressed into the stomach, both lowering stomach acid production to impair digestion, promote ammonia excess, and causing potassium deficiency, which also then disturbs our commensal microbiome. *H. pylori* also actually hides inside *Candida* cells when the environment is unfavorable for its survival, so *Candida* can and does also promote continued *H. pylori* infection and might even be made virulent through hijacking by *H. pylori*. *H. pylori* is a widespread pathogen and probably one of the first catalysts of metabolic disease since it directly impairs digestion.

In addition to white tongue, cracks also often appear in the tongue during colonization by *H. pylori* because it and other pathogens steal the calcium required in *cadherin* proteins which hold together the tongue tissues, thereby disabling cadherin and causing cracks to appear and which may occur even in young children which is erroneously and harmfully often explained (without evidence) by medical professionals as a genetic feature when in fact it is pathogenic and, like many pathogens, *H. pylori* also uses calcium to buffer itself against our immune system. Because it is caused by pathogens like *H. pylori*, severe tongue cracks are usually accompanied by anxiety, depression, or even bipolar disorder or schizophrenia as discussed in the upcoming chapter on depression and immunity because interference in our calcium pathways and toxins produced by these microbes also disturb the endocrine system and nervous system, and the tongue is not evolved to have giant fucking cracks across its surface, and cracks on the tongue are a definite sign of *H. pylori*, if hypochlorhydria (low stomach acid) isn't already obvious.

Another widespread, highly virulent gut pathogen called *Clostridioides difficile* (formerly classified as *Clostridium*) also exploits calcium dysregulation and causes tens of thousands of deaths each year in aged or immunocompromised people as *C. difficile* is harbored by nearly everyone on Earth, but a healthy, intact microbiome and working immune system normally keeps it in check and minimizes or prevents symptoms of colonization. *C. difficile* even colonizes the guts of infants although because of the naturally low iron environment of infant tissue *C. difficile* is generally unable to induce disease in neonates, unless they are given supplemental iron which is alarmingly common in milk replacement products and medical care for premature neonates as if this is somehow physiologically appropriate. Nearly all stomachaches are caused by *C. difficile* because it produces very harmful toxins to destroy our tissues and access blood sugar which it also stimulates from release of glycogen by synthesizing the adrenaline analog *phenylethylamine* to harvest an intermediate of the polyol pathway called *sorbitol* created during the interconversion of glucose and fructose. Because of this, long term colonization by *C. difficile* underlies conditions like gut cancer, diabetes, and severe mental health disorders like schizophrenia and bipolar disorder due to the excessive production of phenylethylamine which acts like adrenaline in the body and causes wild fluctuations in mood and blood sugar. *Clostridioides difficile* is a sporulating bacteria so it is utterly impossible to avoid exposure as spores are everywhere in food, on unwashed hands, in the mouths, gut, and feces of infected individuals, and even on food laid out at the grocery store because spores are indestructible and able to survive extremely high temperatures, antibacterial compounds, all disinfecting agents, and even radiation, and absence of infection is never, ever due to cleanliness, sterility, or absence of exposure but from of a healthy commensal microbiome and working immune system.

But while many such pathogens cause severe disease our immune system would normally be able to easily eradicate them, and instead most metabolic illness is first catalyzed by colonization with *parasites*, because parasites are especially evolved to inhibit the immune system after which secondary infections occur from opportunistic microbes that exploit reduced immunity. Yes, if you have any health problems you are colonized with any of the many thousands of possible parasites distributed throughout our environment in spite of our modern medical systems and sanitation, because we are still a megafauna, vertebrate species and a target for a great many parasites which are not in fact effectively controlled even by the most thorough sanitation standards. Many people confuse their ignorance of parasites for the absence of them, which is made worse by the fact that most parasites also do not cause outright, obvious disease but simply inhibit the immune system so they can feed on our sugar and other nutrients and are thus easily distributed throughout the population without causing occasion for treatment or raising alarm. Parasitism is in fact more wide-spread in developed, industrial countries with adequate sanitation because of complacency from medical treatment of more serious and obvious parasites like hookworm, malaria, giardia, etc., in both humans and livestock (especially livestock), and colonization is strongly supported by highly refined, industrial diets low in protective antimicrobial factors and thus greater distribution of drug resistant, microscopic, and less obvious parasite species that remain undetected in the general population.

For instance the microscopic tapeworm *Hymenolepis nana* is widespread in developed countries like the United States which produces almost no symptoms during colonization, so their infection is never addressed unless it leads to more serious secondary infections by more other more obvious pathogens. There are also protozoan parasites that can live in the spleen and bone marrow, sexually transmitted parasites that live in the reproductive organs and mucosal tissue, and nematodes and flukes that can infect the blood, lungs, and even many that can and do live in the brain while producing very little symptoms of parasitism. Waterborne parasites like *schistosomes (Schistosoma)* are spread globally and enter human bodies from the skin after exposure in lakes and reservoirs and produce mild rashes which can be mistaken for bug bites, and live inside blood vessels and migrate to organs like the lungs, spinal cord, brain, or the nervous system and can and do cause symptoms like diarrhea, abdominal dissension, and enlargement of the liver and spleen. While parasites often freak people out they are so common that being scared of them is really dumb and unprofitable in efforts to be well since willful ignorance actively makes us more vulnerable to disease, not less. It has also been shown in studies that *Toxoplasma gondii*, the most widely distributed parasite, is an etiological factor in the development of Alzheimer's and is very likely a candidate for migraines as discussed in the upcoming chapter on cancer and migraine. There are also *Cryptosporidium, Babesia, Taeniidae, Trypanosoma, Echinococcus, Cyclospora, Trichomonas, Trichinella, Leishmania, Ascaris, Taenia, Entamoeba*, and most people have heard of *Giardia* which are also common waterborne parasites—That's *parasites*, plural, as like many parasitic organisms *Giardia* are not a single species but a genus of many different species and strains which are all specialized in the colonization of organisms like ourselves, which have also become resistant to chlorination, and *Giardia* colonization specifically causes gut distension and anal itching, and anyone who experiences bloating or itchy butt is colonized by *Giardia* (it is NOT normal for the butt to itch, ever).

There are also more than a dozen species of *Blastocystis* which is a sort of parasitic algae (stramenopile) which colonizes human and animal guts, with one study putting the infection rate of humans in the United States at an enormous 23%, but still being widely considered asymptomatic even though there are studies which demonstrably show their potential to cause illness. *Blastocystis* isn't actually after our tissues but instead feeds on our bacteria thereby indirectly causing disease, gut dysbiosis, and deficiency of nutrient. Studies show *Blastocystis* correlates with an increase in microbial diversity which is prejudicially considered a good thing by researchers but is occurring because blastocystis is literally eating our commensal microbiome and thus disturbing populations of commensal species required to protect us against colonization by other opportunistic microbes. Lyme disease is often characterized as colonization with the bacterium *Borrelia* but ticks also transmit *Babesia* parasites which enjoy far less medical surveillance and colonize red blood cells much like *Plasmodium* (which causes malaria) and thus systemic distribution throughout the body. Even giardiasis can show little symptoms in those who are well fed and healthy so parasites easily contaminate and persist without being recognized by the medical industry, and especially not the larger public. One study even identified *Blastocystis* infection being misdiagnosed as irritable bowel syndrome and symptoms can include abdominal cramps, nausea, constipation, diarrhea, bloating, excess gas, and anus itching. In fact most parasites which infect the gut cause anal itching as a symptom, and any anal itching definitely means you have parasites (sorry). *Blastocystis* is also entirely immune to chlorination so it can and does easily spread through municipal water systems in direct opposition to assumptions and prejudices of modern sanitation.

Because of their medical and sanitation systems, capitalist, industrialized countries stupidly consider parasitic diseases to be exotic and foreign problems to exist only in those countries we exploit for natural resources, cheap labor, and political power to support our wasteful, exploitative, and bloated consumer markets as if those countries we impoverish have chosen to be poor rather than forcefully oppressed and exploited by our predatory corporations and governments raping them of resources, capital, and labor, even as populations in industrialized societies present with epidemic symptoms of chronic and widespread parasitism. These frankly xenophobic and racist sentiments about parasites causes we who live in developed countries to be willfully ignorant to parasitism in our own communities and their significant impact on our health, which are in fact the primary factors responsible for the unchecked epidemics of obesity, metabolic disease, and mental illness so common to industrialized societies and industrial food systems, because it is extremely easy to become infected by unwashed hands, food contaminated by rodent, mollusk, insect, and human feces, sexual intimacy with an infected person, swimming in damned lakes and reservoirs, undercooked meat, or exposure through at-risk professions such as nursing, dentistry, childcare, farming, hunting, teaching, sex work, etc. Relying also on impoverished, underpaid, and exploited laborers to run the food industry and harvest produce and meat as we do in countries like the United States further increases risk of parasitic contamination of the food supply because exploitation of labor prevents impoverished people from affording healthy food, sanitary living conditions, and medical care which would otherwise protect them from also contracting and spreading microorganisms, and studies on parasites and opportunistic bacteria contamination of produce and other food sources always return alarmingly positive samples for this very reason.

ALL animals, including humans, are and will always be vectors for parasitic microbes because most parasites are also NOT species-specific, meaning parasites that infect birds, dogs, cows, and snails also infect us, and in our increasingly industrialized societies which destroy the health not only of humans but also livestock, pets, and wild ecosystems increase the exposure risk to parasites, not in spite of our access to chemicals and industry but because of it. The damming of rivers for instance increases waterborne parasites by destroying local populations of snail-eating prawns which would otherwise keep mollusk host populations in check, and snails, slugs, clams, and oysters are a major vector for several waterborne parasites which in turn increases contamination of fresh water reservoirs from which our drinking water comes because of environmental destruction. Married, monogamous couples are also the most frequent carriers of pathogens because couples continuously pass microbes back and forth to each other and their children for decades and decades without realizing their health problems are rooted in colonization with pathogenic microbes like parasites, wrongly thinking because they are monogamous they don't in fact carry disease in spite of plainly obvious evidence to the contrary, unlike single persons who have increased occasion to get treated if they catch sexually transmitted disease for which medications can and do incidentally treat other opportunistic pathogens.

Parasites inhibit the immune system in part by also producing toxic ammonia, primarily from the amino acid *arginine,* using enzymes like *arginase* and *arginine deiminase,* to both disturb our immune system and destabilize and supplant the commensal microbiome. Because ammonia is derived from protein (and used to make protein) it also occurs during normal digestion, but ammonia is normally acidified by stomach acid into *ammonium* which is then packaged into metabolic pathways like the synthesis of *glutamine* and *urea* or excreted in urine as ammonium chloride. Besides being generally toxic, ammonia is highly alkaline and is most harmful in the gut because its alkalinity neutralizes acid and prevents dissociation (digestion) of chloride from sodium in dietary salt (which is composed of sodium chloride) by strongly alkalizing chloride which strengthens its bond to sodium (and other elements) to thus prevent absorption into the body. Many other nutrient absorption pathways such as for zinc, sulfur, vitamin C, citrulline, etc., are in turn dependent on sodium and thus ammonia excess and dysregulation causes significant metabolic disease by directly or indirectly interfering with absorption of many nutrients by preventing their dissociation and instead promoting their polymerization.

Studies show that the enzymes which catabolize arginine in the intestines required for these processes is inhibited by lactate, which means that domination of the gut by lactic acid producing microbes such as what are used in the manufacture of yogurt and kefir (but which also occur regardless of these foods) causes metabolic illness by directly inhibiting arginine catabolism which then increases the circulation of free arginine. This higher circulating arginine or deposition of increased arginine into tissues thence makes us more susceptible to colonization by ammonia producing microbes which then blocks important pathways such as the absorption of salts, vitamin C, sulfur, etc. In fact, studies show that excessive arginine promotes pancreatic necrosis and death of the acinar cells which produce and store digestive enzymes, which is likely caused by these opportunistic microbes, and those with conditions like diabetes, cancer, autism, Crohn's disease, etc., are indeed also shown to present with far higher lactic acid in feces in ratio to short chain fatty acids than healthy people and problems like pancreatic insufficiency and inflammation. Because pectin oppositely shifts the gut toward acetogens it helps activate arginine catabolism to help reduce arginine access by parasites. Fruit and vegetables contain lots of pectin, but it is locked behind plant cell walls which requires that commensal microbes have access to vitamin B12 which, as discussed in the chapter on gut health, is derived from Thaumarchaeota archaea when they have access to vitamin D, so it is impossible to benefit from fruits and vegetables without getting enough sunshine and during metabolic disease a supplement of pectin and use of supplemental B12 with fruits and vegetables can be required until vitamin D repletion is restored as discussed in that upcoming chapter.

Surprisingly, the enzymes arginase and arginine deiminase used by microbes to produce ammonia from arginine also use *water* as a cofactor, which means that during colonization by parasites the simultaneous consumption of protein and soda or other drinks such as is so common in industrialized diets directly fuels production of ammonia from dietary arginine, which easily explains the rampant rates of metabolic disease that accompany industrialized food systems in which high protein intake and commercial beverages are so common. Thankfully these enzymes are actually inhibited by polyphenols called *tannin,* which are common to foods stereotypically associated with good health like coffee, tea, chocolate, nuts, berries, olives, olive oil, wine, etc., (most commercial wine contains sulfites, however, which can kill off your microbiome and promote disease). During the course of my research I purposefully infected myself with oral pathogenic microbes in order to better understand and cure them. But I was overconfident after discovering the cures to alcoholism and depression and cured my cancer and thought it would only take a few months, maybe a year at most, but after several years had grown tired of being ill and was just going to use and recommend anti-biotics. To my surprise, experimenting with several antibiotics including powerful *clindamycin* not only failed to resolve these infections it also wiped out my commensal microbiome and catalyzed acute *C. difficile* infection in my gut which in less than a year moved into my liver and gallbladder and was so uncomfortable I nearly went to the hospital. I realized serendipitously that the hazelnuts on which I had been occasionally snacking which retained their skins and not the naked nuts seemed to restrain the symptoms of infection. Knowing that nut skins were a potent source of tannin I then experimented with daily, consistent, high intake of tannin fully resolved the *C. difficile* infection in a matter of days which otherwise requires weeks or months using specialized antibiotics and even sometimes a fecal microbiome transit (and even that sometimes doesn't even work).

Most justification for supposed health effects of tannin is erroneously attributed to its antioxidant action (guys, not everything is an antioxidant!), but tannin complexes with the hydrogen atoms in the water molecule and the true role of tannin is that it is the most effective, protective, and selective *prebiotic* in nature intended by plants for the cultivation and management of the soil microbiome which then happens to have that same effect in our bodies by regulating the activity of pathogenic microorganisms by inhibiting processes such as the enzymes used to produce ammonia from protein. There are many pathogens which live in soil which target plants, and tannin is an evolutionary medicine to control soil and plant pathogens, but because tannin is very tart in flavor (sometimes even bitter) it has long been thought to be an antinutrient and deterrent against browsers, which it can be in high concentrations, but tannins from seeds, leaves, and other plant litter slowly leaks into the soil when exposed to water from rain, ponds, and streams where it saturates water like steeping tea and thus conditions the soil, conveyed downward through gravity, and over long periods of time eventually forms common soil compounds like humic acids, all of which has nothing to do with browsers but everything to do with microbes in the medium where plant roots grow. Tannin is the reason forests smell so clean and not like sulfurous rot though there is an abundance of decay, and consuming nuts, seeds, flowers, fruit, leaves, or other source of tannin performs this same function in our gastrointestinal system, binding and protecting micronutrients from intercepting pathogens while promoting commensal access to those micronutrients, and we are also dependent on the role of tannin in the maintenance of our gastroinestinal and metabolic health because we have always lived in tannin rich environments and, until the advent of modern technology, drank from tannin saturated water sources such as vernal pools, small brooks, or springs littered with fallen plant matter and thus our evolution as always been constrained to the presence and function of such environmental factors in our development as a species.

This role of tannin is already recognized by aquarium enthusiasts, for instance, because fish and amphibians kept in freshwater aquariums and paludariums will get sick and die if plant litter is not added to the water. Famously, commercial beverages first developed during the early industrial revolution like colas and root beer were actually made from real leaves, spices, and herbs which are high in tannin, though the people making them didn't believe they were actually healthy and simply interested in profit, later changing the formulas to be nothing more than flavored sugar water and preservatives. Ironically many of those first beverages were not only tonics that did provide medicinal assistance through the presence of polyphenols like tannin, changing the formulas served to actively increase parasitism in the general population now conditioning to consume beverages with meals which, once tannin was removed from beverages, actively promotes parasitism through the simultaneous consumption of tannin-free water accompanying dietary protein.

Many market gardeners and organic farmers also use a cultivation technique called *weed tea* in which plant material is allowed to steep in water for an extended period of time to produce a solution which actively helps plants grow. This is often erroneously attributed to its 'nutrient' content but plain dirt contains many magnitudes greater nutrient than compost and this benefit comes instead from tannin saturation which then helps to inhibit pathogens and promote commensals that support plant health. While modern water treatment prevents some parasite and microbial diseases like cholera it also ironically promotes other parasites like *Toxoplasma, Trichomonas,* and *Blastocystis* because of the total absence of tannin in drinking water. Unsurprisingly, studies also show that tannin added to the diet of livestock or directly to manure strongly reduces the formation of ammonia, methane, and hydrogen sulfide, and the problem of excess methane production by livestock is a consequence of low-tannin diets fed to industrially raised animals which then directly promotes the growth of methanogens and parasites. While most cattle are kept on restrictive, overgrazed, barren fields and feedlots cows are actually forest dwelling animals descended from the mighty aurochs and do best in a semi-wooded environment such as is replicated in the practice of *silvopasture* specifically because of access to tannin sources such as twigs, tree leaves, seeds, nuts, fruit, and tannin saturated water. Grazers like cows and sheep are often seen gleefully munching on fallen leaves in preference to grass because grass is low in tannin and access to natural tannins by livestock treats gut pathogens and increases their health, and the unnatural diets of industrial meat production for animals confined in pens and stalls is antithetical to producing high quality meat and increases the requirement for antibiotics and other harmful husbandry practices to then increase disease pressure in humans. Free grazing pigs, cows, chickens, turkey, and sheep with foraging diets produce higher quality meat, but overgrazing and free-ranging damages the environment and further reduces sources of tannin for them to consume. Instead the purposed cultivation of trees and other tannin sources for livestock, even producing tannin-infused drinking water like "weed tea" (make sure to use non toxic plants), can replace the use of antibiotics and antiparasitics since water is also the primary cofactor required in the production of ammonia which first facilitates parasitism and secondary opportunistic infections.

Because we are also animals and vulnerable to parasitism which catalyzes all metabolic illness the similar use of tannin in *all* sources of fluid intake from water to milk to watery foods like soup and sauces during treatment of metabolic disease can and does also protect our gut from parasites and other harmful ammonia producers. Options for dietary tannin are those already associated with good health like tea, coffee, cocoa, olives and olive oil, herbs and spices, wine, most fruit, and nuts if they retain their skins (coffee is not very potent, however, and for instance is not strong enough to protect all the milk in a latte). The diets of populations like those who live around the Mediterranean which gave rise to the eponymous dietary fad produces better health not because they are high in things like fish or olive oil but for their abundance of tannin, and leaves of bay and curry commonly used in cuisine also imparts tannin to foods in which they are used and should be generously increased especially in watery foods like soup and sauces (ten or twelve bay leaves instead of the usual one or two is also fucking delicious—why the hell have we been using so little?). While grapes contain tannin their leaves are much higher, and the oak barrels in which wine is aged also imparts even more tannin during the winemaking process, and tannin is far more common than is appreciated. Tea is the most potent tannin source in the human dietary arsenal, and its long tradition of healthful properties is a direct result of blocking pathogenic arginase and related enzymes, and tea can be simmered or allowed to steep for longer periods of time to extract greater tannin content. Indian bay leaf (not bay laurel, which is better for soup) makes a great non-caffeinated tea but must be simmered for more than an hour to fully extract its tannin (herbal teas are not really useful for this purposes and can even be harmful, for instance camomile tea blocks sugar absorption and as such can increase stress hormones and lower respiration).

The most potent sources of tannins for the resolution of opportunistic gut microbes (especially bacteria) are high-tannin fruit, because tannins in fruit are generally the more bioavailable forms than what occur in leaves, because fruit has evolved in nature along with its animal patrons as a natural medicine to help promote the wellbeing of the organisms which help distribute their seeds, in share evolutionary cooperation against opportunistic microbes which would otherwise harm this symbiotic relationship. For instance blueberries are shown in studies to result in high quantities of urinary tannin metabolites, which proves their bioavailability, but fruit which is highly hybridized by agricultural development often contains less tannin than their natural counterparts, since tannins are tart and sour, and the most effective choices are those fruit which are highly astringent like chokecherries, sloe berries, aronia (also called chokeberries), gooseberries, crabapples, persimmon, currants, pomegranate, lingonberries, etc. The mouth-puckering, dry, tart sensation of those fruits are the tannin, which makes it easy to identify its usefulness, and can be used medicinally to help more strongly inhibit opportunistic pathogens and should be used immediately by those whom are very ill. I have not tested all of these fruit but after only a day consuming preserved chokecherries (the whole berry is probably better than only the juice) it completely resolved symptoms of *H. pylori* colonization (bloating, belching, and low stomach acid), although several days of consistent intake were required for more persistent resolution. Because we can always be reinfected with these pathogens these medicinal berries should be eaten regularly and kept around as a regular part of the diet and in storage (dried) for any occasion in which they may be required to treat new or recurrent infection. Most of these fruits are very difficult to acquire, so it is a good idea and may even be required to plant them on your property or in pots if at all possible, and could even be grown under lights indoors if there is not other space to do so, while large scale operations to produce those fruits should be used to help more widely treat the general population, using these fruits in smoothies, salads, breads and pastries, jams and preserves, dried, frozen, juiced, etc., using the symptom of belching after meals as a primary diagnostic for this requirement, since that symptom originates mostly from SIBO induced by *H. pylori* inhibition of stomach acid.

One study I saw demonstrated that tannin can bind iron and lattice over exposed dentin in rotted teeth and promotes enamel regeneration, so while tannin from tea can stain teeth it also helps preserve teeth and reduce tooth decay (staining actually occurs to biofilm and plaque, though, not the enamel, as addressed in the upcoming chapter on oral health). Because tannin does bind some nutrients it has sometimes been considered an antinutrient, and there are some tannins which are excessively strong and can potentially cause deficiencies of iron or copper, and strong sources like tea should also not be given regularly to children for long periods of time as this can result in stunting of growth (by the way, obligate carnivores like cats are not adapted to tannins and may be harmed by those which are very strong). But studies also firmly establish an association of high tissue iron and high-iron diets with diabetes such as occurs from diets high in heme-iron (high meat intake). Iron overload of the pancreas causes significant oxidative stress and promotes excess collagen which reduces circulation to prevent healthy pancreatic function and promotes microbial overgrowth in the pancreas. Because iron in meat is heme iron it is highly bioavailable which then makes it easier for pathogens to colonize the gut. For children, an increase in fruits and vegetables, especially high-polyphenol fruit like purple grapes, other berries, or their juices are good sources of tannin (don't dilute their juice!), but studies on food sources of tannin almost never show nutrient deprivation nor interruption to growth and development because we have evolved in concert with the biological function of tannin through the entirety of our evolution. Our mucous proteins are even shown to actually react with and bind tannin, and having a high tannin diet while also anchoring the diet in fruits and vegetables instead of meats and iron-fortified food can strongly begin to resolve diabetic symptoms. Some sources of water and protein combination which require tannin protection are quite inobvious, such as sauces that are thickened with roux or starch like what accompany macaroni and cheese which will result in as much ammonia production as drinking a glass of unprotected milk, so when presenting with metabolic illness care should be taken to evaluate every single food item for protein, water, and tannin content to prevent the combination of unprotected water and protein which is the substrate for ammonia production by parasites. For this reason it can be more simple to have tannin in or with all food and beverages if illness is very severe, although it's perfectly fine to occasional drink plain water if you get really thirsty, but care should be taken to include tannin as often as possible.

Tannin's role in our biology is also primarily enteric (only going through the intestines), simply to regulate access to nutrients by oral and gastrointestinal microbes, because most tannins are not well absorbed into the body, nor should they be, and wild ideas like administering tannin intravenously or using synthetic tannic acid as have many poorly done studies are both dangerous and misguided. There is no such thing as 'tannic acid,' as tannins are many and varied and only effective from natural sources, not synthetic supplements. After regular inclusion of tannin in my diet I noticed regrowth of thinning eyebrows and thickening of nails which began to naturally look like I had a manicure, as it so effectively promotes the uptake of many nutrients required for good health while also suppressing pathogens. Because of their expense nuts were hardly ever a part of my diet, but my grandad subsisted mostly on nuts and though he spent most of his life as a horse rancher in the blazing hot Arizona sun eating a general Western diet he didn't become invalid until very shortly before his death in his nineties, still with a full head of hair. Baking with tannin like high quality cocoa powder, nuts which retain their skins, cinnamon, nutmeg, teas, etc., can also be used to make delicious deserts or beverages high in tannin such as cinnamon raisin bread, tea infused pastry, or high quality chocolate milk to protect protein from ammonia producing pathogens in ways that are delicious, gratifying, and especially useful for children (most commercial chocolate milk contains harmful emulsifiers like carrageenan, though, so remember to always read labels). Many cultures such as in India and Pakistan have brewed tea in milk for generations which happens to then protect milk protein from opportunistic pathogens and thus the gut from ammonia producers, and I also love making milk tea or cinnamon milk in which I add sugar, cinnamon, and nutmeg as a bedtime tonic. Especially since many fruits also contain tannin (berries, grapes, olives, sumac, etc.,) there is no shortage of options, which only requires planning, curiosity, and consistency, and just having a good cup of strongly brewed, regular tea is always an easy and effective option. As regular plant leaves from shrubs and trees or grapevines usually contain tannin they could even be used as an option (do not use any that are poisonous!), but because the most effective are the astringent varieties of fruit (also make sure you don't eat any poisonous berries!) it might be required to plant your own since they are not widely available for purchase.

It is not only important to block microbial production of ammonia through the generous use of tannin but also to restore and support our body's normal detoxification of ammonia. The most effective and relevant pathway is through production of *glutamine* which not only sequesters ammonia but is also used as an energy source and fuel by the body and is taken up by the citric acid cycle along with carbohydrate in the processes which produce energy. So not only is para-sitism harmful for the production of additional ammonia which actively inhibits necessary pathways but the impaired production of glutamine then deprives us of a valuable energy source. Glutamine synthesis is rather easy for the body to accomplish and is most strongly caused by deficiency of the B vitamin *biotin* (vitamin B7) not because it is directly involved in glutamine synthesis but because biotin is needed to break down the *branched chain amino acids* (BCAA) which are required as substrate for glutamine synthesis, and conditions in which ammonia is elevated such as diabetes and autism present also with high circulating levels of unmetabolized BCAA, and studies show that high BCAA is associated with diabetic symptoms, which is not likely caused by branched chain amino acids but by the inability of cells to metabolize them as necessary substrates for pathways like the synthesis of glutamine and sequestration of ammonia. Biotin is requisite for many other pathways, so its deficiency is catastrophic for our health in general and because elevated ammonia is one consequence of biotin deficiency a common diagnostic symptom is brain fog such as what commonly accompanies metabolic conditions.

But biotin is not only quite high in the diet such as from eggs, nuts, and root vegetables, it is also produced in abundance by our own microbiome, and biotin deficiency which impairs glutamine synthesis *never* occurs from dietary deficien-cy but is in fact a problem of anti-biotin factors in our diet and environment. Although egg yolks are one of the highest sources of biotin in the diet, egg whites actually contain a potent anti-biotin factor called *avidin* which irreversibly binds biotin and thus impairs its participation in dependent pathways. Avidin in eggs is meant to prevent bacterial colonization if an eggshell is breached, to protect a developing embryo, but the avidin-biotin bond is one of the strongest in nature and cannot be broken once bound. As such it has long been established but not widely known that excessive consumption of egg whites is actually toxic to humans and can induce catastrophic biotin deficiency, so frequent consumption of eggs, especially just the whites, is actually a catalyst for many metabolic condi-tions and disturbance of the gut microbiome since our commensal microbes also rely on and produce biotin for their own needs.

Even less well known is that microbes also produce avidins, and common bacteria called *Streptomyces* produce an even stronger form of avidin called *streptavidin* which even more powerfully binds biotin than that found in eggs, which is saying a lot, and it has escaped the attention of researchers and medical professionals that such avidin producing microbes colonize the human gut which then easily causes chronic biotin deficiency to chronically impair ammonia sequestration into glutamine to cause toxic ammonia accumulation which then disrupts many crucial biological pathways both by causing ammonia excess and deficient energy production. Microbes like *Streptomyces* which produce avidin are not inhibiting biotin to compete with us, but instead to compete with our commensal microbes for space inside our gut, but this causes disease by then disturbing our commensal microbiome and causing biotin deficiency.

During my research into the toxicity of ammonia I realized that colonization by microbial avidin producers like *Streptomyces* are the cause of *autism spectrum conditions,* because the resultant inability to sequester ammonia due to chronic biotin deficiency impairs growth and development, disturbs the normal human gut microbiome, and results in toxic accumulation of ammonia. Those of us with autism indeed present with ammonia excess, biotin deficiency, and strongly disturbed gastroinestinal microbiome. Because of the ubiquity of microbes like *Streptomyces,* all humans eventually acquire them at some point in our lives and for those who are already fully grown their presence results only in symptoms typical to aging such as brain fog, weight gain, insomnia, muscle wasting, erectile dysfunction, reduced immune function, etc., as the body is slowly depleted of B vitamins, short chain fatty acids, and other products of the commensal microbiome. In those of us with autism, colonization by avidin producers occurs while the body is still developing and because glutamine is so important for both development and ammonia detoxification this then impairs growth and development, and the degree of ammonia excess is directly causal to the degree of autism severity because ammonia toxicity impairs neurological function in a dose-dependent manner. This even includes feeling the urge to pee or other control of the bladder or bowels which is why both young people with autism and very aged persons experience varying degrees of incontinence. Enuresis (involuntary peeing at night) beyond the age of five is a common symptom of autism because of excess ammonia which must be rapidly removed from the body in urine also impairs the neurological sensation of a full bladder which would otherwise wake or alert a healthy person, and because of stupidity, prejudice, and insecurity the fact that I wet the bed until I was fifteen-years old was treated as my fault and an embarrassment to my family instead of a medical condition requiring attention and treatment. Rather than take me to a doctor my arrogant father tried to "cure" me of it himself through insane and even dangerous abuse like forcing me to drink a lot of water without letting me pee in order to "stretch" my bladder, which is one of the most fucking stupid things I've ever heard in my entire life and not at all how any organ in the body actually works. Doctors might not have been much help anyway since this was before the widespread recognition of autism, and enuresis does not always present in autism because ammonia excess can become so great as to even impair the normal function of the kidneys in the first place and timely formation of urea, and then ammonia instead accumulates even further to thus cause even worse developmental impairment such as what occurs in the most severe of cases.

Because biotin helps our body break down the branched chain amino acids to then sequester ammonia into glutamine, biotin supplements have been shown in studies to help alleviate symptoms of autism, but without recognizing this mechanism of action since *Streptomyces* are not yet recognized as a cause, and can be used supplementally to help reduce symptoms not only of autism but of many other metabolic diseases since ammonia dysregulation is a primary mechanism by which most microbes cause disease. A biotin supplement is best dissolved in water then added to food (such as in water used to make tea, coffee, soups, pasta sauce, etc.) and is especially useful in tea, coffee, or fruit juice, where, when eaten, the biotin and abundance of tannin not only contributes to our own biotin supply but also helps promote commensal biotin producing microbes to help restore normal, microbial biotin production (because biotin producers are dependent on biotin) to help supply biotin long-term and in spite of dietary biotin.

Biotin is also required for the synthesis of insulin in the pancreas for *pancreatic glucokinase* which phosphorylates glucose for use in metabolic pathways including the production of *insulin* disturbed in conditions of diabetes. Pakistan, the country with the highest rate of type-two diabetes in the world though they are hardly plagued by junk food or excess sugar, commonly use large amounts of eggs and have also adopted the prevalent, misguided attitude spread by global misinformation about the nature of cholesterol and preference to egg whites. Heat denatures some avidin but the cooking times and temperatures normally used for eggs is not even close to what is required to fully neutralize avidin, so diets high in eggs and especially those high in egg white rapidly destroy colonies of microbial biotin producers to thus enable colonization by *Streptomyces*, and during any metabolic disease eggs should only be consumed if hard boiled or baked into other foods which results in total cooking of the egg white, and children should never be given eggs as food until they develop an established and robust microbiome, which probably occurs after months of eating lots of solid food, especially lots of fruit.

Exposure to *Streptomyces* occurs because they are integral to both plant growth and decay and thus accompany all food sources, so exposure can never be avoided. Interestingly, *C. difficile* also requires biotin for its survival, and biotin deficiency such as is caused by avidin is shown in studies to increase *C. difficile* virulence which means that colonization by *Streptomyces* or high egg white consumption enhances the virulence of *C. difficile* which produces toxic adrenaline analogs to force release of sugar from glycogen stores, and the combination of *Streptomyces* and *C. difficile* in autism and related disorders is the source of the severe emotional stress, insomnia, and coping behaviors like repetitive motion or even self harm seen in those with autism and psychological illnesses like bipolar disorder and schizophrenia because these coping behaviors help to distract the mind from unrelenting, torturous, physical, emotional, and neurological stress through the release of endorphins which help dull pain and suffering caused by *C. difficile* toxin and relentless adrenaline expression.

While many people have mischaracterized autism and treated those with autism as a problem, the spectrum of neurodivergence seen in autism and related conditions is in fact the body's adaptive response to colonization by these microbes, which ranges from the extremely impaired, obvious cases to those like myself whom are not even perceptibly affected whom are just considered a little odd or different who may even have heightened cognitive ability due alteration of the *kynurenine pathway* as discussed in the upcoming chapters on niacin therapy and hair loss. I once saw a post in an autism support forum by a young man of sixteen who just wanted to stop having to wear a diaper, but when I tried to help I was attacked and shouted down by more able-bodied persons and so-called advocates who then also made fun of my symptoms and personal experience. Although my own condition was easily masked by the abuse which existed in my home and my skill at trying to fit in I was occasionally ridiculed for my odd gait and inability to speak correctly, and learned at a very young age that if I just kept my mouth shut people would assume I was the same as them. I did not do this because anyone was especially cruel, as most children and people I experienced growing up were very kind and loving, but because I had been taught by my family and religion to be embarrassed of being weird or different or of drawing attention to myself, so doing so brought me intense stress and negative experiences amplified by having autism in the first place, and even attention from telling a funny joke or making funny voices as I once did during lunch in high school when everyone cheered for me to do it again were developmentally debilitating instead of affirming. Being wholly unable to understand how people were supposed to relate to one another, intuitively and intellectually, making friends was only something I could ever do by waiting for others to come to me, letting them create their own idea of who they thought I was and never being my real self which I had no concept of since this entire function is inhibited by the condition to begin with. When I was a young man experiencing stomachaches so severe I would have to regularly call in sick to work or avoid going to restaurants or on dates, and depression so extreme I cried myself to sleep every single night, without the tools or support to cope with such utter hopelessness suicide began to seem the only recourse for relief. It was not until my life entirely fell apart in my mid-thirties that I realized it was pathogenic microbes and a dysfunctional endocrine and nervous system, not lack of effort or religion which was responsible for my long suffering, and for the first time in my life started experiencing relief through changes in my diet and caring for my body instead of resenting it as I had been taught to do.

Avidin-induced biotin deficiency is the reason why vegetarians or vegans initially experience health benefits when adopting such diets, because a lower protein, high polyphenol diet strongly reduces microbial ammonia production. But this also simply masks the problem of biotin deficiency, and long-term protein deficit is extremely dangerous and why these diets, especially extreme versions such as fruitarianism, can cause severe health consequences such as wasting and cancer because protein is so crucial to all systems in our body. As discussed in the chapter on gut health, we also cannot break down most plant foods without cobalamin produced by vitamin D dependent *Thaumarchaeota* archaea, so it also does no good to eat most plant foods when also suffering from vitamin D deficiency, as we simply cannot break them down without the help of commensal microbes. Factors which compromise commensal gut microbes such as occurs from dieting, exposure to toxic agrochemicals, frequent antibiotic use, and high egg white consumption can promote colonization by opportunistic microbes to initialize these conditions, but since we inherit our microbiome from our parents and other family members a healthy microbiome can also be impaired even before we are born, since our microbiome must come from somewhere and does not generate spontaneously. Anyone who's been around infants have seen them shoving handfuls of dirt into their mouths which is actually an instinctual human biological survival strategy meant to acquire microbes from the environment, since adults can often have compromised microbiomes due to the stresses of diet and disease (but which now can be dangerous in areas like lawns and gardens which contain toxic 'lawn-care' chemicals that actively destroy microbial life). This behavior is also why babies drool an ungodly amount because saliva is an effective way to filter opportunistic pathogens while allowing in those which are beneficial. It has also been stated that rates of conditions like autism seem higher than what appears usual and the answer is that, yes, it is, because apart from increased awareness and diagnosis the commercial dieting industry became a cultural epidemic promoted by mass-market consumer predation through television, magazines, and the internet promising self-esteem through skinniness by amoral businesspeople taking advantage of fears and insecurity leading to millions and millions of women starving themselves even as they conceived and bore children during a time when food is also increasingly lacking in nutrition and contaminated by toxic chemicals, pesticides, and herbicides, and deficient in protective dietary polyphenols like tannin. There is in fact no faster way to destroy the commensal microbiome than by avoiding carbohydrates, and *Streptomyces* primarily feed on cellulose and so are promoted precisely by the kinds of diets typical of dieting and weight-loss culture high in protein, tough plants lacking in protective polyphenols like tannin, and low quality beverages like diet soda.

Streptomyces are themselves a major source of antibiotics used to treat disease by the pharmaceutical industry, which brings up the point that antibiotics do not exist in nature to benefit human health at all—indeed we didn't even know about them until recent history—but instead function as chemical weapons used by microbes to compete with one another and only incidentally can be used to benefit human health when used appropriately, and frequent, undisciplined use of antibiotics thus also cultivates a gut which is hospitable to those microbes which make them (or related compounds) such as *Streptomyces*. This complexity of the gut microbiome and factors which can destabilize it is also why vaccines have appeared to be associated with autism—and yes while there are people who incorrectly characterize vaccines as dangerous many parents including some I personally know who are not against vaccines have still observed correlations of vaccination with the onset of autistic spectrum symptoms. This occurs because vaccines temporarily stress the immune system—that's how they confer immunity—and an already weak microbiome due to aforementioned factors can be more completely eradicated by the immune reaction vaccines trigger. Vaccines *do not* cause autism, and vaccines and antibiotics are often necessary for immunity and treatment for other diseases like mumps, measles, strep throat, etc. (Mumps is an especially devastating disease, far more awful than autism, and frequently kills children by causing their throat to swell up so much they die by asphyxiation or from meningitis or encephalitis). But vaccines *can* cause autism when children are fed poor diets low in fruit, kept away from sunlight, born to parents with a preexisting poor microbiome, or exposed to antimicrobial factors like agrochemicals or antibiotics or when parents diet and starve themselves or fail to provide their children with protective foods. My own experience having autism was a likely consequence of my mother's lifelong dieting behaviors and starving herself like many women indoctrinated to believe their body is the only way to achieve value as a person, while also being exposed to an abundance of toxic, industrial chemicals and factors like avidin in eggs which then prevents recovery of a protective, commensal microbiome and allows the ingress of those which cause metabolic illness.

Making things worse, *Streptomyces* do not only inhibit biotin, and other species also produce an analogue of *riboflavin* (vitamin B2) called *roseoflavin* which competes with riboflavin for flavin dependent pathways, and since flavin pathways are especially common in the body the presence of roseoflavin also disrupts many biological systems. Our commensal microbes use riboflavin in their own immune defense and riboflavin binds to free iron helping our body absorb and sequester it away from pathogens. Some microbes also produce an enzyme called *thiaminase* which outright destroys *thiamine* (vitamin B1) which is required for the production of insulin and metabolism of fats and carbohydrates but also in glutamine synthetase which packages ammonia into glutamine and thus thiaminase is also highly destructive to our health and accompanies metabolic illness like autism and diabetes by preventing glutamine detoxification of ammonia and production of insulin. Because thiaminase is produced by many organisms including *Candida, Heliobacter, Clostridium, Staphylococcus,* and *Bacillus* thiamine deficiency is extremely common, for instance diabetics are often found to be deficient in thiamine as one ridiculous study I saw which claimed a 75% reduced thiamine concentration in the blood plasma of diabetics was not a deficiency, even when it occurred in those taking a supplement, characterizing 25% of normal as enough which is absurd and further evidence of why the medical industry hasn't figured out any of this fucking shit. Some plants like tea, coffee, ferns, horsetail, bamboo, and fish also contain thiaminase, although it is also destroyed by heat so these are not as concerning a factor, but a cold-extraction of tea or green coffee beans would for instance contain thiaminase. Then the consumption of carbohydrate more quickly depletes the body of thiamine which then impairs further metabolism of carbohydrate, which can be especially catastrophic since this then results in problems like metabolic lactic acidosis which can affect breathing, energy production, and leads to problems like sleep apnea and diabetic necrosis. Thiamine supplementation is thus often used for treatment of diabetic complications because restoring sufficient thiamine suddenly enables the body to properly metabolize carbohydrate, indicating that not only insulin is at issue in diabetic conditions. But like all B vitamins (except niacin) thiamine is primarily produced by commensal gut microbes, especially from foods high in indigestible carbohydrate such as root vegetables, and colonization by opportunistic pathogens, not dietary deficiency, is the primary cause of deficiency. Another toxic anti-thiamine called *oxythiamine* is also produced from cooking thiamine in an acidic pH, and flour is commonly fortified with *thiamine mononitrate* which thus results in oxythiamine mediated thiamine deficiency ironically caused by thiamine fortification (one study found those with end stage renal disease present up to 15 times the normal amount of oxythiamine).

As if it couldn't get worse, the research industry has for decades also used *Streptomyces* bacteria to mass produce streptavidin for the research and medical industry in the manufacture of laboratory tests, and have developed mutant strains which produce molecules which are even more powerfully effective at binding biotin than streptavidin, and it may be likely that these strains now circulate in the population and make conditions of autism and metabolic disease more severe or more common. The discovery of *Streptomyces* and their role in plant growth has also led to their purposeful cultivation in agriculture in coordination with artificial fertilizer which strongly promotes their growth due to its high *nitrate* content, as *Streptomyces* respirate by reducing nitrate, which is the entire point to the use of artificial fertilizer which also contaminates industrially grown food and thus more easily sustains gastroinestinal colonization by *Streptomyces* which also happen to metabolize nitrate into ammonia to increase ammonia burden and excess. Where they used to be healthier, agricultural communities are now regularly plagued by morbid obesity and other metabolic disease because such agrochemicals destroy their commensal microbiomes and promote colonization by *Streptomyces* and other harmful species, where traditional farming and principles of regenerative agriculture which prioritize soil microbial health and refuse the use of chemicals are oppositely associated with a healthier human microbiome.

Because it's water soluble, nitrate can and does also contaminate drinking water and at one point nitrate contamination around agricultural communities was so bad it caused fatal methemoglobinemia in young children until nitrate was finally regulated by the government. Since the entire point of artificial fertilizer is the application of synthetic nitrate the eating of organic food as much as possible significantly reduces nitrate exposure and can greatly help in recovery or prevention of diabetes, autism, and other gut-related metabolic illness. But many foods also contain purposefully added nitrate in forms like *sodium nitrate*, *celery powder*, or *thiamine mononitrate*. Uncooked, processed meat products would despoil rapidly on store shelves and nitrate is toxic to microbes of spoilage so foods like raw sausages or bacon can and do contain added nitrates (cooked meats usually don't but still read labels, and smoking is an effective preservation technique that then reduces the need for toxic chemical preservatives), and thiamine mononitrate added to flour in foods like pizza, pasta, sandwiches, and cookies not only risks formation of oxythiamine but also nitrate excess to help sustain nitrate respiring microbes which inhibit biotin and riboflavin and produce excess ammonia. Because nitrate also causes methemoglobinemia, fortification of food with added nitrate accounts for a great deal of metabolic disease and mental health disorders, and the addition of thiamine mononitrate to the grain supply is the single worst example of food, scientific, and medical incompetence and malfeasance since Harvey Wiley's efforts to reform the food industry and establish the FDA, and because nitrate excess is so toxic to so many systems of the human body and promotes harmful opportunistic pathogens its purposeful addition to foods or supplements should be considered poison.

Nitrate also does occur in nature, even forming naturally in our own bodies from oxidized nitric oxide, and is very important for plant growth and so occurs in most plants. Besides avoiding excess nitrate by eating organic as much as possible, nitrate is also highly water soluble and the practice of simply immersing them in water for a few minutes, even without boiling, then discarding that water is also effective and should be done with fresh leafy greens, especially when making meals such as salads, especially for those whom are very ill. It can be difficult to feel or evaluate nitrate toxicity but as health improves the consumption of excess nitrates can and might result in more obvious symptoms such as nausea or migraine due to conversion of nitrates to ammonia by microbes.

Because acid also neutralizes nitrates the alternative addition of dietary acid like a vinaigrette dressing on salads or vinegar on sautéed greens are highly effective neutralizer of nitrates in foods, so the two primary options for treating nitrate is water immersion and draining or dressing with dietary acids like vinegar, lemon juice, etc., which should be practiced consistently *with no exception* if there is *any* metabolic illness.

Diabetic models in mice and rats for clinical studies are also NOT developed by feeding excess sugar to rodents, but instead by destroying insulin producing beta cells in the pancreas through the administration of a bacterial toxin called *streptozotocin* made by—guess what?—*Streptomyces* bacteria! And here is the smoking gun for the development of diabetes staring scientists scientifically right in their scientific faces more scientifically than any evidence has ever done in the scientific history of science, which is that the cause of diabetes is fucking microbes, not sugar, which produce biological molecules to manipulate our physiology for their own benefit. As discussed in the chapter on misleading science the results of studies which explore hypertension in rats from the intake of sugar recklessly extrapolated to human diabetes are also induced by other factors than sugar such as traumatic, invasive surgery or the purposed infliction of torture. I am not being hyperbolic here—scientists will torture rats by hanging them by their tails, restraining them in place, or putting them in a vat of water until they drown. Rats whose bodies were more able to respond to that stress due to sugar were observed to be hypertensive as if having a fucking shunt sticking out of your neck has nothing to do with hypertension, reflecting both professional and moral incompetence which then has serious ramifications for the understanding and application of that information in humans and the spreading of disease as evidenced by the fucking current state of things. The consequences of denying the emotional intelligence of other creatures and their merciless exploitation without regard for their wellbeing results in dire consequences for us in the failure to understand disease as we lose parts of our own humanity. We are by nature omnivorous and eating some meat is a part of our biology, but we do not need much and torturing animals in the name of science or food production is nothing more than psychopathic, amoral torture of other living creatures which produces direct and harmful consequences for our own health and wellbeing like widespread misunderstanding of metabolic disease and increase in human suffering as an immediate, karmic consequence.

Dysregulation of carbohydrate metabolism is not only a feature of diabetes, and while sugar as *sucrose* or *fructose* and "sugary" foods like sweets, candy, and desserts are often blamed for diabetes it is the sugar *glucose* which is actually elevated in circulation. We cannot even absorb sucrose and indeed diabetics usually have no problem consuming natural foods like fruit which are high in sugar and fructose because, unlike glucose, fructose does not require insulin to be metabolized. In fact, as discussed in the chapter on sugar it is not well known even to doctors and scientists that the great majority of all glucose taken up by cells *is first converted to fructose* before use in biological pathways, even when those pathways require glucose, in complete antagonism to all ideas of diabetes being a problem of fructose consumption. This fact seems redundant and wasteful but likely serves to maintain fructose pools since glucose must be converted to fructose before it can be catabolized by *aldolases* in the citric acid cycle for the production of energy, and because fructose leads directly to energy production it actively assists cells to use glucose, and prior to insulin treatment diabetics were usually prescribed an *increase* in table sugar (sucrose) because it was observed that inclusion of sucrose actually reduced sugar loss in the urine (guess how they measured that?).

This highlights another overlooked problem in diabetes, which is that lots of sugar is actually lost in the urine of diabetics, where fructose and glucose are normally reabsorbed in the kidney which prevents loss of valuable caloric energy, and fructose reabsorption in the kidney is specifically mediated by dietary *anthocyanin* which are the dark purple, blue, and red pigments common to foods like berries such as blueberries, chokeberries (also called aronia), blackberries, strawberries, raspberries, red and black currants, purple cabbage, purple sweet potato, purple corn, etc., highlighting again the incomparable importance of berries and other fruits as a requisite staple of the human diet and wellbeing. Anthocyanin is also a tannin, and because fructose actively raises the metabolic rate and foods like berries are only available during certain environmental conditions this is likely a direct adaptive survival mechanism to lower the metabolic rate during conditions of food scarcity by dumping fructose, because fructose directly raises the metabolic rate, and without fructose we cannot actually metabolize glucose, and without fructose and anthocyanin many pathways in the body stay perpetually in adaptive survival modes of low metabolic function. This is also why it is so emotional-ly difficult to abstain from fructose consumption, as it is a primary nutritional substrate for human biology and high metabolic function, which normally occurs from fruits and other plants which also contain anthocyanins commonly missing or deficient from industrialized diets high in processed foods and food products.

Inhibition of sodium absorption by ammonia also causes even more problems in these conditions because when salt is not absorbed into the body guess what happens? Yes, it remains in the gastroinestinal tract, and this not only destroys our commensal, healthy microbiome but also actively promotes salt-tolerant opportunistic microbes of *putrefaction* (decay) which thrive in high in salt, high protein environments and produce toxic biogenic amines like histamine, putres-cine, cadaverine, tyramine, tryptamine, and phenylethylamine which then cause significant damage to the body and exhaust our enzymes like monamine oxidase which which normally process them. The presence of salt-tolerant pathogens is the reason why high salt diets are shown in studies to correlate with condi-tions like hypertension, diabetes, and autism, not because of high salt diets but because of *salt malabsorption* which then disturbs the microbiome on which we are dependent while also causing ironic deficiency of sodium and chloride in spite of high consumption. *C. difficile* itself actually possesses a toxin which removes the sodium/hydrogen exchanger from epithelial cells which directly impairs uptake of sodium and increases sodium in the intestines to destabilize commensal micro-bial populations and promote *C. difficile* which then produces other toxins to also eat away at our tissues. Failure to absorb salt such as occurs in these conditions increases cravings for salt, since we are not actually absorbing it, and results in over-consumption in attempts to instinctually correct deficiency but which typi-cally leads to further gut dysbiosis, metabolic illness, and even appendicitis and leading to incorrect analysis of causality.

Failure to absorb sodium also results in higher adrenaline production because adrenaline *increases* sodium flux through cells to drive metabolism, and when sodium falls adrenaline increases in order make cells more sensitive to reduced quantities of sodium, but adrenaline also releases glucose from glycogen storage so this results in excessive circulating blood sugar as seen in diabetes and related conditions which then causes glycation of hemoglobin (Hb1Ac) which then impairs oxygen delivery to tissues, causing a state of hypoxia in which tissues suffocate and become necrotic and diseased. Phenylethylamine and tyramine produced by gut pathogens like *C. difficile* in the presence of unabsorbed salts are adrenaline analogs and also additively compound our own adrenaline excess and increase glucose circulation. Tiny quantities of amines found in fermented foods like cheese and bread are the primary reason why cheese is so fun to eat because a tiny bit of adrenaline stimulates a small increase in excitement and metabolic stim-ulation, supported by its dense nutrition (these do not need to be avoided). But because adrenaline mobilizes sodium it is also inhibited by sodium, which is why healthy people with normal sodium status do not have problems with adrenaline and high blood sugar, and why taking extra salt is often therapeutic to metabolic stress and an instinctual craving. But effective absorption fails in the presence of ammonia excess, requiring then resolution of ammonia excess, and because tannin inhibits ammonia the use of tannins also taken with supplemental salt or food that is salted (such as soup in which bay leaves can be used to impart much tannin), or the use of dietary acids like lemon juice with salt, greatly increases salt absorption which not only promotes salt repletion to help lower adrenaline but also removes it from the gut thus reducing the formation of microbial biogenic amines. It also very useful to first boil supplemental salt in water along with dietary acid like lemon juice, tannins, or citric acid powder in order to utilize hydronium formation to increase the dissociation of chloride from sodium, and boiling about 1/2 tsp of salt in a few cups of water for a minute or two with lemon juice, tea, and a little sugar is not only highly efficacious but also somewhat pleasant (allow to cool before taking, and if you are very large this recipe can be doubled).

Type-one diabetes thus seems to be catalyzed by antibiotics, agrochemicals, and egg white which eradicate the commensal microbiome and invite *Streptomyces* colonization which impairs insulin production in the pancreas, while type-two diabetes is caused by a diet high in inflammatory polyunsaturated fats and low in vitamin E which then allows pathogens to synthesize oxylipin to disrupt the commensal microbiome and normal metabolism of carbohydrate. To further demonstrate this latter point, every single study which has attempted to find a benefit for the famous, polyunsaturated omega-3 fats in the treatment of diabetes have actually shown an increase in severity of diabetic complications, proving its etiology as harmful inhibition of sugar metabolism by polyunsaturated fats and related compounds, leading researchers to perform amazing feats of copium trying to reconcile the discrepancy of the results with their biases favoring polyunsaturated fat, mischaracterizing polyunsaturated fats as healthy in spite of direct evidence right in front of their eyes to the contrary. The highest rates of type-two diabetes around the world also show an obvious correlation with climate, not sugar consumption, with generally higher rates occurring in tropical latitudes which are home of a vast amounts and variety of parasites and yeasts that better survive in warmer climates such as the southern, hottest, and most humid parts of the United States which in this country has the highest rates of type-two diabetes even though more northerly regions have the same poor dietary habits. One study found half of commercial yogurt samples analyzed were contaminated with *Candida*, which is immune to lactic acid, refrigeration, and even most preservatives, implicating the role of technology also in the distribution of pathogens and disease. Before the advent of industrialized food systems and the proliferation of diabetes fat consumption in the South was not yet adulterated by high rates of vegetable oil which instead came mostly from lard from pigs fed scrap or forage including access to foods like nuts, fruit, roots, and mushrooms (and animal fats also concentrate fat soluble vitamins like vitamin E). But even pigs are now mostly fed soy, corn, cotton seed, and rapeseed (rapeseed is where canola oil comes from as there's no such thing as a canola), and Southern cooking which has always been high in fat has simply changed composition to those high in unstable polyunsaturated fats and thus excellent substrate for the production of oxylipins, lipid peroxide, malondialdehyde, and other toxic byproducts of polyunsaturated fat which damages human metabolic health and increases susceptibility to diabetes causing organisms.

Oxylipin most consequently blocks chloride channels to promote chloride deficiency, and since chloride is one of the most important elements in the body, responsible for things from the regulation of metabolism to production of stomach acid to the basic function of the immune system, so this problem can be best reversed through the use of a natural vitamin E supplement along with dietary and supplemental salt (sodium chloride). Do *not* use synthetic vitamin E, which is not the same, as vitamin E is not one thing but a collection of 8 different tocopherols and tocotrienols, and the synthetic is not identical to any of them and can possibly cause problems, and the label should also state its source of origin, such as sunflower oil or wheat germ (I also avoid soy derived vitamin E as it doesn't seem to work the same as other sources). If a vitamin E supplement is not available it is possible to use high vitamin E food sources like sprouted nuts (sprouting increases vitamin E up to 600%), wheat germ oil (it has a lot of PUFA but also has more than twice the amount of vitamin E of the next most potent source), wheat germ, etc., and when vitamin E accompanies dietary or supplemental salt it can restore chloride absorption to help reverse many of the symptoms of diabetes and other metabolic disease. But tannin also helps protect vitamin E from oxidation and saponification, and having something high in tannin like tea as a medium for dosing vitamin E followed afterward by a supplemental dose of salt is so effective in reversing these problems that its effect can be felt almost immediately.

The element *lithium* which is so often prescribed for treatment of mental health disorders is an analog of sodium and also just happens to paralyze parasites. This does not kill them outright, but paralyzation helps our immune system to better eradicate them, and although the medical profession is not aware of this the effects on parasites and inhibition of ammonia is the primary reason for the therapeutic effect of lithium in treatment of severe psychological illness, which is in truth caused by parasitism, which is also why no other, better intervention for mental health disorders has yet been discovered or developed, because lithium is in fact *required* for resistance to parasitism, and without a high lithium diet such as from an abundance of leafy greens, fruit, legumes, or water supplies which also contain lithium we are made highly vulnerable to parasitism and become easily colonized on exposure. There are interesting correlative studies on lithium deficiency and rates of violent crime and suicide which prove our dependency on lithium and which similarly implicates untreated parasitism as the underlying causal factor for those problems as well, which makes a great deal of sense since disruption of the normal metabolism of sugars and ammonia then leads to severe neurological and emotional stress, even to the point that people lose complete control of their mental faculties.

Lithium strongly reacts to ammonia, which is also a reason for its therapeutic effect, but also that ammonia can and does deplete lithium. Studies also show lithium to be required in the regeneration of intestinal tissue and organs and reduces the rate of gastric emptying, which means that food remains in the stomach longer to be better digested to thus prevent undigested food from reaching microbes in the intestines and promoting SIBO. However, lithium is the third lightest element and strongly affected by environmental pH such as is determined by ammonia or acid, and from my research I believe the short chain fatty acids like butyrate, required by the enterocytes of the gastrointestinal system (the lining of the gut) for production of energy, also strongly promote lithium bioavailability and thus promoting gut regeneration and resistance to parasitism. Lithium is widely available in plant foods, especially things like fruit, tea, and legumes, and part of the reason for recovery when fixing the gut and restoring short chain fatty acid producers is likely in large part from a boost in lithium homeostasis due to the increase in short chain fatty acids from commensal microbes feeding on potent polyphenols and other indigestible carbohydrates. One of the primary benefits of a high tannin diet is thus also its promotion of lithium repletion since foods high in tannins, which help inhibit microbial ammonia production, also tend to contain lithium, so for instance the addition of lithium to a diet is not effective in the resolution of parasitism without also the strategic use of tannins from healthy foods. Tannin also complexes with lithium, and natural sources of water containing tannin and lithium was probably a major health resource which became lost once we started drinking water low in tannin such as from wells and reservoirs.

Lithium is also shown to improve the function of the pyloric sphincter (the muscle which releases food from the stomach to the intestines) and to prolong gastric emptying, which is good because food spends more time breaking down in stomach acid. Rapid stomach emptying (frequent hunger, even after eating) is thus also a useful diagnostic symptom for lithium deficiency, as microbes scheme to impair our digestion through such factors as induced lithium deficiency, but any metabolic disease will present with lithium deficiency or dysregulation and anyone with any metabolic disease should eat a high lithium diet as well as a low-dose, daily supplement such as 5-15 mg *lithium aspartate* or *lithium carbonate* in the morning with food (those are my preferred sources but they are not always available). Always mix a supplement into fluids like juice, coffee, or tea to drink alongside a large meal rather than taking dry, as dissolving into water (protected by tannins) will also improve its absorption (do not do this with the high doses common to medical treatments, as those are excessive and can and will cause toxic lithium overdose). A meal of root vegetables (such as a sweet potato for breakfast) will result in enormous quantities of butyrate production by microbes, so taking this dose of lithium alongside such foods will very strongly help to rid the gut of parasites like giardia, even in a matter of days (improvement in gut distension and itchy butt should be very obvious and rapid). Children easily produce butyrate from foods like fruit, but once colonized by parasites only root vegetables like sweet potatoes or yam can be sufficiently effective for butyrate production in adults required for benefit from lithium in restoration of the gut. Lithium's benefits and behavior is far more complex, however, and more required information on its use, function, and therapy is discussed in upcoming chapters such as immunity.

Most people also do not know that the majority of hydrogen atoms which compose stomach acid originate from carbohydrate, so conditions of metabolic disease and diabetes become extremely difficult to resolve since our ability to even absorb or use sugar is impaired which thus promotes long term hypochlorhydria that would otherwise scavenge dietary nitrate, suppress microbial avidin producers, and prevent SIBO. Obviously many people associate sugar consumption with diabetes, and some diabetic studies do show negative effects of high fructose feeding in rodents such as when 60% of calories are nothing but fructose, but studies which feed an excess of any nutrient in this manner demonstrate ignorance of biology since taking excess of any nutrient would always result in harmful side effects—even water can be poisonous in excess, and high doses of pain killers will outright kill a person but nobody infers they should be avoided entirely as is done with things like sugar.

Fructose also is not absorbed into the body in the absence of glucose, so feeding even low amounts of isolated fructose can and does result in negative changes to the gut and microbiome, as fructose *never* occurs in nature absent of glucose. Sugar absorption in the gut also requires a neutral pH and, because ammonia excess disturbs the normal pH of the gut, diabetes is also actually a condition of *fructose malabsorption* (or deficiency) in which the body also becomes unable to absorb dietary fructose just as it is unable to absorb sodium and magnesium which then ironically causes fructose deficiency in spite of fructose consumption, and the worse the malabsorption the greater cravings for sugar become, and the resulting intake in response to cravings which then appear as a causal factor in those who do not understand what is actually going on. Disparate studies prove this to be true because some show that fructose inhibits the hyperglycemic response caused by adrenaline, but diabetics present with both hyperglycemia and high adrenaline, where if fructose absorption were efficient it would inhibit liver phosphorylase and thus prevent excessive glucose release from glycogen stores.

Fructose deficiency is also caused by insufficient production of the *sucrase* enzyme which breaks down sucrose into fructose and glucose, due to deterioration of intestinal microvilli caused by gut dysbiosis, which is even worse because this allows sucrose to remain in the gut, undigested, which further promotes pathogenic growth and impairs all our biological pathways which are dependent on fructose. Another reason fruit consumption is so healthy for those with metabolic illness is that well-ripened fruit contains mostly invert sugar rather than sucrose or starch, which is sucrose that has been 'pre-digested' during the ripening process which then results in free fructose and glucose that does not require digestion and is thus more easily absorbed into the body. This is not an accident of nature but likely one of co-evolution from parasitism pressure on animal patrons where fruit which ripened to invert sugar better promoted survival of the animals which distribute seed for plants since invert sugar can and does bypass the interference on sugar absorption caused by opportunistic pathogens. Invert sugar only occurs in well-ripened fruit, however, and much of the underripe fruit which is common to industrial supermarkets and food production prematurely harvested to survive distribution will not have this benefit, and growing your own fruit or buying direct from market gardeners who produce high-quality, well-ripened fruit before harvesting (regardless of fresh, frozen, dried, or juiced) is a great way to achieve long term recovery from diabetes, autism, and related conditions. Any abnormally elevated heart rate (which often occurs when trying to sleep) or other effects of hyperglycemia are thus a symptom of impaired fructose absorption and impaired sucrose digestion which then results in excess release of glucose from glycogen storage from high adrenaline and its analogs.

Invert sugar is in fact used in industrial production of foods and beverages and is also available for sale, but it can also be made at home by boiling 2 parts sugar to 1 part water with a small amount of acid (such as 1/2 tsp lemon juice) for about ten minutes (allow to cool before using). Part of the reason people with metabolic disease consume processed sugars like invert and high-fructose corn syrup is because these simple sugars bypass impairments to absorption to reverse fructose deficiency and ironically lower blood sugar by inhibiting glycogen release and excess adrenaline, but these don't end up resolving the illness due to an otherwise poor diets high in protein and (tannin free) beverages but low in fruits, vegetables, tannin, and deficiency of sunlight. Interestingly, studies also show that tannins actually have insulin-like effects on our cells, and since they also inhibit pathogenic microbes are extremely useful in helping to restore normal pancreatic function and thus helping restore functions like digestion and stomach acid. Combining tannins and invert sugar together helps so strongly to promote stomach acid, in fact, that even one serving of sweetened tea (brewed strongly) can and does cause acid reflux. This occurs because stomach acid (hydrochloric acid) is not, in fact, secreted from the stomach but hydrogen atoms and chloride atoms which compose stomach acid are secreted separately by parietal cells and combine after secretion, which means that imbalances of chloride and hydrogen ratios can and do occur if deficiencies of either are an issue, which is usually the case in metabolic conditions due to inhibitory ammonia, and restoration of stomach acid production from restoration of sugar absorption will cause excess hydrogen atoms in ratio to those of chloride which then causes leaching of chloride from surrounding tissues, including the esophageal sphincter muscles which then forces them to relax and allow stomach contents to rise into the esophagus.

Acid reflux is actually great confirmation that this restoration of sugar absorption is working, but in those with severe illnesses like cystic fibrosis or GERD a deficiency of chloride can be so severe that it makes acid reflux life threatening such as occurred to me several times in my adult life in which I woke from a dead sleep choking on aspirated stomach contents. The first time this happened I thought I was going to die, but standing upright allowed it to drain back into my stomach and I was able to breathe again in about thirty or forty seconds. Instead of using antacids which neutralize acid in complete opposition of the goal of restoring stomach acid, reflux should thus be treated with a small dose of salt (about 1/2-1 tsp, depending on size) in some juice or tea, and supplementing salt during acid reflux also acidifies chloride and sodium in opposition to ammonia to increase their bioavailability. Of course, combining both the use of invert sugar and salt into one beverage can and will also preempt this effect and is quite pleasant (DO NOT use salt in excess as it can cause nausea, but instead take more doses later as required). Repletion with chloride will then restore contraction of the esophageal sphincter (and other sphincters) to resolve reflux and GERD, and those with GERD, cystic fibrosis, acid reflux, or incontinence should preemptively treat this problem by always using salt in the invert sugar and juice used to make lemonade, sugared tea, etc., especially before bed since laying down makes acid reflux more likely, until such time that these problems are obviously resolved in the long term. Decaffeinated tea would be a good option for very ill children since children should not generally have caffeine (especially in large doses), but tannins such as from astringent fruits or Indian bay leaf mixed into the lemonade can be especially delicious, and fruit is plenty good a source of tannins for healthy children *Thaumarchaeota* and local B12 production).

Avidin also happens to be neutralized by acids like stomach acid or acetic acid which is the primary constituent of vinegar, which is why healthy people don't have many health effects even when eating poor diets, as robust stomach acid production and a healthy microbiome strongly protect us against avidin and avidin producers, since our commensal microbiome also can and does produce biotin. Not many people are aware that the stomach also secretes ascorbic acid (vitamin C) during digestion, which even more powerfully neutralizes avidin and nitrates than other acids. But many people take biotin as a supplement hoping this reverses deficiency but studies show that avidin even accumulates in the kidney and remains there for up to four days (and is a likely cause of kidney failure), so the constant presence of avidins from microbes or the diet (from frequent consumption of undercooked eggs) promotes chronic, systemic biotin deficiency such that a supplement cannot do much to resolve long term disease until *Streptomyces* and parasite colonization is fully resolved, which requires other information such as in the upcoming chapters on vitamin D, immunity, and hormones.

During diabetes and other metabolic disease the increase in circulating sugar is generally also considered a side-effect of the condition, and both sugar and ammonia leak from the skin, in sweat and other skin secretions, which can and does make skin sticky, and those with diabetes are also more likely to sweat than those without the condition (which can all be diagnostic symptoms). But this is in fact a great misunderstanding and the secretion of sugars through the skin is not an accident but a purposeful adaptation meant to cultivate commensal skin microbes. Most people are not aware that the skin in fact contains its own helpful microbiome just like the intestinal system, and on every square centimeter of skin at any one time there will be about *one billion* bacteria or other commensal microbes. In fact, studies show that the skin also hosts *Thaumarchaeota* archaea, which oxidize ammonia as an energy source, and during severe metabolic disease ammonia quantity in the skin can increase such that it is readily odorous.

There are several reasons for resident microbes on the skin, one of which is to primarily protect us from pathogenic organisms, because it is impossible for the body to mount an effective immune response to the outer layer of skin which is instead performed by helpful, friendly microflora. But the skin is actually a primary site of steroidogenesis (producing steroids), which is shown in studies to produce pregnenolone, androgens, estrogens, and even the glucocorticoids which help manage and maintain electrolytes and water. This process even uses acetic acid and other short chain fatty acids which very likely originates from microbes like Propionibacterium residing in the pores, glands, and hair follicles of the skin and feeding on secreted sugars and fatty acids which is then absorbed into the glands and endocrine cells of the skin. While this sounds quite incredible studies have conducted much research on the connection of the skin microbiome and diabetes such that many researchers already suspect that skin dysbiosis, rather than gut dysbiosis, could in fact be the cause of diabetic conditions. If this were the case, the increase in circulating sugar is actually an adaptation meant to help capture, cultivate, and help restore commensal skin microbes to support and restore the function of the skin in opposition to those opportunistic microbes which derange the metabolic state.

The solution to this problem then also implies that the commensal microbes targeted by our physiology must be acquired in order to fully reverse diabetes and related metabolic conditions. Throughout my research I often experienced resolution of symptoms when getting plenty of sunshine and thought that sun exposure and vitamin D were the primary mechanisms, since vitamin D directly supports a healthy commensal gut microbiome, and often recommended that people with metabolic illness engage in activities like gardening which place them out of doors more often. But after realizing the skin microbiome directly affects metabolism it became apparent that activities like laying in the grass while getting sun was actually recruiting environmental microbes such as *Thaumarchaeota* to reside on skin, produce B12, and even migrate into the body and mucosal tissue. This behavior too is widely seen in nature, with most terrestrial animals, from cattle and bison to birds and primates, even rolling on the ground or giving themselves dirt baths, often understood by researchers to be a self-care and healthful behavior that protects the skin of those animals, but never thinking that we humans, which are also animals, should also be engaged in similar behavior in order to keep and maintain a healthy, commensal skin microbiome, even as our own infants instinctively even eat dirt as a mechanism for acquiring microbes.

It turns out my guidance for gardening (or similar activities which put us in contact with healthy soils) is not just a suggestion, but a requisite for recovery, because this behavior brings us in contact with soil microbes that can and do colonize our skin to provide the skin with protection and nutrients like short chain fatty acids. In fact, there are studies which directly investigated gardening's benefit on diabetes specifically, although it was considered exercise and not a benefit from exposure to useful microbes, and found that only 16% of those whom gardened had ever been diagnosed with diabetes while 20% of those who exercised but did not garden had (and 30% in those who did neither). Anecdotally searching social media I found only TWO gardeners in the entire world who also had diabetes, although both reported much improvement, but both *were wearing gloves* in every photo in which they directly interacted with soil. Effectively, there are no gardeners in the entire world that have diabetes, because the combination of getting sunshine, eating homegrown and healthy plant foods and directly interacting with the soil microbiome prevents skin microbial dysbiosis and thus the elevation in sugar circulation which is the response to diabetic conditions. So, getting sunshine daily without using sunblock (do not get sunburned) while also interacting with earth in activities like gardening, playing on the lawn, or laying in the grass while sunbathing is required to make a full recovery from any metabolic illness, and this behavior should be requisite for all children in all stages of development in order to prevent and resolve systemic metabolic illness which plagues industrial societies (more information on the function of sun exposure and vitamin D are discussed in that upcoming chapter, which is also requisite to benefit from sun exposure).

While B vitamins are often discussed in this book their supplementation is never a long term solution to health problems since most B vitamins should come primarily from our gut microbiome. That being said it can be therapeutic to symptoms of metabolic disease to supplement the B vitamins and the best, natural source of all B vitamins (except B12) is the commonly available *brewer's yeast* or *nutritional yeast* (they are the same yeast, *Saccharomyces cerevisiae,* just different product names), which is also high in biotin and can also be an acceptable source for that as well. *S. cerevisiae* is the yeast used to make bread, beer, and wine, and yeast are prolific producers of all B vitamins (except B12) which is why beer, bread, and wine are so fucking good but also why cultures which prohibit alcohol consumption are not necessarily healthier than those who take it since yeast fermentation of foods actually does provide supplemental dietary B vitamin. For instance the religious cult in which I was raised is famous for their strict prohibition against alcohol and tea but are also plagued by obesity, depression, and have a shorter life expectancy than the general population of places like France and Japan which take an abundance of wine and tea. Brewer's yeast is also very high in selenium, mannose, glutamate, protein, manganese, copper, and zinc, but its taste is a bit offensive but can be tempered when taken in milk, and long term resolution of gut health will restore normal repletion with B vitamins thus eliminating the need to supplement, although it should be used for those whom are very ill, reasons for which will be clearer in upcoming chapters.

As discussed in the first of this chapter, autism, diabetes, cystic fibrosis, and other metabolic disease are all essentially the same illness and only appear separate due to differences in ratios of specific pathogens, age of onset, and differing diet and lifestyle behaviors which then result in differing dominant symptoms but which are all essentially part of the single condition of non-health that is rooted in lacking sun exposure, dietary requisites like tannin, anthocyanins, lithium, and sugar, and deficient interaction with the natural world and natural biomes in which we evolved as an animal organism. As the skin and its microbiome is fundamental to our overall health, exposure to fluoridated water in showers, bathing, and swimming (and even highly chlorinated water such as chlorinated swimming pools) is a likely accelerant to many metabolic conditions.

It is also *extremely* important to know that the dietary and pathogenic stress underlying these metabolic illnesses will also have caused significant mitochondria dysfunction which greatly increases risk of cancer, and even if you do not think you have diabetes or cancer we all risk these illnesses since we are all human, and these diseases are primarily caused by abundant opportunistic microbes in our environment which can and do colonize all humans, differing only in the time and age of onset, and the chapter on cancer is required to address mitochondrial dysfunction and prevent cancer and further improve metabolic health in all persons that are not without illness or age.

The nutritional quality of all food has declined considerably in the last several decades as the agriculture industry breeds for size and shipping which dilutes the nutrient density of plants and animals alike. One study showed that the vitamin C content of garden vegetables has declined by 50% since 1950 (and is likely even worse now since that study was done the year I graduated high school, in 1999). Even organic farmers can use bad farming practices and produce nutrient-poor food or grow nutrient diluted crops, and because agrochemicals are also used on lawns of homes, parks, and public spaces they can be a source of exposure and microbiome disruption. A telltale sign of chemical use on public spaces is grass with no dandelions during spring and summer because dandelions are very susceptible to toxic herbicides and are normally prolific colonizers of open space. The job or niche of weeds in nature is to colonize soil poor in microbial life and help establish and promote a better soil microbiome, and growing and sustaining healthy soil is the key to low weed invasion for farming, lawns, gardening, and farming operations without the use of chemicals such as is achieved by no-till farming and other regenerative practices.

You can stop buying conventionally grown food, petition or sue your local government to stop using chemicals in public spaces and the food supply, or run for office and do it yourself, or start cooperative operations to grow and distribute high quality food and cut out predatory systems that degrade the environment and quality of goods and services we require for our survival. Studies have confirmed a direct correlation of increase in herbicides and rates of autism as well as deaths to Alzheimer's disease which shares many similar morbidities to autism, because there are direct and immediate consequences to our wellbeing when we are inconsiderate even to that of lowly weeds and microbes in the complex web of interdependency that is all life on this planet. Conventional farming and the use of toxic agrochemicals and monoculture is only necessary when farmers don't understand soil and the microbiome, and learning about and practicing regenerative agriculture can eliminate the need to use toxic chemicals in the first place which also makes farming easier (no tilling!) and more profitable and gratifying through production of higher quality products and preservation of land, farms, and the environment.

Conditions like diabetes and autism are at their heart a problem of industrial food systems and if access to requisite food is difficult it's always possible to grow your own fruit, nuts, and vegetables on your property or in public spaces wasted with ornamental landscaping. Even if you only have space for some pots near a sunny window there is no reason we shouldn't have access to good foods, especially when useless lawns and ornamental gardens take up so much land which could otherwise provide abundant access to nutrition, and even if you don't have direct access to land there are often cooperative or community gardens in which you can grow food, or set up a home grow system or green wall to grow fruits and vegetables using artificial light. The care and maintenance required of gardening will also get you out in the sun for regular vitamin D, and children will love digging in the dirt and being taught how to grow plants and in the process get plenty of vitamin D to support their own health (do avoid times and duration which risks sunburn since sunblock impairs vitamin D synthesis). After treatment with these specific strategies, maintaining commensal microbial homeostasis through an abundance of these required behaviors and dietary requisites can entirely prevent recurrence or development in the first place and relegate diseases like diabetes to the bin of history where they belong.

CHAPTER 10
VITAMIN D AND VASCULAR DISEASE

I have known many women with varicose and spider veins which caused them no small degree of discomfort aesthetically or physically, and when I grew up the discomfort in my testicles that occurred for several years which my doctors failed to diagnose was a similar condition called *varicocele* in which blood flow out of the testicles is not sufficient and can pool to cause pressure. I also developed a minor case of spider veins on the insides of my feet, and though insignificant was enough to become an worrying focus of my failing health, even when I suffered from more serious health issues, because it appeared concurrently with more unfortunate developments and was a constant reminder of my constantly poor state of being. The medical profession has no recourse for healing any of these issues anyway, and likewise three months before my cancer diagnosis an inept doctor told me the hairy leukoplakia on the side of my tongue was nothing even though healthy people do not have leukoplakia and it appeared at the same time my energy began to plummet. It turns out leukoplakia is a hallmark of either HIV or cancer, due to severe immune dysfunction, and since I did not have HIV the pain in my body made a lot more sense once I was diagnosed with tumors growing on my thyroid.

Vascular insufficiency also causes a condition called *soft glans* which I didn't even know I had or was even a thing until the therapies I devised in this book reversed it (if you have a glans you will find this relevant as discussed in the chapter on erections). Vascular insufficiency really becomes a question of comfort and health rather than aesthetics, even though aesthetics are also a legitimate cause for concern, dismissed only by doctors and pharmaceutical companies because they have no idea how to treat it because you know if they did it would be given a stupid name and advertised ad nauseam like every other bullshit pharmaceutical. In fact, the aesthetic protuberances of vascular insufficiency are quite dangerous because they are caused by the same factors which catalyze serious cardiovascular issues, and any asshole can see that people with these conditions never suffer them in isolation but always with a host of other comorbidities. To say they are unrelated is to perceive the body as a disparate collection of entirely independent systems which have nothing to do with each other, which could not be further from how the body really works, and these should be as much concern to medical practicians as it is to those who bear them because they are evidence of developing or established cardiovascular stress that affects the whole system. These vascular conditions have intrigued me for some time in part because though much of my body healed during the first few years of my recovery the spider veins and varicocele showed absolutely no sign of improvement. The hormone progesterone is protective of the cardiovascular system and yet many women develop varicose and other vein abnormalities during pregnancy when progesterone production is highest, which should in theory protect against such conditions, which it does not. Like most of the health problems I suffered, trial and error and some exhaustive research finally helped me confirm the cause and cure to these various conditions of venous insufficiency which has implications then for the health of the entire cardiovascular system.

On the cellular level the functional derangement common to vein disorders, whether they are small like spider veins or large like varicose, all originate from the failure of tiny valves inside veins which prevent back-flow of blood during the resting phase of a heartbeat which is in turn caused by fatigue of the inner smooth muscle lining which slacks and expands outward from the downward pressure of gravity pulling on blood and causing the valves to misalign which then allows even more blood to fall backward and downward which in turn stretches veins further and becomes a self-fulfilling cycle. In healthy individuals these valves and the surrounding tissue are strong and resist the immense pressure blood exerts on the system, but over time metabolic stress causes these structures to weaken and the back-flow of blood further stresses the tissue and causes blood stagnation and thus reduced delivery of oxygen and nutrients to affected tissues.

The real failure in these conditions is the inability to heal and regenerate tissues rather than the actual physical stress produced by blood pressure, gravity, etc. But what makes cardiovascular health so difficult for most people to understand is first the difference between *blood pressure* and *blood volume*. When we are young, before the onset of adulthood, we have much less hormone activity and thus a much easier time assimilating and storing nutrients and greater resistance to pathogenic colonization, since for instance parasites colonize us in part to exploit sex hormones for their own reproductive cycle. The entire point of childhood and why children even exist as a thing in nature is to grow a skeleton of mass which, besides keeping us upright and providing a rigid structure, also stores nutrients like calcium, phosphorus, boron, magnesium, etc., which can be recalled later during adulthood when—not if—we experience nutrient stress and deficiency caused by eventual colonization by opportunistic microbes which then actively promotes the increased loss of elements from the body which then eventually results in disease and eventually death. This loss of nutrients throughout adulthood is further exacerbated by behaviors such as dieting or excessive exercise and, most consequential for the health of the cardiovascular system, is the loss of *sodium* which the body uses to manage and control water, and without sufficient sodium in the bloodstream water is actually lost from blood plasma to surrounding tissues which not only reduces the volume of blood but dilutes electrolytes in cells and the extracellular space which are otherwise required for proper cellular metabolism, and so this water efflux and influx promotes water retention in tissues and lowers the metabolic rate of the body. Most people don't understand that *inflammation* is mediated by water, which is why good inflammation helps cells and tissue grow and repair as it facilitates the movement of cells and organelles and other components, but also why bad inflammation oppositely causes disease as water dilutes electrolytes and lowers metabolic respiration. This is also why chronic use of powerful inflammatory inhibitors like *ibuprofen* or *acetaminophen* can actually inhibit healing and recovery such as from a workout, post-labor, surgery, and general healing because inflammation is required to trigger tissue remodeling and regrowth after injury which powerful NSAIDs also suppress (they should only ever be taken if absolutely necessary).

Abstaining from fluid intake during problems with water metabolism is also not helpful as it only serves to further dry out the bloodstream, not reduce water retention, making blood even more viscous to the point of risking heart attack, while consuming excess does nothing but promote even more edema, water retention, and potential catastrophe. Though it may seem kind of obvious it is worth pointing out that the bloodstream is also a reservoir for water. Excessive translocation of water from the blood to tissues stimulates fat deposition, and the mechanism of action by which adipogenesis is stimulated is by the increased influx of water into fat cells. Because excess water retention is inflammation (and inflammation is water) which can slow down important organs like the heart, brain, and liver, fat also protects us by sequestering water away from internal organs and this also means fat functions also as a backup storage site for water, and very few people understand that when fat is metabolized by the body it is not 'burned' as fuel but is instead converted into CO_2 and water (H_2O), a process which releases energy but also water for use by the body so, like blood, fat also functions as a water reservoir. *Edema* which is chronic swelling and water retention in the extremities to the point that tissues begin to resemble bags of water rather than human limbs is a state of severely impaired ability to properly manage water, which then begins to simply hang around in tissues and so severely impair cellular metabolism it can result in necrosis (decay) of tissues and is a common problem in diabetes due to severe inability to produce energy.

Blood pressure, which is different than blood volume, is the force that blood volume exerts on the cardiovascular system, and when blood volume is optimal the cardiovascular system has no problem maintaining blood pressure because the volume of blood sufficiently fills the space of the cardiovascular system much like a fully inflated inflated water balloon. Oppositely, when blood volume falls the cardiovascular system must instead contract around a reduced volume of blood to compensate for the loss of pressure else the heart would not be able to pump, and the more water lost from the bloodstream the greater the cardiovascular system must contract to maintain adequate pressure. This is why medical tests are not often useful since a person can present with good blood pressure but this does not indicate volume of blood nor conditions in which the cardiovascular system may actually be chronically contracted to maintain that pressure which will be stressful to the cardiovascular system as chronic contraction around chronically reduced blood volume fatigues cardiovascular tissue which then begins to result in hypertension, angina, and eventually heart attacks, stroke, embolism, etc., as the vascular contractile tissues fatigue and fail. Thus, cardiovascular health is, above all, dependent on the volume of blood which fills it, to reduce water loss to surrounding tissue and relieve the cardiovascular system from chronic contraction.

The traditional attribution of cardiovascular problems to sodium is entirely misguided and dangerous, as cardiovascular problems are instead caused by the excessive loss of water from blood, and water follows sodium (and sodium follows chloride) and the increase of sodium in the bloodstream seen in cardiovascular disease is not a cause of cardiovascular disease but instead an effect of it, where the body is attempting instead to draw water back to the bloodstream through a higher concentration of salts. The fact that researchers and doctors don't realize that loss of water from any solution also concentrates dissolved solutes also makes this issue extremely ridiculous, because test results would show higher sodium when blood volume is reduced, so higher concentration of sodium in the blood-stream during disease is evidence of bloodstream water deficiency, not dietary sodium excess. Reduced blood volume also makes blood more viscous which increases the workload of the heart and coagulation potential (usually measured as 'prothrombin time') and thus also the threat of sudden cardiovascular trauma due to clots and blockages.

This misunderstanding about sodium is reinforced by the fact that sodium is one of the easiest elements for the body to manage, and would have no problem resolving excess if the problem in cardiovascular disease was truly excess. Instead, the body actively expresses *aldosterone*, *angiotensin*, and *renin* to *prevent* sodium loss from the bloodstream, while medical treatments like dialysis, diuretics, or beta blockers do the exact opposite of what the body is actively trying to do and instead cause removal of sodium as if the expression of those hormones is a mistake and not purposeful, which most people don't understand because we have been condi-tioned to distrust the body even though it has evolved for literally millions of years to literally perform these functions in the goal of keeping us alive, to do amazing things like spontaneous regeneration of tissue and synthesis of molecules in the coordinated management of trillions of atoms for the construction of life. It is not the body which is mistaken.

Loss of water from the bloodstream cannot be reversed by simply drinking extra water since this process is biochemical and requires working pathways in order to actually use water biologically, and chronic stress, no matter the cause, contributes to the chronic loss water from blood volume to surrounding tissues in spite of fluid intake because of derangement of the pathways which normally regulate this process. Stress hormones like adrenaline also worsen this problem by increasing sodium flux through cells to increase energy production in response to stress, so chronic stress causes disease by promoting increased loss of electrolytes through their increased use in the stress response. Intracellular potassium opposes sodium and is used by cells to get sodium get to the outside of the cell in order to maintain constant flux homeostasis and prevent excessive intracellular sodium, but stress hormones like adrenaline increase the flux of sodium by dumping potassium to reduce this inhibition and increase the metabolic rate. Over time the chronic expression of stress hormones (especially from dieting, since reduced intake of carbohydrate and salt lowers the metabolic rate and thus stimulates an increase in adrenaline) results in severe deficiency of potassium so cells are less able to withstand metabolic stress and prevent excessive intracellular sodium.

Calcium flux is in turn dependent on sodium flux, and calcium regulates synthesis of proteins, peptides, enzymes, etc., so buildup of sodium caused by low potassium also slows calcium flux, which not only slows production of required metabolic products and pathways but also promotes calcification of cells, and this is the basic mechanism by which metabolic disease occurs. As such, studies show that diets high in potassium but *not* reductions in sodium protect against cardio-vascular disease, because potassium then keeps sodium in constant flux which then also keeps calcium in constant flux to maintain constant cellular metabolism.

Extracellular potassium reverses the electrochemical gradient which maintains cellular metabolism, actively preventing the flux of sodium and calcium required to maintain these pathways, so too much extracellular potassium can actually be very dangerous and even stop your heart, so instead of storing potassium which is dumped from cells the body instead pees it out, which is why urination often accompanies an increase in adrenaline, and the effect of stress hormones increasing the ratio of sodium to potassium is the feeling we experience during the fight or flight response during interpersonal conflict, excessive exercise, catastrophically low blood sugar, drinking caffeine on an empty stomach, or even colonization by parasites and bacteria which mimic or hijack our hormones, and why behaviors like fasting or arguing can often feel good or exhilarating because they stimulate adrenaline release which in turn enhances sodium flux and increases glucose circulation to thus increase the production and consumption of energy.

But this is also why stress depletes us of energy and stress hormones are aggravating because we must also consume sources of energy in order to fuel the rise in cellular metabolism, so we crave foods that are sweet, salty, or full of carbs not because we are undisciplined but because sugar and sodium are the chemical resources mobilized and consumed by adrenaline stimulus, so providing more in the diet reverses the deficiency caused by stress and avoiding them during stress more rapidly depletes us of fuel which then damages the body which is unable to produce the amount of energy required to respond to stress.

The main problem with sodium and potassium imbalance is that when stress subsides the body must reestablish homeostasis to reset the body's metabolic rate back to normal, otherwise the cellular metabolic rate would remain elevated and quickly fatigue cells and waste nutritional resources, but since potassium is lost due to stress dumping of potassium the only recourse is for the body to *also* dump sodium in order to reach a state of equilibrium. This repeated pattern of sodium loss after potassium loss chronically over years and years from dietary stress, physical and emotional stress, and pathogenic stress eventually causes severe deficiency both of sodium and potassium, with too little sodium to maintain sufficient blood volume and too little potassium to protect cells against activation by sodium thus catalyzing chronic cellular stress and fatigue of cardiovascular tissue that leads to cardiovascular stress and illness.

The exchangers responsible for transporting calcium, sodium, and potassium through cells and sustaining cellular respiration, metabolism, and homeostasis are also dependent on adenosine triphosphate (ATP) in the function of *adenosine triphosphatases* (ATPases) because they consume ATP as a required cofactor. Because ATP production is entirely dependent on food consumption, imbalance of potassium to sodium ratio is most deranged by fasting, insufficient carbohydrate intake, other dieting, or conditions like diabetes because reduced carbohydrate directly impairs the production of ATP required to move electrolytes. This is one of the reasons why exercising in the morning before eating as I did throughout my youth strongly contributes to early metabolic demise, because exercising on an empty stomach and low blood sugar (especially if you have existing metabolic disease) is the single most powerful way to deplete the body of energy and exhausts spare nutrient stores and why studies show things like leakage of chromosomes into the bloodstream in those who exercise before eating as cells literally fall apart due to the extreme deficiency in energy and high stress.

Many studies show that caffeine increases ion exchangers, which is why caffeine can and does help people feel an increase in energy as it thusly increases the flux of ions through cells, driving an increase in energy production. But this only occurs as long as there is sufficient energy (ATP) to supply those exchangers, and while caffeine is primarily dopaminergic, adrenaline is also made from dopamine, and using caffeine without a source of fructose due to dieting behaviors, avoiding sugar, or impaired sugar digestion and malabsorption of fructose as discussed in the chapter on parasitism and metabolic disease results then in massive release of glucose from glycogen stores to cause hyperglycemia, racing heart, and serious glycogen depletion, and since the body cannot use all that circulating glucose but also cannot again store it as glycogen due to fructose deficiency that glucose is instead deposited as fat, and in anyone struggling with metabolic problems the use caffeine without calories, carbohydrates, and fructose such as is common to dieting culture, industrialized diets, diet drinks, and chronic metabolic disease like diabetes it directly contributes to weight gain, chronic glycogen depletion, and loss of electrolytes which over time causes catastrophic loss of blood volume as the body loses the ability to retain water to the bloodstream, blood thickens and is less able to transport nutrients, and loss of water to surrounding tissues dilute electrolytes in cells to further lower their electrical conductivity and electrochemical gradient potential to promote heart failure, stroke, embolism, senility, edema, Reynaud's, erectile dysfunction, osteoporosis, etc.

Sodium in turn follows *chloride*, and chloride channels are also primary mediators not only of water management but many other biological pathways in the body, and while increasing salt intake is in opposition to accepted ideas on hypertension and diabetes, those with metabolic diseases like diabetes are shown in studies to present with deficiency of circulating sodium and chloride, proving that dietary salt is not actually absorbed or retained during these states of illness, which instead causes derangement of the gut microbiome and promotion of putrefying microbes in the gut which thrive on high salt and protein environment and producing harmful biogenic amines like histamine, tyramine, phenylethylamine, etc. This makes a great deal of sense because many people with metabolic illness crave salt but cravings should be satiated by repletion, and persistent cravings in spite of dietary consumption is a primary symptom of malabsorption. A case report of a diabetic woman who experienced cardiac arrest from diabetic ketoacidosis on a high potassium diet after stopping insulin medication was continuing to take an *angiotensin* blocker for high blood pressure. These medications work by increasing potassium retention and promoting loss of sodium in direct opposition to the normal function of angiotensin (but exactly as prescribed in conventional treatment of diabetes) which then reverses the chemical gradient of cellular metabolism and prevents cells from producing energy. While such misfortune seems to demonstrate problems with diabetes it actually demonstrates how messing with electrolyte channels with pharmaceuticals can be very, very dangerous even if recommended by a doctor, because in all cases the body is always, always already trying to maintain homeostasis and fix what is wrong, but the medical industry is merely exploiting disease for profit and working against the body will always be a losing strategy. Blocking angiotensin or aldosterone or having a low sodium diet not only fails to prevent heart disease, it potentiates it, since this impairs the ability of cells to produce energy and manage water.

The pathway which takes up sodium from digestion and promotes its reabsorption in the kidney, lungs, sweat, etc., called the *epithelial sodium channels*, is itself upregulated by *fructose*, so having extra salt with something very sugary such as juice, a smoothie, or sugary lemonade with added salt can more strongly promote sodium uptake to help restore blood volume. This works so well in fact that it is well studied in the context of hypertension, which is not caused by sodium but by insufficient potassium, poor sun exposure, and low-quality diets. Since sugar is required to uptake sufficient sodium to maintain cardiovascular health, heart disease is the number one cause of death because people frequently starve themselves in misguided and self-destructive efforts to uphold patriarchal attitudes of sexual attraction and personal worth, harmful attitudes about maleness or femininity which are not even achieved by these strategies that destroy and weaken the body and ironically end up becoming fat and diseased or disfigured by steroids or plastic surgery, or mentally insane as their minds and bodies cope with the extreme stress caused by unrelenting abuse of the human body such trauma motivates. When women starve themselves it's often called an eating disorder but for men or athletes we instead call it diet and exercise. In reality ALL DIETING IS AN EATING DISORDER because it is not healthy nor normal for an organism to purposefully restrict nutrient or caloric intake, and a person who chronically consumes diet caffeinated soda and actively engages in dieting behavior which restricts carbohydrates, fats, and electrolytes is actively draining their blood volume to invariably cause cardiovascular failure, and because other functions of the body such as erections or hair growth are also directly connected to the bloodstream the consequences of such abuse are not limited to the cardiovascular system but affect the entire body, because the body is one integrated organism and not simply a collection of disparate systems.

Because diet sodas strongly promote adrenaline release they are often used as self-medication for depression and emotional malaise since the combination of low carbohydrate and stimulants very strongly forces adrenaline release and thus also hyperglycemia and sodium flux which then gives a sense of excitement and motivation otherwise lacking in we who abuse our bodies and suffer unresolved psychological trauma, and those who consume diet sodas are similarly often given to volatile emotional behavior, outbursts, and interpersonal conflict because of the stress of unresolved trauma and destructive behaviors on the mind and body. There is nothing wrong at all with wanting to feel good—in fact thinking there is a problem with wanting to feel good contributes to these behavioral problems and it is often mentally difficult to give up these coping mechanisms because we do not have other tools for real self compassion and self care which can and must be addressed through *inventory therapy* as discussed in the upcoming chapter on spirituality, or my other book on trauma and psychology. The truth is our body wants to be alive and healthy just as much as we do, and is always trying to take care of us in spite of our efforts to undermine that. This is one reason why getting well can often be surprisingly easy because the body is already trying to heal us and take care of us and only requires knowledge, proper care, environment, resolution of harmful coping behaviors, and nutrition, such as always making sure to have something with fructose such as well-ripened fruit or invert sugar before using caffeine, to prevent hyperglycemia and exhaustion of glycogen (and restoring sugar digestion). But much science and medicine overcomplicates biology and fixates on minutiae such as receptors, signaling, DNA, etc., because people spend far too much time and effort fixating on disease rather than understanding health. People are often so fixated on killing pathogens, for instance, they have no idea they also eradicated their own healthy microbiome, and almost never consider diet in a manner that is actually productive due to harmful attitudes about food, sugar, self-worth, and sex appeal, and so are ineffective in resolving their constant struggle for wellness.

For these same reasons it has eluded most people's attention that the single most important factor for a healthy body is the simple blood protein, *albumin,* which is also the most abundant protein in the blood and primary regulator of osmotic homeostasis. Albumin is also the primary transporter of most nutrients and products of detoxification, and reaches every single part of the body to promote and assist cells and tissues to obtain and balance nutrients, including water. During albumin deficiency nutrients like sodium, calcium, copper, magnesium, and fatty acids are still released freely into the bloodstream because the body still needs those nutrients even if they cannot be properly chaperoned, so researchers and medical professionals have largely dismissed the importance of albumin except in extreme cases of illness such as end stage kidney failure, not understanding that free elements in the bloodstream are more rapidly lost through the kidneys and liver or prematurely react with other components as a direct consequence of albumin deficiency because albumin would otherwise act as a reservoir, buffer, and chaperone for these nutrients which then prevents filtration of nutrients by the elimination organs and uncontrolled reactions with other elements.

Because albumin controls electrolytes it is the most powerful osmotic regulator in balancing the water content of the bloodstream and preventing its loss to surrounding tissue, and a decline in albumin is the most injurious deficiency which impairs our ability to constrain water to the bloodstream and prevent diseases caused because without albumin the body cannot effectively distribute electrolytes throughout the body or retain them to the bloodstream and prevent their loss in urine. Considering albumin's profound importance in human health it is very curious that almost no attention is paid to the fact that diseases like diabetes present with low albumin except during emergency procedures where albumin might finally be administered intravenously to keep people alive, and there is otherwise no effort to address or resolve album deficiency in general treatment even though it has been known since 1970, for instance, that those with cystic fibrosis present with albumin deficiency. The measurement and testing of albumin in the treatment of all metabolic disease would lead to far improved prognoses and could prevent serious harm. Infamous studies which show aged animals benefitting from the transplant of young blood, which motivates insane and stupid rich people to harvest blood from young people, is simply an effect of albumin repletion, which is also why blood transfusion does not have long term benefits (it also serves to overload the body with iron which actively promotes aging and illness) nor can it actually reverse disease because albumin only has a half-life of about nineteen days, and repletion of albumin can only ever be persistent from the restoration of the body's natural ability to produce it.

Most people also reasonably consider the heart and cardiovascular tissues as being similar in function to skeletal muscles such as biceps or abdominals, thinking cardiovascular muscle is strengthened by exercise and tires and fatigues from excessive use and believing then a slow heart rate characteristic of high performance athletes facilitates greater rest of the heart muscle and thus a healthier heart. This is not actually at all how cardiovascular muscle works, however, and a low resting heart rate is instead indicative of cardiovascular fatigue and insufficient ATP to move electrolytes because the heart is designed to pump constantly without resting, and contractions of the heart are stimulated not by effort or exertion but by the entry of electrolytes and nutrients inbetween beats through those ATP dependent pathways. Adulation of slow resting heart rate is entirely a bias fallacy originating from the undeserved adulation and idealization of athletes due to our personal control desires of sexual appeal and youthfulness, with absolutely no basis in science or biology, which instead demonstrates increased risk of sudden cardiovascular incidents in overly lean or overtrained athletes. Common heart failure in overtrained athletes is usually then excused (every time!) as inherited weaknesses, but are in fact a consequence of the dangerous depletion of ATP and electrolytes due to excessive physical stress which also overconsumes ATP required to sustain electrolyte flux, especially during concomitant disease such as impaired carbohydrate metabolism by opportunistic pathogens. The heart pumps blood to sustain delivery of oxygen and nutrients to the body so why would a slow heart rate be beneficial? That would mean reduce flow of oxygen and nutrients. Cardiovascular muscle is designed by nature to contract indefinitely, autonomically, in a stair-step pattern where it beats harder as it beats faster in order to increase blood circulation and delivery of oxygen and nutrients, and cardiovascular tissue does not fatigue so long as it is supplied with adequate ions and ATP, which is also why heart attack is treated with glucose, steroids, and electrolyte infusions and not *by putting patients on a fucking treadmill!*

Albumin is synthesized in the liver from every single meal if it contains requisite nutrients and is then released directly to the bloodstream where it transports other nutrients, and albumin sufficiency is the primary and ultimate reason for effortless health in those who are young and healthy. One of the most important requisites is *potassium* which, though not made of potassium, is required to release albumin to the bloodstream in the first place, so the first and primary catalyst for albumin dysfunction and the initiation of metabolic illness and cardiovascular disease are dieting behaviors and excessive stress since this inherently reduces potassium homeostasis. Grains and meat are extremely low in potassium, so industrial diets are the most common cause of heart disease, besides dieting behaviors, simply due to their low potassium content (sorghum is one grain high in potassium, and potatoes are very high).

But because cells require ATP to take up potassium, carbohydrate is also required for efficacy of dietary or supplementary potassium and release of albumin to circulation, otherwise potassium remains in the extracellular space, to then be eliminated in urine, which ironically increases stress and promotes cardiovascular disease rather than reversing it since potassium must be located in cells to be effective. While there are many high potassium food, in those who are very ill a low-dose supplement of *potassium citrate* can make it much easier to achieve potassium sufficiency since citrate feeds directly into ATP production, but this must be supported by generous carbohydrate and sodium intake and supplementation can actually stop your heart if not accompanied by sugar and sodium, so supplementation is always secondary to a diet high in potassium and carbohydrate (never use potassium chloride, which is shown instead to promote potassium loss).

Albumin itself is most dependent on the element *selenium*, which is extremely important for human health, and selenium is normally quite abundant in any diet, but just as *Streptomyces* reduce nitrate for their energy source (and humans and other animals reduce oxygen), some pathogenic microbes reduce selenate forms of selenium used in selenium-dependent proteins to its *selenide* form which is also highly toxic to our biology and causes selenium deficiency, even before dietary selenium is absorbed into the body.

Albumin is also a *sulfated* carrier of fats and fat soluble nutrients because sulfation makes fatty nutrients more water soluble in the watery environments of our bodies and thus assist in the transport, but other microbes similarly reduce sulfate to sulfide, which not only causes sulfur deficiency but the resulting hydrogen sulfide (and related compounds like methyl mercaptan) is also highly toxic.

Without sulfate fats congeal and block pathways such as occurs in atherosclerosis and cardiovascular disease, hypogonadism, and immune dysfunction. So sulfur deficiency either caused by too little intake or, more commonly, its reduction to hydrogen sulfide not only disrupts sulfation dependent pathways but hydrogen sulfide (and related molecules) is also highly reactive to many elements and chelates sulfur, copper, iron, molybdenum, boron, and selenium out of the body to then strongly impair dependent functions like albumin.

Although this chapter is also long and complex, understanding the reduction of selenium and sulfur to hydrogen selenide and hydrogen sulfide is also not difficult to understand or diagnose because they are the highly offensive malodors present in bad breath and smelly feces and flatulence, and the reason they are so offensive to our sense of smell is because they and the microbes which produce them are so toxic to our wellbeing that our biology evolved to give us the ability to detect and avoid them as a means for our evolutionary survival.

Oftentimes simply increasing consumption of sulfurous foods like brassicas (kale, broccoli, cabbage, collards, mustard) or garlic will result in significant health improvements for young people who are not ill due to the increase in sulfate, selenium, and dependent products like *taurine, glutathione, and glutathione peroxidase* which protect cells from stress, calcification, and oxidative damage, but during metabolic disease sulfate and selenate reducing microbes will instead cause production of smelly hydrogen sulfide and even more offensive hydrogen selenide which can then be used as a diagnostic for the underlying dysregulation of albumin and other dependent pathways.

What's worse, the lining of the cardiovascular system and all cells in the human body have a sulfated cholesterol later which blocks water passage, because sulfur and fats are highly hydrophobic (repels water) which in turn also prevents potassium leakage from cells, so after infection by opportunistic bacteria (especially oral, gingival pathogens as discussed in the upcoming chapter on oral health) which gain access the bloodstream as made obvious by bleeding gums they begin stripping this protective lining of the cardiovascular system of its cholesterol sulfate which then destroys this regulatory barrier and begins allowing leakage of water from the bloodstream into the rest of the body, not only reducing blood volume but causing water retention and bloating in tissues.

Cholesterol is also the precursor to vitamin D and most hormones, and cholesterol is a highly sulfated protein required to prevent fats from congealing in the cardiovascular system and evenly supplying dietary fats and fat soluble nutrients to cells as needed. There also exist amino forms of both dietary sulfur and selenium in the forms of methionine, cysteine, and selenomethionine and selenocysteine which, because they are already in their sulfate and selenate forms, are primary targets for these opportunistic pathogens than other forms of dietary sulfur and selenium. The epithelium of the digestive tract is also similarly sulfated, however, and lined with cholesterol and other lipid-dependent protective defenses, and colonization by opportunistic pathogens similarly impairs the osmotic regulatory properties of the gut, to promote an increase in water uptake which results in bloating and water retention and slows gut transit of food and allows pathogens and opportunists to grow out of control and result in gut distension, sluggish posture, and eventual heart and liver disease from systemic dysregulation of water and deficiencies of sulfur and selenium.

Hydrogen sulfide also reverses the function of vitamin B12 (cobalamin) in promoting adhesion of commensal microbes to the mucosal layer to thus let sulfate reducers outcompete our commensal microbiome, including of the oral cavity and other mucosal tissues like the lungs, thus also contributing to bad breath as well as smelly feces and flatulence from feeding on the mucosal secretions meant to otherwise promote commensal mucosal microbes. Sulfate reducing microbes are also why some people think they have sulfur intolerance, as consuming sulfurous foods can and does then result in significant production of toxic hydrogen sulfide (and selenide) when colonized by these opportunistic pathogens.

As sulfur and selenium are so, so vital for the normal function of many pathways and the health of the gut, cardiovascular system, hormones reproduction, and even immunity, foods high in sulfur and selenium are *not* optional for recovery (from any illness). But most people get the bulk of their sulfur and selenium from animal products and thus the amino acid sources of sulfur and selenium which are primary targets of these pathogens, so once metabolic disease sets in those sources are the least ideal, and unaccompanied by protective phytochemicals are not only stolen by pathogens but actively contribute to disease due to the formation of toxic sulfide and selenide.

By weight, high sulfur vegetables like kale and collard greens have more sulfur than meat, making them ideal sources to help reverse this problem of sulfur dysregulation, and nuts are not only high in selenium but contain protective tannins and other phytochemicals that help to impair access by pathogens and thus suppress the production of malodorous hydrogen sulfide and hydrogen selenide.

Pathways which absorb sulfur and selenium into the body are also dependent on sodium, which means that their absorption is also strongly inhibited by ammonia produced by ammonia producing pathogens which inhibit sodium uptake through the alkalization of chloride as discussed in the previous chapters. This then causes dietary sulfur and selenium to remain in the gut, contributing to even more to malodor production than would otherwise occur and thus easily identified as highly smelly feces, flatulence, but also the loss of elements like copper and molybdenum which strongly react to sulfur. Making matters even more complex, our body also uses sulfate to detoxify things like polyunsaturated fats, used hormones, xenobiotics, and other products of detoxification through the liver and bile which are eliminated through feces, and sulfate reducers which steal sulfate from detoxification products then causes the reabsorption and recirculation of toxic factors back into the body endlessly which then sustain metabolic disease and make recovery very difficult, so any hint of malodor in feces is also a sign of dysfunctional detoxification which sustains metabolic dysregulation and prevents recovery even when eating a good diet.

Yes, this does in fact means that shit, gas, and your breath should *not* actually smell bad, and if they do it portends metabolic disease and is in fact not normal nor healthy and *must* be addressed. Even consumption of high quantities of sulfur such as an entire head of roast garlic should *not* actually result in sulfurous malodor of feces or flatulence, which instead indicates failure to absorb dietary sulfur, due to sodium deficiency caused by ammonia excess and dysregulation, and the presence of hydrogen sulfide and hydrogen selenide producing pathogens (by the way, raw garlic has no advantage over cooked but can harm mucosal tissues, so only consume garlic in large quantities when cooked).

The problem of resolving sulfate and selenate reducing pathogens took over six years of research until finally one day I found a paper describing *carotene* as not only an antioxidant but also an *antireductant*. Carotene are terpenoids responsible for the red and orange colors found in fruit and vegetables, and while it was well known that carotene is a potent antioxidant the potent antireductant (reduction is the opposite of oxidation) properties of carotenoids are so unknown and so rarely discussed even in scientific literature I did not learn about it until nearly ten years of academic research, consuming thousands of scientific studies, even when several of those years were directly focused on carotene. This function of carotene is so strong in fact it can entirely prevent malodorous hydrogen sulfide and hydrogen selenide not only in bad breath (also known as *halitosis*) but also in feces and flatulence if it accompanies all consumption of dietary protein, sulfur, and selenium. Even if you don't brush with toothpaste breath should *never* smell malodorous, and carotene is so effective at inhibiting microbial reduction it is actually *more* effective than toothpaste at inhibiting oral malodor and keeping breath fresh.

I had suspected carotene could be useful for the resolution of illnesses but its efficacy for resolving reducing pathogens came not from quantity, which is what I had been trying, but entirely from *frequency*, so past experiments using carotene did not reveal this usefulness because I did not consume it sufficiently often to be noticeably effective. For instance, it will not matter if a previous meal was very high in carotene, as if the following meal is high in sulfur or selenium but absent of carotene the previous ingestion of carotene will no longer be present to provide its protective effects.

Because all protein is also a source of a sulfur and selenium all meals containing any protein or sulfur *must be accompanied by carotene* to achieve this effect such that no malodor of the breath, feces, or flatulence occurs at any time, and if a meal does not already contain carotene the chewing of several bites of high carotenoid food like carrot, peaches, sweet potato, tomato, watermelon, apricots, dates, etc., before, during, or after a meal can strongly prevent production of microbial hydrogen sulfide and hydrogen selenide, especially if sodium status and excess ammonia are resolved, which will promote the increased removal of sulfur and selenium from the gut, and the presence of malodor can thus also be used effectively as a diagnostic to confirm effective sodium repletion and ammonia inhibition, as if those efforts have not been effective carotene will be digested by the time feces are excreted and any remaining sulfur or selenium will still result in malodor (meaning that if fecal malodor still occurs when consuming carotene with meals this indicates continued sodium deficiency caused by continued ammonia dysregulation).

To be clear, this antireductant effect of carotene is a function of carotene, not all carotenoids, the other class of which are *xanthophylls* which tend to be more commonly yellow and occur in leafy greens which, while also very important for our health, do not have this specific antireductant function, which is instead largely achieved through red and orange fruit and vegetables, although high xanthophyll foods like broccoli or kale will still contain some carotene to protect their own sulfur content and won't require additional intake, but won't be high enough for instance to protect an additional head of garlic or serving of protein.

Because carotenoids are terpenoids they rapidly penetrate the mucosal layer and mucosal tissue to directly inhibit oral and gastrointestinal hydrogen sulfide microbes and can even be felt doing so as they impart a slightly minty, fresh sensation when chewed throughly, so the effects can be felt in the oral cavity much the same way that toothpaste feels on gum tissue. Because these pathogens colonize the oral cavity, resolving oral disease as discussed in that upcoming chapter will be required for full resolution of cardiovascular disease and restoration of sulfur and sulfate status which affects hormones, albumin, etc.

One of the most important functions of dietary carotene is also the formation of *vitamin A* from pro-vitamin A carotenoids which, as a fat-soluble nutrient, is also primarily transported by albumin and other sulfated proteins like chylomicrons and cholesterol. Many people believe that preformed vitamin A such as from a supplement or eating of liver is healthy and useful but, while some preformed dietary vitamin A is fine, vitamin A is also highly metabolically active and taking too much can actually poison the liver and contribute to metabolic disease. For instance human liver contains about 30 micrograms of vitamin A per gram of weight but polar bear liver is famously toxic to humans and can contain up to 10,000 micrograms per gram, which also demonstrates that we are not actually evolved to handle high quantities of vitamin A, and thus preformed and supplemental forms being physiologically inappropriate for human health. The endogenous formation of vitamin A (retinol) from dietary carotene also occurs primarily in the mucosal layer, not in the body after absorption as is commonly thought, and this reaction also consumes reactive oxygen in the process thereby also helping to keep the gut in a properly hypoxic state which in turn supports healthy gut microbes, a function that does not occur from the consumption of preformed vitamin A.

Since vitamin A is also required for things like production of hormones and healthy eyesight, conditions like diabetes and cystic fibrosis commonly present with hyposteroidogenesis, night blindness, and poor immune function. But because carotene foods are delicious it is not difficult to get carotene with every meal, and can even take the form of fruit pies, jams and preserves, ice creams, smoothies, sweet potato fries, generous use of carrots, oranges and orange juice, peaches, nectarines, apricots, papaya, mango, peppers, cherries, dates, chontaduro, tomatoes, watermelon, cantaloupe, etc. Some fruit is preserved using harmful forms of sulfur like sulfur dioxide, however, which can entirely wipe out the microbiome, so take care to avoid any foods and beverages preserved with sulfur additives like sulfur dioxide, sulfite, etc., (wines are often treated with sulfites which cause those problems and should be avoided by drinking only organically produced wine).

Hydrogen sulfide also actively destroys *thiamine* (vitamin B1) because thiamine is a sulfurous B vitamin (as is biotin), and studies in ruminants show that excessive production of hydrogen sulfide can result in fatal thiamine deficiency which results in the formation of lesions across the brain and nervous system (because ruminants have foreguts where greater hydrogen sulfide synthesis can occur), so thiamine deficiency such as occurs in diabetes can also be caused by excess microbial hydrogen sulfide, but because humans are hindgut fermenters this is not recognized as a mechanism of action which causes thiamine deficiency, though it very much is as evident by the presence of hydrogen sulfide and selenide malodors. Because both biotin and thiamine are made using sulfur, our commensal microbes require dietary sulfur also to synthesize them, not to mention our own needs for sulfur, so the active consumption of dietary sulfur such as from brassicas, onions, cooked garlic, and protein, protected at all times by carotene, must occur to reverse these deficiencies.

As might be obvious, fatty liver which accompanies metabolic illnesses which is thought to be caused by sugar consumption is in reality a deficiency or dysregulation of sulfate required to detoxify fat from the liver. Sugar intake is only correlatively associated with fatty liver because sugar is a signal of abundant environmental nutrition to which the body responds by releasing fat for detoxification and elimination through feces. Fat is metabolically expensive—it literally adds weight to the organism and requires calories to maintain—but since detoxification of fats occurs through sulfation a fatty liver is a symptom of impaired sulfate-mediated detoxification such as from the presence of sulfate reducing microbes, not sugar excess, which then causes those fats to be reabsorbed back into the body. Considering that pathogens disrupt normal fat metabolism anyway, it becomes clear how problems like fatty liver are a result of pathogenic colonization and not the macro-composition of the dietary.

Supplemental sulfate might also seem like an option to reverse sulfate deficiency but the nature of sulfate is to resist spontaneous diffusion through membranes, which is why it is used in detoxification and transport pathways as this helps prevent reabsorption, so direct sulfate use does not really resolve the problem of sulfate deficiency or dysregulation. Instead, dietary *sulfur* must be processed into sulfate at sites of sulfation in the body and this step in turn requires the enzyme *sulfite oxidase* which oxidizes dietary sulfides and sulfite into useable sulfate. Sulfite oxidase is in turn dependent on the element *molybdenum,* and molybdenum deficiency also then prevents conversion of dietary sulfur into sulfate which not only causes sulfate deficiency but increases toxic sulfite and sulfide which cause metabolic dysregulation which also manifest as irritation and agitation, as sulfite is highly oxidizing (and the reason why sulfite additives to food can cause health problems). Higher circulating sulfide and sulfites also strongly react with iron and are secreted through the skin to cause familiar sulfurous skin malodor several hours or more after eating food high in sulfur, so body malodors which occur after eating sources of sulfur (including protein) are also an excellent way to diagnose molybdenum deficiency. Sulfur in fact has a high affinity for molybdenum, which is why the body uses it to process sulfur, and it would not be mentioned in this chapter if not for the fact that hydrogen sulfide also strongly reacts to molybdenum to not only contribute to molybdenum deficiency but also to form toxic *thiomolybdate* which itself also has a high affinity for copper which then actively poisons copper dependent proteins in the body, and the formation of thiomolybdate due to unaddressed hydrogen sulfide formation is a major catalyst of many metabolic diseases since copper enzymes are fundamental to many basic biological pathways. Thiomolybdate induced copper deficiency is a common problem for livestock because of foregut fermentation, and can rapidly develop fatal copper deficiency if their diets are too high in sulfur and molybdenum simultaneously, but because we humans like to consider ourselves better than our fellow animals we ignore these kinds of mortal problems in our diets to our peril, and the presence of hydrogen sulfide malodors also indicates poisoning of copper enzymes by thiomolybdate and thus deficiencies of sulfur, copper, and molybdenum.

It has long also been known in the medical profession that infusion with sodium chloride such as from intravenous saline as what occurs during medical emergencies can and does increase circulating *vitamin D* to such a degree it can actually cause temporary hypercalcemia. And though it has long been known that vitamin D is strongly beneficial to cardiovascular health this knowledge of sodium's effect on vitamin D has never been used to help address general vitamin D deficiency or cardiovascular disease in the general population. Vitamin D also directly benefits the gut microbiome through support of *Thaumarchaeota,* which require vitamin D and actually produce it themselves in wild populations, as it is found in their effluence, and deficiency of vitamin D is one of the primary causes of gut dysbiosis and immune dysfunction because, as one study described, "we share vitamin D with our commensal microbes and they in turn share their B vitamins."

But our microbes also make other nutrients like the short chain fatty acids, amino acids, hormones, and even protect us from opportunistic microbes, so vitamin D is far more important than its typical attribution and oversimplification and absolutely vital for good metabolic and cardiovascular health. Unfortunately, taking a supplement of vitamin D rarely resolves health problems, however, because vitamin D metabolism is also far more complex than most people understand, and simply taking a supplement *will not* result in the reversal of vitamin D deficiency related symptoms because this does not solve the underlying problem which creates the deficiency in the first place. Studies show, for instance, that vitamin D use by our body is entirely dependent on butyric acid produced by our commensal microbes (remember that root vegetable are most reliable for butyric acid), and without butyrate our cells do not activate or utilize vitamin D, and studies also show that during butyrate deficiency the metabolism shifts from carbohydrate metabolism to that of fat. To health and appearance obsessed persons this may sound like a benefit, but when the body shifts to fat metabolism it also stores more fat, converting dietary carbohydrate to fat storage. Because carbohydrate oxidation is the more efficient metabolic state this also then means we cannot achieve the higher cellular functions required for healing.

Vitamin D is also chaperoned through the body by a variant of albumin called *vitamin D binding protein,* which is structurally almost identical to albumin and can be thought of as a specialized form of albumin which facilitates more efficient and effective transport of vitamin D (albumin also transports some vitamin D). So the same deficiencies which cause low albumin, especially of potassium and selenium, also cause vitamin D dysfunction *regardless* of how much sunshine or vitamin D is taken, and this is the primary reason vitamin D function is often so difficult to address. Because vitamin D is a fat soluble nutrient sulfation is also one of the most important factors, likewise requiring dietary sulfur and molybdenum protected by carotene to suppress microbial hydrogen sulfide and hydrogen selenide. Unsurprisingly, polyunsaturated fats irreversibly compete with vitamin D for vitamin D binding protein, and during metabolic disease and diets high in polyunsaturated fats or problems detoxifying fats through the liver due to hydrogen sulfide producing microbes which interrupt detoxification these fats then actually block vitamin D binding protein from binding, protecting, and delivering vitamin D throughout the body. One of the functions of albumin and other protein chaperones like vitamin D binding protein is to prevent kidney filtration of the nutrients they bind, so when absent of working vitamin D binding protein our vitamin D is then just peed out in the urine, showing again a very specific reason how high dietary polyunsaturated fats can and do contribute to metabolic disease, requiring the avoidance of refined and concentrated intake of dietary polyunsaturated fat sources like vegetable oil, canola oil, omega-3s, fish oil, etc., and to protect liver detoxification of PUFA with ubiquitous carotene intake.

While a supplement of vitamin D can occasionally help some people if these functions are working (those whom live in places with long winters should use one), it really only serves to mask problems with making our own, and endogenously produced vitamin D is also more potent and lasts longer in the body. It has long been known that vitamin D is primarily made in the skin from *cholesterol* during exposure to sunlight, not achieved from a supplement or even dietary sources, although some dietary sources like animal fats will contain some vitamin D (fish oil is often marketed for its high vitamin D content, which it has, but fish oil is also extremely high in polyunsaturated fat and will result in high peroxidative stress). But this means that working cholesterol is required to produce vitamin D, although this is not much more complicated as, like albumin and vitamin D binding protein, cholesterol simply also requires amino acids, sulfur, and selenium, but also dietary fat since cholesterol functions primarily as a vehicle to transport important dietary fats for synthesis into bile, vitamin D, hormones, or cellular integration into cellular structures and metabolic function. It is commonly understood that cholesterol is sulfated and thus requires sulfur for proper metabolism, but selenium is right next to sulfur on the periodic table and has very similar chemical and physical properties to sulfur which is why it is often interchangeable in biological functions, but has a slightly different charge and behavior and its active integration into sulfur pathways *increases* their stability and efficacy, and though it is not currently demonstrated by studies I believe that selenium is *required* for good function cholesterol, to substitute some of the sulfur atoms, as studies do show selenium improves cholesterol profile, so taking care to consume sources high in selenium like brewer's yeast, Brazil nuts, cashews, shellfish, or a low-dose supplement of selenium with dietary fats and remembering to protect selenium with carotene will promote better cholesterol synthesis and lead to profound improvements in cholesterol dependent pathways (more on cholesterol is discussed in the upcoming chapters on immunity and hormones).

The skin is actually also a reservoir for sodium, erroneously considered a buffer of sodium excess rather than storage site since sodium has for so long been vilified, the skin requires sufficient sodium to function properly and to participate in metabolic pathways like vitamin D synthesis, the formation of sweat, and proper skin hydration since sodium helps move and manage water. This also means that ammonia excess which disturbs sodium absorption also disturbs skin health and vitamin D status. During a brief period of access to a saline swimming pool I once experienced profound and entirely unexpected improvements to many of my symptoms since saline pools (also called brine pools in some places) electronically separate sodium and chloride which then promotes the effortless uptake of sodium and chloride through dermal sweat reabsorption channels where they then actively promote greater vitamin D synthesis, and access to the sea or saline pools is often therapeutic probably for its direct facilitation of vitamin D status.

Sunlight deficiency is the simplest and most primary cause of vitamin D deficiency since sun exposure is required to convert cholesterol into vitamin D, but the form of vitamin D made in the skin or taken as a supplement is also the inactive form, called vitamin D3 or *cholecalciferol*, which is often regarded as if it were active vitamin D, which it is not, which must first be *hydroxylated* to its two active forms *calcifediol* and *calcitriol* in the liver and kidney, respectively, or by other cells such as in macrophages during an immune reaction. This activation occurs either through the enzyme *25-hydroxylase* or by our copper-dependent respiratory enzyme *cytochrome oxidase* (which can be poisoned and inhibited by formation of thiomolybdate from toxic microbial hydrogen sulfide). Studies also show that magnesium is also required for activation of vitamin D, as magnesium is a very common enzymatic cofactor, though its deficiency is not usually so acute as to prevent this, since magnesium is quite widespread in a healthy diet.

Because vitamin D is synthesized from cholesterol, vitamin D is not actually a vitamin, but a hormone, and knowing that cholesterol is the precursor to things like bile, vitamin D, and hormones makes the vilification of cholesterol as has been the case for several decades extremely problematic, as without cholesterol many metabolic pathways like vitamin D production in turn become impaired. Aldosterone and other mineralocorticoids which prevent sodium loss and excess extracellular potassium are also made from cholesterol, so impaired cholesterol homeostasis from low-fat dieting, use of pharmaceuticals, or poor digestion of dietary fats due to factors like saponification in the gut is highly consequential to the health of the body, and cholesterol instead supports many pathways, rather than impairs them as has been so errantly and catastrophically misunderstood. Contrary to popular belief, cholesterol is also almost entirely made within our body and does not come from dietary cholesterol, and lipid dysregulation such as elevated triglycerides or deranged LDL and HDL cholesterol levels indicate fundamental disturbance of normal fat digestion or cholesterol synthesis that must be reversed to restore vitamin D and cardiovascular health, not simply treated chronically with the use of pharmaceuticals—some of which (like prescription fish oil) actually *destroy* the parts of the liver which make them as their mechanism of action, which in the long term can be fatal.

As mentioned in the chapter on gut health, cravings for easily digestible foods like meat or starches is the easiest way to diagnose deficiency of vitamin D and local B12 production by *Thaumarchaeota*, since B12 is required for microbes to break down tough plant foods, and when replete with vitamin D there can and should be very strong cravings for fruits and vegetables, especially fresh, leafy greens, in preference of meat because although these foods are more healthful for us they are also impossible to break down without a healthy microbiome capable of digesting cellulose and releasing plant nutrients. So a lack of cravings for leafy greens, cravings for meat, and abundant flatulence is a reliable way to diagnose deficiency or dysfunction of vitamin D which in turn means problems with vitamin D metabolism, even if exposure to sunlight occurs daily.

Most people are also not aware that our skin *accumulates* carotenoids. This is often discussed as an aberration or defect of the body, such as occurs during *carotenemia* when the skin can turn orange from too much carotene. But carotenes are transported to the skin in the first place for the same functions they provide plants, which is to absorb *high energy wavelengths* of light like ultraviolet and the blue spectrum, to protect our tissues and DNA from damage by those high-energy wavelengths. As would thus then be the case, studies which investigate skin cancer find highest correlations not with sun exposure, which we do require to be healthy, but with low dietary carotene (and air pollution), because even marginal exposure to light, even artificial lights and ambient light, can still excite molecules and DNA in cells missing protective carotene in the absence of significant sun exposure, which is why older people, whom are highly deficient in skin carotene due to malabsorption and transport issues, sometimes don't even like having their curtains open. Being that we as humans do not have protective body hair or fur, carotene is even more important for human skin than other animals, and increasing dietary carotene (and its transport by albumin) greatly improved and restored the caramel color of my skin from summer sunbathing which for several years had been waning during the aging process.

Carotene carotenoids absorb light and slowly release its energy, but *xanthophyll* carotenoids, which are the more yellow carotenoids typical of leafy greens, actively *direct* that energy into the process of photosynthesis and would not lose this feature when being incorporated into human skin, which means that xanthophylls are in fact *required* for vitamin D catalysis (synthesis). This function has never been investigated by studies, but it also doesn't make sense that cholesterol should spontaneously convert to vitamin D simply from light exposure without some catalyst directing and controlling that light energy. One ridiculous study on cattle supposed they got vitamin D from licking their fur on which was deposited vitamin D from cholesterol reacting alone in sunlight, which obviously found its premise entirely wrong, never mind the ridiculousness of having to lick your fur to get an essential biological nutrient. Without the ability to direct light energy it would and does go anywhere and everywhere it pleases, to react with tissue, proteins, DNA, etc., and cause ionization damage to the entirety of our cells rather than controlled synthesis of a necessary prohormone. Without intending to, studies which investigate correlations between vitamin D and carotene prove a *dependency* on carotene for vitamin D synthesis, because if carotenoids merely absorbed high frequency light and did not also discharge it for use in systems like photosynthesis of vitamin D this would block vitamin D synthesis, not facilitate it, and they would compete with vitamin D for light the same way melanin does, and there would be an *inverse* association with carotene and vitamin D, not *association* as is demonstrated in studies. Therefore xanthophyll directly participates in vitamin D synthesis and is required from generous consumption of leafy greens and other chlorophyll associated foods in advance of sun exposure, to ensure the most efficient and effective production of vitamin D.

Anecdotally, lacking carotenoids in the skin results in feeling irritated and restless from sun exposure, due to the irradiation damage of sunlight, consuming high xanthophyll foods like leafy greens prior to sun exposure instead produces a profoundly enjoyable and relaxing experience since this protects the skin and body from high intensity wavelengths of light, and it should be possible to sit in the sun even in excess of an hour (not at times which risk sunburn) without feeling overexposed and restless but calm, warm, and pleasant, which indicates repletion with carotene and other antioxidant factors (like vitamin C) required to benefit from sun exposure.

As carotene accumulates in the skin for protection and harnessing ultraviolet radiation this also accounts for old, racist stereotypes toward people like indigenous Americans or East Asians, as diets high in specific carotenoids can and do impart a strong red, orange, or yellow hue to skin such as from the deep orange-reds of pumpkin or the bright yellows of leafy greens. This occurs in all humans since we all have the same DNA, and if carotenoid transport is working properly the increased consumption of carotene can and will also result in changes to skin pigment and greater tanning from sun exposure, as well as staining of clothes and bedsheets as increased carotene is secreted in sweat. Until recent times it was usually customary to wear undergarments beneath clothing to protect nicer pieces from discoloration, and I think this practice has declined primarily due to western industrial diets low in carotenoids, so undershirts can be helpful to avoid staining nicer tops or other clothing articles and showering before bed to reduce staining of sheets and blankets. Because carotene increases tanning, a reliable symptom then of carotene deficiency is reduced tanning of the skin after sun exposure, caused either by low intake or malabsorption.

Exact mechanisms of vitamin D synthesis are still not fully understood by science, however. For instance there has never been a study which purifies dehydrocholesterol and exposes it to UV radiation, but instead such studies are performed on human skin or animal secretions like lanolin from sheep. As discussed in chapter on pathogens and metabolic disease, resolution of metabolic diseases as diabetes, cystic fibrosis, and autism require exposure to commensal microbes in our environment such as is achieved through activities like gardening, playing in healthy dirt and soil, or swimming in natural swimming areas which have high density of plant life and other healthy sources of commensal microbes. Practicing this behavior results in resolution of symptoms related to vitamin D deficiency, and it is my belief that no animal on Earth actually does make their own vitamin D, but which is instead synthesized by resident *Thaumarchaeota* archaea in and on the skin. Vitamin D likely originated as a mechanism to 'detoxify' ultraviolet radiation, and helps certain species of of microbes like archaea survive exposure, but then around which other forms of life evolved to exploit and benefit from commensal association.

The primary reason I believe this to be the case, however, is that vitamin D is shown in studies to extend the lifespan of *earthworms* up to three times their normal life span, which in fact does not demonstrate the health benefits of vitamin D but instead their *dependency* on vitamin D and how their lifespan is *reduced* up to one-third its normal length when lacking vitamin D. Earthworms notorious-ly avoid light exposure, however, and lack defense against ultraviolet radiation, so they are obviously unable to produce vitamin D themselves and this begs the question, where does their vitamin D come from? Earthworms also feed on plants, but also soil microbial life, and help cultivate and change the soil microbiome to those which also directly benefit plant growth, and if their physiology is designed to benefit from vitamin D this means they must get their vitamin D from wild *archaea* populations when coming to the surface at nighttime or rainstorms to feed on archaea effluence for their vitamin D supply, since they lack any mechanism to produce it themselves.

All animals (including humans) are essentially worms with extra appendages, as we share 70% of the same genes with worms and share a common evolution-ary ancestor, and it appears to me that we also *do not* actually make vitamin D at all, but instead share carotene and cholesterol with commensal archaea in the skin whom instead make it when exposed to ultraviolet radiation, and then we absorb the vitamin D from their effluence where it is then picked up by vitamin D binding protein and distributed throughout the body. Anecdotally, the act of exposure to healthy soils (plant roots, soil earthworms, tannins from plant litter, dark from carbon sequestration), including the spread of soil microbes over the body, followed then by sun exposure results in markedly obvious and immediate increases in symptoms of vitamin D repletion compared to sun exposure without this behavior, just as our wild ancestors would have experienced when foraging for roots, insects, and even sleeping behaviors which would have occurred with direct contact to the ground, soil, and plant litter.

To be clear, this *is not safe*, as there also exists potentially pathogenic soil microbes, which is why exposure to healthy soils is part of this recommendation, to reduce the chance of pathogen exposure. But our commensal microbes are also our first line of defense against pathogens, and when supplied with adequate nutrients our body purposefully tries to cultivate such commensal species specif-ically also for protection against those which are pathogenic. These microbes can even be collected from contact with other humans such as through touch, sex, inoculation of food, etc., but eradication of these requisite, commensal, skin microbes occurs very commonly in our contemporary environment separated from healthy soils, earthworms, plant roots, etc., as well as when showering in fluoridated or highly chlorinated water, swimming pools, dieting behaviors, or lacking a diet high in carotenoids which are required to protect skin microbes from irradiation by high energy wavelengths of light. Reversing these impedi-ments then through activities as gardening, which actively cultivates soil health through plants, tannins, earthworms, etc., (earthworms can be purchased online) or swimming in safe, natural swimming areas can easily restore vitamin D and all its associated metabolic benefits.

Light deficiency, however, does not only impair vitamin D synthesis from simple lack of ultraviolet exposure, but also through active downregulation of vitamin D through the concomitant rise in the torporific hormone *melatonin* in response to light deficiency which then increases the enzyme *24-hydroxylase* which, opposite to 25-hydroxylase, *actively destroys vitamin D*. This is obviously a survival mechanism originating from ancient evolutionary traits to promote survival during times of insufficient food availability like winter, but it is also not common knowledge that harmful gastrointestinal bacterial species are more active at night, in the presence of *melatonin*, which rises when light is unavailable, and studies show various microbial species are able to engage in swarming behavior once levels of melatonin rise, activating the ability to aggressively translocate across surfaces by active movement rather than just growing outward the way normal bacteria do. The bacterium which cause *appendicitis* are more active during darkness, though strangely no one has yet made the observation that appendicitis only develops at night, and the far majority of appendicitis attacks (probably all?) occur at night or early morning which means appendicitis also promoted by both chronic light deficiency and dieting behaviors too. Darker and malodorous urine and discomfort or pain in the middle-right of the abdomen are primary symptoms of appendicitis, and quickly using the strategies in these chapters (especially the upcoming chapter on immunity) can knock out appendicitis pathogens and avoid rupture and surgery if disease is not too advanced (it can also be treated with anti-biotics). So prolonged darkness exposure such as occurs in our modern lifestyles also actively depletes us of vitamin D regardless of supplementation and sun exposure due to the active downregulation of vitamin D stimulated by the rise in melatonin that accompanies light deficiency.

Indeed many people with diabetes, autism, and other metabolic diseases like cancer have lifestyles or environments which do not facilitate daily and generous exposure to sunlight, being largely sequestered indoors, sometimes never getting any sunshine at all. During the great tuberculosis furor of the early nineteen-hundreds when researchers were close on the heels of a cure they had previously observed that galavanting in a natural environment tended to greatly improve tuberculosis prognosis and survival, so a great raucous was made about escaping to higher climes with purer air in which to recuperate which, I learned, is the reason for the great many old sanitariums to which many people were also forcibly relocated (sanitarium is a play on the word sanitize, to prevent the spread of disease, and not mental sanity which I had assumed from the many horror films and books demonizing the mentally unwell at such landmarks). Unfortunately they were mistaken and the true benefit of exposure to nature was actually exposure to sunshine, not fresh air (although fresh air is nice). As mammals we original-ly evolved in colder climes away from large dinosaur populations which is why hibernation responses, milk production, and body hair are common features of all mammals, and excessive indoor sequestration artificially replicates conditions which trigger metabolic hibernation mediators like 24-hydroxylase and melatonin, thus lowering the metabolic rate and impairing the high-metabolic functions of vitamin D as what results from long term sunlight deprivation (not to mention the loss of commensal skin microbes too). Glass also inhibits UVB rays which make vitamin D, but windows are often manufactured with more light-blocking technol-ogy in misguided attempts to promote energy efficiency which instead harms our health (and doesn't actually block much heat transfer and is a stupid exercise in meaningless and disingenuous conservation by industry since infrared light, not visible light, would need to be inhibited for tinting to be effective), so it is possible to develop severe light deficiency from the interference of windows, especially when light contact is not direct as ambient light does not do much to address any of these problems.

While we only need a minimum of thirty minutes of UVB exposure per day for vitamin D sufficiency, a minimum of *two hours* of general sun exposure is required to sufficiently suppress melatonin, 24-hydroxylase, and raise the metabolic rate, so anything less than two hours a day of sunlight exposure constitutes deficiency and more effort should be applied to building habits and lifestyles which facilitate sufficient, daily exposure to the outdoors. This is extremely important because vitamin D3 is not the only product of sun exposure, but which results also in isomerized variants like lumisterol, tachysterol, and 7DHC which result from prolonged exposure to UV radiation and heat which are proven by studies to alter biological pathways and actively activated by specific genes which affect the body in ways which we don't yet fully understand (some for instance have been found to have anti-viral effects). If light deficiency does occur (and even if it doesn't) it can be helpful to get a very bright, warm-colored lamp to supplement additional light exposure to the eyes and head to better suppress melatonin and 24-hydroxylase as much as possible. It will not reverse the effects of sunlight deficiency, only mitigate harm, and will be especially necessary for those in regions with long winters or very hot summers which prevent access to the outdoors. Because so much exposure is required it should also always be at times and durations which *do not* risk sunburn because sunblock impairs vitamin D synthesis (but sunblock can be used during very long exposure if its unavoidable), where sunburn is highly destructive to skin health. No matter the time of day direct sun exposure to the body is highly beneficial, but not only the face and hands which will not be helpful and as much skin should be bared as possible, so even getting sun first thing in the morning or late afternoon when low in the sky will still be productive.

Another yet unexpected and equally potent regulator of 24-hydroxylase is also dietary *boron* such as from fructoborates commonly available from fruit and is most abundant in *Prunus* species like apricots, peaches, plums, and nectarines, although grapes are an equally good source and thus also grape juice and wine. For a long time I couldn't imagine why the body would actively destroy vitamin D when it is so necessary for so many functions except that it might be a way of downregulating the metabolic rate, but boron is also important for commensal microbes in *quorum sensing* and *autoinducer protein* which allows microbes to communicate with each other and also our own body, which prevents our immune system from eradicating commensal species. Because we share vitamin D with microbes so they can then produce vitamin B12, the downregulation of vitamin D during boron deficiency may be a mechanism to induce greater storage of fat for thermoregulation during potential times of famine and to downregulate the metabolism that we can instead better survive by suppressing commensal microbes which help instead sustain a high metabolic rate.

While this chapter is quite complex, most of these requirements are entirely satisfied through just one food—the *Prunus* species of fruits like apricots, plums, cherries, nectarines, peaches, etc., which are high in carotene, anthocyanins, potassium, sulfur, boron, molybdenum, selenium, magnesium, etc. Prunes (dried plums) are well known to improve digestion and are commonly recommended for improved bowel function especially in those whom are older, but this is wrongly attributed to their fiber content which, while high, is not any higher than many other fiber foods (legumes have several times more fiber but do not provide this service). This benefit is instead due to the high fructoborate, anthocyanin (tannin), sulfur, selenium, and carotene content of *Prunus* species which achieve every requisite in this chapter. Our dependence on so many nutritional elements available in *Prunus* fruit in fact demonstrates its participation in our evolutionary history and thus requisite as a human food, as all animals evolve to fit a specific environmental niche which they can exploit for their nutritional needs, and not one aspect of human biology, morphology, or even psychology are independent of our evolutionary history as an animal fitting into our own specific ecological niche. Specifically, the evolution of clawless, dextrous, prehensile fingers and relatively larger hands and arms than other mammals is no accident—Many animals climb trees very well with claws which are far more efficient for locomotion in both arboreal biomes as well as flatter terrain like grasslands than our wimpy, flat little nails. The kind of hands and fingers we possess are instead specifically evolved for grasping and harvesting fruit, and not just any fruit either but specifically that of the *Prunus* genus, which are widespread across the entire Northern Hemisphere, including where we originally evolved around the Mediterranean region before becoming human. Animals with claws or without hands are not able to digitally grasp fruit, and either waste fruit trying to tear into it or must wait for fruit to fall to the ground where it quickly despoils and is not a dependable food source. Being able to directly access the fruit of trees like those in the *Prunus* genus promoted the evolution of hands which specifically evolved to help our ancestors colonize an underutilized environmental niche after the disappearance of larger dinosaur species from the landscape and thus also evolve alongside those food sources to become the animals we are today.

Plants also do not possess efficient pathways for elimination, and fruit probably evolved originally not as a reproductive strategy but as a system for waste disposal, structures into which were sequestered elements not useful to the plant such as excess of halides, boron, and salts to be shed or discarded but which animals and insects discovered and exploited as a source of nutrition which plants thereafter in turn exploited as a means also of propagation and cooperation. Our first use of tools (even before becoming human) was also likely the use of rocks to smash open the pits of *Prunus* fruit to access the delicious seeds inside, which are almonds because almonds are also a *Prunus* species specifically bred by humans for the sweeter kernel, and all *Prunus* seed is high in healthy saturated and mono-unsaturated fats as well nutrients like protein, molybdenum, lithium, selenium, copper, calcium, oxalate, and even cyanide which is required by our immune system as discussed in that upcoming chapter (never feed children high quantities of other *Prunus* kernels, however, as their cyanide content can sometimes be extreme). It is anecdotally apparent that populations which lack regular consumption of *Prunus* fruit also tend to present with greater cardiovascular and metabolic disease while those with regular consumption do not. The exception is economies which use toxic *sulfur dioxide* to preserve dried apricots and other fruit which oppositely wipes out the microbiome in opposition to the benefits of a diet high in boron and carotene, so regions of the world like the Middle East which would otherwise be healthy from high dietary *Prunus* consumption instead have higher rates of cardiovascular disease than places dominated by industrial food systems like the United States which still has abundant consumption of fresh peaches, nectarines, and plums due to widespread cultivation, and endemic species like black cherry.

This fact of the necessity of *Prunus* fruit in our evolutionary past is also confirmed by the unmatched sensory euphoria of eating good peaches, apricots, plums, and nectarines, which is not arbitrary or subjective, as every biological function we have is a direct design of our evolution and the function of instinct intended to support our exploitation of our environmental niche which does not similarly occur from any other type of food on the entire planet. These fruit do not need to be fresh to be beneficial, however (although fresh is better) and can be juiced, dried, frozen, and preserved so long as preservation lacks toxic chemicals like sulfur dioxide (ascorbic acid or citric acid would be good choices to replace sulfur dioxide). The consumption of *Prunus* fruit daily as much as possible leads to rapid and persistent improvements in health and wellbeing when accompanied by other principles in this book, and those with any metabolic disease such as diabetes, autism, cystic fibrosis, etc., should prioritize the consumption of apricots, peaches, cherries, chokecherries, nectarines, pluots, etc., even planting your own if possible since access to these fruits is often limited or cost prohibitive.

During sun exposure, vasculature in the skin is also stimulated by light to produce *endothelial nitric oxide* which dilates blood vessels and increases blood flow directly to the skin to help collect sulfated vitamin D for distribution throughout the body. After generous sun exposure it is common to feel cold more easily, even if your skin is burned by the sun and feels hot to the touch (*do not get sunburned*), because the dramatically increased blood flow to the skin also causes increased heat loss. The reason this only occurs during sunlight exposure is because the sun also keeps us warm and there is less risk of dangerous heat loss during times when it is warm enough to get sun exposure. Nitric oxide is in turn made primarily from the amino acid *citrulline*, after amination to arginine, and you will remember from the chapter on parasitism that arginine is the primary target of ammonia producing pathogens, so dietary arginine is rapidly converted to many other substrates, including citrulline, to prevent microbial access and then resynthesized back to arginine as needed. Though citrulline can be synthesized in the body from arginine and proline, many so-called non-essential amino acids are often discussed in circular logic as if they come from an infinitesimal pool of substrate and not interchangeable amino acids which in reality must all be got from the diet. Citrulline in fact is the greatest rate limiter for production of endothelial nitric oxide due to the *arginine paradox* in which the body will not use arginine for nitric oxide synthesis when deficient in citrulline, which likely occurs because citrulline is required to condense ammonia back into arginine for elimination in urea, and which shows how citrulline is the primary substrate for this cycle and nitric oxide synthesis.

But nitric oxide helps dilate all blood vessels, and chronic nitric oxide dysregulation is also a common feature of cardiovascular disease, as the immune system also employs nitric oxide to inhibit pathogens and during chronic disease this can and does rapidly deplete citrulline and arginine from the body to cause nitric oxide deficiency which then results in hypertension, high blood pressure, and other complications of cardiovascular disease. Citrulline sufficiency is typically only possible (in an evolutionary sense) when there is abundant food in the environment during warm weather, but fruits of the *Cucurbitaceae* family, commonly called *cucurbits*, are the absolute highest dietary source of citrulline and include cucumbers, watermelon, chayote, melons, squash, pumpkin, etc., which can be eaten all year to maintain citrulline sufficiency (which also helps promote elimination of excess ammonia through urine and often result in an increase in urination for this reason after consumption).

As mentioned earlier, cucurbits are also high in molybdenum, as are other refreshing foods like peas, nuts, and even spring water, as the taste of refreshing things like spring water, peas, and cucumbers is in fact the taste of molybdenum, and the reason molybdenum tastes so pleasant is in part because the *molybdenum cofactor* required in enzymes like sulfite oxidase is actually one of the oldest biological molecules on Earth and is found in nearly every life form in existence. In those who are ill it is *required* to consume cucurbits daily to support sulfur metabolism and ammonia metabolism, and will directly support recovery and cardiovascular health in general after consistent suppression of microbial hydrogen sulfide and hydrogen selenide with carotene. Pathogens which respirate on nitrate (which can be made from nitric oxide) also use molybdenum as a cofactor, which another reason molybdenum deficiency occurs during disease, but toxic agrochemicals like glyphosate also bind molybdenum, and molybdenum deficiency can thus become so toxic that is causes severe sulfur-deficiency symptoms like profound insomnia, mood disorders, and trouble detoxifying toxic products from the liver.

Studies also show that anthocyanin (purple, blue, and dark red pigments in fruits like berries, plums, cherries, etc.) promotes the increased production of endothelial nitric oxide, which likely reflects the protective effect of anthocyanins against pathogenic microbes, so consumption of *Prunus* fruit or other sources of anthocyanin also increases the dilation of blood vessels during sun exposure to increase collection and distribution of vitamin D and improved cardiovascular function when consumed on a daily basis as possible.

Because of its intense demand for blood flow and high neurological tissue, our brain is the highest consumer of nitric oxide in the body, and our evolutionary proximity to watermelon in eastern-central Africa at the time we later evolved into humans seems to imply that our brain size is a direct consequence of access to watermelon and other cucurbits high in citrulline rather than any other environmental or behavioral theory (red watermelon is also high in carotene and anthocyanin). After the disappearance of dinosaurs from the landscape, large cucurbit fruits were just sitting around waiting to be consumed and were rapidly exploited by animals which also grew very large such as the *Proboscideans* (elephants and related ancestors), but in we wily humans this excess of dietary citrulline relative to body size allowed our brain to increase considerably instead, and I believe it was access to both fire and watermelon specifically which caused us to become the evolutionary humans we are today. Considering that citrulline is required for healthy blood flow and many other metabolic pathways and that watermelon is also a potent source of carotenoids and molybdenum many metabolic illnesses could be accurately described as a '*watermelon deficiency*.' Consuming watermelon outside in the summertime is a rite of passage for most children on the planet, but it is not simply hedonistic and does in fact fulfill basic physiologic pathways required for human nutrition which many of us fail to practice now as adults in our cloistered and industrial lifestyles, and daily consumption of cucurbits, especially first thing in the day before sun exposure or consumption of dietary protein, is highly effective in promoting human health.

As illnesses like tuberculosis and rickets began to be treated with exposure to the outdoors and sunshine it naturally led to a culture of sun-bathing and outdoor recreation across Europe and South America and the establishment of a more easy-going and recreational approach to life which includes generous, paid time away from work and indoor seclusion which places like the United States and other materialism obsessed cultures have yet to adopt, but is also precisely why places like the United States are burdened with high rates of diabetes and other metabolic disease because the human body never evolved to spend life indoors away from sunlight and soil, eating diets low in fruit, sugar, and high in grain and animal products. Failing to appreciate the benefit of sun exposure and the healing effects of recreation we in the U.S. and other stridently overworked societies continue to suffer the consequences while the rest of the world builds access to their outdoors with walkable cities and safe biking infrastructure, flocking to beaches, mountains, and swimming pools to soak up the healing rays of the sun to create healthy and happy populations. Our ancestors used to spend most waking hours walking around in direct sunlight, farming or gathering which exposed them to the microbiome environment, and eating nutrient dense foods like nuts, fruit, roots, and shellfish, especially before the time we wore clothes, and our biology is still exactly the same as theirs and thus suffers when deprived of this environmental niche in which it evolved. If places to fulfill these requisites do not exist it is likely you live in a car-dependent hellscape destroyed by capitalism, and you can move somewhere with parks, trails, nature, gardens, swimming holes, and an abundance of third places even if it means making less money because what is success anyway if you're too ill to enjoy it. Or you can organize, petition government, run for office, boycott businesses and people who prevent change, or start a non-profit and get these made in the place where you live.

The hormones *pregnenolone* and *progesterone* are also widely available as supplements (only use natural forms) and can temporarily help make up for deficiencies in cholesterol and expand blood volume by helping to regulate electrolytes and water as discussed in the upcoming chapter on hormones, and will be necessary for anyone who is very ill or very aged to recover more effectively. Like most hormones, these are also a casualty of cholesterol dysregulation and can be restored as discussed in that chapter. The upcoming chapter on immunity will also further assist in the removal of pathogens which contribute these problems required to make a full recovery.

CHAPTER 11

CALCIUM, PAIN, RESPIRATION

By the time I was sixteen I was already six-foot four and still growing. People gawk and ask about my height whenever I step foot out of my house which, when I was younger, also gave me a bit of agoraphobia. When I lived in Utah questions about my height were always followed by wondering if I was a basketball player. I couldn't hide or blend in *anywhere,* and people strangely assumed that because you're tall you also possess other traits they desire such as an absence of insecurity and fear, better basketball skills, or a thirteen-inch penis. As a teenager my clothes never fit right, either too short if they came from normal stores or billowed like church bells on my thin frame if from a big and tall retailer. Thankfully some stores finally began to make tall sizes that fit properly, and as a young adult I taught myself to sew and amateurely tailor my clothes and for a few years I got to dress really well until I realized the reason my skin always felt weird after touching their products was due to toxic, endocrine disrupting chemicals used to promote stupid marketing points like "no-iron" and "soft-washed," which really just means the company doesn't care at all about our physical heath nor their impact on the environment, making synthetic fibers like polyester and nylon which contaminate our bodies with plastic toxins and cause microplastics to show up even in male testicles.

One question to arise in a conversation about my height is often *why.* I usually respond with a tired joke about eating all your vegetables or drinking milk or something, because to most people achieving height seems an illusive and mysterious lottery and issue of supreme import. In truth if we were half the size we are the world would be twice as big for us, and desiring to be large is simply a desire for security borne from experiences of powerlessness as children which does not actually bring any of the imagined benefits. But height is a very simple formula and there are exactly two reasons for large growth. The first is that being very tall is not actually healthy. Anyone over six-foot-four (I'm now six-foot-seven) is usually tall because their thyroid function didn't fully mature in a timely manner as it should have. Thyroid in an adult causes maturation and a change from *quantitative* growth into *differentiated* growth (or *qualitative* growth), which means that rather than increasing the amount of cells in the body it begins changing and maturing those cells into secondary and specialized traits possessed by adults, which is why shorter people are often more healthy than those who are very large as it is a result of environmental and nutritional stress in which a larger body grows in order to better compete in a stressful environment but which also compromises the health of the individual. A study on tadpoles once administered thyroid very early in their lifespan and the tadpoles developed into fully mature frogs in appearance but at the tiny size they were currently, producing very mini versions of adult frogs. The opposite happens when thyroid is delayed—organisms grow larger and adult differentiation is late because they grow for a longer period of time. Those with gigantism should take thyroid hormones and address their thyroid health which will arrest quantitative growth and promote cellular differentiation.

Additionally, most gay boys experience adolescence on the same timeline as girls, between eleven and thirteen years of age, and grow early just as girls do, so I was *always* tall and never really had a growth spurt the way heterosexual boys do who more often start adolescence later between thirteen and fifteen and continue growing sometimes even into their early twenties. I started adolescence between eleven and twelve and grew early and was often lauded for my height as if it were something I chose, where my straight brother didn't begin growing until about fourteen which, to him and others, seemed like I was maturing into a man more quickly when in reality it was because I was homosexual (this is not always the case but is usually the case). In addition to this very early growth my thyroid disorder, caused by a poor diet and metabolic disease from pathogenic colonization, delayed my thyroid function and the combination created a situation in which I continued to grow past my determined height which would have been about six-foot four (you can double the height of a child at two years of age and that will be their approximate adult height if there is no interference).

But even with deranged thyroid function I would never have been able to grow to such height without the second factor in growth, and that is *calcium*. Cultures with traditionally low calcium intake (or factors which block calcium absorption) are all shorter in stature. Although this has a lot to do with bones which are made largely of calcium and provide structure to the body, calcium is also required in the *endoplasmic reticulum* which is an organelle in all cells where proteins, enzymes, and other components required for growth and biological functions are actually synthesized. So calcium deficiency not only prevents robust bone growth but also the function of every cell which thus affects overall growth.

Asian and American demographics are a good dichotomic example of this growth function. Because of passively racist attitudes, Americans think of people with Asian heritage as being shorter due to race. But there is no such thing as race, and features of homogenous groups of people are no different than having brown hair or blonde hair and are just physical differences mediated by *epigenetics*. Height has less to do with genes and more to do with the nutritional composition of diets during the growth phase (and even gestation). This is why so many people of pure Asian genetic descent (and yes I mean all residents of what is colloquially considered geographic Asia from those in the Indo-Pacific to Indians in the subcontinent to Afghans on the Western side) who grow up in America end up just as tall as other Americans. I have a friend whose entire ancestry is Chinese, whose parents and grandparents are all well under six-foot, who is also six-foot seven-inches tall like me because he also grew up on a similar American diet with generous access to milk and pasta. Calcium from dairy is the primary driver of the height in Western cultures and all nations with above-average height trends are generally large consumers of some kind of dairy products (though there are plenty of other calcium sources like leafy greens, nuts, etc.). The Maasai of Africa, for example, also use milk as a cornerstone of their diets. I had milk every morning when growing up and also as a snack of sorts between meals, after school, swim practice, and late-night cereal with friends. Leafy greens such as are consumed by cultures that do not rely on milk have really great calcium content, but leafy greens are harder to break down and require a healthy microbiome and often contain factors like oxalic acid or phytic acid which can potentially limit calcium absorption. Indians actually consume quite a bit of dairy but their diet is also high in legumes which contain an abundance of isoflavones and phytate which likely limits the effect of high dietary calcium. Like fruit, milk is *intended* by nature to be consumed as a food, so it not only lacks anti-nutrients but can contain other helpful factors like lactoferrin and oligosaccharides which help manage a healthy microbiome and inhibit pathogens.

Dairy fat is also good for us because cows and other ruminants harbor populations of specialized bacteria for the disarming of antinutrients as well as the conversion of polyunsaturated fats to monounsaturated and saturated fats. This is why dairy milk is higher in saturated fat than the plants they eat (and thus so delicious), because bacteria in the guts of ruminants chemically convert fats to those which are healthier for the animal, and thus ourselves, which we sadly lack. Often when experiencing digestive stress with dairy foods a person is quick to identify lactose or dairy as the culprit, but lactose intolerance is actually the effect of unhelpful bacteria feeding on undigested lactose in our own guts rather than any problem with lactose itself, and simply avoiding dairy does nothing to eradicate or control for those opportunists which continue to persist in the gut and cause illness regardless of dairy consumption.

Often the problem with dairy is that American breeds of cattle were bred to overproduce milk, because this hybridization mutated the casein protein in A1 type dairy cow milk to substitute a *proline* amino acid with a *histidine* which is the precursor to *histamine* which is then used by histamine producing microbes to overload our body with excess histamine, which is a highly stimulatory biogenic amine which then causes symptoms like excess mucus and phlegm production, neurological overstimulation, and chronic immune activation. Because of the effect of A1 dairy it is very helpful to consume only sources that are *not* from A1 cattle, which can mean the use of other types of dairy like goat milk, sheep milk, buffalo, or milk from cows that do not typically carry the A1 gene like Guernsey cows (Jersey cows typically have far less A1 than American Holstein but still do have some) or milk from A2 identified cattle.

Pasteurization of dairy products is fine and does help prevent the spread of food borne pathogens like tuberculosis without destroying much of the nutrition quality of milk (it's pasteurized when you cook it anyway), but the *homogenization* process which combines the fat and water portions of milk is extremely harmful to milk and human health because the process both destroys helpful milk proteins like lactoferrin and introduces massive quantities of oxygen into the final product which oxidizes the milk and promotes aerobic microbial overgrowth in the gut. Studies have shown that homogenized milk does not last as long on store shelves, because the oxygen better promotes despoiling microorganisms.

Whipping cream or half and half are also often cheated with gums and binders to make the product appear thicker than it really is, to cheat consumers so the extra fat can be siphoned off for use in other products like butter, but which can lead to digestive stress which is then blamed on dairy. Fat products like cream and butter are also the reason for low-fat milk, which tastes revolting due to its deficient fat content, which is not a healthful food but was instead shopped onto the consumer using false health claims in order to sell the otherwise useless byproduct of cream and butter manufacture. The dairy industry itself is solely responsible for their own decline over the intervening decades due to their incompetence and malfeasant adulteration of their own products, because who the fuck wants to consume disgusting low-fat milk, but of course people are going to buy it because of ridiculous dieting behaviors but whom then grow to hate milk because of the awful taste of these products. Milk also contains trace amounts of *chlorophyl*, so storage and transport of milk in transparent or translucent cartons results in the *active* oxidation of milk, as store lights react with the chlorophyl particulate to oxidize milk as it sits on store shelves to produce an even grosser-tasting product. Fucking hell clean up your industry, you weirdos.

But access to such amounts of calcium and foods like milk can also be a double-edged sword because although calcium is extremely important for our health its excess or dysregulation of calcium metabolism can cause significant metabolic distress, promote soft tissue calcification, and encourage colonization by microbes like *Candida* and *H. pylori* which thrive in an alkaline or neutral pH environment and use calcium to buffer themselves against our immune system to cause conditions like white tongue which can and do persist for long periods of time. In more severe states of calcification these microbes cause life threatening *calciphylaxis* or *milk-alkali syndrome* which almost entirely impairs the immune system and promotes necrosis and infection—A famous comic book artist once died from this type of immune inhibition wrongly attributed to their drinking of raw milk—he in fact died from severe *candidiasis* which caused a heart attack, and the milk was a very likely factor not for being raw, as pasteurization does not kill *Candida* (most people harbor *Candida* anyway), but for absence of acidic factors like vitamin D and vitamin K required to metabolize calcium which, when deficient, can then result in death from excessive calcium consumption.

Vitamin D is required for proper calcium metabolism because the presence of vitamin D increases extraction of *citric acid* from the citric acid cycle (yes, the same kind of acid in lemons and other citrus) and citric acid strongly binds free calcium to prevent calcification of soft tissue. During vitamin D repletion greater zinc influx into cells slows the enzyme *aconitase* which in turn slows citric acid consumption (for the production of energy) to produce an accumulation of citrate which then reacts very strongly to also decalcify soft tissue. Endogenous citric acid is the primary factor used by the body to prevent chronic calcification which causes chronic pain and promotes pathogenesis, but citric acid is also directly synthesized from carbohydrate, so failing to get sufficient sunlight, eating low-carbohydrate diets, carotenoid deficiency, zinc deficiency, or impairments to cholesterol production from which vitamin D is synthesized under exposure to sunlight directly promotes calcification, pathogenesis, and chronic pain, while resolving those issues will instead help to reverse it. Studies show that a citric acid deficiency specifically causes stress to the endoplasmic reticulum, the site of protein synthesis in cells which requires lots of calcium, which then impairs synthesis of enzymes, proteins, immune factors, and other components important to cell function and resistance to disease and pathogens. Citrate has also been shown to suppress tumor growth by inhibiting glycolysis (meaning glycolysis as the energy source since glycolysis also directly feeds into the citric acid cycle), which is the process by which cancer cells produce lactate from carbohydrate which promotes cancer and metabolic disease, because the citric acid cycle instead drives mitochondrial respiration. But I also believe citric acid prevents calcium from reacting inappropriately with phosphorus, which then keeps more phosphorus free to function in specifically phosphate dependent pathways like ATP, ADP, AMP, and protein phosphorylation which drives metabolism. Studies confirm that an increase in citrate improves phosphate status in the body, so restoration of vitamin D function directly promotes energy production and resolution of pain by increasing energy production from an increased availability of phosphorus. Cancer often presents with hypophosphatemia (phosphate deficiency) but phosphate status is shown by studies to be poorly correlated with dietary phosphate, meaning that other factors influence phosphate status more strongly than the content of dietary phosphate, which in this case is related to vitamin D and endogenous citric acid.

Though it is also well known that vitamin D promotes increased absorption of calcium from the diet the exact mechanism has not actually been elucidated. Since citric acid is highly reactive to metals like calcium I believe it is simply the extraction of citric acid from the citric acid cycle under the influence of vitamin D which promotes increased absorption of calcium from food. Because of its relationship to calcium, citric acid made by our body also participates in the growth of bones, teeth (but not enamel), and prevents calcification of soft tissues such as the cardiovascular system, mucosal tissue, and kidneys, and bone is actually the densest site of citric acid concentration in the body, especially craniofacial bone, and citric acid is the primary agent responsible for holding bone together. This means that (endogenous) citric acid production is the primary protective factor against *osteoporosis,* which is why vitamin D supplements sometimes but not always help treat osteoporosis, because it is citric acid made under the influence of vitamin D which mediates bone health and other calcium and phosphorus related functions and not vitamin D directly. Because citrate is synthesized from carbohydrate, this also means that low-carb dieting also impairs citrate production, regardless of vitamin D status, and low carbohydrate diets directly contribute to osteoporosis and other calcium related disorders. During the era when *rickets* was a common disease of children, which is characterized by fragile bones and poor bone development caused by deficiency of sunlight and thus vitamin D, an enterprising doctor showed rickets could be cured by administration of dietary citric acid alone, regardless of vitamin D status. This is also why vitamin D is shown to help support the cardiovascular system, because citric acid helps decalcify the soft tissues of the cardiovascular system to keep cells free of calcium crystals. For this reason, urine is also high in citric acid (which is why peeing can sometimes sting, if there are lesions or infection of the urinary tract), which primarily functions to prevent kidney stones, and kidney stones are also thus a consequence of deficient citric acid production, dieting, and sunlight deprivation (dietary citric acid and magnesium can help rapidly resolve kidney stones).

Populations which don't traditionally consume large quantities of calcium also don't develop bodies which are as dependent on calcium, and nor are they prone to obesity because their calcium intake tends to be properly balanced by proportional intake of vitamin K which is the primary factor required for healthy calcium metabolism through the function of *vitamin K dependent proteins* made in the body which acidify calcium through carboxylation (carbonation). Many people rarely consume leafy greens, which are the highest source of dietary vitamin K, and quickly descend into metabolic illness because such extreme deficiency of vitamin K leads to rapid calcium dysregulation and exploitation by calcium-dependent pathogens. Not only this, but our gut microbiome which also produces nutrients and protects us from pathogens are also highly dependent on vitamin K and produce more potent forms of vitamin K (phylloquinone) called vitamin K2 (menaquinone) which are even stronger than vitamin K1.

One of the most consequential problem of calcium dysregulation is that opportunistic microbes use calcium to cause *saponification* of dietary fats, which is the formation soap from reaction of fatty acids with alkali elements like calcium, sodium, and potassium, and the formation of these biosoaps then have a surfactant effect on our protective mucosal layer and the biofilms of commensal microbial populations, dissolving them away and allowing pathogens unfettered access to underlying mucosal tissues. This also blocks the absorption of dietary fats, which is also catastrophic because most hormones are made from cholesterol which is itself made primarily from dietary fat. As discussed in the chapter on vitamin D, it is also made from cholesterol which means that disruption to normal fat digestion and metabolism due to calcium dysregulation also impairs vitamin D synthesis to worsen calcium dysregulation and prevent recovery from disease. There is no current science which adequately investigates the role of saponification of dietary fats by pathogens in the gut, but it is well known that soaps form spontaneously in the presence of strong alkali, and since pathogens harvest of calcium from our tissues and produce highly alkaline ammonia the formation of soaps from dietary fat is inevitable and likely a purposeful mechanism by which pathogens cause disease. Studies do show an increase of methane production by 250% in the gut of rats from saponification of dietary fatty acids.

While soaps can form from reaction with any alkali, calcium is also far worse than sodium or potassium because it results in the formation of metallic *grease*, and during metabolic disease many people then present with fatty, greasy stools which are indicative not only of this saponification and calcium dysregulation but then also of malabsorption of fats, fat soluble nutrients, calcium, and severe disruption of the commensal microbiome. It is also well known that all cells in the human body accumulate cholesterol, which is both incorporated into the membrane of cells and used in the synthesis of hormones, proteolipids, phospholipids, lipoproteins, etc., and required for the metabolism of electrolytes, water, and mitochondria and other cellular organelles, and the saponification of fatty acids by opportunistic microbes is thusly the most fundamental disruption of metabolism which underlies all metabolic disease, both by shielding pathogens from the immune system and disturbing the normal digestion of dietary fats (especially healthy saturated fats). Saponification of dietary fats and fat malabsorption always leads to obvious symptoms such as *steatorrhea* (fatty stools) and *hyposteroidogenesis* (low hormone production), but steatorrhea is easy to identify, since fatty stools are very obvious, and hyposteroidogenesis (as discussed in the chapter on hormones) always occurs in anyone with long term, chronic metabolic illness and is the reason for loss of secondary sex characterics, energy, vitality, etc.

Since pathogens use calcium to cause this problem, there is a very useful tool in dietary *oxalate* which ca be used to restrain their calcium, since oxalate strongly binds calcium and can help rob opportunistic intestinal pathogens of the calcium they use to cause fat saponification and inhibit the immune system. Oxalate is greatly misunderstood, often considered an antinutrient because it binds to calcium, but is actually generally protective against disease simply because it prevents pathogens from accessing the calcium they require to cause illness, even if it does compromise some calcium absorption. Calcium oxalate is also often a factor in kidney stones and joint pain, so health advocates frequently recommend avoiding dietary oxalate and characterize it as harmful, and indeed some people with poor health can experience problems like kidney failure from suddenly consuming large doses of dietary oxalate. But dietary oxalate is also metabolized to acetic acid by commensal microbes like *Bifidobacterium* and *Oxalobacter* which not only helps to normalize the gut microbiome and support commensal species but also restores intestinal pH, bile, and nutrient production by commensals while protecting calcium from pathogens. Oxalate is rapidly absorbed into the body, but calcium oxalate is not absorbed at all, so this benefit of promoting commensal microbes is achieved from the formation of calcium oxalate in the diet itself, or what occurs when oxalate scavenges calcium from the environment of the gut. Consuming too much oxalate and too little calcium will definitely result in calcium deficiency, though that is more a function too little calcium intake, and while studies on oxalate in rodents show reduced absorption of some calcium in the presence of oxalate they also show an *increase* in bone mineralization and reduced soft tissue calcification, demonstrating improved calcium bioavailability and better calcium status, which is far more important to our health than the total absorption anyway.

Most tellingly, our body itself purposefully produces oxalate from glyoxylate, oxaloacetate, glycine, and vitamin C, a fact which many proponents of low-oxalate diets seem incredibly confused, as more than 90% of oxalate secreted in the urine *does not come from the diet*, but from production in the liver, and microbes can also convert vitamin C to oxalate, which entirely demonstrates that problems with oxalate metabolism are not usually a problem of dietary intake, since our own body can and does produce it. Studies also show an increase in endogenous oxalate production during parasitism irrespective of dietary oxalate consumption, and knowing pathogens use calcium as a strategy to infect our bodies and rebuff our immune system this seems to indicate that oxalate is *not* a cause of disease but a purposeful biological defensive response to invasive parasites meant to scavenge the calcium they otherwise exploit for colonization and infection. Those with autism are found to have higher circulating oxalates, which leads many people to recommend a low oxalate diet for those with autism, but a low oxalate diet does nothing to address symptoms of autism, and may even make it worse since this increases calcium availability for pathogens. Those with cystic fibrosis also have higher rates of osteoporosis, even in childhood, which is the manifestation of calcium dysregulation as an underlying etiology of immune dysregulation. Advocating for low dietary oxalate in conditions like autism and cystic fibrosis is even more ridiculous considering they begin in very young children whom absolutely do not have high dietary oxalate as oxalate is highly distasteful to children whom require higher calcium intake to promote greater bone growth and development. My own diet growing up was *extremely* low in oxalate, primarily from potatoes once or twice a week (which are only moderate in oxalate), but many children with high oxalate diets do not have autism, cystic fibrosis, or other common childhood diseases, and considering the body produces the far greater quantity of oxalate it is clear that oxalate is an adaptive response to parasitism meant to scavenge free calcium, for which dietary sources can be similarly used.

As discussed in the chapter on vitamin D, the formation of calcium oxalate crystals in the kidney or other organs of the body is also a symptom of vitamin D deficiency, as vitamin D is required to make *citric acid* endogenously from dietary carbohydrate (yes, the same kind of acid found in lemons and other citrus). Citric acid is a significant component of urine and primary regulator of calcium which prevents kidney stone formation, and problems with oxalate such as stones and kidney disease are instead a problem of vitamin D deficiency or other impairment of endogenous citric acid production (such as low-carb dieting or diabetes which impairs carbohydrate metabolism). But since vitamin D is made from cholesterol which is made from fat which can be saponified by opportunistic microbes, vitamin D cannot be restored anyway during chronic saponification of dietary fats, making dietary oxalate a crucial tool in restoration of normal metabolism of dietary calcium and fat (using a vitamin D supplement in those who are very aged or ill can possibly help restore some citric acid production).

Further evidence that oxalate is actually useful for the body and used to inhibit pathogens is that mucosal tissues *actively transport* oxalate to the mucosal tissue and secretes oxalate through the mucosal barrier. While this could be construed as elimination there's not much reason for this to occur in non-digestive mucosal organs like the lungs and reproductive systems, and given oxalate's promotion of commensal microbes and binding of calcium otherwise exploited by mucosal pathogens is highly suspicious and instead seems to indicate the body using oxalate to actively curate populations of healthy commensal microbes while protecting calcium from microbes which are harmful.

Dairy is thus a primary reason for the high rates of metabolic disease in Western cultures, not because there is anything wrong with dairy but because these diets are also typically low in vitamin K, oxalate, vitamin C, tannins, and other nutrients which are required to properly metabolize such high dietary calcium as dairy provides, while industrialized societies also frequently suffer from chronic deficiency of sun exposure and thus also vitamin D deficiency. Dairy also contains lots of phosphate, which also helps metabolize calcium, but grass-fed dairy has a much higher vitamin K content than from dairy animals constrained on feed lots fed only grain and hay. Certain cheeses like parmesan are very high in vitamin K2 due to the presence of certain microbes used to make the cheese and are an excellent source of calcium for this reason. While foods such as leafy greens are our primary sources of dietary vitamin K, vitamin K2 made by our commensal microbiome are far more powerful and thus more effective in promoting normal calcium metabolism, so problems of calcification of soft tissue which underlies metabolic disease is a direct consequence of gut dysbiosis and derangement of the commensal microbiome and colonization by opportunistic microbes. While dietary vitamin K is a major requisite for our health, its greatest benefit in fact comes from promoting *vitamin K2* production from our commensal microbiome. Some people think we can take a supplement of vitamin K1 or K2 and while this may be helpful there are at least eleven different types of K2 made by the microbiome, all of which are very poorly understood by science, and a supplement of vitamin K1 or K2 can never, ever replace the function of dietary vitamin K in support of the microbiome and production of vitamin K2. Places like France continue to consume sufficient vitamin K and oxalates in their normal diets and have higher standards of food production such as for milk and cheese from cows naturally low in A1 protein grazing in pasture rather than feed lots and so do not have such metabolic health epidemics as countries like the United States. Places like Japan and China still consume immense amounts of vitamin K and oxalate foods, even for breakfast, so they also have very low rates of metabolic disease since they also don't consume much dietary calcium in ratio to dietary vitamin K and oxalate, which strongly promotes vitamin K2 producing commensal microbes to benefit health even greater than vitamin K1 alone.

Pathogens which produce ammonia also find milk an ideal substrate because of its high protein and total absence of tannin. Young animals, including human children, do not require strong tannins (those in fruit are usually sufficient) because their physiology prevents excessive absorption of iron, and lack of adult sex hormones generally prevents colonization by some parasites that otherwise derange the commensal microbiome to more easily benefit from milk as what occurs in adults. So adults with any degree of health problems will find that milk contributes to production of ammonia, hydrogen sulfide, and histamine if not protected by tannin, carotene, and oxalate at the time of consumption. This is not too difficult to achieve since tea is very high in tannin, carotene, oxalate, and vitamin K, and tea brewed in milk is very delicious. In fact, most of India and Pakistan have prepared their tea in milk for generations, but this is not the same as preparing tea in water then adding milk after, because vitamin K is fat soluble and oxalate reacts to calcium, and not much of either are imparted to water extraction of tea, so tea must be prepared in hot milk, which will result in significant migration of vitamin K, carotene, and oxalate into the milk while the tannins will bind the protein and water to inhibit microbial ammonia production, and should be allowed to steep for at least 15 minutes for best results (this will not work well with reduced-fat milk either, and milk boils over very rapidly, so watch the pot!). Chocolate (cocoa) is also high in tannin and oxalate, and homemade chocolate milk or the use of cinnamon or berries or other spices in milk are also very effective for children (store bought chocolate milk usually contains highly allergenic emulsifiers like carrageenan or gums which should be avoided, however). One of the reasons my consumption of milk and casein in my early recovery was so successful was that it nearly always occurred in fruit smoothies with generous quantities of frozen organic berries which added plenty of tannin, carotenes, and anthocyanin to protect its digestion in my gut from opportunistic microbes even before I knew about any of those phytochemicals or the pathogens they inhibit.

Because many leafy greens high in vitamin K like spinach, kale, broccoli, basil, parsley, etc., are quite common it is very easy to get more than enough daily vitamin K, even through indulgent foods like pesto or creamed spinach. But vitamin K is very poorly absorbed into the body, with studies often showing only about 5% on average from plain leafy greens, but an increase of up to 15% absorption when prepared in dietary fat, since vitamin K is fat soluble. Many leafy greens like spinach and purslane are also high in oxalate, which makes the task of protecting dietary calcium an easy thing to accomplish. While there are plenty of options for dietary oxalate there is little consistency in food types, so choices are limited to specific options, for instance cooked spinach is one of the highest with about 1500 mg of oxalate per cup but only about 2 mg per cup in kale, so not even all leafy greens are reliable sources, and dietary oxalate can be included in meals or taken before or during a meal. Some high oxalate options are spinach, guava, star fruit, amaranth, purslane, collards, sorrel, beet greens, okra, rhubarb, parsley, silverbeet, radishes, plantains and banana, black pepper, chives, parsley, and cassava (the whole root, not refined flour). Some moderately high options which can be included but will not on their own be sufficient for therapy are potatoes, nuts like almond and hazelnut, raspberries, pineapple, corn, whole grains, asparagus, green beans, snap peas, ginger, garlic, broccoli, brussels sprouts, lettuce, and cocoa (and thus also high-cocoa chocolate). Delicious high oxalate fruits like guava, raspberries, and pineapple make great additions to foods high in calcium or fats to easily achieve these benefits.

Many people who have severe calcium dysregulation likely find high oxalate foods instinctively offensive to taste, because of our body's instinctual regulation of dietary cravings which are moderated by its nutritional status, and in this case it will be required to also consume more dietary calcium simultaneously to vitamin K and oxalate foods, using tea or other preferable sources effectively. Because neonates consume only milk, children of mothers deficient in vitamin D, vitamin K, and oxalate can also become colonized by *Candida,* causing *thrush,* which also often affects the mother simultaneously since the rise in prolactin during breast-feeding mobilizes large quantities of calcium (which mostly comes from bones if the diet is too low in calcium or high pathogenic saponification of the gut which disturbs calcium uptake), and is likely a consequence of the mother not consuming sufficient dietary vitamin K, calcium, oxalate (studies confirm there is oxalate in human milk), or not getting enough daily sunshine, or engaging in low-carb dieting which impairs production of citrate, and it is required for mothers actively bearing children to consume calcium daily, protected by dietary vitamin K and oxalate, and to get sufficient carbohydrate and sunshine (decaffeinated milk tea taken in the morning while getting sunshine for instance can accomplish all these requirements).

Calcium problems get even more complicated, however, because all physical pain is actually also mediated by cellular calcium regulation. Calcium is normally contained mostly to the extracellular space where it helps promote osmotic regulation and functions like the fluid volume of blood and lymph, and only small amounts of calcium are fluxed through cells to run organelles like the endoplasmic reticulum, and immediately effluxed as soon as its function is achieved. But this management of calcium is ATP dependent, through the *calcium, sodium ATPase exchanger,* and injury or insult to cells impairs the production of ATP required to keep calcium out of cells which then causes rapid and uncontrolled intracellular calcification which is then relayed as a pain signal to the brain. Chronic pain often originates from injury, scar tissue, and even pathogenic organisms, which is due to chronic inhibition of normal cellular respiration and the production of ATP, and reversing dysfunctional energy production as discussed throughout this book helps to restore the ability for cells to reverse intracellular calcium excess and to thus not only resolve chronic pain but also heal and regenerate tissue through the normalization of calcium function.

While medicines like ibuprofen and acetaminophen are effective pain relievers (analgesics) they also delay cellular healing and actually worsen clearance of intracellular calcium and increase the duration of pain and injury because they too strongly impair inflammation, as good inflammation is actually required to stimulate repair and regrowth of damaged tissue, which cannot occur without that inflammation. They also powerfully deplete sulfate required for synthesis of *taurine* and *glutathione* and sulfation of cholesterol and hormones which also help protect cells from calcification and excessive cellular excitation caused by excess calcification. Since microbial hydrogen sulfide production also depletes sulfur, the use of medications while also colonized by hydrogen sulfide producing microbes can rapidly deplete sulfur and thus promote significant chronic pain ironically because of the frequent, overuse of painkillers and resultant deficiency of sulfates.

Many women I know have experienced delayed, slow healing after labor because the use of ibuprofen and acetaminophen so powerfully slows the healing process, by excessively inhibiting inflammation required to allow cells to grow and regenerate in the process of *mitosis.* Instead, aspirin is a much better tool to address pain as although it is not as effective an analgesic it does accelerate healing and clearance of intracellular calcium by acidifying mitochondria which increases respiration and thus the production of ATP required to help cells normalize calcium, so the time spent in injury and pain is greatly reduced, even if it is not fully inhibited. Of course, it's not ideal to have aspirin circulating in breast milk (but not other NSAIDs either), so they should be used as little as possible after labor, and aspirin is always a better choice for adults than any other pain reliever (although most aspirin is also contaminated with many ingredients, to make them look fancier to justify higher prices, and should be very simply made and cheap, and aspirin should be kept on hand in every home for emergencies).

Sugar also strongly reduces pain and accelerates healing because it so strongly promotes mitochondrial respiration and the production of ATP required to maintain normal flux and efflux of calcium from cells, so long as mitochondria are working properly as discussed in the upcoming chapter on cancer and migraine, which for many people is not the case, and when mitochondria are dysfunctional the production of energy is not sufficient to support fully reversing intracellular accumulation of calcium. Eating sugar and fruit should promote rapid resolution of pain and injury, and if it does not this is a great diagnostic for dysfunctional mitochondria which can and should be addressed by the steps in the chapter on cancer which will help a lot during recovery from labor, pain, surgery, etc.

The ATP molecule is also stabilized and buffered by *magnesium*, and in fact ATP always occurs as ATP-magnesium, not just ATP, which then prevents ATP from dissociating from itself prematurely or reacting to proteins and pathways inappropriately, and an ideal treatment for any kind of pain which also promotes rapid healing, especially of injuries like breaks, tears, sprains, and surgery is the topical application of *magnesium chloride* in some water to the area of the skin around locations of pain. Whenever I assist someone with a broken bone they are amazed at how rapidly the application of topical magnesium chloride solution both helps resolve pain and accelerates bone regeneration (it effectively doubles the healing rate). Someone I know nearly died in a biking accident from a broken neck, and using topical magnesium even just a few times promoted such rapid healing their doctor wondered why they weren't already back to running and jogging after a mere few months. The magnesium chloride solution should not be so strong as to cause skin irritation, which is a sign of excess, but not too little it cannot be tasted strongly in solution (magnesium chloride is also sold as 'magnesium oil,' which must be diluted before use). Because of its role in stabilizing ATP, magnesium directly helps resolve calcification, pain, and injury, by increasing ATP-dependent calcium efflux, and painful conditions caused by calcification of soft tissue such as arthritis can directly be improved by regular use of topical magnesium chloride when supported by the other requisites of calcium homeostasis as discussed in this chapter (arthritis is caused by ammonia producing bacteria feeding on connective tissue which disrupts mitochondrial respiration as discussed in the chapter on cancer). Magnesium chloride solution can dry out quickly, so it can also be helpful to soak a small rag or towel in the solution and hold it to the area for several minutes, giving the solution sufficient time to be absorbed in sweat resorption pathways. Magnesium chloride will sting open wounds and should not be used directly on cuts or lesions, but can be used around them.

Blood coagulation is also a function of calcium through calcium dependent *thrombin* proteins and vitamin K, and aging often presents with conditions like thrombosis, stroke, heart attack, etc., due to dysregulated (increased) coagulation and the dysregulation of calcium which, being dysregulated, spontaneously stimulates coagulation even when it is not needed. Many aged people with cardiovascular disease are also on anti-vitamin-K blood thinners (or beta blockers to stop adrenaline production) to supposedly prevent stroke and heart failure, but these medications also accelerate aging and metabolic decline through vitamin K loss which increases soft tissue calcification, as vitamin K carboxylates calcium metabolizing proteins (adds carbonic acid, or in other words carbonates them) to also assist in metabolism of calcium, and vitamin K dependent proteins are the most important calcium chelator without which tissue calcification then becomes too great for vitamin D and citric acid to have much benefit and becomes overwhelmed by excessive calcium. Citric acid also thins the blood, however, by inhibiting calcium dependent coagulation, and daily consumption of citrus fruits, juice, or a supplement of citric acid could likely replace pharmaceutical blood thinners which otherwise cause vitamin K deficiency and severe health side effects, and problems with coagulation and viscous blood like thrombosis and stroke are instead also a result of cholesterol dysregulation from the formation of calcium soaps (grease) in the gut, as cholesterol is one of the most powerful regulators of water, electrolytes, and blood volume through the function of mineralocorticoids made from cholesterol, so restoring normal digestion of calcium and fats through the use of dietary vitamin K, oxalates, and vitamin D also helps address cardiovascular disease at its root. Unknown to medical professionals, vitamin K does not only promote coagulation but simply regulates it, and studies have shown that high vitamin K intake actually *normalizes* coagulation, not only promoting it, as without vitamin K we cannot use calcium biologically at all, and it then simply circulates freely around in the body, reacting errantly and causing more calcification and aging which also increases susceptibility to pathogenic colonization, where citric acid and endogenous citric acid production are the primary mediator to prevent coagulation which thusly requires the normalization of fat absorption and daily sun exposure.

Studies also show that perturbation of vitamin K directly impairs pancreatic function and production of insulin, and the immediate availability of both vitamin K and calcium together such as occurs from whole food sources rather than taken separately is likely required for the pancreas to produce all the enzymes and insulin and other factors required for good metabolic health (because the endoplasmic reticulum, where most biosynthesis occurs, is highly dependent on calcium), and the reason many people seem to be effortlessly healthy even when they don't eat diets especially high in vitamin K is that vitamin K is normally recycled many thousands of times in a healthy body, so even small quantities of vitamin K can be enough to sustain health in those who are already healthy, especially when the microbiome produces potent vitamin K2 derivatives of vitamin K1. Oxalates also prevent calcium from reacting to vitamin K, which is why foods like spinach high in both vitamin K, calcium, and oxalate can be so good for our health (a reminder that leafy greens are often high in nitrates as discussed in the chapter on parasitism and metabolic disease, which can be removed by first soaking greens in some water for a few minutes then discarding, or the use of dietary acids such as a vinaigrette salad dressing).

If dairy is a problem generally, sautéed leafy greens like kale, spinach, collard greens, or broccoli in fats like butter, olive oil, or coconut oil can be effective since leafy greens are already high in calcium, but could be made more effective with the addition of a little extra calcium such as from a supplement, mixed into the food or taken immediately with it, such as *calcium citrate* or *calcium carbonate*, careful not use excess since calcium overdose can actually cause seizures and other harmful side effects. By the way, the reason adding dairy to leafy greens makes them taste better such as in creamed spinach is because the added calcium binds the oxalates which then increases calcium ratio to oxalate, where calcium oxalate is not absorbed into the body but instead directly feeds the gut commensal microorganisms. So adding calcium to leafy greens sufficiently to neutralize their oxalate is a useful way to purposefully balance calcium with oxalate for this strategy, using taste as the guide and indicator. Make sure to always prioritize taste over function since eating must be pleasant to facilitate compliance, and calcium supplements should generally never be taken or used separately from dietary sources of vitamin K and oxalate which will otherwise only serve to worsen pathogenic colonization due to high free circulating calcium.

It is well known that calcium can inhibit zinc uptake which can effectively cause zinc deficiency during severe calcification, and this occurs because regulation of zinc is highly controlled by calcium pathways, and free calcium directly causes inhibition of zinc regulation, where vitamin K or oxalate-reacted calcium and carboxylated proteins which manage calcium instead help to promote zinc status. Zinc is most important in the function of *zinc finger proteins* which read DNA to transpose DNA information into the production of enzymes, proteins, peptides, etc., so zinc deficiency caused by pathogenic dysregulation of calcium is also a primary etiological mechanism of metabolic disease, and restoring calcium homeostasis and regulation also helps restore effortless zinc repletion from a healthy diet without requiring a supplement (although a low-dose zinc supplement can be taken weekly if needed). Studies also show that oxalate increases zinc absorption, and that zinc deficiency underlies conditions like diabetes and metabolic disease, confirming this dysregulation of calcium as the underlying factor which causes those illnesses.

Calcium deficiency also ironically causes calcification of tissue as low circulating calcium increases *parathyroid hormone* expression which then mobilizes calcium from bones to replace that which is absent from the diet, and parathyroid also increases calcification of soft tissue, so avoiding dietary calcium is never a solution for problems with calcium dysregulation, but instead actively promotes calcification since the bones are always there to provide calcium when the diet is deficient.

Parathyroid function is not only regulated by calcium, however, and just as lithium is related to sodium and participates in sodium pathways but with a stronger ionic charge, calcium function is also replicated strongly by the element *strontium,* which also participates in calcium pathways and can and does enhance calcium related functions. A medication with strontium has long been used as a therapy for osteoporosis, as bones are also a storage site for strontium. An older study I found in the course of this research showed a doctor using strontium to treat epilepsy, and I personally noticed that dosing strontium helped to eliminate a slight tremor in my hands which accompanied my other symptoms and conditions for several years. This effect of strontium is likely simply alleviating the problems caused by calcium dysregulation, however, as strontium is usually quite abundant in the diet and is especially high in mollusks like clams, mussels, oysters, and snails, but is also found in most plant foods. Because strontium is such a powerful analog of calcium it can actually inhibit calcium regulatory pathways excessively and cause severe side effects when taken in excess. For instance strontium can entirely inhibit parathyroid expression which is required to maintain calcium homeostasis, to then ironically also cause calcium deficiency, and strontium is most effective when used during and after resolution of calcium dysregulation, not as a replacement for this requisite, because the normalization of calcium function will then also promote strontium deposition in bone to restore the normal supply and function of strontium, and because of this it only required several moderate doses of strontium over a few months to eliminate my tremor for years afterward. Very specifically, a pointed finger should not tremor, and if it does is an effective diagnostic for severe calcium dysregulation resulting in strontium depletion which can be reversed with a low-dose of strontium but only after the restoration of at least some calcium homeostasis, with this principle applied to more severe states of tremor and seizure such as in epilepsy, Parkinson's, muscular dystrophy, ALS, cerebral palsy, stroke, Tourette syndrome, etc.

Similarly, endogenous deficiency of citric acid also likely underlies seizure disorders due to excessive, uncontrolled free calcium. For instance, olive oil is often a constituent of diets used to address epilepsy, as *oleic acid* stimulates and promotes mitochondrial respiration which results in production of energy and CO_2 used in the carboxylation of vitamin K dependent proteins to properly bind and control calcium, but oleic acid does not fully reverse epilepsy since oleic acid is only one factor which supports respiration and the citric acid cycle and does not on its own provide vitamin D, carbohydrate, zinc, or citric acid which are the other requirements for normal calcium metabolism. All seizure conditions involve excessive influx of calcium into nerve cells which then specifically causes stress to the endoplasmic reticulum and inhibits normal production of neurotransmitters, proteins, peptides, enzymes, etc., which are required to maintain normal neuronal function. Indeed, anti-epileptic drugs function by blocking calcium influx, and why seemingly paradoxical states of hypocalcemia (as measured in the blood) also induce seizures because hypocalcemia *increases* parathyroid hormone which also promotes intracellular calcium influx, which is also why strontium can also help treat tremor and seizure conditions, by helping to lower parathyroid expression, but only if calcium regulation is also normalized. It has been mentioned many times, but these problems are all pathogenic in origin, so all seizure conditions are also rooted in these pathogens which dysregulate calcium and impair the absorption of dietary fats since fats also help to insulate nerve cells. But since healthy saturated fatty acids which are incorporated into cholesterol required for normal cellular function are often low or absent in the diet anyway, the introduction of pathogens which disrupt fat digestion make those with low dietary saturated fats more prone to neurological conditions like seizure due to catastrophic deficiency of protective and regulatory saturated fats. Conditions of seizure can thus also be treated by the daily consumption of citrus foods and juices, especially accompanying dietary sources of saturated fats such as butter, coconut oil, cocoa butter, etc. One useful example for children of this strategy would be something like strong raspberry lemonade with a little added cocoa butter, butter, or coconut oil (the fats should be melted and the lemonade at room temperature to avoid solidification of fat particles, for taste), because the oxalate, citrate, sugar, polyphenols, anthocyanins (tannins), and good fats would most strongly promote commensal gut microbes and absorption of good fats which then protect the nervous system from overexcitation and promote normal vitamin D synthesis which would be most effective when accompanied by daily sun exposure (without the use of sunblock and avoiding sunburn). Raspberries in chocolate, and raspberries, dates, pineapple, or guava in ice cream, milk shakes, or milk smoothies would also be very effective, especially since milk is already high in healthy saturated fats and calcium.

Because CO_2 is required to carboxylate calcium proteins the most important aspect for normal calcium homeostasis is cellular *respiration* itself since, along with ATP, CO_2 is also a primary end product of the respiration pathway. While this terminology may sound strange to lay persons since respiration is normally associated with the act of breathing the term respiration simply means gas exchange, and in humans is associated with the uptake of oxygen not only by the lungs but also by cells for use in mitochondria in the respiratory oxidation of carbohydrate (primarily) for energy production, where oxygen acts as the terminal electron acceptor at the end of the *mitochondrial electron transport chain*. Adenosine triphosphate (ATP) is how our body uses the energy harvested from food, sunlight, and stretching (as discussed in the chapter on sleep) required for pathways like the transport of ions through cells to drive metabolism. But the process of respiration also results in ample carbon dioxide (CO_2), which is often described as a waste gas but which in fact is a requisite substrate for many biological processes such as carboxylation of vitamin K dependent calcium proteins or maintaining normal oxygen pressure, because oxygen and carbon dioxide displace each other from their shared transport vehicle, *hemoglobin* in red blood cells in a phenomenon described by both the *Haldane* and *Borh* effects discovered by John Scott Haldane and August Krogh, respectively, which in reality are the same, single effect where different concentrations of CO_2 and oxygen displace each other depending on concentration and is absolutely required for the normal transport and exchange of oxygen. This means a person can breathe all they want and even take up oxygen into hemoglobin but if there is insufficient CO_2 production by cells that oxygen remains trapped in red blood cells which effectively suffocates tissues regardless of the O_2 status of blood, and impaired O_2 delivery to cells such as occurs in disease also lowers the production of CO_2 required to maintain respiration and CO_2 pressure since CO_2 is produced from pathways driven by oxygen delivery to the respiration pathway. When respiration is interrupted cells then lose the ability to keep ions like sodium and calcium in flux, which then causes cells to accumulate calcium which slows cellular machinery to promote tissue calcification (and pain) due to declining CO_2 production, and since CO_2 is required to maintain respiration by balancing O_2 (oxygen) pressure breathing becomes shallow and causes conditions like shallow breathing, breath holding, sleep apnea, anxiety, and panic attacks as the body becomes deprived of oxygen and does not respirate sufficiently to both drive metabolism and maintain oxygen pressure, then opportunistic microbes take advantage of the low oxygen environment and exploit the increase in calcification to make conditions more severe.

Mitochondrial biogenesis (the increased population of mitochondria) is entirely dependent on vitamin A, so low intake of dietary carotene or problems converting to vitamin A as discussed in the chapter on vitamin D and vascular disease prevents adequate production of both energy and CO_2 simply due to insufficient population of mitochondria. Although mitochondria produce CO_2 they are also called into existence by CO_2, and high CO_2 production from adequate intake of carbohydrate (especially fructose) causes mitochondria fission (dividing) to produce even more mitochondria, ATP, and CO_2. Oppositely when respiration is inhibited mitochondria fuse and become less in number, to produce less and less CO_2 and ATP, which is a characteristic feature of low metabolic rate which occurs during wintertime (light deficiency) or dieting behaviors that restrict carbohydrate. This is the primary reason why dieting is so destructive, because it literally impairs our cell's ability to produce energy, respirate, and produce citric acid required for the maintenance of calcium bioavailability. When I was dying of cancer and cystic fibrosis it felt like I was drowning in the air and burdened with debilitating amounts of anxiety because this functional hypoxia (low oxygen) produces such profound anxiety and hyperventilation as the body desperately attempts to increase oxygen delivery, and I would wake in the dead of night (when I could sleep, which was very rare) gasping for air (sleep apnea causes breath holding while asleep). The only way I could get a breath was to practice bag breathing, which helps by increasing CO_2 concentration by preventing ventilation through rebreathing of exhaled air. But this only works while doing it, and manually increasing CO_2 is never effective in reversing metabolic CO_2 deficiency because this is instead a biochemical problem of deficient oxidative respiration from impaired carbohydrate metabolism, requiring functional mitochondrial, dietary carotene, carbohydrate, boron, etc. Later when I began eating lots of carbs, fruit, and used other tools to increase respiration my breathing returned to normal due to the increase in mitochondrial CO_2 production which resulted in greater production of energy and accompanying feelings of wellness and relaxation and finally the ability to sleep without apnea.

As discussed in the chapter on gut health concerning problems with water filtration, CO_2 spontaneously dissociates into both *carbonic acid* and *bicarbonate* when dissolved in water, according to pH balance, which also occurs in our cells when they produce CO_2, though this process is also accelerated by the enzyme *carbonic anhydrase*, and carbonic acid pulls oxygen from hemoglobin while the bicarbonate helps transport CO_2 back to the lungs where bicarbonate is transformed back into CO_2 for exhalation, or bicarbonate is used in other processes like neutralizing stomach acid after digestion or activating mucus proteins in goblet cells. This interconversion of CO_2 and bicarbonate is the primary mechanism by which the body maintains pH in tissues and fluids, and carbonic anhydrase which accelerates interconversion between them is also zinc dependent, so the dysregulation of calcium which impairs zinc homeostasis also directly impairs the normal maintenance of pH required for normal respiration by impairing the function of carbonic anhydrase. When we are young and healthy our body can produce so much CO_2 from the metabolism of carbohydrate or fat the maintenance of pH and respiration is very easy to accomplish. Infants produce so much CO_2 after eating they must breathe very, very rapidly to properly ventilate all the CO_2 and avoid excessive displacement of oxygen, which can be surprising to first time parents whom understandably think the high rate of breathing is abnormal, though it is expected.

Metabolic disease and aging present with the opposite problem and thus reflect with symptoms like hyperphosphatemia and calcification of tissues with low rates of respiration. This is not yet understood by science or medicine but, because breathing and respiration are the utmost priority for carbon dioxide, what little CO_2 is produced during metabolic disease is directed to maintain the ability to breathe at the expense of all other functions which normally use CO_2, since breathing is paramount to survival, but because a primary function of CO_2 is also the maintenance of pH this lost function is then also replaced by elements like calcium and phosphorus to cause and contribute to states of *hyperphosphatemia* and tissue calcification frequently seen in conditions like kidney disease, diabetes, heart disease, etc., which is normally attributed to high dietary phosphate since many foods like grains, potatoes, dairy, meat, and commercial beverages like cola are significant sources of phosphate. While dietary ratios of phosphate and calcium can and do contribute to calcium and phosphate status, phosphate is primarily supposed to be located *intracellularly,* and its elevation in circulation is a reflection of its backup function assisting in pH maintenance due to insufficient rate of respiration. CO_2 also reacts with ammonia to form urea, which means high extracellular phosphate is also a consequence of ammonia excess (since ammonia is highly alkaline) from ammonia producing pathogens and the resultant decrease in CO2 saturation. Those with conditions like renal failure and tooth decay (discussed in the chapter on oral disease) are strongly advised to limit dietary phosphate and consume more dietary calcium, but phosphate is required to produce energy, and calcium excess without protective factors like oxalate, vitamin D, and vitamin K leads to further promotion of pathogens which exploit dysregulated calcium.

A healthy body can also easily regulate phosphate, and young people with high phosphate diets do not present with hyperphosphatemia because in reality this condition is caused by disruption to respiration and CO2 saturation due to factors like low dietary carotene or low-carbohydrate diets which diminish mitochondrial biogenesis and respiration to result in the decline of carbonic acid and bicarbonate which then causes a myriad of other health problems including and especially states of hyperphosphatemia. Most people are almost never aware of shallow breathing that accompanies states of anxiety, panic attacks, sleep apnea, and general metabolic disease until, as what occurred in my experience, it develops to very severe conditions. Having sleep apnea at the age of thirty-four was extremely demoralizing, as many health problems can be endured with patience but the inability to sleep is simply excruciating, but like many others I tried to treat my sleep apnea with behavioral practices like bag breathing, breathing exercises, mediation, behavioral changes, and medication such as carbonic anhydrase inhibitors (which increase circulating CO2). Many others use CPAP breathing machines to keep them alive during the night, since sleep apnea can be fatal, but none of these solutions solve this problem because it is entirely a function of biochemistry and the cellular respiratory production of carbon dioxide from working mitochondria and dietary carbohydrate that requires consistent and healthy diets and eating habits and not anything that can be managed by medicine, manual intervention, or specialized supplements.

The primary respiratory enzyme in the mitochondrial electron transport chain, *cytochrome oxidase*, is most strongly stimulated by fructose, so starting every day with sweet carbohydrates, especially generous intake of fruit, is the strongest stimulant of mitochondrial respiration because fructose immediately feeds into the citric acid cycle which runs mitochondrial respiration. Vitamin C also activates respiration (as discussed in the upcoming chapter on immunity), which can easily also be satisfied by fruit consumption. Cytochrome (or one of its neighbors in the electron chain) is also sensitive to light, so sun exposure first thing in the morning also starts up respiration and raises the metabolic rate, and when these behaviors are done consistently the body will more easily rehabilitate than when inconsistent, as these are fundamental requirements of our evolutionary biology which evolved in the open environment, constantly exposed to sunshine, feeding on abundant fruit and other foods in our environment.

Studies also show that the cytochrome enzyme is stabilized by *oleic acid,* which means that consumption of dietary oleic acid such as from olive oil and olives, tiger nuts, hazelnuts, almonds, macadamias, pistachios, etc., potentiates the cytochrome enzyme to function longer and better before having to be recycled and remade, which means cells can produce more energy and carbon dioxide in support of metabolic respiration when the diet contains oleic acid on a daily basis. This is also why oleic acid helps treat conditions of seizure, because it promotes an increase in respiration and thus CO2 which further helps the body carboxylate proteins that manage calcium (using vitamin K in that process).

Cytochrome is also directly inhibited by hydrogen sulfide, which also chelates iron and copper, so resolution of microbial hydrogen sulfide through the ubiquitous use of dietary carotene also strongly promotes metabolic respiration by freeing cytochrome. It is even extremely easy to over-promote respiration after resolution of excess hydrogen sulfide, ammonia, and consumption of sugar and vitamin C by over-consuming dietary sources of oleic acid which can lead to significant output of so much CO_2 such as occurred to me one day eating from a bag of hazelnuts causing the lungs become involuntarily obligated to breathe deeper and faster to vent excessive quantities of CO_2. When first recovering from metabolic disease this increase in CO_2 from increased respiration even caused temporary heart palpitations (the heart skipping a beat), which was at first alarming since I had been so used to being ill, but this effect of high CO_2 is a residual consequence of breath holding as an instinctual adaptation to low CO_2, due to excess displacement of oxygen by such high CO_2, but high CO_2 is actually protective of mitochondria and less dangerous than low CO_2 induced hypoxia, and simply breathing normally resolved the problem which completely disappeared after long-term restoration of normal mitochondrial oxidative respiration through these strategies. Whole milk, cream, butter or ghee (clarified butter), olive oil, most nuts, and high-oleic sunflower oil (but not regular sunflower oil) are also useful sources of oleic acid, and without sufficient dietary intake of oleic acid cytochrome oxidase instead becomes destabilized and experiences high turnover which exhausts nutrients and limits production of CO_2 and thus respiration.

It is this function of oleic acid in supporting cytochrome by which oleic acid has its long established benefit to human health, and as an evolutionary human being much of our diet would have consisted of nuts and other foods which contain plenty of oleic acid. Our body can synthesize oleic acid from carbohydrate or the saturated fatty acids *steric acid* and *palmitic acid* which can also be got from the diet and good sources of fat or even made endogenously from dietary carbohydrate, but the body only makes enough to keep us alive and not enough to raise the metabolic rate since this helps preserve calories and nutrients at times when such nutrients are scarce in the environment (evolutionarily). Our Celtic ancestors believed hazelnuts imparted wisdom, because they actually do, by strongly increasing cellular respiration, CO_2, and thus heightened mental cognition as the brain is able to acquire more oxygen and produce more energy and function better. Oleic acid isn't merely healthy, it is an *essential* nutrient on which our physiology evolved and without it being healthy is impossible. While many high-oleic acid foods are easy to use, the production of homemade mayonnaise using high-oleic sunflower oil or olive oil is also a really simple and delicious way to get oleic acid into the diet more frequently, to raise metabolic respiration, and it will be noticed after consuming some along with carbohydrate that the volume and rate of gas exchange from the lungs (breathing) will increase for a few hours afterward, which will be the increase in CO_2 which helps reverse these problems of calcium dysregulation.

Because oleic acid is also a fat it too can become saponified by free calcium and pathogens in the gut, which then prevents its absorption. Taking high selenium foods along with fats helps to more rapidly promote their digestion and packaging into cholesterol which removes them from digestion and thus reduces the rate of saponification. But because saponification is also primarily a problem of calcium dysregulation and acquisition by pathogens, foods high in oxalate can also be used to further protect dietary fats like oleic acid and steric acid from saponification, when eating alongside things like mayonnaise, salad dressings, butter, cream, etc., and should be actively practiced by anyone with severe metabolic problems. Nuts like hazelnuts do contain some oxalate, so they are especially useful, but this can be increased such as with the use of guava, raspberries, banana, rhubarb, spinach, etc., as required. Hazelnuts which are especially useful are an easy to grow shrub, and high-oleic sunflowers not only produce an abundance of seeds to eat for this same effect but are also very beautiful, and anyone that has property can grow these themselves for a free source of healthy oleic acid.

As discussed also in the chapter on vitamin D, one of the most important and thus debilitating problems in vitamin D homeostasis required for citrate production and normal metabolism of calcium is the deficiency of *boron*, which is required to inhibit the excessive hydroxylation of vitamin D (24-hydroxylase) which otherwise destroys vitamin D as a mechanism to lower the metabolic rate during times when food is scarce in the environment, so boron deficiency also debilitates the normal metabolism of calcium and promotes calcification and metabolic disease. Many foods like *Prunus* fruit (peaches, cherries, plums, prune, etc.) and grapes are very high in boron and normally can be plenty for healthy people so long as their diet is anchored in fruits and vegetables, although the use of a low-dose supplement of boron can also be helpful to more rapidly reverse deficiency. But another unsolved biological problem related to respiration is exactly how oxygen actually reaches mitochondria for use in oxidative respiration after release from hemoglobin in red blood cells. Oxygen cannot freely diffuse through cells as it would react with and oxidize anything it touches, and so must have a chaperone which binds and transports it to mitochondria for participation in oxidative respiration and production of energy. Studies show that boron can and does also raise mitochondrial respiration, and being boron replete can and does also strongly result in an increase in the volume of gas exchange from the lungs and rate of breathing, sometimes even to the point of being disruptive. Unlike other elements boron also forms stable complexes with reactive oxygen species, and boron repletion is also shown to dramatically prevent the loss of calcium as well as other elements involved in cellular metabolism such as sodium, potassium, etc., which is probably a result of more efficient production of ATP and inhibition of oxidative stress, in spite of an increase in oxidative respiration. I believe there exists a boron-derived ligand which thus chaperones oxygen after release by hemoglobin to mitochondria and thus boron is also required as a factor for effective respiration. Boron repletion can occur easily from a high fruit and vegetable diet (especially from *Prunus* species and grapes), but for those whom are very ill a low-dose supplement could be required for more rapid resolution of illness. Poor libido and erectile dysfunction are also a consequence of boron deficiency as discussed in that upcoming chapter, which can be used as a further diagnostic for the requisite of supplemental support and necessity to restore boron homeostasis.

Cytochrome is also made of iron and copper, so foods like nuts and leafy greens, which contain plenty of iron and copper, also directly support respiration. Meat contains very high quantities of heme iron, but this can actually mask impaired synthesis of endogenous heme by effectively supplementing extra heme, to mask problems with respiration due to impaired iron metabolism that are not made obvious unless abstaining from meat consumption. As discussed in the chapter on iron, sulfur is required for the normal metabolism of iron through the formation of iron-sulfur clusters, and iron regulation is in turn regulated by vitamins A and D, so deficiencies in dietary carotene and sunlight as well as colonization by hydrogen sulfide producing pathogens are the primary contributors to this iron dysregulation which can and should also be addressed as discussed in previous chapters. Kale and collards are higher in sulfur by weight than meat, and along with other high sulfur foods like garlic and onions, protected by consistent use of carotene to suppress microbial hydrogen sulfide production, can strongly help restore normal heme synthesis to support normal cytochrome function.

But one final problem with the consumption of dairy comes from the aging of the body and a slowing metabolic rate, wherein a fast, young metabolism with high respiration receiving plenty of sun exposure will tend to convert its tryptophan mostly to niacin (vitamin B3) which directly potentiates NAD which also participates in the mitochondrial electron transport chain as discussed in the upcoming chapter on niacin therapy, to assist in transport of electrons derived from energy production and promote great metabolic health. Niacin is essential for our wellbeing and generally we get enough from food or what is synthesized endogenously from dietary tryptophan, but pathogenic microbes which colonize the gut steal dietary tryptophan and convert it to toxic derivatives like indoles, and the body redirects what tryptophan it does receive into more hormones of torpor like serotonin and melatonin, slowing the metabolic rate and preventing high cellular respiration. This fine line between the nature of tryptophan metabolism to either niacin or serotonin is why milk can either be a lifesaving food for some or illness causing for others, and in order to maximize the health benefit of tryptophan it is required to understand niacin and tryptophan pathways as discussed in the upcoming chapter on niacin.

High quality dairy also contains both vitamin A and carotenoids which are derived from grazing green plants and are what give milk and butter their yellow tints, but because the dairy industry often feeds their animals only grain-based diets such dairy often lacks these helpful nutrients (as well as vitamin K). There are also dairies which will add anatto to cheat the yellow color, though anatto is also a carotene so it's kind of funny their cheating actually kind of fixes that problem when it wasn't intended to, but milk should always be purchased from highly reputable businesspeople and taste incredible, because animals cannot produce great tasting milk without a good diet. The same is true for eggs which, when industrially produced, result in pale yolks with less nutritional content instead of the healthy, deeply orange color they should be, which are also absolutely fucking delicious and far healthier as a result. Animals also require daily sun exposure, so chickens raised in the darkness of mass-farming factory sheds produce poorly nutritive eggs and are at increased risk of contracting diseases, since vitamin D and sun exposure are also required for immune function as discussed in that upcoming chapter. If you consume poor quality food products like pale eggs and low quality dairy you *will not* get well, and the money you save now in buying cheap, poorly produced food will cost you later in health problems, medical bills, and quality of life.

Dairy and calcium can help people improve overall health as long as it is protected by tannins, carotene, vitamin K, and oxalate, and the restoration of vitamin D, endogenous production of citric acid, and restoration of metabolic respiration. All disease is mediated by dysregulation of calcium since this strongly alters pH and promotes opportunistic pathogens which is not resolved either by too little or too much calcium but instead its biological regulation. Early in my recovery when milk was problematic I instead primarily used casein protein, but in my fruit smoothies it was also protected from microbial producers of ammonia and hydrogen sulfide by an abundance of tannin, carotene, anthocyanin, and oxalates which promoted its healthful properties before I even understood the function of these important dietary factors. Because casein is used to make cheese, cheese can be used as a source of casein instead of buying it as a supplement (but which still requires a diet high in protective factors), but not those blocks of orange crap which usually contain additives like gums and carrageenan and don't get me started on that pre-shredded crap coated in shitty non-stick fucking shit that you shouldn't be fucking eating if you can shred cheese yourself you lazy fuck God stop putting that processed shit into your body the fuck do you think your health problems come from?

CHAPTER 12

IRON, ANEMIA, AND INFECTIOUS DISEASE

One day when still living in Utah I was floored by a sudden onset of flu-like symptoms, but which included a very sore throat. I had just returned from living in Hawaii after my suicide attempt and, though recently begun a new job, I did not yet have medical insurance and so I went to a city clinic. On admittance a nurse only a little older than I asked questions about my health history. After I answered that yes, I did have sex with other men, none of which had been penetrative in recent months, she promptly announced that I had an STD though she had run no test, but would need to test me in order to prescribe me antibiotics. To my horror she returned shortly with an oversized cotton swab about eight inches long. It looked like a Q-tip made for a giraffe.

"What's that for?" I asked.

"To test you for STDs," she replied. I imagined her swabbing my ear for chlamydia with this comically-sized cotton swab, or perhaps a throat swab

"But—where?"

"We have to swab your urethra."

"With that?" I said, feeling the blood drain from my face. Before I really knew what was happening my pants were down and this giraffe-sized cotton swab was being shoved up my dick and spun around inside my urethra where the dry fibers scraped the inside of what I now know to be extremely sensitive tissue. It was so painful my knees buckled and, giving a shout, I grabbed reflexively and embarrassingly onto the shoulders of the nurse to avoid falling over her. One of my friends actually passed out during this test, because it's that invasive.

Afterward they gave me a prescription and sent me home. I immediately got better, but a phone call six days later informed me that the test had come back negative, but supposedly that was common and they said I had definitely contracted an STD. I thanked them for their help, vowing never to return to that place again, and went on with my life.

Unfortunately about two weeks later I began to feel woozy again, and my throat got scratchy just as before. After I had finished the antibiotics and gotten better I had met a boy and gone home with him and engaged in some pretty raucous sex. Berating myself for yet again having contracted some disease because of my behavior and accusing myself of every stereotype gay men have been condemned I returned to the clinic with my head hung in despair. I met with the same woman and told her the symptoms had returned (leaving out the sex part) and insisted she give me some more medication. She refused to do so without another test. I asked if there was any other way we could get them for me, as it was extremely painful and invasive. She said no.

Once again I found a giant cotton swab shoved up into my penis. But I got new medication and took it home, grateful at least for access to some healthcare, however archaic their methods. Suspiciously the follow-up call once more failed to confirm any sexually transmitted diseases, and once more I was ensured of the frequency of errors in these tests (why were they giving them then?) and the accompanying but unspoken prejudice toward those like me. I locked myself away from even looking at other boys after that, afraid of the embarrassment and guaranteed torture of having to return to that place again.

But a few weeks later my symptoms returned *yet again*. This time I called the clinic crying and begged for them to get me better medication without testing and summoned every ounce of self respect left in me to demand better treatment. Thankfully the woman waived the test and called in another prescription, also for STDs.

A few weeks went by and the time-limit for my new work-based health insurance was drawing near (because I live in the United States which does not give it's citizens health care). If anything happened again I would soon have access to a real doctor in a few days so I didn't think much of it when a beautiful boy asked me over one night after a night out at the club. AAAAAAnnnnd sure enough I started to feel sick a week afterward. Finally equipped with proper insurance I made the next available appointment with my new doctor. I have never been one to enjoy lying and though I suspected this middle-aged white man of harboring conservative sentiments I was upfront about my sexual activity. "What symptoms are you having?" he asked as he felt up my throbbing tonsils. "Sore throat," I said, "tired and achy, the same symptoms I have been experiencing for months. I didn't have health insurance and went to a state clinic and they kept telling me I had an STD even though the test results kept coming back negative. They gave me antibiotics but the symptoms keep coming back."

The doctor opened my mouth and looked at the back of my throat, gagging me with a tongue depressor while I fearfully eyed the bottle of cotton swabs on the formica counter. "Looks like you have *strep*," he said.

At that moment I wanted to get in my car, drive to the clinic, and shout obscenities at the nurse who had twice shoved a giant, giraffe Q-tip up my dickhole for no goddamned good reason. But I was raised to be nice, to neglect my own wellbeing for the sake of others, and that wouldn't be a very nice thing to do. "No way," I said in disbelief. The doctor took a swab from my throat, prescribed a different antibiotic, and sent me on my way (and the tests did indeed confirm strep infection). I got better in a few days and did not get sick again for years, in spite of a raucous sex life, and it seems that the tests for STDs at the clinic are not likely to be as inaccurate as is often repeated but that medical staff often mistake diseases because they are instead informed by bias and prejudice. Because of that nurse, who either wanted to play with my dick or was obligated by antiquated health care policies imposed by an authoritarian state that thinks causing people pain during testing prevents sexual activity which it absolutely does not and only prevents them from being tested, not only had I been subjected to unnecessary pain and humiliation but she inadvertently helped spread *Streptococcus pyogenes* around the community in which we lived. Certainly, the bias of her environment prevented her from doing her job properly, because she still could and should have recognized the obvious symptoms of fucking strep throat. If I had known then what I now know about infectious illnesses and that *painless urine tests have been around for years* I would not have had to rely on the mercy of an inept medical clinic nor subjected to the prejudice and failure of religion-infected social services (it was not specifically religious, just existed in a state dominated by religious bigots which control these services).

A decade later during the worst decline of my health (before discovering my cancer) I contracted flu every year, every trip home for Christmas getting whatever my eighteen nieces and nephews were carrying, then spending all of January in recovery. After my cancer discovery and learning how to truly take care of my health I didn't again contract the flu even when I continued to suffer through severe health problems and immune challenges, because my efforts to improve my health also removed some of the entry points used by infectious agents to cause disease, the most consequential being that of *iron.*

Much fuss is made about iron as if it is a panacea of health. It is added to flour, cereals, and children's food products, supplements, and even infant formula. Some brands even claim more than 100% daily recommended values of iron. People talk about being anemic, or menstruating, or whatever, as if they "*get*» iron. You don't. You have no idea what iron is capable of. If we were Hobbits in Middle Earth iron would be *Sauron.* Iron is everywhere, and it is powerful. Growing children need iron, but adults who have finished growing need very little to maintain health, and certainly not the kind of raw metal shavings which are added to fortified foods. Iron is highly unstable. It's a messy drunk at a party. Unless properly managed and bound by proteins like *transferrin* it bumps into and destroys everything it contacts. Iron is a heavy metal like arsenic, mercury, cadmium, and lead. To think that iron is benign in the diet is to die of it. Although overuse of antibiotics is a problem for so-called antibiotic resistant bacteria, the real reason for antibiotic resistance is factors such as iron excess from dietary fortification. Many antibiotics function simply by binding nutrients like iron which then deprives pathogens of the nutrients they use to cause disease, then the body gets the upper hand and fights off the pathogen. There are studies and demonstrations which directly show iron availability in vitro where antibiotic resistance is greater in a medium higher in iron.

Diet has a lot to do with getting sick, as pathogens need optimal conditions in order to infect a host. Iron is used in biological systems because it can so easily switch redox states from oxidation to reduced states of oxidation, and viruses and bacteria also need iron for their own growth. Iron is also used by pathogens to defend themselves against our immune system by cleaving hydrogen peroxide into the hydroxyl radicals which not only impairs the immune response by impairing the function of hydrogen peroxide but also reverse-Uno-cards that oxidative stress back onto our own bodies to destroy our tissues and causes us massive oxidative stress. The reason stomachaches so often occur from eating foods like pizza and pasta is the iron fortification common to wheat in most industrialized food systems (but which also occurs in rice and other grains or supplements) is not whole-food bound iron but little more than iron shavings and is extremely useful by gastrointestinal pathogens to buffer themselves against our immune reaction by changing hydrogen peroxide into the hydroxyl radical which then destroys our gastrointestinal tissue and facilitates pathogenic ingress into our body which then requires quite some time and resources for the body to remedy. Since many people consume food made from iron fortified flour or other grain or supplements stomachaches are a regular occurrence. For the first decade of my adulthood the regular stomachaches I experienced became so debilitating I had to regularly call in sick to work and often spent that time just sitting in a hot shower. When I finally learned at the age of twenty-six that gluten was potentially harmful and contributed to inflammation and immune dysfunction, changing my diet to avoid wheat incidentally also prevented me from consuming food fortified with iron, and my almost daily experiences of stomachaches miraculously lessened to about once every few weeks.

While the hydroxyl radical causes significant oxidative stress it is most damaging because it also attacks the ATP binding sites of the ATPase channels which transport elements like sodium, potassium, and calcium through cells as discussed in the chapter on vascular insufficiency, so one of the primary causes of aging and metabolic disease is excess iron accumulation and dysregulation which then causes oxidative stress and inhibits the transport of many elements required in both normal metabolic function and immune reactions. Unfortunately we also do not possess a natural mechanism to extinguish the hydroxyl radical. Instead, inhibition of hydroxyl radical stress comes from the diet in the form of phytonutrients called *cinnamic acids* common to fruits, spices, and vegetables. Yes, as the name sounds cinnamic acids are a primary constituent of cinnamon, but in fact cinnamic acids and their derivatives occur regularly in most plant foods and are even found in coffee, celery, potatoes, and leafy greens. Cinnamic acid is actually one of the oldest plant chemicals and is the precursor to most other plant compounds, even lignin (wood) but also ferulic acid, caffeic acid, gallic acid, coumaric acid, curcumin (in turmeric), chlorogenic acid, etc., to which I am all referring when saying 'cinnamic acids,' since these other acids are related, derived from, and behave similarly to their parent cinnamic acid, and tannins and cinnamic acid are the primary reasons why a diet high in fruit is required for health and wellness because tannins suppress ammonia producing pathogens while cinnamic acids prevent the production of the hydroxyl radical by pathogens.

Cinnamic acids are in fact the euphoric flavors in fruit and spices and are so stimulatory to our sense of taste and smell, most especially Prunus fruit, because of their primary function of protecting us from the hydroxyl radical, so a diet high in fruit and other sources of cinnamic acids are required for a well functioning immune system. Spices like cinnamon, turmeric, or ginger can also be used in foods or tea or juice as a very convenient way to replicate this function, and inhibition of hydroxyl radical stress by the generous consumption of dietary cinnamic acids is also a natural benefit of a diet high in fruit, vegetables, and spices but also imperative to reversing metabolic disease, immune dysfunction, and other problems associated with ATPase dysfunction and copper status. Indian bay leaf, bay laurel, and other laurels are also in the same family as cinnamon, the *Lauraceae*, and using bay leaf tea (*Cinnamomum tamala* is sweeter) likely promotes health and wellbeing by generously contributing cinnamic acids when steeped for long periods of time. *Sassafras* is a laurel species common to North America which is the original ingredient in real root beer (commercial root beer is now just artificial flavoring), which is extremely delicious because of its likely high cinnamic acid profile and thus likely provides a similar benefit (although it contains safrole which may be carcinogenic in high doses), and Northern spicebush (*Lindera benzoin*) is similarly widely distributed, even used as a lawn ornamental, which also makes an excellent herbal tea high in cinnamic acids (many laurels are toxic so do not assume they are all safe, and plants like cherry laurel are not laurel but *Prunus*, the leaves of which are toxic).

It is hard to avoid iron even if we try. Other vitamins and minerals don't carry the consequences of iron. If we overdose on magnesium our body can flush it very quickly and we probably wouldn't even notice. This is not the case with iron, because iron is so important for growth, tissue repair, and even immune function the body sequesters iron rather than discard excess, not least of all to protect that iron from acquisition by pathogens, so exposure to excess iron easily contributes to iron excess toxicity. Iron added to foods in fortification is especially toxic because it is not already bound by chaperones or proteins. It contributes to all sorts of diseases from hypothyroidism to cancer and fuels bacteria and virus growth in the body, and studies in rodents have shown that high iron intake impairs growth and promotes copper deficiency anemia. Reducing excess iron helps remove excess weight gain, heal cancer, restore hair-loss, stop insomnia, raise energy levels, and extend lifespan.

Nature has been aware of this vulnerability of iron for millions of years and is one of the reasons why mammalian milk is nearly absent of iron, to protect vulnerable babies from pathogenic infection in the gut. Milk also contains proteins like lactoferrin which powerfully bind free iron, further reducing the risk of bacterial infection, and then you go and feed your baby replacement formula or baby food fortified with iron and directly circumvent what millions of years of nature has designed to protect your baby. Tragic problems like sudden infant death syndrome is likely caused by iron supplementation to neonates and infants, and early ingress of bacteria which cause autism, diabetes, and cystic fibrosis can be promoted by consumption of iron fortified foods or iron fortified infant formula, especially if those are also high in harmful polyunsaturated fats, because pathogens use those nutrients to colonize our bodies.

The reason our food is fortified with extra iron in the first place originated from well-meaning efforts to cure disease. Years ago the FDA mandated the addition of iron to refined flour in an attempt to rectify small populations burdened with anemia. Anyone who eats even one large portion of meat just once a week would get an *excess* of the required iron for good health, yet even more was added to food with no evidence it actually benefitted anyone, especially the anemic populations it was meant to address. After the initial fortification proved unhelpful the FDA increased the amount in foods again, but it still did not have the intended effect so they raised it *yet again*, and then a fourth time before scientists and health professionals finally spoke up and warned against the potential harm so much added iron would do the population. The added iron made no difference for the populations it was meant to address, and even appeared to contribute to other diseases like hemochromatosis, but instead of removing the iron which proved a failure the iron is maintained to this day without any evidence for benefit and even an excess of evidence that it causes harm. In most countries iron is now added to corn and rice and other grains, countries who have also shown dramatic increases in metabolic diseases ever since the introduction of fortification, while countries like France, which never adopted these scientifically unsupported policies, have been spared the severity of these devastating pandemics.

The fortification of foods with iron shows an alarming lack of understanding about biochemistry and nature from those who are supposed to understand it. If a person is iron-deficient anemic even when eating an excess of iron, wouldn't that suggest a causative factor which is *not* iron? Most anemia in fact is not actually caused by a lack of iron exposure at all but is in fact a deficit of the vitamins and nutrients involved in the metabolism of iron such as zinc, B12, vitamin A from dietary carotene, and vitamin D. This should be pretty obvious since iron supplementation never helps anemics get better, only altering test results, often making symptoms worse, and clinicians are more likely to increase iron dosage until it forces physiological changes such as the increase of ferritin in the bloodstream. Ferritin is mainly an intracellular product, which means the amount measured in the bloodstream occurs with cellular leakage, caused by the harmful destruction of cells due to excess iron.

Generally, the only test used by doctors to measure iron only measures iron in the blood, but most iron in the body is tissue-bound and in disease states there is even less iron in the blood because during disease the body preferentially sequesters iron away from places like blood where pathogenic microorganisms can more easily access it. Doctors are routinely mistaken as to the state of iron in the body because without a biopsy there is no way to tell if iron is high or low in tissues, and they do more harm by prescribing iron supplementation when they should instead be measuring and treating vitamins involved in the metabolism of iron. Tests should not even be required to diagnose such diseases and instead demonstrates very poor understanding of diseases like anemia and its associated symptoms and dietary causes, which can be diagnosed and treated without running a single test by evaluating a patient's symptoms, diet (as measured by standards in this book), eating behaviors, and sunlight exposure. The primary factor which regulates iron homeostasis is a liver protein called *hepcidin* which is in turn regulated by both vitamins A and D, and a deficiency of these vitamins stimulates iron storage in tissue because the body perceives these deficiencies as problems of wintertime or famine when these nutrients are naturally unavailable, so the body sequesters iron for storage and future use, and it is only when normal amounts of dietary carotene and sunlight exposure return that the body once again lowers hepcidin and release iron from storage.

Supplementing iron even when there is sufficient iron in the diet is simply loading excess iron into the gut and tissue storage and eventually overburdening the body with toxic levels of iron or fueling the growth of harmful gastrointestinal pathogens which use that iron to cause oxidative damage and inhibit the immune system (seriously, how do doctors not know this?????). Transferrin is dependent on the amino acid *tyrosine,* so a deficiency of tyrosine due to caloric stress, emotional stress, or deficient protein intake as discussed in the chapter on depression directly impairs transferrin and thus iron metabolism. The copper dependent protein, *ceruloplasmin* is a molybdenum dependent ferroxidase which oxidizes iron for binding to transferrin which helps protect it from interception by pathogens and from forming the hydroxyl radical in reaction with hydrogen peroxide, so ceruloplasmin deficiency caused by deficiencies of dietary molybdenum (cucurbits and legumes) and copper (nuts) is a bigger driver of anemia than dietary iron.

Riboflavin (vitamin B2) also helps regulate iron transport and readily forms a complex with iron, so gut dysbiosis can strongly interrupt iron homeostasis through interference with riboflavin by *Streptomyces* which produce the riboflavin analog *roseoflavin* which suppresses commensal riboflavin producers and thus causes us riboflavin deficiency. So long as there is some iron in the diet, which is nearly impossible not to do, the restoration of a healthy diet and environment will always resolve iron related issues without the need for inappropriate and harmful interventions such as iron supplementation, which should never itself be used, not even in pregnancy or anemia, and iron should *always* come only from whole-food, non-fortified sources. Riboflavin strongly complexes with iron and using a temporary, daily dose of riboflavin helped to scavenge a lot of the excess iron in my gut and fully arrest any remaining stomachaches, and it can be very useful to more rapidly rescue severe gastrointestinal distress such as what occurs in autism, diabetes, Crohn's disease, etc., while also promoting normal iron metabolism from whole food sources until such time as the commensal microbiome can reestablish itself and once again produce riboflavin.

Because iron is required for growth, the hormone estrogen, which is a hormone of growth, stimulates the uptake of more iron (and copper) into the body. One of the reasons women have elevated estrogen is to facilitate the growth of structures related to the reproductive cycle such as the endometrium or the corpus luteum which completely dissolves and regenerates every cycle, or for growing a fetus in the womb when pregnant. Progesterone and testosterone work in opposition to estrogen, to protect against its growth stimulation when growth is not necessary such as in the body of a fully grown adult. During metabolic disease estrogen is elevated higher than normal because of a lowered metabolic rate and increased aromatization also portends a future need to regrow and regenerate tissue for which estrogen and iron are necessary, but long term and chronic metabolic disease caused by diets low in fruits and vegetables and thus protective nutrients like cinnamic acids, tannin, carotene, etc., often never reaches the healing phase so a body can both continue absorbing iron and producing estrogen excess indefinitely. If the diet also contains iron fortified food the uptake can be so excessive to strongly catalyze disease, and it is especially important that children avoid iron fortified food which will otherwise cause them long term health problems due to premature promotion of opportunistic microbes, and over time the regular consumption of tannins, cinnamic acids, and other phytonutrients from a diet high in fruits, vegetables, nuts, etc., and restoration of a healthy microbiome will naturally balance iron status.

One of the primary produces made from iron in our body is called *heme*, which is iron bound with a protein called *porphyrin*, and acts as a cofactor for many biological processes like hemoglobin, respiration, thyroid hormone synthesis, and immune factors discussed in the upcoming chapter on immunity. Most dietary iron is actually difficult for the body to absorb but heme is far more bioavailable (about twice as bioavailable, depending on the study), so diets high in meat greatly increase iron absorption and high meat diets are shown in studies to be associated with diabetes because organs like the pancreas become oversaturated with iron which then increases vulnerability to pathogenic colonization. After learning about the damage caused by iron I began a regimen of iron chelation to improve my prospects for surviving my cancer and to heal my body, but it took a long time and was based on incomplete understanding of how iron excess is caused in the first place, because there is not much helpful knowledge about iron's function even from educated medical professionals, let alone the internet. The real key to restoring proper iron balance is to not be afraid of food. Plants do not contain heme iron, so their iron content is not nearly as bioavailable as heme iron found in animal products, and some plant foods high in iron like leafy greens are also high in nutrients such as phytate, sulfur, tannins, cinnamic acids, and other phytochemicals which also help control iron, prevent oxidative stress, and block iron access by pathogens, which is not the case with meat. It is not necessary to avoid meat and animal products but heme can actually mask problems with iron metabolism and iron excess, by providing preformed heme (which is extremely important to our biology) will substitute for our own heme production if that is deficient and in the process sustain our heme supply even if we cannot make our own.

The primary problem which causes iron excess and iron dysregulation is that of *sulfur* deficiency as discussed in the chapter on vitamin D and vascular health, because iron is firstly bound to sulfur in the formation of *iron-sulfur clusters* requisite to the endogenous synthesis of heme and other iron-dependent pathways. When we become deficient in sulfur due to opportunistic sulfate reducing pathogens we then lose the ability to properly metabolize iron which then not only causes iron overload and excess iron saturation of cells but also deficiency of products like heme which would otherwise use iron stores. Not only this, but the accumulation of iron then also causes systemic oxidative stress such as in the increased production of the hydroxyl radical from reaction to hydrogen peroxide, and during iron overload iron even interferes with the insertion of manganese into superoxide dismutase (because manganese and iron are highly similar) which renders the enzyme inactive and thus also increases superoxide. So restoration of sulfur status through the management of hydrogen sulfide malodor with carotene and frequent consumption of high sulfur plant foods like kale, collards, broccoli, etc., (because the sulfated amino acids common to meat are primary targets of sulfate reducing pathogens) is the most important step in restoring normal iron homeostasis.

Because vitamin A powerfully stimulates the release of iron from tissue storage for use in the body, supplemental vitamin A can be quite harmful because preformed vitamin A can overwhelm tissues with free iron or even deplete iron stores if iron status is actually low, especially in those who are metabolically comprised. High free iron circulation then leads to the formation of more hydroxyl radical as iron reacts with reducing agents like vitamin C or hydrogen sulfide in the blood stream to then cause significant metabolic disease as the hydroxyl radical shuts down ATPase pathways. Severe hypervitaminosis A can even result in liver damage hemorrhage, or even coma because of the effect of vitamin A on iron homeostasis. My own experience with supplemental vitamin A resulted in losing the regrowth of hair in the thinning spots on my scalp which I had regrown during my long recovery from cancer, and some significant acne which I had not had in many years. For this reason vitamin A, in my experience, should only come from dietary sources, especially from pro-vitamin A carotenoids.

Alcohol, being estrogenic, artificially stimulates the increased uptake of iron by tissues and increases the elimination of zinc, and this effect is one of the primary reasons for the deleterious effects of excess alcohol consumption, and if alcohol excess is a problem (drinking regularly is excessive) this is not a problem of willpower or self control but an underlying neurological condition as discussed in upcoming chapter on alcoholism and addiction which can and must be addressed to avoid the consequences of excess consumption. Alcohol metabolizes into aldehyde which the body then uses molybdenum to detoxify, which also increases the loss of molybdenum and thus reduces protective molybdenum-dependent ceruloplasmin which is required to manage iron (especially if products like wine are not organic or contain added sulfites which could potentially chelate molybdenum).

True iron excess is easy to diagnose. Obesity, dull skin, greying hair, degenerative eye conditions, fatigue, bloating, and stomach/digestive problems are all signs of iron excess. Severe diseases like Leukemia, Alzheimer's, and Parkinson's all involve elevated levels of iron and its deleterious role in health has been unaddressed for far too long. The most important thing in avoiding the destructive effects of iron is to avoid iron-fortified foods. READ LABELS. Anything labeled with the words iron, ferrous, or ferric in the ingredients list should absolutely be avoided—especially common wheat flour or grains like rice. Fortified iron is nothing more than rusted metal in our food. As long as you follow these few guidelines and address hydrogen sulfide producers the body will even out levels of iron naturally.

It is also well known that *cobalamin* (vitamin B12) is required by our body to make both red and white blood cells, as B12 is required as a factor for DNA synthesis (which occurs when cells divide) so anemia then also results from deficiency of B12 either from low dietary intake or impaired microbial production such as the loss of *Thaumarchaeota* activity resulting from vitamin D deficiency as discussed in the chapter on gut health. What's worse, however, is that B12 deficiency also prevents the recycling of red and white blood cells, so a deficiency also prevents efficient use of nutrient resources for blood cell synthesis and faster exhaustion of them. While true B12 deficiency comes from vitamin D deficiency and impairment of *Thaumarchaeota*, many people find it difficult to reverse vitamin D deficiency, and it may be required to use a B12 supplement, but during thyroid disease the body actively destroys proteins that capture and transport B12, so those whom are very ill will not even be able to use a supplement effectively (though it will still advantage our microbes) as vitamin B12 is must be captured by the haptocorrin glycoproteins. Cobalamin metabolism also very likely includes ATPase dependent pathways, so if the general use of B12 or restoration of microbial B12 production does not also improve anemia symptoms (low breathing rate, low tissue oxygenation, severe insomnia, etc.) this likely demonstrates poor absorption due to hydroxyl radical production in the gut and B12 should be accompanied by (mixed into) potent sources of cinnamic acids like cinnamon, turmeric, ginger, or tea of Indian bay leaf, or northern spice bush, sassafras, etc. Because B12 can be stored in the liver, even one dose will begin restoring blood cell synthesis, although it takes a few days for them to mature, after which there will be greater energy and faster recovery from metabolic illness.

Also, when treating infections like the flu, strep throat, or sinus infection one of the best things I have discovered is (besides making an appointment with your doctor) to gargle *coconut oil*. The pain from strep throat is almost unbearable, and until those antibiotics kick in we have typically suffered through it, perhaps with a little bit of that shit spray that only works for five seconds until you can't resist the urge to swallow. Coconut oil can help relieve sore throats rapidly, and other infectious diseases, even some sexually transmitted ones because the types of pathogens that cause such diseases are instantly killed by the fatty acids released from the enzymatic treatment (saliva) of coconut oil and other good fats. Because the types of fatty acids in coconut oil triglycerides are antiseptic it has antibiotic properties, but even more so when the oil is held in the mouth for some time to allow the salivary enzymes to break apart the triglyceride bond and separate the individual fatty acids, which are far more reactive when released from those triglycerides. Merely swallowing coconut oil with eating and cooking does have some antibiotic nature, but in order to leverage its full potential for acute infections the triglycerides *must* be broken down, and in those with metabolic disease there will not be sufficient enzyme activity in the gut to accomplish this, which can instead occur in the mouth via salivary enzymes by swishing it for several minutes until it becomes watery (not just melted—don't be impatient), then gargling helps to distribute the fatty acids across the membranes of the back of the throat and up into the nasopharynx. This oil should also be swallowed after so those fatty acids circulate through the bloodstream, and can be done by children as long as they don't risk choking on it. Do not gargle coconut oil unless it has been enzymatically liquified by saliva, as this could risk choking since it is so thick.

It is well known that vitamin C influences illness and recovery, and vitamin C is often recommended for prevention of the common cold. Unknown to most medical professionals, this occurs because vitamin C is a powerful regulator of immune function as described in the upcoming chapter on immunity, and in spite of my many years experimenting with infectious pathogens I only had one cold in the last decade due to my frequent consumption of vitamin C, where before that period I often got at least several colds every year. But this does not work well after infection occurs, only for prevention, as vitamin C regulates many pathways in the body which are required for an effective immune response which, at the time of infection, cannot be activated quickly if previously deficient in vitamin C. As heme iron is a primary factor in the immune response, vitamin C helps coordinate iron for use in the immune system. Vitamin C should primarily come from the diet, but absorption and regulation of vitamin C is in fact very complex and can be impaired in chronic illness which, because vitamin C is required in so many other pathways, can also result in many other symptoms besides dysfunctional immunity, and more information on vitamin C can be found in the upcoming chapter on the immune system, while the daily intake of high vitamin C foods like leafy greens, straw-berries, *Prunus* fruit, etc., can help promote recovery and prevent many types of illness.

A boyfriend of mine once contracted appendicitis which required emergency surgery and two hospital stays because his appendectomy incision became infected and required to remain open to prevent him contracting sepsis and dying. But in spite of copious amounts of antibiotics and constant medical supervision his inci-sion continued to deteriorate. After much worry I finally insisted on treating his open, infected wound with coconut oil and honey since I had begun to understand things about human biology and discovered the traditional use of sugar to treat wounds and coconut oil's antibiotic properties. This sounded crazy, I know, and it took a frightening return trip to the emergency room before he decided to try it, but because of coconut oil's antiseptic properties and the sugar in honey fueling tissue growth (honey is also antiseptic) the three-inch long incision, which went all the way down to his abdominal wall, finally began to heal and stop producing puss. I had gotten this idea after using coconut oil in a little finger condom to regrow the tip of my finger which I had accidentally sliced off on a mandolin while making potato gratin. My finger grew back without *any* scarring, and coconut oil works like this because of its lubricating, antibiotic, and pro-hormone properties which in the skin results in an increase in local production of the parent hormone pregnen-olone. In spite of our success over my protestations my love refused to continue application after the wound closed, and it then resulted in an enormous scar which otherwise would have been quite diminished from both application by coconut oil and covering with plastic or other barrier to prevent drying. Coconut oil is a great food but it's also a great medicine, and more households need to know of its healing properties and how to leverage it in times of disease and injury (butterfat is a decent alternative if coconut oil is not available but should have all milk solids removed first, such as in the production of ghee). Scar tissue is highly influenced by bacterial ingress into a wound as well as simply drying out which impairs migra-tion of new cells to the regenerating area and all incisions or wounds should be covered with coconut oil and airtight seal like with some plastic wrap or wax paper. Sugar also promotes more rapid tissue healing and is also antibacterial, and can also be used to strongly inhibit bacterial infection such as what my boyfriend experienced, to hasten wound healing. Sugar has long been shown to improve wound healing, and studies on sugar demonstrate significant promotion of healing for conditions like burns, surgery, and wounds healing.

Aspirin is also extremely effective during infections (although it should not be used in young children), and there are many studies about the usefulness of aspirin on healing, wounds, and protection against pathogenic bacteria and virus infection discussed in the upcoming chapter on viruses and immunity, and aspirin can be used any time infection becomes present as long as other conditions your doctor has diagnosed won't interfere with its use. Incidentally, aspirin can be used to banish warts and HPV of all kinds, including genital warts and anal warts, painlessly and quickly. In fact, wart remover solution or strips are often just aspirin, called by its chemical name, *acetylsalicylic acid* or its metabolite, *salicylic acid*. I will not relate to you the entire horrifying story of contracting HPV while living in a conservative community, but that topical aspirin could have spared me scarring and the same kind of embarrassment as happened with the cotton swab by inept and prejudiced medical practitioners. HPV can cause cervical and rectal cancer, and aspirin can be a very helpful tool applied topically to directly resolve growths or taken orally in support of cancer as discussed in that upcoming chapter. Viruses which cause wart growths do so because the extra dermal tissue is colder than the body and facilitates the environment in which these viruses thrive. Aspirin increases oxidative respiration and reverses the conditions that viruses engineer in our tissues which then causes them to die off.

To be clear, antibiotics are useful and oftentimes necessary to prevent serious illness, and a person should always follow the advice of a competent medical professional. But more information on how the immune system works is discussed in the upcoming chapter on viruses and immunity and safer alternatives such as iodine can be effective in resolving illness. The tradition of following antibiotics with yogurt can negatively and permanently shift gut bacterial populations toward those which produce large amounts of harmful lactic acid and concurrent and post-antibiotic diets should instead consist of foods high fruits such as dried apricots, apples, raisins, prunes, berries, etc., the use of real kombucha, or organic, unfiltered apple cider vinegar, apple pectin, bifidobacterium probiotic, Swiss cheese, and foods high in vitamin K which support populations of our most healthy native species rather than food industry strains.

When it comes to our health, eating a proper diet is the best defense against not only metabolic disease but also the communicable ones which plague humans even in this age of modern health. Coconut oil is a powerful relief agent for pain and infection, as well as other sources of good fat like butter (butter oil, cocoa butter, and shea butter can be used if coconut oil is not available), not only helping to disinfect but to reinforce cells against the vulnerabilities which lead to infection. Other immune support like iodine, aspirin, and vitamin C as discussed in the upcoming chapter on immunity are also powerful aids in fighting infections, so long as iron excess and dysregulation have been resolved.

CHAPTER 13
NIACIN THERAPY

Niacin (vitamin B3), is arguably the most important of the B vitamins. But that is also like saying the head is more important than the body—one cannot exist without the other—and all vitamins are essential for life (that's why they're called vitamins). As living mammals we basically are B vitamins. They make all the enzymatic and energetic processes that govern the creation and direction of energy for the purpose of sustaining life, niacin being the driver of that metabolic energy once it is converted into the form *nicotinamide adenine dinucleotide*, or NAD for short.

NAD's function in the body is to shuttle electrons from processes which obtain energy from food to those which then use that energy. It is basically a helper which plugs the gap between eating food and using that food as energy and is required in many enzymes, reactions, and other metabolic processes. When niacin is insufficient in the body, and thus NAD because niacin is needed to form NAD, the metabolic rate falls and backup modes of metabolic function kick in.

Generally, deficiency of NAD does not really occur until we begin to age or suffer from metabolic disease, especially gut dysbiosis, and if this does happen there are ways to improve levels of NAD and thus the overall state of health. In fact, the quality of health is a direct reflection of our endogenous production of NAD because without NAD our body cannot run the higher metabolic systems which define wellness, or even run the immune system as discussed in that upcoming chapter. When NAD synthesis is impaired so too is health, and when NAD synthesis is repaired, so too is health. Real niacin therapy is a lot more complex than just supplementing niacin, however, and while using supplemental niacin can be very helpful it never reverses chronic deficiency because the problem is our ability to produce it, not lacking a supplement.

Unlike many B vitamins which are normally gotten from the diet or beneficial microbes our bodies actually produce niacin and in the *kynurenine pathway,* and while niacin can occur in the diet (or supplementation) endogenous production is our primary and most important source of this crucial vitamin. The kynurenine pathway begins with the amino acid *tryptophan* from dietary protein and is a nine-step metabolic process which also producers other metabolites like *kynurenic acid* necessary for other biological processes, but when all nutritional requirements for this pathway are present the final step in the pathway results in the synthesis of niacin and thus NAD.

In the years before the advent of scientific nutrition a devastating disease called *pellagra* was very common in certain parts of the world, which is caused by a deficiency of niacin due to dietary deficiency of tryptophan. European colonizers who committed genocide against Indigenous Americans in what is now the Southern regions of the United States subsisted on corn which they obtained from the Americans they had killed and displaced but because they killed and displaced the very people with knowledge of how to properly use this food the colonizing settlers did not know corn must be submitted to the process of *nixtamalization* by soaking and cooking in an alkaline solution such as lime (lime as in calcium hydroxide which indigenous Americans mined from limestone). Nixtamalization frees tryptophan from corn grain and makes it digestible which, by the way, your popcorn is not, for this reason. It's fine to consume corn occasionally that is not nixtamalized, but it is most nutritious when properly prepared and many misguided producers of corn products like tortillas and chips fail to properly process corn so these foods do not contribute well to nutritional status, and properly prepared corn products will usually identify nixtamalization, lime (again, not the fruit), or calcium hydroxide as an ingredient.

Although pellagra is no longer common in developed countries the same type of low-grade niacin deficiency is a major contributor to metabolic disease because of other factors which actively inhibit the kynurenine pathway instead of deficiency of niacin or tryptophan as was caused in the past. What's worse is that one of the primary functions of the kynurenine pathway is to catabolize tryptophan which then reduces its deposition in tissues, and when kynurenine pathway activity declines tryptophan instead remains in tissues and promotes greater quantities of the hormones of torpor serotonin and melatonin which, as discussed in the chapter on depression, oppositely downregulate the metabolic rate. Although it can and should be used when needed, supplementation of niacin is not entirely a replacement for endogenous synthesis of niacin because high niacin intake in turn inhibits the kynurenine pathway as a feedback mechanism which then causes greater tryptophan deposition since the kynurenine pathway also functions to catabolize tryptophan. This pathway is often characterized as a poorly efficient pathway for production of niacin since it takes a whopping 60 milligrams of tryptophan to produce one molecule of niacin, but in reality this demonstrates how robust the kynurenine pathway is in limiting tryptophan excess by very efficiently catabolizing tryptophan and thus protecting our body from its potentially harmful influence. When properly restored, niacin therapy utilizes the body's own kynurenine pathway to leverage the best outcome from dietary tryptophan by both reducing tryptophan deposition and increasing synthesis of niacin to stimulate dramatic healing and improvements in metabolic health.

The more NAD cells have the faster and hotter they run, which means more energy, health, and relaxation for the organism. This does not mean it is healthy for cells to run non-stop, however, and doing so causes cells to become depleted of their structural and nutritional integrity, which is what happens to many health seekers and "biohackers" who overstimulate their cells in their quests to get well. The body alternates between states of excitation and inhibition, and keeping one or the other on too long results in imbalance of metabolic systems. But low levels of NAD mean less energy and more agitation, fatigue, and disease, and an inability to meet the demands of daily stress. The sweet spot of NAD synthesis is one which can be naturally sustained by the body through proper diet and nutrition rather than supplements, and most metabolic diseases exist precisely because NAD production is too low to support mitochondrial respiration and other NAD dependent functions. Failure of the kynurenine pathway thus increases deposition of tryptophan in tissues to promote increased torpor from increased serotonin and melatonin which accelerates the aging process by inhibiting energy dependent pathways. While glutamine is required to synthesize NAD from tryptophan or niacin it is *not* required to synthesize NAD from *niacinamide,* as niacinamide is a spent form of NAD which is easily recycled back into NAD through other pathways, so the use of low-dose, supplemental niacinamide (about 250 mg once or twice a day is usually enough) to rescue metabolic illness and address problems like insomnia, depression, anorexia, and hair loss is extremely useful until the diet, microbiome, and metabolic rate can be restored.

A primary inhibitor of NAD synthesis is deficiency also of *glutamine* as described in chapter on pathogens and metabolic disease and autism, because glutamine made from arginine, glutamate, and ammonia is required as a cofactor in the kynurenine pathway and, besides dieting behaviors which starve the body of nutrition, is most commonly caused by opportunistic microbes which interfere with arginine-ammonia-glutamine cycle.

As discussed in the chapter on gut health, tryptophan is also a major target of pathogenic microbes which produce harmful tryptophan derivatives which not only depletes tryptophan but also causes active metabolic harm to our body as microbes disturb the normal metabolism and regulation of tryptophan and gut serotonin. Any symptoms like constipation, bloating, water retention, insomnia, intermittent diarrhea, SIBO, etc., are symptoms of opportunistic microbial interference with tryptophan and gut serotonin which results in toxic tryptophan derivatives which must be restrained through the ubiquitous, strategic, and consistent consumption of foods high in pectin like fruit, especially apples, apple butter, apple sauce, other cooked apple products, marmalade, or use of a pectin supplement with foods if fruit on its own does not sufficiently restore these functions since microbial B12 is also required for microbes to break down the plant tissue matrix to release its pectin content, as pectin inhibits opportunistic microbial catabolism of tryptophan by advantaging our commensal acetogens.

While dietary tryptophan is necessary for normal endogenous NAD production most people do not realize that our commensal microbiome also produces amino acids like tryptophan, lysine, alanine, serine, etc., and that a non-zero supply of amino acids comes directly from a healthy and functional population of commensal gut microbes. As discussed in the chapters on gut health and parasitism, problems like vitamin D deficiency which impair local microbial cobalamin (B12) production required by microbes then invites opportunistic microbes to instead colonize mucosal tissues, especially the mouth, stomach, and intestines, which then outcompete our commensal microbiome to then interfere with the production of B vitamins, short chain fatty acids, amino acids, vitamin K2, and other nutrients for which we are dependent on our microbiota. Studies show that the gut microbiome can produce up to 20 grams of protein daily, which probably occurs best from high quality, healthy foods like fruits and vegetables when we are also replete with vitamin D, and although there is no science which yet explores this I believe that our tryptophan supplies are in part supported by gut microbial synthesis which, when it occurs, directly supports the kynurenine pathway and endogenous NAD synthesis since the conditions for successful kynurenine pathway activity are also largely those also required for a healthy, functional microbiome, so that microbial synthesis of tryptophan is also more likely to occur during times when it will also be directed in greater ratio to NAD synthesis than hormones of torpor.

Unfortunately, studies also show that *fluoride* inhibits the microbial enzyme tryptophan synthetase which synthesizes tryptophan, and studies show that fluoride exposure such as what often occurs from fortification of municipal water, salt, milk, and oral care products with fluoride can and does cause mental health disorders which very likely occurs from this interference from swallowing xeno-biotic sources of fluoride. Studies also show that glyphosate, a common herbicide, also blocks the shlkimate pathway which is the precursor to synthesis of microbial folate (B9) and the aromatic amino acids, tyrosine, phenylalanine, and trypto-phan, so many contemporary industrial toxins can also participate in kynurenine pathway dysfunction and much effort should be made to avoid fluoridated water, salt, milk (anything swallowed), and agrochemicals.

Studies also show that the omega-3 fats DHA, EPA, and ALA, which are found in many inferior fats such as canola, soy, vegetable oil, and fish oil, and added to commercial products for their supposedly health-promoting properties not only halt the kynurenine pathway, they do so at a point which produces a toxic neurological stimulant called *quinolinic acid*, so the diet can and does also direct-ly regulate production of NAD separately from the microbiome. Quinolinic acid is a neurostimulant meant to increase mental cognition in order to facilitate better creative problem solving in stressed organisms such as ourselves when we encounter environmental or nutritional challenges. It is a strategy which tries to better help our mind find solutions when our survival or wellbeing is in danger, but because this neurostimulant is also stressful to the nervous system it also causes psychological stress and when expressed in excess for long periods of time is the a mechanism of action for causing severe psychological disease such as schizophre-nia, mania, anxiety, and other forms of insanity. The production of quinolate due to dietary omega-3 fats is the reason why those fats produce heightened cogni-tive function in studies which are then marketed as advantageous for increasing mental cognition in children and added to things like milk or eggs or other prod-ucts targeted toward parents, but because quinolate functions in stress pathways it also causes psychological stress and results in problems like ADHD, restlessness, and irritability in children (and adults). This dual function of the kynurenine pathway is why children with autism spectrum disorder such as I experienced as a child and young man can and do present also with increased intelligence but also restlessness, depression, anxiety, and self-harm behavior because the nutrition-al deficiencies which impair the kynurenine pathway result in both an increase in intelligence, as an adaptation to that stress, but also severe emotional stress and reduced ability to endure stressful stimuli like abuse, mistakes, loss, or even seemingly little things like loud noises and interpersonal conflict, and this psycho-logical effect of chronic quinolinic acid and deficiency of NAD and the discomfort it causes is the reason for high rates of self harm, suicide, and suicide attempts among neurodivergent people because, speaking from experience, it is torturous to endure.

Quinolate excess due to kynurenine pathway dysfunction is also the primary causative factor of most hair loss, especially male-pattern baldness, which not only deprives the scalp of NAD required for normal hair follicle function but, since quinolate is a neurostimulant, also overstimulates the nerves of the scalp which overexcites surrounding tissues to overconsume nutrients during deficiency to catastrophically impair their ability to function, so diets high in polyunsaturated fats are also more likely to cause hair loss. Because fats are highly temperature sensitive the body uses desaturase enzymes in the skin to reduce saturation of more saturated forms of fatty acids, since the skin is always at least several degrees cooler than the core of the body in which fats can and do get stuck if they are too saturated. One such condition caused by this problem are *styes* or *chalazion* of the eye which are usually treated by lancing or other minor surgery by doctors since they do not understand the underlying biology. Styes and chalazion occur when the body is literally too cold to melt saturated fats, but also so deficient in zinc which is the primary cofactor in desaturase enzymes that desaturase activity is also deficient. The blockages caused by solidified fats in the skin then cause buildup of fluids and can then become infected, and treatment of these conditions is specifically raising the metabolic rate through things like sugar, vitamin C, sun exposure, niacin, aspirin, etc., using a few, low doses of zinc, and applying a constant hot compress to the area until the fat is finally melted and enzymatically processed.

Normally fatty acids are also detoxified through the liver and bile when conjugated with sulfate which reduces fat retention and promotes carbohydrate oxidation and increase in endogenous niacin (if there is sufficient dietary protein). But fatty acid detoxification also requires desaturase enzymes because the more unsaturated fats are the more water soluble they are which makes their elimination in the gut through bile and conjugation with sulfate more effective. This becomes a problem when colonized with sulfate reducing microbes which produce hydrogen sulfide as discussed in the chapter on vitamin D because they can and do remove sulfate from products of detoxification in the gut like polyunsaturated fats which then causes their recirculation back into the body, and now being highly unsaturated these fats as products of detoxification further interfere with kynurenine pathway function to promote disease even if the diet is low in polyunsaturated fats. This is why supplementation of niacinamide can help therapeutically because it circumvents the deficiency of NAD caused by increased circulation of polyunsaturated fats due to an increase in gut pathogen colonization or lowered metabolic rate, and suppression of hydrogen sulfide production through the consistent consumption of carotene with meals and restoration of a healthy microbiome can prevent the recirculation of polyunsaturated fats and thus restore better kynurenine pathway function.

Good dietary fat oppositely serves to stabilize the metabolic rate by insulating the kynurenine pathway from the influence of harmful fats, so limiting dietary fat to those which are mostly saturated (and monounsaturated) such as occur in butter, cream, tallow, coconut oil, hazelnuts, almonds, cocoa butter, olive oil, etc., helps protect the body from metabolic decline by preventing interruption of endogenous niacin synthesis. This positive effect of saturated fats is the reason why many centenarians like Jeanne Louise Calment often cite foods like chocolate as a reason for their longevity, but in those who are already very ill the ability to even digest and absorb these fats can be impaired, and simply consuming them is not likely to directly provide this function necessary for the kynurenine pathway since many gastroinestinal pathogens impair fat digestion and bile function. In this case salivary lipase can be used to break down these fats to better promote absorption by first swishing some dietary fat like coconut oil or butter in the mouth

before swallowing as discussed in the chapter on self therapy. During any metabolic illness this is far more effective than simply having fat in food because the
introduction first of liberated fatty acids will enter circulation before food to thus
activate and support the kynurenine pathway to insulate the kynurenine pathway
from polyunsaturated fats to thus increase catabolism of tryptophan to niacin.

Activation of the kynurenine pathway may seem like something nebulous or
imperceptible but in fact there are very obvious and immediate effects its activation produces on the body which can be used to confirm kynurenine pathway
completion because niacin is highly bioactive and produces immediate effects
on our biology. Anyone who has used a niacin supplement (not niacinamide) will
be familiar with the "niacin flush," which is a fairly uncomfortable flushing and
tingling sensation on the skin because niacin so strongly increases peripheral
blood flow and neurological activation. Males are especially likely to notice the
niacin tingle in the forearms from niacin because in the presence of testosterone
niacin actually reduces grip strength from the forearms. When I saw the study
which found this effect from niacin it was quite perplexing, but I later realized this
is a method by which the human body achieves features of sexual dimorphism
(when males and females present with differing features), by reducing the contractile strength of forearm muscles or jaw muscles causes them to increase in size
and vasculature, which is a common feature in human males. The tingle sensation
from natural, endogenous niacin production is not nearly as severe as that from a
supplement and can be barely noticeable (it might feel like simply an increase in
blood flow to the skin) but failure of the kynurenine pathway also means little or
no niacin production and thus no tingling. Sometimes between meals this niacin
tingle can also happen spontaneously, even without a recent food source of tryptophan, when cortisol is released and liberates amino acids from tissue storage which
are then used as a source of tryptophan for niacin synthesis (which also helps
remove tryptophan from tissues which is beneficial to increased metabolic health).
This tingle occurs between forty and ninety minutes after protein consumption
and will fade thereafter but niacin production and sufficiency will continue for the
remainder of the day. Because niacin immediately increases the metabolic rate and
blood flow the other obvious symptoms of completed kynurenine pathway are a
rising temperature and heat production as well as increased color to the fingertips
and toes as they receive increased blood flow. This absolutely should occur and
if fingers are pale in color after any meal it indicates impairment to endogenous
niacin production and kynurenine pathway (and likely toxic quantities of quinolate
or excessive hormones of torpor) which accompanies or portends metabolic illness
which must be reversed.

While an increase in niacin will increase the metabolic rate, the metabolic rate must absolutely first be activated and raised before consuming dietary
tryptophan. In severely compromised metabolisms it will be necessary to use such
things as sugar, coffee, vitamin C, getting sunlight or other light exposure to turn
on the metabolic rate, for if the metabolic rate is not already risen the production
of torporific hormones like melatonin will be engaged which will divert dietary
tryptophan to serotonin instead of niacin. It is most advantageous to turn on the
metabolic rate every morning anyway with foods such as fruit which are high in
sugar, carbohydrate, and vitamin C so by the time we are practicing niacin therapy
later in the day the metabolic rate is already well activated as measured by the
pulse and temperature diagnostic (the metabolic rate does not need to reach ideal
numbers, only that it be noticeably elevated from inactive as occurs on waking).
The success of this practice will raise the temperature and pulse even more, and in

fact niacin therapy is one of the best ways to restore the most healthful and robust metabolic rate as prescribed in the chapter on self therapy, but only if the metabolic rate is already active and not inhibited. While its principles should generally inform dietary behaviors and choices, specific practicing of niacin therapy is not beneficial more than three times a week as niacin and NAD does persist in the body, so doing it every day is not necessarily very useful.

The metabolic rate and kynurenine activity can be further stimulated by factors like coffee and tea for their caffeine content if desired before consumption of dietary tryptophan which will also better help activate the metabolic rate if needed. But the amino acid *taurine* is the most powerful way to increase kynurenine pathway activity and directly increases the conversion of tryptophan to niacin because taurine improves the effective use and metabolism of all amino acids by protecting cells against excessive cellular excitation and calcium stress, and the supplementation of taurine is usually required for this therapy if the metabolism is very poor and does not activate easily by the consumption of carbohydrate, vitamin C, and light exposure, or there are other symptoms of obvious taurine deficiency such as insomnia, depression, or significant weight gain. Taurine is a casualty of sulfate reducing microbes as discussed in the chapter on vitamin D which then produce toxic hydrogen sulfide, and restoration of normal sulfur metabolism and suppression of sulfate reducers through the consistent use of dietary carotene can help restore normal taurine synthesis and homeostasis. Similarly, any malodor of the breath, flatulence, and feces are symptoms of taurine depletion for this reason.

Besides the role of fatty acids in kynurenine pathway, the B vitamin *riboflavin* (vitamin B2) is also a major nutrient required for successful niacin synthesis. Supplementation of riboflavin is not always necessary since our gut microbiome is our primary source of riboflavin, but if there is any gut dysbiosis and metabolic disease this likely reflects the presence of *roseoflavin* producing microbes which, you will remember from chapter on pathogens and metabolic disease, is an anti-riboflavin antibiotic which interferes with flavin dependent pathways. Just as microbial avidin producers are not necessarily competing with our body but with biotin producing microbes these opportunistic roseoflavin producers are competing with our commensal riboflavin producers for colonization of the nutrient rich interior of our bodies and all the yummy food we eat. So taking a source of riboflavin preceding food can be helpful to reactivate and promote the kynurenine pathway and greatly improves conversion of tryptophan to niacin, while long term restoration of riboflavin sufficiency and thus the kynurenine pathway will occur from resolving parasitism and gut dysbiosis.

Synthetic B2 is more convenient (and less expensive) than natural forms and only requires a very small amount (like 5-10 mg) where most supplements come in far too large of doses (like 100 mg) and can be thusly divided into much smaller doses for efficiency. Brewer's or nutritional yeast can provide more than enough natural riboflavin for this purpose as well and using brewer's or nutritional yeast in these beverages (is gross tasting but effective) or with food can also be a great option. *Pyridoxine* (vitamin B6) is also required for this pathway (several different vitamers are classified as pyridoxine), but the body also cannot use B6 without B2 and B6 deficiency is not at all as common as B2 deficiency so it's not usually required to supplement B6, and synthetic forms of B6 are also not as helpful as natural forms and in high doses can damage the nervous system. If your gut microbiome is working the subtle niacin tingle and increased peripheral blood flow will be obvious from the previous steps and riboflavin will not be required, but if this does not occur it absolutely reveals the presence of roseoflavin producers and necessity to use riboflavin to overcome its inhibitory effect.

To be clear, for this specific process of activating the kynurenine pathway supplemental niacin or niacinamide should *not* be consumed on the days of practicing dietary niacin therapy as a high dose of supplemental niacin will stop its endogenous production from tryptophan which is the entire point of this therapy, but which is fine to use at other times when niacinamide is needed. In terms of protein sources, poultry is a great source to use when starting this practice, not only for the large amount of niacin it contains but also because of its high arginine and tryptophan content which potentiates the activity of the kynurenine pathway and makes its result more obvious. The feeling of warmth and sleepiness which often accompanies poultry, especially turkey, is from the resultant rise in NAD since an increase production of energy also promotes relaxation and lowering of stress hormones. This practice works with anything naturally high in niacin and protein, however, and can even occur from using grains, dairy, and nuts so long as the same steps are followed to promote the kynurenine pathway. pathway.

After restoration of a healthy microbiome their constant supply of tryptophan synthesis is the primary source for our tryptophan and niacin, and will help to restore normal and effortless hair regrowth and maintenance so long as all the other requisites are also addressed. But there remains one major problem which is that our own immune system also destroys tryptophan as a mechanism to protect our body from opportunistic microbes and which in turn can and does cause chronic tryptophan deficiency even when there is plenty in the diet or plenty made by the commensal microbiome. This occurs in chronic metabolic illness and aging and in fact is one of the reasons why older people experience cachexia (wasting), as to fight chronic colonization by opportunistic microbes the immune system oxidizes their target amino acids like tryptophan and tyrosine which then in turn causes their deficiency as well as of their metabolic products like niacin, NAD, serotonin, melatonin, dopamine, adrenaline, etc. This problem is then only resolved by also resolving chronic infection and colonization of the gut by opportunists as discussed in the upcoming chapter on immunity, especially the problems of oxidative stress which result from chronic immune activation. Quite unexpectedly, the niacin tingle/flush would sometimes occur spontaneously, even after it had been some time since consuming protein, but was because gut microbiome tryptophan production or scavenging of tryptophan from tissue storage.

Boron also affects NAD by binding to its oxidized form, and while science does not yet understand why this occurs my research leads me to believe this prevents NAD from prematurely activating calcium channels or reacting to other molecules and becoming reduced before NAD has a chance to accept electrons participating in the mitochondrial electron transport chain. Indeed studies show that repletion with boron is associated with reduced calcium loss and higher ratios of oxidized NAD to its reduced form, so the consumption of foods high in boron such as Prunus fruit like apricots, peaches, nectarines, or grapes and raisins directly supports the kynurenine pathway by stabilizing the NAD end product which thus lowers the required production of NAD and helps the body more easily maintain normal NAD levels and function. If boron foods are difficult to acquire, the occasional, low-dose supplementation of boron can help.

Some fructose is also required for the enzymes which enable the kynurenine pathway and while healthy metabolisms can produce some endogenous fructose a diet which does not include fruit or sugar can actually inhibit the process altogether when the ability to synthesize sufficient fructose is lost (which it is during any kind of metabolic disease). A healthy diet should include fruit every single day anyway if possible. Sugar's support of the kynurenine pathway is precisely why cultures which have protein accompanied with sugar produce such beautiful and healthy populations because the tryptophan in the protein is then easily and consistently metabolized into niacin and thus NAD, thus facilitating an optimal metabolism and resistance to aging and metabolic disease. For NAD synthesis, fructose is essential. Fruit or dessert could immediately follow dinner, or followed by a coffee with sugar added, or dinner could be brown sugar chicken, which includes sugar in the recipe, or sweetened tea, etc. If boron foods are difficult to acquire, the low dose, occasional supplementation of boron can help (and is also more readily absorbed when premixed with taurine).

Alcohol depletes niacin and destroys and blocks the absorption of vitamin B2 and B6 (and depletes zinc), so this therapy cannot function during alcohol use. It is also not possible to overemphasize how sunlight deficiency, which raises melatonin, or supplemental melatonin, strongly downregulates the kynurenine pathway because the body's response to light deprivation (which it mistakes for wintertime) is to downregulate the metabolic rate. This not only stops the synthesis of niacin and NAD but also that of the robust healing and restoration of youthful qualities. Generous light exposure reduces melatonin and so enables more robust function of the kynurenine pathway and restoration of niacin dependent metabolic pathways. For those with depression, PTSD, and alcoholism and addiction it will be required to heal the dorsal raphe nucleus with targeted light therapy as described in those chapters because the dorsal raphe nucleus is the serotonergic center of the brain and trauma to the raphe nucleus automatically causes sustained redirection of tryptophan to serotonin synthesis. During the winter or times when natural light exposure is impossible, bright artificial lights in the warm spectrum (no fluorescent) can be used to help lower chronic melatonin and promote kynurenine activity. Light exposure immediately lowers melatonin and the effect lasts for a few hours, so it is best used to interrupt long stretches of low light such as first thing in the morning and later in the evening.

Studies also show that degradation of tryptophan by pathogenic gut microbes is inhibited by dietary *anthocyanin* which are the purple, blue, and red colors common to fruits like berries, which directly implicates dietary anthocyanin as the primary protective factor of the kynurenine pathway by preventing toxic microbial activity in the gut (this is a reason why red wine or purple grape juice can have significant health benefits). Because pathogenic interception of both dietary and microbial tryptophan is the greatest problem in endogenous NAD synthesis the daily consumption of high anthocyanin foods like berries, grapes, or plums along with a dietary source high in tryptophan like pumpkin seeds is one of the most therapeutic behaviors possible and can result in obvious improvements to metabolic health literally within hours though the effective promotion of NAD. Since dietary anthocyanin is correlated with the seasonal availability of food, specifically berries and other fruit, it would make sense that this pathway should also downregulate during the absence of sufficient environmental nutrition since the increase in NAD increases blood flow to the skin which risks heat loss, and other high anthocyanin options like purple cabbage, purple onion, purple sweet potato, etc., could also be served with protein meals to promote this benefit. The conditions which promote microbial tryptophan synthesis are also those which raise our metabolic rate (sun exposure, vitamin D, local microbial B12 production, green vegetables, etc.), so it seems that the primary source of tryptophan should in fact be the microbiome and not supplemental or even major dietary sources like meat, which during times of light deficiency will cause an excess of torpor and serotonin and melatonin to cause depression, inhibit sex hormones, and promote gut dysbiosis. As discussed in earlier chapters, we require a healthy microbiome to digest plant foods, however, so this is not a function of willpower or force, but knowledge and understanding of biology and listening to cravings to work with the body rather than against biology.

Fruit also contains *malic acid* which enters the citric acid cycle right at a point which also regenerates NAD. While citric acid is directly supportive of this cycle too, malic is slightly more effective. For this reason malic acid enhances the sweetness of sugar and fruits like pineapple, apples, guava, peaches, nectarines, grapes, strawberries, tangerines, and watermelon where citric acid slightly blocks sweet flavors and makes them taste more tart, so extremely sweet tasting fruit or juices not only promote NAD levels better with their sugar content but also potentiate the duration of NAD activity in the body, further promoting tissue regeneration, cellular respiration, energy, and blood circulation. But because NAD also promotes mitochondrial respiration, taking niacin or niacinamide as a supplement can actually, potentially, be harmful during states of cancer which is a problem of mitochondrial dysfunction as discussed in the upcoming chapter on cancer, and resolving that dysfunction can then cause niacinamide to aid in recovery from cancer and other metabolic disease more safely and effectively.

Getting our body's own niacin pathway working can result in very good metabolic restoration, helping to reverse metabolic diseases, reduce unwanted body fat, improve the quality of sleep, regrow hair, and restore youthfulness, among many other benefits. After health is improved by such therapies the process begins to come back more or less as naturally and easy as it is in youth, and the body will, with proper nutrition and supportive behaviors, engage the kynurenine pathway without having to think about it so long as environmental and dietary interruptions to the kynurenine pathway are avoided. Incidentally, yeasts produce a special form of vitamin B3 called *nicotinamide riboside* which is even more supportive of NAD synthesis than niacin. It is one of the reasons why we crave bread, beer, and wine, and as discussed in the upcoming chapter *Good Bread* it can be restorative to health and directly promote NAD activity if made from safe grains.

There is also evidence that NAD is a light sensitive molecule and doing this therapy in the daytime and getting sun exposure afterward can be more productive than doing it at night and going to bed afterward (but it takes time to wake up the metabolism in the morning, so don't practice it until the metabolism has had a few hours to wake up). In review, the niacin therapy process involves stabilizing metabolic pathways through the use of a good fat source like coconut oil or butter (pre-digesting with saliva), then preceding a protein source with supplemental taurine and riboflavin if required, and using sugar to accelerate and sustain the kynurenine pathway which will support the body's natural tendency to get well.

Look Brightly, Little One

Look brightly, little one
And take your place out in the sun,
Run and play and have some fun
And work until the day is done,
Love all those you pass among,
Give thanks when waking every dawn
And when upon the end you come,
You'll celebrate those here and gone
And all the happiness you've won,
All the pain that made you strong
And then to others pass this on,
Look brightly, little one.

CHAPTER 14
CURING DEPRESSION, PTSD, ANXIETY, ETC.

I never dreamed that a place like *Club Axis* in Salt Lake City actually existed. I was nineteen-years old and for the first time I saw people just like me who were not only open about their sexual orientation but were having a damn fine time showing it. Hordes of gorgeous boys and girls my age danced and socialized as if the entire world was like us. Clubs like *Axis* were a haven in a world that showed little compassion and a lot of hatred.

Axis had an underage side and a legal-age side in which you needed a wrist-band to order drinks. Not daring enough to hunt for a fake ID I would usually join my friends before the club to do some pre-drinking. The first night I got drunk to Alice Deejay and remixes of Tiffany and danced in front of a speaker nearly as tall as me I knew the rest of my life was going to better than it had been. To my great surprise I ran into a few High School crushes at that club, from a time when I had never even suspected others boys were also gay, who kindly filled me in on all the gayness from our High School which had somehow passed right beneath my nose, and I realized that all those boys stealing a glimpse as I showered in P.E. had not in fact just been comparing sizes. It seemed if only I'd been brave enough to come out earlier, or had even a single friend with whom I could have confided and been supported I would have found many boys I could have dated, even gone to prom with, some of them the most handsome and wonderful in our school and ones with starring roles in my dreams and fantasies.

One such night at the club while leaning against a wall having a drink and talking with my friends, a cute, kind boy approached me unhesitatingly, standing very near as if there was already some fraternity between us.

"Hey—" he said.

"Hi?" I replied.

"Is your name Nathan?"

On account of my height I was used to people knowing who I was, so I was not alarmed. "Yeah."

Then he asked about my mom, by name, and it was getting weird. Or interesting. "My name is Brian—we were friends when we were eight."

My jaw hit the floor. Standing in front of me was my best friend from childhood from whom I had been unceremoniously ripped away. My first real loss (and the first person to show me oral sex, lol). I couldn't believe it. We caught up for a while. He was actually living out of state and was there visiting, and had gotten a boyfriend (with whom he is with still to this day). Life was coming full circle, and coming out was beginning to pay dividends to my happiness, and another night several months later while traipsing across the dance floor I spied a devastatingly handsome boy with stone-white skin and short auburn hair. His eyes were wild with adventure, haze colored, lips hovering slightly apart as if whispering all the while his lust for life. I smiled at him but naturally unsure of myself continued on to the bar (our side only serving soda, water, and Red Bull). Passing back on my return through the crowd the same boy caught my arm. "Do you have a problem meeting new people?" he asked.

"What?" I replied, thinking he was being humorous. Apparently he had tried to say hi as I passed earlier and thought I ignored him. Always afraid of offending everyone, I struck up a conversation, but our shared obsession with each other was soon too obvious to ignore. I asked if he'd like to go on a date. He agreed. "Where do you live?" I asked. "In this little town up north you've probably never heard of," he replied. It turned out he was in the Air Force and stationed at the base near that dry, dusty hillside neighborhood when I was friends with Brian. Our first kiss happened while hiking an island in the Great Salt Lake, and thereafter fucked like rabbits almost every day for the next year. If we had been an opposite-sex couple one of us would have surely gotten pregnant. Three months in I fell in love with him, but it was right before the holidays and he went home to Louisiana for Christmas and would not return until exactly one hour after I left for the Caribbean on a New Years cruise on with my conservative family. I had never longed for someone so severely, and left a message written in glow-in-the-dark stars above my bed to see when he would slip in alone later that night, but I was caught putting it up by my family who had arrived earlier than expected to take me to the airport and when asked what I was doing mumbled something incoherent and avoided eye contact. I felt like the first person to ever hate being in the Caribbean, bearing the suffering of separated lovers in secret, condemning myself for spending my very first New Years with a boyfriend away from him and further resenting my family, forbidden to share even a hint of my happiness with them.

But ours was not to be an ever-after story. My melancholy brooding and his mercurial temper proved quickly incompatible, and I mistook a silent departure one morning where he didn't even say goodbye and failure to phone for a week as a sign he was done with me. He would later get diagnosed bipolar, which would have been helpful information for the both of us (and my depression as well). So I slept with someone else, surprised and horrified when he called a few days later as if we were still fast boyfriends and nothing had been amiss. The fallout from my honesty was further compounded by a surprise infection with HPV, which I had not even known existed thanks to my religiously oppressive upbringing, and caused him some much undeserved heartbreak.

Dealing not only with the tumultuous newness of a relationship between two young, excitable, mentally ill and abused boys I continued to battle the demons of my youth and that all consuming crisis deciding whether or not I was loved by God. I knew my family had abandoned me, and the circles in which I was raised, what had heretofore claimed God appeared to confirm that I was indeed unwanted and unloved. That boy was my only joy, the warmth and comfort from his embrace unmatched in its tenderness and passion to anything I had ever experienced, but because of my upbringing and the poison of religion did not see that my prayers for salvation had very much been answered, it just was not the answer wanted by my family and religion (nor then myself). Tormented by this life, with no one in which I could confide I broke apart on the inside. Old friends and family were not only emotionally absent, but physically as my family packed up and moved back to Hawaii and left me alone in a State where danger seemed to spring from every corner. Inconveniently during the midst of this relationship I realized I had committed to one person too soon, with whom I probably could not live the rest of my life. If I did I would also miss out on the opportunity of dating other people. It also seemed my waning affection for him was punishment for unnatural emotions over which I was powerless, so I resolved to end things with him and give religion one more go. But I was cowardly in how I approached it, having no real skills at all by which to live life and navigate relationships, overstating my belief in a religion which had plainly rejected me to avoid responsibility for the heart I was break-ing. This boy is such a good person and loved me so much he actually took me to church meetings and entertained missionaries because of my frenzied endorse-ment. It was not entirely dishonest, because I found that I could not reconcile the hurricane of shame and heartache in me. Eventually we split for good.

The most senior church official in my area was younger than they usually came. He had a debonair, masculine quality that instantly made me feel at ease. The last church official I met with, a bishop, was bent with age and scowled even more when I told him I was gay, before ghosting on me though I asked for help in getting reacquainted with the church. I didn't let his behavior deter me from finding answers, though, and now sought help from this more senior person who oppositely considered me with warmth and compassion the other lacked entirely. He didn't blink when I revealed being gay, and we met a few times and he listened to my heartache and confided in me about his own struggles coping with the tragic death of his darling wife from ovarian cancer. Though this man was a more senior official than many I had known over the years he was the first person in all my life to tell me sometimes people are the way they are for no particular reason, that God loved me the way I was, and counseled me not to join the contemptuous conversion therapy groups that had infected the region because he had seen how it destroyed men like me. It was the first time an adult, knowing full well my deepest secret, had ever indicated I was worth loving as I was, something not even my own parents had done.

One night while ruminating on my situation I realized unhappiness would forever be my prison if I continued to sit the fence between religion and being openly gay, and that I should make a decision and stick with it. Continuing in religion meant more lying and dishonesty, and I was desperately sick of it. Love in the arms of a boy had been more precious than anything ever given to me by any religious conception of God, so I chose to fully accept I was gay and live with those consequences, rather than the others.

When I was twenty-one and could legally entertain my growing alcoholism I went straight for it. Most of my friends were also ruined Mormon boys expelled from their families, and all of us loved to drink. One night before I learned to monitor my drinking I found myself at *Club Axis* with the world spinning wildly. I'd been enjoying myself, but in the middle of the dance floor I was suddenly overcome with the realization of just how much I missed my parents. Not only had I lost them to the middle of the Pacific Ocean, I had lost them to eternity, having moved away from home without ever really getting to know them in the first place. A suffocating sob rose to my throat. I was the tallest person in the middle of a dance club and about to start crying. I escaped before the tears could come to my eyes, but found it difficult to walk the many blocks home, the city, spinning, more than once jumped out from under my feet. To this day I don't know how I made it home but opening the door to my apartment I rushed to my computer, ignoring my dog, Angus, who pined at me from his crate and began searching for plane tickets to Hawaii. I would call in sick and spend some time out there to repair the rift that had made me an orphan no matter what resistance they put up.

But I was too drunk to navigate the ticket system. Tears poured down my cheeks as I realized that my plan was stupid anyway, that they hated who I was, and even if I got to the island everything would end in as much heartache as it had before. After all, I was not the one who left.

The pain was overwhelming. I wanted it to stop. I was tired of being depressed. For years my life had only ever gotten worse. The depression which had begun around the age of twelve had matured right alongside me. Now that I was on my own I could see no future for myself which did not involve an avalanche of unbearable sadness. I was exhausted, and lost. I could not do it anymore. There was a bottle of vodka left in the freezer. I could drink it and killing myself would not be hard to do. So I downed the rest of it straight from the bottle, then pulled out a serrated bread knife. I put it to my wrist and gave a quick test-slash. It didn't hurt, but a small divide opened on the skin. At first it was white, but it quickly turned pink and then red as a trail of blood ran down my arm. *Good*, I thought. *This is going to be easy.* I pressed the knife hard against my wrist and slid it with determination. But the pain was as if the knife had suddenly become searing hot. Unexpected, it made me drop it. For a moment my vision popped into clarity. The skin separated in a wide yawn and thick red blood spilled out like yolk from a cracked egg. It was much darker than I had expected, dull, almost like a shadow, and it ran down my arm like an open faucet.

I don't remember picking up the phone to dial 911 but suddenly I had the receiver to my ear and the person on the other line was asking me to stay calm and that paramedics were on their way. Just as suddenly my apartment was filled with four or five medical personnel. Embarrassed at causing so much a ruckus I alternated repeatedly between drunken apologies and thanks. I lost consciousness in the ambulance and awoke later while lying on a hospital bed as a doctor put stitches through the open wound. "Thank you," I said, purposefully servile from so much embarrassment. "Why did you do it?" he asked. Even in this drunken state I was too ashamed to admit I missed my mom and dad. No, it was more than that. How do you tell someone you have lost your family while they yet live? *How pathetic I was*, I thought. "I think I have HIV," I said instead. It was also not a lie since for the last year I had lived in constant fear of the disease, fueled by both the shame of my conservative upbringing and indoctrination but also the alarmist conditioning from LGBTQI+ leaders. "Have you been tested?" was his reply. I shook my head, and blacked out once more.

I finally came to in a small room with windows looking out to the hospital reception, spread out on a couch with my arm wrapped in clean bandages and identification bands around my wrist which confirmed that this was indeed entirely real and not a stupid dream. My head was swimming, but the world was no longer in free-fall. I felt embarrassed at my behavior and my failure. Failure to avoid suicide, failure to do it right. What I wouldn't give to have someone who loved me at my side.

Soon a frumpy woman entered and greeted me with a tepid, condescending smile. "Before we can release you," she said, "I need to ask you a few questions." I confirmed that I was not a danger to myself or others (what a stupid question to ask someone who just slit their wrist). She accepted the lie without any prodding, because she knew as well as I her only job was to protect the hospital from liability, and when asked for a motive I repeated the answer about HIV. The woman gave me a card with some resources for counseling and said I was welcome to call someone to come get me.

My friend Frederick had been waiting in reception all night, said one of the receptionists, but had gone home to get some sleep and left a message that I should call him when I was released. He appeared at the hospital ten minutes later, but seeing me offered no greeting and promptly turned around as if I should simply follow him out. I reached out and grabbed him and began crying into his neck. He had come to my apartment looking for me, horrified to see the ambulance departing, and my apartment covered in blood. He cleaned it up for my return and taken my Angus to his house, and for two days made me stay with him while he cooked, rubbed my back, and let me sleep in his bed, teaching me how to sculpt clay while we traded stories about our family and coming out.

But weeks later no matter what I did the malaise had not disappeared, and I was afraid of falling back into a place from where I knew I would not return a second time. To add insult to injury my insurance wouldn't cover my ambulance ride to the hospital and sent it to an aggressive collections agency which employed a peer from high school who used our connection to harass me for payment when I couldn't (both the hospital and insurance were also subsidiaries of the religion I was trying to escape). My sister had come to stay with me after returning from her religious mission but, like myself, had no life skills with which to survive and had spent the weeks on my couch trying to make sense of being loosed into the world while saddled with debilitating depression and hopelessness. After revealing to my dad what happened he agreed, contemptibly, to let me come to Hawaii, upend my life and spend time recuperating. I quit my job, sold my belongings, and gave my beloved Angus to a friend whose brother had a large farm in the middle of Utah.

Landing at at the Kahului airport the fragrant, wet air hit me in the face like a warm kiss, filled my lungs with a calmness that nowhere else on earth comes so easily. But stepping out onto the curb I did not see my family anywhere.

"Oh," said my mom when she picked up the phone, "we forgot you were coming."

I dozed on the curb in the bright Hawaiian sun, happy at least to be in paradise, though uncertain of my future, content that it would at least not be any worse. Two hours later my parents finally arrived.

"We don't mind you being here," said my dad after we got into the car on the long drive into Lahaina. "But there are a couple rules."

"Rules?" I laughed. I was twenty-one and had not lived at home for three years and already they were treating me again like a child. "Under no circumstances are you allowed to bring your lifestyle in our house—"

"Lifestyle?" I started, feeling the heat of shame rising within me much sooner than expected. This was the last thing I thought to endure on an island paradise reconnecting with those who raised me after a year of separation and attempted suicide. But of course they would. "It's not a lifestyle—" I replied, trying not to let them see how choked up I had become. "What about pedophilia or murder, Nathan?" said my mother. "It's not any different."

The gravity of my mistake buried me like a landslide. I was not on my way to recover, nor to win back the love of my family. I was like a man who pleads guilty without understanding his fate until the prison door slams shut behind him, trapped far away from any semblance of an adult life. Everything that belonged to me which had enabled the small bit of freedom to live on my own was now sold or given away. I was trapped on a literal island, unable to even drive or walk away from here, least of all to afford a plane ticket somewhere else or place to live, not realizing this until I could do nothing about it.

The rest of the drive was quiet, my reunion with my siblings dry and emotionless, my sisters concerned more with the politics of sharing a limited wardrobe and tight living quarters than my visit after being separated for so long. No doubt they felt some uncertainty around the reason for my return and unsure how to approach me, having heard in every prayer and inquiry about me since my departure that I was a deviant living in sin and quiet rumors of what I was.

A few days later my parents introduced me to some new friends of theirs—A handsome couple, slightly younger than my own parents with almost as many kids and each of whom near in age to one of us. Their eldest was a girl name Helena, beautiful and intriguing they wasted no time in making her acquaintance on my behalf. When we were alone I wasted no time letting her know I was gay, not because she had any interest in me, which she did not, but to dispel the obvious imposition on her which had right away burdened our friendship. We did not become fast friends, as I think she was quite adhered to her religious sentiments. That's the way it is with religious people—we would be their friend but for the fear and hatred in their hearts.

One day while my family was at church and I was asleep in a cot behind the living room couch a knock came to the door. Surprised, I opened it to find their friend Adam, Helena's father. I immediately suspected a conversion scheme.

"Hey Nathan," he said.

"My parents aren't here," I pithily replied, hoping it was not too thinly veiled.

"I wanted to talk to you," he continued. "I heard about your condition and I hope you don't mind me saying but I wanted to let you know I suffer from the same thing."

The shame which had threatened to surface turned suddenly to surprise. I relaxed a little and opened the door wider. "It's part of why we moved down here," he said. "The weather helps."

"I'm okay," I lied. Adam hesitated.

"Do you want to go kayaking?" he said. "I thought we could go out on the water."

"Oh," I stuttered. The last time an adult had expressed a desire to hang out with me was many, many years ago. Or maybe never.

"Sure," I said. "Let me get my suit."

Adam's kayaks were already on his car, apparently quite confident in his success with me. We drove out of town and headed toward the inside of the southern bay on Maui. It was well into January but the air was warm, the ocean content. The kayaks were the river sort, short and broad, not at all suitable for ocean going. The paddling was tough and required no small effort to put some distance between us and the shore, but it was magical with the waves lapping at the sides, the clear blue ocean beneath us, and I poured all my despair and sadness into each stroke, the strength of my own arms taking me further and further from shore.

No more than a few minutes into deeper water an explosion suddenly shot up from the surface a few yards away, a blast of mist that sounded both alive and breathing. Whales do that, appearing out of nowhere. Lurching to my left at another sound of breaking water I saw the back of second humpback break the surface no more than five feet from my boat, an enormous, bumpy, grey ridge rising higher than my head as it undulated slowly through the calm water. The fluke of its tale barely broke the surface as it gently glided beneath me, as if taking care not to harm the small and fragile life in it. A third whale then bobbed behind us, spy-hopping, where a whale rises high enough to look across the water at whatever has caught its interest, which in this moment was us, and yet a fourth whale came rocketing from the depths a little ways off, his entire bulk leaping fully into the air as if all its many tons were weightless. It seemed to float for a moment before crashing down with a tremendous splash which nearly swamped our kayaks.

Adam was all smiles and so was I. At rest in the midst of a peaceful ocean, the salt on my skin, the free air in my lungs while the majesty of life literally encircled us and the companionship of one kind person I began to cry at the wonder of it all. On the water in the midst of this experience I realized suddenly there were probably answers to be found, it was only that I had not yet found them. Clearly my family and religion had no answers to give me, but perhaps I only needed to search somewhere else. I wanted to live, and in spite of my wounds I was going to figure out how.

If you don't know depression you don't know the limits of mortality. A condition made worse by the stigma of dark ages mental health abstraction and religious indoctrination I tried as many ways to heal as there are books about depression—medication, drugs, therapy, socializing, alcohol, food, sex, abstinence, self-will, yoga, meditation, religion, love, entertainment, journaling, exercise, being super nice, being a jerk, working, reading, not working, praying, asking for help, taking control, losing control. Getting sober in my thirties helped me gain a change of mentality and purpose but it did not relieve my depression. Many religious friends and family, and sober fellows in spite of their best efforts and spiritual wrestling continue to suffer from depression. I deeply respect the abstinence of drinkers despite such a struggle, and unlike most of the world know a compassion for those who cannot abstain. Alcohol was a welcome reprieve from the monster of despair. Medication was hardly better since it caused as many problems as it was meant to help, and robbed me of more than alcohol ever did but never actually brought happiness. When it comes to depression, cure is a dirty word.

These days when I have sadness it is a beautiful, June Cleaver sadness. It is neither suffocating nor depressing. Having faced the black dragon, sadness now actually makes me happy, because it feels so normal, so safe. I have not had depression for a long time now, save for a few days spat at the first of my recovery which was pretty mild by my usual standards. I spend my days in happiness, content to be alive even when things are in the shitter or loneliness makes me want to crawl into bed. I know it is gone because I also no longer have swings to the higher spectrum, those rare moments of fleeting euphoria which are not the opposite of depression but its conjoined twin, the condition of mania which is unbalance in the soul of a depressed person, not just the depressive troughs which over time grow lengthier than the crests to which those who are depressed cling desperately with hopes that maybe this one will last.

I would never have survived to find these answers had it not been for Madonna, Erasure, Cher, Annie Lennox, and Jennifer Saunders and Joana Lumley who fought for people like me, and the handsome men with whom I occasionally had sex and made friends which brought me comfort when I could not find it anywhere else. But firstly in my depression I somewhat enjoyed it—My life took on a melodramatic depth and intensity of feeling that matched and justified my experiences, and indeed many people when faced with a possible cure to such problems will actually reject it since the pain of suffering serves to validate the loss and heartache we have endured. But this is not a way to live, and initially my path back to health was motivated by righteous vanity, done being overweight and sick I didn't think much about how it would affect my inner conflict, until one day in Los Angeles's hearing the chatter of immigrant flocks of lorikeets coming in my open window I suddenly realized that though I was utterly alone I was, for the first time in my life, content. I fell down crying from sheer happiness, realizing that twenty years of suicidal depression had finally ended and would no longer be my constant shadow.

"*The opposite of depression is not happiness, but vitality—*" my favorite quote, by Andrew Solomon, was a key moment in my recovery which helped inform my understanding of depression not as a problem of pharmaceuticals or discipline but of biology and knowledge, which illustrates exactly the dilemma faced by those suffering depression in that we lack nothing that can bring happiness, merely the energy to live for them. But if vitality is what a depressive person lacks, is vitality the cure? How can I get it? What would I do to get it? What even is vitality? Do I even want it?

Anyone who has spent time with children knows how close to the surface their feelings lie. From an early age we learn what makes us happy, what makes us sad, and all the other complex emotions of the human experience but have little experience in their control or meaning. Before we have an inkling of reason these emotions drive us with as much instinct as any animal. Then we spend the rest of our lives operating from this perspective, seeking stimulus for the feelings we like and relief from those we don't, keenly aware of the effect each emotion has on our wellbeing but deranged from our childhood and trauma that makes us resent our feelings and afraid to express them.

Our brains aren't able to sense their own existence. Or, more precisely, we do not consciously perceive the action of the brain because the brain is the very thing which is doing this perceiving and cannot perceive itself. The mind is what the brain does and how well it does that function is the measure by which we experience life. Senility, autism, even youth are all states of the brain which compromise an individual's relationship to other adults, and a great deal of my trouble making friends and understanding life as a young person was due to undiagnosed autism and the failure of my family and others to understand and help. The more insidious states of rage, violence, and mental disorders further complicate human relationships and make the finding of peace and happiness seem elusive indeed.

Medicine has for decades inculcated the names of hormones like *serotonin* and *dopamine* into the bourgeois lexicon, and people drone on about them as if they're of no more consequence than a license plate or a flavor of soda. For most of the recent history of mental health research the hormone serotonin has been considered the happiness hormone, but this stemmed from a misunderstanding of the effects and purpose of serotonin on the mind and body. Experimenting on those presenting with mania, researchers saw the administration of serotonin-regulating pharmaceuticals to cause alleviation in the manic, depressive symptoms and inferred properties of serotonin with hypothetical explanations, then through medical and lay discourse serotonin eventually evolved to possess supposed properties never actually supported by scientific research. In fact serotonin is not at all the happiness hormone, but a hormone of torpor which regulates metabolic pathways (torpor means to slow things down), and to demonstrate this role serotonin is most abundant in the gut where it serves to regulate water absorption by the gut which in turn regulates the transit of food through the gut, not too little so that food doesn't remain stuck but not too much so that the body has time to absorb nutrients without risking microbial overgrowth. Serotonin also regulates the general metabolic rate, and in all animals which hibernate serotonin and its more powerful derivative, *melatonin*, also a hormone of torpor, triggers the hibernation response at the onset of wintertime. This function of torpor hormones is to similarly slow down the entire metabolic rate so animals don't tear through stores of valuable nutrients during hibernation, not so bears and squirrels will be super happy at the approach of winter.

Without serotonin (and melatonin) hibernating creatures like frogs, turtles, bears, and dormice would probably not exist, nor any mammals at all. Though we do not hibernate as a species (wouldn't that be something?), serotonin still has this same function in humans, and instead of losing our hibernation response our ancestors instead evolved an *anti-hibernation* response which keeps us from going into actual torpor, by responding to elevations in serotonin and melatonin with a concomitant increase in adrenaline which forces an increases the metabolic rate. Pharmacological intervention in manic depression had the appearance of benefit to patients because forcing a state of torpor by higher serotonin dampened manic symptoms. To an agitated, anxious sufferer of depression the tranquilizing effect of serotonin can appear to be a cure in comparison to the alternative, but since it achieves this effect by keeping the metabolic rate low and torpor hormones high this also eventually leads to new and worse developments of psychiatric diseases and physical health because a body in a state of torpor is never able to return to the robust state of healthy metabolic rate which supports vitality and enjoyment of life. This is why so many pharmaceuticals do not relieve depression and why they often carry an inexplicable increased risk of suicide, homicide, and sexual and metabolic side effects, because they further derange an already deranged metabolism and mental state. After all, how could the hormone of happiness carry the increased risk of suicide?

Depression is a hormone deficiency, but rather than serotonin it is a deficiency of *dopamine*. This is often fairly easy for people to understand since dopamine is already colloquially associated with the understanding of *reward*, but because of widespread, religious desecration of the human experience and prejudice against reward and 'reward seeking behaviors' the concept of reward often implies a lack of self discipline, risk taking, or undisciplined indulgence, which also prejudices medical research preventing the proper understanding of dopamine as the actual hormone of happiness. Yes, dopamine is the hormone of reward because reward is how biology communicates to an animal the importance of successful and productive behaviors most likely to improve our wellbeing and chances of survival. Reward is not only confined to risk or indulgence but also comes from love, from close bonds, from achievement, from eating, sleeping, moving, fulfilling responsibility, from sex, from intimacy, talking to someone nice, from learning new skills, expanding our understanding, and overcoming hardship. Finishing your homework literally stimulates a reward response and dopamine release, but nobody denigrates studiousness as 'reward seeking behavior.' The purpose of dopamine is not to impress upon a person the ways which can gratify us but to instead emphasize behaviors which build the successful life of a social animal and increase wellness and vitality—behaviors like honesty, togetherness, accomplishment, food choices, eating patterns, useful resources, etc. It is nature's way of motivating creatures to do things which bring us the resources we require to survive.

But in the depressed individual dopamine is deficient because the stress hormone *adrenaline* is actually made from dopamine, which means that increased stress, no matter its origin, actively depletes a person of dopamine. Depressed individuals lack motivation and vitality because there is not sufficient amounts of dopamine to provide stimulus for reward behaviors like relaxing, or talking to a loved one, or doing a good day's work, no matter what a depressed person does it fails to raise dopamine, so those who are depressed close the curtains and crawl into bed rather than go out and face the world.

Veterans who prefer the military and a battle-ready unit to normal life fail to see how dopamine enmeshes us with military brothers and sisters in the replication of a more natural human tribal existence, confusing the closeness with others facilitated by the military as a function of the military and not closeness with other humans and thus resultant dopamine, something we could easily duplicate at home with our own friends and family if the prison of emotional constipation and personal insecurity and ineffective control behaviors could be banished. Dopamine is also why things like video games can appear to be 'addictive,' which they are not, because a young person's environment may be absent of opportunities for fulfillment growing up in car dependent societies lacking third-places to meet friends and burdened with the trauma of past generations, where dopamine release is then easily achieved by beating the final boss with online friends. Without dopamine there is no mechanism for reward accomplishing behavior in the first place, and thus no happiness.

Of course, because dopamine is a hormone it can be hacked by taking drugs or engaging in thrilling exploits (which actually increases adrenaline, which is the hormone of excitement, since adrenaline is made from dopamine) but these are not evidence that dopamine is harmful but that our lives are often lacking in those things which bring true fulfillment and permanent contentment. The characterization also of hormones as being mere mechanisms of biology, keys which fit into certain locks to elicit a biological response, cheapens the nature of hormones and prevents the understanding of what hormones really are and what they do. Hormones *are* the feeling which accompany them just like a rock is hard or a feather soft, or fire is hot and snow is cold. There is no receptor for fire or receptor for hardness. Something burns because of plasma and something is hard because it is hard. If a hormone could be anthropomorphized into an actual person that person would embody the quality of that hormone because of what it is, not what it does. Hormones are not signalers or keys or locks or receptors. They are the very thing that they do. Cortisol is the hormone of anxiety, adrenaline is excitement, testosterone motivation, progesterone empathy. Serotonin being that which mediates torpor is also the hormone of remorse, shame, and guilt, which is why SSRIs have increased risk of suicide but also why serotonin antagonists like cocaine are also associated with antisocial behavior since remorse serves a functional purpose to motivate moral behavior. If dopamine were a person it would be insufferably happy, and in fact this is exploited by parasites called *Toxoplasma* which, when infecting mice, cause an excessive rise in dopamine which alleviates mice of fear to increase chances of predation by cats on which *Toxoplasma* depends to complete its lifecycle. Humans can and are colonized by *Toxoplasma* which causes the same kind of endocrinological disturbance and contributes to symptoms of mania by disturbing normal dopamine function.

If we believe the illusion that our thoughts determine emotion and not the other way around then our brain is functioning exactly as it should. The most basic illustration of hormones are as the catalysts which compel the course of our lives. Did you notice you were hungry before the thought came to you? Of course not. First the hunger must occur, then the signal is conveyed to the brain. The same happens with sleep and the need for physical intimacy. Feelings must rise first and then the thought follows. With the higher emotions the illusion of being led by thought is stronger, yet no less an illusion. Compare two persons equally inclined to react to a negative stimulus, such as making a choice between polarizing political candidates. One person in our example who has a full stomach will have a much milder reaction than the other who hasn't eaten for some time. If thoughts lead emotion then why a variable with blood sugar? In fact, populations in poorer health tend to be more susceptible to political fear and agitation because less stimulus is needed to raise already high stress hormones caused by poor diets, metabolic illness, and stress of insufficient nutritional and material resources. It is no coincidence that populations generally exposed to better diets and resources as those who are educated, metropolitan, and wealthier are less likely to succumb to fearmongering and deceit, because those with more stable diets, better nutrition, and material security have a more stable endocrine system and thus more stable emotions, which are hormones, less susceptible to oscillation. Those who suffer from poor diet also suffer from extremes of emotional wellness precisely because our bodies are not able to deal with stress due to the absence of requisite nutritional resources, and so suffer from more extreme consequences, having more fear, depression, and unhappiness than those who have healthy endocrine systems because adrenaline is made from dopamine which then causes dopamine deficiency and thus more unhappiness. Hormones are the sole arbiter of our thoughts and motivations. Pump a man with enough drugs and he may soon act more like an animal because the alteration of hormones by those drugs alter his thought and motivations, not the other way around. Yet we treat addicts and sufferers of psychiatric disorders as if they chose that fate or actually have control over their own biological systems, which is fucking insane, expecting them to do what no other person in their place could do either.

During a visit to see family a sister of mine was easily excitable and I later found her crying in secret. She confessed that she'd been short tempered and mean to her new husband, as if for no reason at all. I had a hunch, her being newlywed, and asked if she was on birth control. That the alteration of her behavior and emotions could happen by pharmaceutical intervention had not crossed her mind, and she'd have continued to suffer had I not caught her crying or if she had not been willing to share her problem with me. She switched products and the turbulence resolved. Similarly, my long battle with depression could have ended much sooner had anyone pointed out that repeatedly starving myself in my attempts to be lean and fit were driving my stress hormones through the roof, because the primary stimulants for adrenaline are low blood sugar, low sodium, and emotional conflict. Yet in such situations we expect ourselves to find relief or change through our thoughts, striving to force by will the resolution of emotional hardships, but since the origin of our suffering is in our bodies, with hormones which affect our mind which is also part of the body, this approach never works except to further frustrate and impair effectiveness. For how can we expect to be happy when we don't even fulfill the first requirement for happiness, which is a full stomach?

When I first learned that adrenaline is made from dopamine I immediately knew the cure to depression because it makes sense that dopamine's opposite which increases from stress to catabolize dopamine should cause the opposite of happiness, to prevent a reward stimulus from experiences which oppositely threaten our wellbeing. A little adrenaline can give a sense of excitement but adrenaline release is extremely sensitive and occurs from a wide range of stressful stimuli both physical, nutritional, psychological since it is through the brain that we perceive and experience life. Dopamine (and all of the *catecholamines*) is in turn made from the animo acid *tyrosine* (which is also made from *phenylalanine*) and so chronic elevations in adrenaline from stress stimuli not only deplete dopamine but also tyrosine from which dopamine is made, eventually and depleting not only dopamine but also its precursors which is why chronic stress results in long-term emotional and chronic emotional turmoil because pharmaceuticals do not resupply tyrosine nor stop its excessive loss from the body. Once when I was a child I happened upon a skunk in an alleyway behind our house, and the flood of adrenaline propelled me instantly and instinctually away from the risk of being sprayed by the so-called *flight or fight response*, which is the massive surge in adrenaline release which occurs in response to threats. Adrenaline releases glucose from storage in *glycogen* and increases sodium flux through cells to drive greater cellular activity and power the needed response to potential threats. But adrenaline is also more strongly stimulated from interpersonal conflict than any other reason because threats to our lives comes most often not from wild animals, disease, or disaster, but other humans. That feeling when a stranger yells at us for not bringing their food on time or when a crazed driver slams on their breaks to teach us a lesson for not driving faster than the speed limit is the action of adrenaline, and when we grow up in a consistently volatile environment, with years of chronic adrenaline expression due to the tumult of abusive parents or other harmful experiences, this conditions a stronger and more sensitive adrenaline response which more rapidly and chronically depletes tyrosine and dopamine to thus sustain conditions of depression.

As discussed in the chapters on gut health and diabetes there are also pathogens which force the release of adrenaline or act like adrenaline and consume tyrosine and phenylalanine to produce the harmful amines *tyramine* and *phenylethylamine* which not only exaggerate the adrenaline response and deplete us of tyrosine but cause even more severe mental health problems like schizophrenia, bipolar disorder, and PTSD, because they cause excessive depletion of glycogen storage which then depletes our body of sugars required to keep adrenaline low, and the combination of stress, high adrenaline, and carbohydrate deficiency is so harmful it actually starts to damage the brain and endocrine system and unrelenting stress and suffering. Colonization with amine producing microbes like *Clostridioides difficile* are major catalysts for depression, anxiety, bipolar disorder, anhedonia, schizophrenia, sociopathy, and psychopathy because pathogens even more strongly derange endocrine and neurological function than environmental stress. *C. difficile* is highly infectious and resolution of gut stress and pathogenic colonization as discussed in chapters on gut, diabetes, and immunity are requisite to resolving these psychological conditions. Also unknown to most is that catecholamines like dopamine and adrenaline require vitamin C as a cofactor, so vitamin C deficiency can also greatly contribute to depression by impairing the rate of dopamine synthesis or even causing adrenaline deficiency which then causes extreme adrenaline rebound when vitamin C becomes available, so daily consumption of high vitamin C foods can greatly contribute to catecholamine homeostasis and balance.

As the primary role of adrenaline is to release sugar from glycogen storage, during the night when we are asleep adrenaline is also expressed in small quantities to keep our organs alive and metabolism running, but metabolic decline, behaviors like chronic fasting and dieting, and colonization by amine producing microbes impairs glycogen storage which then causes other problems like mania (temporary euphoria) but also insomnia caused by hyperglycemia. Dieting or fructose malabsorption, which both cause fructose deficiency, strongly contribute to mania because even a little adrenaline will then cause massive release of glucose from glycogen, causing temporary elation as cells are overwhelmed with glucose (and produce high amounts of CO_2 and ATP, which is relaxing and invigorating) but then experience glucose deficiency shortly afterward as glycogen stores become depleted. Because it sustains blood sugar, adrenaline takes biological priority over dopamine, so depression begins to occur from chronic depletion of dopamine, tyrosine, and glycogen, especially during behaviors or conditions which promote adrenaline like avoiding sugar, low-carb dieting, and emotional conflict. Non-sufferers of depression take for granted that they are inspired to go to work, be chummy with old friends and new, the conceiving and execution of plans, discipline, and ambition—things which become inexplicably impossible to the depressed individual because not only do we lack the very mechanism which motivates such behavior but the absence of dopamine oppositely motivates us to isolate and to stagnate to avoid using up spare and valuable nutritional resources. Dopamine is so important to our function as a healthy human animal that when dopamine deficient people discover drugs and alcohol, which temporarily restore or force dopamine function, we become addicted because without dopamine all humans feel hollow and worthless, and our deepest desire is to be fulfilled, healthy, and functional. Being ignorant of this biology or how to purposefully accomplish dopamine repletion, drugs and alcohol become a convenient treatment.

While dopamine made from tyrosine is the agent of joy and happiness, taking tyrosine as a supplement or even getting more protein in the diet is more likely to just promote excessive adrenaline since adrenaline takes preference over dopamine, to continue exhausting glycogen stores, and the primary treatment for this problem is getting fructose daily through high-quality fruit, fruit juices, or other sources of highly bioavailable fructose like invert sugar, to suppress the release of glycogen by adrenaline, and restoring the normal digestion of sugar as discussed in the chapter on parasitism and metabolic disease since fructose inhibits hyperglycemia caused by adrenaline and its (microbial) amine analogs. Sodium malabsorption as discussed in that chapter also accompanies fructose malabsorption and studies show that sodium repletion also promotes dopamine and alleviation of depression, since sodium helps to inhibit adrenaline release, which can be felt rapidly through a low dose of salt (about 1/2 - 1 tsp) taken in something very sugary like fruit juice, lemonade, or even just some sugar water, since epithelial sodium channels are activated by fructose. This benefit of salt, however, absolutely also requires restoration of absorption such as the use of tannins to inhibit microbial ammonia production, otherwise sodium remains in the gut where it instead promotes the very amine producers that stimulate hyperglycemia and high adrenaline and interfere with sugar absorption.

Taurine is very effective in support of depression recovery because taurine actively helps to protect cells from excessive excitatory activation and the stress of excitation (such as excessive calcium influx). Studies show taurine helps the body use protein more efficiently, raises dopamine, and protects cells against calcification. Taurine also directly supports the GABA system and prevents the over-consumption of glutamine. When I was first curing myself of cancer I began using taurine daily for these reasons but in turn found that, in addition to regular maintenance of blood sugar by eating every two or three hours, the use of taurine helped to rapidly cure my depression. Taking a taurine supplement helps to rapidly elevate dopamine (if there is sufficient protein intake and steps to reduce adrenaline stimulation) by facilitating the restoration of cells through the GABA pathway which then lowers both the expression of adrenaline and the effect of adrenaline on cells. It should not be required to use Taurine as a supplement, however and, like most health problems, deficiency is caused by gut pathogens like *Bilophila* or *Desulfovibrio* which actually steal taurine from bile and produce toxic hydrogen sulfide. Over time a body in the active state and under stress experiencing taurine deficiency is unable to meet the demands caused by stress and is quickly and rapidly depleted of dopamine via adrenaline excess while glutamine is depleted as an alternative energy source to carbohydrate due to an excessive state of activation. Until gut dysbiosis is resolved taurine can be used to treat severe cases of depression or other mental illness so long as carotene is used simultaneously to prevent microbial conversion of taurine to hydrogen sulfide. Other metabolic diseases like Parkinson's and diabetes are also marked by taurine deficiency and because sulfurous malodor from halitosis (bad breath) or feces or flatulence is the odor of hydrogen sulfide (or related compounds like methyl mercaptan) it is very easy to evaluate and monitor active taurine loss and effective use of carotene to inhibit its depletion, and over time the consistent use of carotene and resolution of gut dysbiosis will result in normal endogenous taurine production from dietary sulfur. Because taurine is a constituent of bile its supplementation can result in temporary over expression of bile and thus a stomachache, and if this occurs from taurine supplementation stop until this resolves and resume after the discomfort has subsided. This may happen several times but will eventually cease as bile expression is normalized.

In addition to dopamine deficiency, social anxiety is uniquely also a specific symptom of *pregnenolone* deficiency because pregnenolone is the master hormone of the body made from dietary fats, B vitamins, protein, and short chain fatty acids produced by a healthy microbiome, so when we are deficient in pregnenolone our body is far more susceptible the release and effects of backup stress hormones stimulated by social interaction (or our perception of it). Because of this deficiency of pregnenolone, social anxiety is very much a consequence of undereating, dieting, excessive exercise, or other nutritional impairment to pregnenolone synthesis as discussed in the upcoming chapter on hormones. Until a full recovery is made pregnenolone can be supplemented daily (25-50 mg in the morning) and several hours before a social event (200-300 mg) to assist in handling social engagements or obligations such as work and to help with depression. Because cortisol (our primary corticoid) is made from pregnenolone the supplementation of pregnenolone can result in very high and uncomfortable levels of cortisol if not properly supported by a diet high in carbohydrate, as taking supplements is never a replacement for good dietary habits and knowledge of biology, but can support changes in diet and care of the body.

Progesterone is also made from pregnenolone and being the hormone of empathy its deficiency along with that of dopamine causes *sociopathy* and *psychopathy* because of the absence of hormonal mediators which normally inform human behavior, and those who suffer these conditions sometimes even purposefully exploit or injure others because the rise in stress hormones like adrenaline from volatile interpersonal conflict is the only feelings they are able to experience. Everything that makes a human being is biochemical, and the higher functions of humanity such as empathy cannot occur without a healthy, working endocrine system. This does not mean that people should be allowed to harm others and use illness as an excuse—consequences are how we as humans learn that certain behaviors are not acceptable—and there are many with sociopathy that do not actually harm others because they recognize the immorality of causing hurt without requiring emotional feedback to know that. But they still lack that emotional experience and so feel empty and emotionless because all emotions are hormones, and normal hormone synthesis can be restored as discussed in the upcoming chapters on calcium, erectile dysfunction, and progesterone and pregnenolone. Steatorrhea is a common consequence of disturbed fat digestion in the gut, and always accompanies emotional dysregulation, and it is very likely that anyone with sociopathy, psychopathy, depression, ADHD, anxiety, PTSD, bipolar disorder, schizophrenia, etc., will present with such symptoms of fat malabsorption which can be reversed by protecting all dietary fat with foods high in oxalate (using more palatable sources like raspberries and bananas for those like children whom are sensitive to oxalate).

ADHD and restlessness in children are early symptoms of depression, bipolar disorder, and anxiety, and reveal colonization of the gut by amine producing microbes specifically and a diet which facilitates their ingress which is made worse since many parents wrongly consider sugar to be harmful which then causes fructose deficiency and thus susceptibility to hyperglycemia induced by high adrenaline and its microbially produced analogs. The reason for symptoms of ADHD is that a primary function of stress hormones is to motivate movement and exploration, to be active in order that an organism might find novel resources and fulfillment. Stress motivated evolutionary humans to seek out solutions to that stress, instinctually, but children suffering stress can hardly be expected to sit still when they are fed diets high in common wheat, iron fortification, polyunsaturated fats, and low in fruit, sugar, carotene, and sun exposure. Many parents mistake the increase in excitement and joy from sugar as "excess energy," when in fact it is alleviation from the stress of adrenaline, and being hateful, judgmental, and irritable themselves don't later notice that the "crash" which comes from having sugar is the resolution of these stress hormones and ADHD they were looking for all along, because sugar (fructose) so powerfully lowers stress hormones and resolves hyperglycemia. If there is any diabetes, fructose malabsorption prevents this benefit of fructose, but ripened fruit contains mostly invert sugar which is easily absorbed and avoids those side effects, so a low-fruit diet is one of the most common catalysts for all mental health disorders and behavioral problems that are not direct consequences of trauma, because it directly promotes hyperglycemia, high adrenaline, and increases stress. Children are extremely resilient to stress, but not immune to it, and the development of ADHD or childhood depression is evidence of just how severe the consequences of dietary and environmental deprivation can be. ADHD is quite easy to avoid and treat by simply feeding children (and adults) a good diet with plenty of ripe fruit high in carotene like apricots, peaches, nectarines, watermelon, grapes, etc., avoidance of food additives like iron and nitrates, getting plenty of sunshine, and avoiding allergenic additives like carrageenan, gums, nitrates, iron, etc., while also facilitating emotionally fulfilling relationships.

The mechanism of adrenaline, dopamine, and sugar in etiology of depression can be demonstrated in the way coffee helps to alleviate depression—coffee (caffeine) is primarily dopaminergic, which is why it makes us feel so good, because it increases the metabolic rate primarily through dopamine pathways. This then improves the metabolism of sugars which results in greater production of ATP and CO2 which in turn promotes relaxation. But if you haven't eaten much food or especially if lacking in fructose, have fructose malabsorption, or dysregulated cholesterol this causes hyperglycemia, high stress hormones, and excessively elevated heart rate and rapid depletion of glycogen stores. Adrenaline also only releases glycogen from the liver and but there is more glycogen stored in lean muscle tissue, so when the body runs out of liver glycogen (due to dieting or excessive release by adrenaline and its analogs) it then produces *cortisol* to catabolize lean muscle into sugar and amino acids and then we become a jittery, anxious, hungry, emaciated mess and the reason those with eating disorders and depression present with wasting is because the body is harvesting muscle for its sugar and glutamine content because not enough sugar and protein is being supplied to the body.

Because it promotes dopamine production coffee can be a great tool to use in the fight against depression so long as you raise your blood sugar before using it or restore fructose absorption if that is not working correctly (this is very easy to diagnose as using coffee should not result in excessive heart rate, sweating, anxiety, etc., which if a source of fructose has been consumed this indicates fructose malabsorption). One of the worst things people do for their physical and mental health is to have coffee (caffeine) first thing in the morning without eating anything (especially avoiding sugar). At the end of a long night glycogen stores are usually completely depleted and stress hormones are already high (this is especially true in people who wake up very early feeling restless), so taking coffee on an empty stomach and low glycogen stores only serves to catastrophically catabolize lean muscle through absurdly high cortisol release. This is also a reason why those who exercise in excess, or in the morning before eating, or who have a caloric or carbohydrate deficiency often develop mental health disorders like anxiety, depression, instability, bipolar disorder, or lose their hair prematurely or even develop metabolic diseases like cancer because the body cannot run metabolic pathways without fuel, and if we have not eaten the body will instead get this fuel by eating itself. Oppositely, coffee supported with adequate blood sugar, dietary fructose, protein, and prepared without aerated water as discussed in the chapter on gut health results in dopaminergic response which in turn facilitates a robust metabolic rate and increased cellular function which can help treat depression and other mental health conditions.

As a young man saddled with body dysmorphia and destructive dieting habits the depression caused by my childhood trauma was made worse by control behaviors like dieting and excessive exercise which are a response to such trauma (which is resolved by inventory therapy discussed in the upcoming chapter on spirituality or in my book on psychology). After a full recovery is made physical activity can be enjoyed but only if it is fun, never for discipline, and not in excess, and dieting should never, ever be practiced. There are many, many, many supplements and pharmacological products which also can and do promote excessive stress hormone expression such as adderall, SAM-e, SSRIs, and herbal supplements. Sometimes people think that pharmacologically inhibiting adrenaline is a good idea, but adrenaline maintains blood sugar so blocking adrenaline actually causes increased cortisol which tears down lean muscle and organs into useable sugars and amino acids. Marijuana functions in this way and provides relaxation by inhibiting adrenaline, and because that tanks blood sugar it then strongly stimulates "the munchies," and potentially an increase in cortisol, and I had to quit using pot long before alcohol because long term use of marijuana during metabolic stress and failing to eat sufficiently strongly causes it to induce paranoia, agitation, and shaking due to significant cortisol expression. For this reason some young people who smoke too much pot or are on too many pharmaceuticals also have a difficult time maintaining muscle mass (discussed in the chapter on muscle) which requires healthy anabolism in opposition to states of torpor or catabolism. No drugs, pharmaceutical or recreational, is *ever* a treatment for depression and anxiety, which is resolved instead by diet, suppression of gastrointestinal pathogens, and self-care behaviors like getting plenty of food, sugar, sunshine, resolving past trauma, and being kind and compassionate to yourself and your body. After that recreational use of marijuana and alcohol can then be just that—recreational—rather than dependence, without experiencing the negative side effects.

Severe conditions of depression, anxiety, PTSD, etc., will also present with actual damage and trauma to the brain due to excessive activation of the primary serotonergic *dorsal raphe nucleus*, which often (but not always) presents with alcoholism and addiction. Melatonin is made from serotonin and has stronger, related functions and rises in response to deficiency of light such as times associated with nutritional scarcity such as at night when we are sleeping or wintertime due to traditionally reduced food availability. But this rise in melatonin is also stimulated by artificial wintertime such as is caused by excessive sequestration indoors, and while many animals respond to reduction in sunlight as a trigger for hibernation humans evolved an anti-hibernation response to a rise in torporific hormones which is also an increase in general adrenaline expression, slightly but chronically, to prevent us from going into the hibernation state. If we did not have this response we too would become lethargic and passive and crawl into caves or burrows to sleep the winter away, but this also means that any increase in serotonin or melatonin which may be caused by environmental, nutritional, or pharmaceutical factors is met by the body with a concomitant rise in adrenaline which is why depression often starts in the wintertime or even presents as so-called "seasonal depression," since reduced light availability triggers higher general adrenaline expression to more constantly drain dopamine, and why medications which promote serotonin excess also promote an increase in suicide and worsen depression because they trigger dopamine depletion through the reciprocal elevation in adrenaline. This is also why we can actually become addicted to adrenaline, because it opposes torpor, and which is why we can become embroiled in volatile relationships, risk seeking, or incessant conflict, because the stimulation of adrenaline counteracts that torpor and helps us feel more invigorated and alive. This is also even why the onset of wintertime can feel exciting, not because of the promise of holidays and joy but because the induction of torpor itself stimulates a little more adrenaline release which in turn counteracts apathy and malaise and gives a slight thrill and sense of excitement.

Bright light, especially sunlight, generally lowers melatonin, but especially in response to chronic patterns of light exposure, or lack thereof. For instance, acute light exposure will immediately lower melatonin, but it will lower it further if light exposure is consistent and generous every single day rather than only administering when it's absolutely needed, and in fact melatonin expression patterns follow daily, weekly, monthly, and even seasonal and yearly patterns, where light exposure one year will also determine melatonin expression the following year. So it is the *absence* of light exposure which causes excess melatonin to rise and thus suppress the restorative metabolic functions, which becomes worse the longer light exposure is deficient, which is conversely resolved by generous exposure to light. Because this shift in melatonin elevation is also delayed in regard to light deficiency, occurring only *after* the stress of light deficiency has begun to take a toll and not concurrently, depression is actually most severe during the spring-time after winter has caused a prolonged light deficiency, which is why depression can be so overwhelming as the world emerges from its great slumber and plants and animals begin to celebrate, the disconnect between demoralizing emotions and the sights and sounds of new life can cause further despair for a person with depression, who is also at their peak melatonin levels which will not begin to drop again until the sunlight deficiency is resolved for several weeks or months. But if a person continues to stay indoors and continues suffering light deficiency after winter has ended this state of metabolic can get even worse, to drive up melatonin and adrenaline so great that it causes real endocrine and neurological impairment to catalyze depression and other related mental health conditions. In combination with other trauma, depression from light deficiency is unavoidable.

The *dorsal raphe nucleus* just so happens to be highly influenced by light. Some researchers are already beginning to confirm this role of the brain and light in studies on PTSD patients, but hampered by bias and limited understanding of the mind their findings have not yet found widespread acceptance among the medical community. During events of heightened stress (nutritional or environ-mental) or intense trauma such as occurs during childhood abuse, military service, being raped, or other traumatic events the function of the raphe nucleus becomes profoundly altered due to the harm caused during "inescapable stress," and as a result begins to chronically and persistently elevate serotonin secretion and the chronic deficiency of metabolic respiration then literally causes lesions and other damage to the brain. This alteration to the serotonergic center of the brain which results in excessive torporific hormone production is also called *learned hopelessness* and is also discussed at length in the later chapter on alcoholism and addiction as this trauma to the dorsal raphe nucleus is the condition which causes all alcoholism and drug addiction. I believe this response of the dorsal raphe nucleus to trauma to be biological reflex designed by nature to lessen the suffer-ing of an animal in predation or other severe trauma as it requires extreme stress to trigger this trauma to the raphe nucleus which then dampens physical pain and feeling to thus spare an animal suffering in its final moments. We no longer experience predation by wild animals and due to medicine and other modern advancements we now easily live through such trauma to find ourselves irrepara-bly harmed by the experience. Some drugs strongly block the effects of serotonin, such as cocaine which acts to inhibit serotonin transporters, and as such can relieve a person of associated traumas which is why drug and alcohol abuse are so common in those who have these conditions, serotonin also being the hormone of shame, guilt, and remorse. But serotonin also plays a role in morality which is why for instance heavy cocaine use can cause a tendency toward extreme amoral and even violent behavior, or why veterans often develop drug abuse problems because the act of killing other humans is not something the mind can just get over (since these drugs also directly affect tissue function they can and do also change body composition, and chronic cocaine users get increased fat deposition in their face). The trauma which occurs to the raphe nucleus directly downregulates dopamine, GABA, lowers the metabolic rate, and even interferes with sleep since it is GABA, not melatonin, which properly mediates sleep. But generous exposure to natural sunlight or other bright light can and does reverse the condition as long as the diet also supports recovery, and recovery from depression, anxiety, bipolar disorder, and PTSD can be permanent through direct bright-light brain stimulation therapy.

Light exposure should largely subsist of natural sunlight without causing sunburn. Many windows today are manufactured with films that block a great deal of light so even being near large windows can change the light wavelength composition reaching the eyes and body and thus stimulate artificial winter adaptations in our biology (glass that appears bluish or greenish is this way). Especially because of our contemporary lifestyles it is not always possible to get sufficient sunlight to reverse this condition (that would be probably six to eight hours total per day, every day) so it can be helpful and necessary for any severe conditions to also acquire a very bright, artificial, low-heat light to supplement extra light. It is important that artificial light be in the warm spectrum, which means it has more red-wavelength light in its spectrum than blue-wavelengths, not its heat temperature, such as a 300-watt incandescent, LED light whose color temperature is 3000k or less, or even a bright halogen lamp (although those get really hot and can present burn or fire risk). Blue spectrum lights like fluorescent, CFL, or LED in the blue spectrum are not helpful because blue spectrum light actually stimulates cellular excitation and energy consumption, where the warmer spectrum promotes cellular relaxation and energy production. Light exposure to the eyes directly lowers acute melatonin production, so any general bright light exposure works to promote this benefit. But specifically for conditions of depression, PTSD, alcoholism and addiction, etc., light exposure to the back of the head or the sides of the back of the head will more strongly stimulate the raphe nucleus with energy production and mitochondrial respiration and thus reverse the chronic and excessive expression of serotonin and melatonin, allowing the raphe nucleus to regenerate and heal by stimulating cellular regeneration of that area of the brain.

The evolutionary reason for targeting this area is the same as would be the case if we spent our days foraging under the sun as did our ancestors, our eyes turned away on account of the brightness the sun and thus the back and sides of the head areas which instead receive direct rays. Light therapy for resolution of dorsal raphe nucleus dysfunction is best targeting these areas instead of the eyes, and because light exposure to the back of head also frees our eyes to be engaged elsewhere this therapy also frees us to do things like watch TV, play video games, work on the computer, or read a book, thus also making it easy to accomplish. There are studies which confirm the sensitivity to light of the brain independent of exposure to the eyes, and it is this sensitivity to light which helps those parts of the brain regulate hormonal function and circadian rhythms, for instance which still continues even for those who have lost their eyes or eyesight. For the resolution of these conditions a course of light therapy with a bright light focused on the sides or back of the head must be completed for *at least* two or three hours *every single day* for two entire weeks without missing a single day, in addition to daily outdoor sun exposure.

Because stimulation by light increases the metabolic rate of the brain, it is also necessary to consume enough dietary *vitamin C* before each session in order to facilitate the increase in metabolic rate, else the brain will refuse to reach its peak metabolic potential, even under light stimulation, since vitamin C is an antioxidant which protects cells during high metabolic rate, and should be taken immediately prior to light exposure. Not much is needed but a serving of high vitamin C foods like oranges, black currants, rose hips tea, bell peppers, guava, strawberry, kale, parsley, papaya, acerola cherry, etc., could help very well, but because vitamin C is destroyed in the presence of ammonia which also inhibits its uptake by blocking sodium transport the resolution of ammonia excess also helps promote vitamin C sufficiency. Because light always stimulates mitochondrial respiration which always produces reactive oxygen species, feeling irritated or restless while in the sun is also a direct symptom of vitamin C deficiency and symptom of oxidative stress. Many old people can't even stand ambient light exposure from open windows because their antioxidant status is so low that even a small amount of light exposure causes them irritation, so inhibition of ammonia and getting plenty of vitamin C is required for this therapy to be successful, and in combination with the use of tannin and sodium chloride will strongly help restore the respiratory metabolism of the dorsal raphe nucleus by light stimulation.

It is very important to know that when effective this therapy will actually cause an *increase* in depressive feelings for the first two days or so after beginning. This is because the rise in serotonin is occurring to supply the excess in melatonin, and because light so strongly stops melatonin production the temporary backlog of serotonin caused by a sudden drop in melatonin will temporarily cause a further decrease in metabolic rate and increase in depression. This is an excellent sign that the therapy is proceeding as it should, however, and after this backlog is resolved a full and permanent recovery of these conditions can be expected forever after so long as the diet continues to support a robust metabolic rate, low adrenaline, and avoid light deficiency (light therapy absolutely will not work if you continue with dieting and behavioral stress, which must be addressed first). If these conditions should ever recur simply practicing this therapy again is a simple task. This practice should not be uncomfortable, so if you experience headaches or other side effects you're probably overdoing light or heat exposure and should take a break, taking care not to overheat. For some reason, a lot of people don't actually attempt this therapy and continue to wonder why they suffer from depression. Light exposure is *vital* to permanently reversing depression. It is required to be healthy. It is NOT OPTIONAL. Light exposure for at least two hours *every single day* is the minimum required to be a healthy human being. If you aren't, then you have a light deficiency and you must take steps to address it. Using an artificial bulb while reading or playing video games is one of the easiest therapies to practice. If you have these symptoms, go outside and get some sunshine or buy a bulb or two and integrate its use into your daily routine.

Many people who suffer from depression and substance abuse may also have eating disorders such as anorexia or bulimia. Ideas about food, weight, and personal worth can sabotage your efforts to get well, because the calories equals fat model of weight gain is not at all how weight loss works, and only serves long term to destroy your health and make weight gain more likely as the body consumes its lean muscle and lowers the metabolic rate, and it is impossible to raise the metabolic rate and cure depression if you are not eating sufficient quantities. But, just like the other conditions addressed in this chapter, anorexia is also a neurological condition which is driven by high torporific and stress hormones. Because the state of torpor is the hibernation response one of its qualities is to suppress the appetite, as hibernation wouldn't be very useful if an animal felt ravenous while waiting out the winter, and anorexia results when torporific hormones are sufficiently high as to disrupt hunger hormones like leptin and ghrelin. Anorexia can easily be treated with light exposure and a daily dose of niacinamide (about 250-500 mg with breakfast should be sufficient) because the absence of sufficient NAD due to excessive serotonin so strongly lowers the metabolic rate it then prevents hunger stimulus. Supplying niacinamide results in greater NAD which in turn lowers torporific hormones and can stimulate normal hunger, making it much easier for those with this condition to eat sufficiently. Many people have anorexia and don't even know they do—if you think of food as a liability for weight gain or engage in any dieting behavior you have an eating disorder, and you must treat it and increase your caloric intake before you can ever expect to make improvements with these conditions, and address your conception of weight gain and personal worth as instructed through inventory therapy.

There are some studies which seem in conflict about the benefits of low melatonin and indeed there is a great difference between melatonin or other hormones which are naturally low due to health and thus little need of its adaptive functions than when they are low because of age or disease and a subsequent *inability* to produce them. The low levels I advocate are that which result from improved health rather than the artificial lowering or blocking of melatonin, since doing so in a stressed state would be damaging rather than helpful. In the elderly and those with advanced disease states it is possible that low melatonin can be a sign of the inability to make it. This apparent discrepancy between studies and medical observation is very relevant for other disease states and biological elements, where there can be a difference between low or high levels of one thing or another in the case of good health, which further supports health and longevity, and the same measurement which might result instead from stress or disease and an *inability* to produce it. Strangely, there does not seem to be much awareness of this nuance in medical studies and certainly not in medical practice, and is why understanding of context is so important in the determination of health conditions and the therapies which restore them, because assumptions drawn from test results can misleadingly correlate and can and does lead to misguided theorizing, prescribing, and diagnoses.

Absence of feeling or motivation is also called *anhedonia*, which is specifically an inability to derive pleasure and reward from experiences which normally provide that, and this is caused specifically by excessive neurological stress from excessive consumption of nightshade plants as described in the chapter on alcoholism and addiction, as toxic glycoalkaloid poisons strongly disrupt acetylcholine homeostasis to stress the nervous system, and many people with mental health disorders, apathy, anxiety, and anhedonia also naively consume large quantities of potato, potato skin, eggplant, or other nightshades which are the highest sources of glycoalkaloid toxins in the diet, and temporary abstinence from potato and eggplant along with other dietary strategies discussed in the chapter on alcoholism and addiction can rapidly help to normalize endocrine and neurological function to help restore emotional feeling and motivation. Even if you have alcoholism or other substance abuse problems, treatment of anhedonia and sociopathy can be begin by having a beer or two to strongly lower acetylcholine, then afterward avoid potatoes and eggplant and directly address depression to prevent subsequent excess of acetylcholine which impairs the nervous and endocrine system. As childhood trauma also greatly determines our psychological response to stress, the inventory therapy in the upcoming chapter on God and Spirituality or my book on child abuse, *The Perfect Child,* will be required to find resolution of traumatic experiences which trigger the stress response. We who have mental health problems have been conditioned our entire lives to cope with stress through ineffective coping strategies such as ignoring or avoiding things we fear or which cause us stress, including our own feelings, responsibilities, love, and other constants of life because the abuse we experienced growing up failed to empower us with the skills required to handle these aspects of life. Empowerment such as is achieved through inventory therapy is the most effective way to alleviate those experiences of trauma. Phobias and intense fear are also caused by higher than normal elevations in stress hormones. For instance, a person with a phobia of flying or spiders will express higher adrenaline release which also has a greater impact on affected organs like the brain due to the long term catabolic effects of chronic stress and as such will experience a directly correlated exaggeration of terror over things which make otherwise healthy people simply a little nervous. Adopting a diet, behaviors, and reforming our environment to naturally drive down adrenaline and cortisol production and reduce hormones of torpor as well as resolving psychological conditioning which triggers such fear through inventory therapy can easily help turn phobias into experiences of simple discomfort.

Early in my recovery a good diet and taurine was enough to resolve my depression, since supplementing taurine so strongly negates the insufficiencies of the metabolic pathways which lead to depression. By using this light therapy and guaranteeing daily light exposure and keeping my blood sugar up my condition became so stable that I have not required taurine to feel happy for many years. My brain chemistry, strangely, has been altered so well that as I recalled my suicide attempt and read my old journal entries I could no longer revisit the feelings which had driven me to such desperation, and began to understand why those without depression cannot comprehend how truly awful it is. Depression indeed is a sinister creature, only understood by those it touches, but it can now be cured with just a little time, understanding, and compassion for the body and our requirements for good nutrition, sunlight, and self-care.

Like most I believed the terms of mortality could be dismissed. Rude was my waking. To work with the limits and logic of human physiology as well as adopting a self-honest attitude toward the factors that influence it has freed me from the darkness of depression and ill-health, and anyone else can do this too. The use of taurine, a good diet and behaviors which supports low adrenaline and normal function of the GABA system, resolution of gastroinestinal pathogens, and targeted light therapy with vitamin C can maintain vitality and provide permanent relief from conditions associated with depression. It is important to have enough carbohydrates, protein, and good fat to fuel the metabolism, so always adhere to the first requirement for happiness which is a full stomach.

CHAPTER 15
THE CURE FOR CANCER (AND MIGRAINE)

My thirties were going to be full of adult realizations and reaching my human potential, finally getting out of life what I expected (most approaching the end of their third decade stupidly think this). I kicked off my thirties with a huge, superhero-glam theme party and invited everyone I knew and loved. So many people came the club asked me to make it a regular night (I did not). I soon discovered, however, that my life was heading in a different direction. For the first three years of my thirties my health and energy slowly and steadily declined. I had been a competitive athlete full of energy and physical ability who was suddenly unable to even get off the couch. I fell away from socializing, hiding my declining appearance and vitality away from the harsh eyes of the world. Eventually I gave up strenuous activity altogether, but even walking my dogs around the block left me breathless and achy and caused my extremities to swell. I developed an infuriating, chronic sensation of which the word *itch* is an insufficient description, which would find its way to my spine whenever I laid down to sleep which whenever I attempted also resulted in a coughing fit that would last for hours and keep me from sleeping all night long. My body ached incessantly, and no matter how much I tried warming my freezing body with baths, blankets, or sitting in the one-hundred-ten-degree Palm Springs sun proved futile, my body breaking out into sweat even when I shivered in the cold of winter and shivering even when sweating from the heat of a desert summer. A lesion on my tongue had appeared a few years earlier too, which I would later find out is called leukoplakia. It seemed an ill omen, a reminder every time I brushed my teeth that something was very wrong with my health. At first I thought I just had a drinking problem, and tried to abstain, with little success. I also suspected a thyroid illness. During this time I visited three different doctors who all said my tests came back "in range", which turns out to be code for *I cheated my way through medical school because I only got into medicine to get rich.* Let me tell you, if I was a doctor and a thirty-two-year-old came into my office looking the way I did, with the symptoms I had, I would consider myself a poor doctor indeed if I ran standard tests and was content with the results, which for the last four years always included the phrase '*You have an elevated white blood cell count, but no infection,*' which it turns out is an obvious sign of cancer.

I finally got to a doctor with enough competence to suggest imaging my thyroid. It was enlarged with *five* nodes, including a large one in the isthmus. I was actually elated because for the first time because after several years of fighting I finally knew my adversary (and my unsupportive fiancé could no longer say I just wasn't trying hard enough). The doctor said it could probably be cancerous, but there was nothing to worry about and that I should make an appointment with an endocrinologist right away to have them biopsied. The only endocrinologist I could get with my health insurance didn't have an opening for *three months.* Hope faded rapidly. How fast did tumors grow? Did I have three months to wait just for a biopsy? Thankfully, I had already started to learn the things which would lead me back to health, and began implementing them into my life. Finally the day came for my next appointment but after getting into the exam room the doctor said it was too late in the day to do a biopsy, that his colleague had gone home, and that I had to reschedule for another appointment in the future. In another three months.

The hoops and hurdles of dealing with indifferent, inept, and condescending medical institutions had now stretched out to years. I was going to die, not from cancer since thyroid cancer is one of the easiest to treat, but from neglect and economic inequality. Making things worse, my terrible relationship finally imploded and my fiancé left for good. I lost my health insurance and found myself utterly without any social or institutional support, having to start my life over in the midst of a devastating health crisis, sleeping on couches and walking to public transit, so tired I could not walk up the one-block hill to an apartment where I was staying without stopping three or four times to regain my strength. But there was a silver lining—the information I had discovered was already seeming to bear fruit. The changes in diet and the various strategies I was using to address my health problems were restoring my sleep, my energy, and lifting my spirits. Eventually my health became more robust and normal than it was even in my twenties. Best of all, because of my lack of access to medical care I inadvertently got to keep my thyroid.

The fundamental flaw of cancer treatment dates back even to early Greek and Roman times. Cancer was rare, but when it did present itself the approach was to cut or cauterize it. This can sometimes be helpful. Often it is not. While cancer today is alarmingly common the view of cancer is still the same—it is considered an alien body, something to be killed and destroyed. This pervasive viewpoint is precisely the reason so many people die from treatment, and why a cure does not exist, and also why cancers return since the underlying causes are not healed in the first place.

Although most cancer is the result of pathogenic microbial colonization, cancer itself is not an invading pathogen. Cancer is made of our own cells, from our own DNA, and as such is not some exotic or foreign adversary, but simply a part of ourselves which is sorely misunderstood. Strangely, it has not yet struck oncologists that all cancer cells "mutate" in exactly the same way, no matter what type of cancer it is, which is either uncanny or simply reflective of the fact that cancer cells are not caused by mutation but by their own inherent cellular programming. Cancer cells are simply cells which are sick and trying to heal, but the processes of self-healing employed by normal cells has become stuck in the "on" position due to the immediate environment of those cells which can no longer support normal cellular function. Cancer does not want to eat you alive. It is the body trying to repair itself but unable to do so. This fundamental misunderstanding is why we pump people full of toxic chemicals, zap them with ungodly radiation, or cut off important body parts and discard them in the trash instead of employing healthy, therapeutic means of resolution and prevention. A friend of mine had to take thyroid medication all his life, because his thyroid was removed as treatment for thyroid cancer when he was only a child, and he later died of liver cancer during conventional treatment at the tragic age of thirty-seven. Millions of men with prostate cancer find an end to their sex-life when the prostate is removed. Women all over the world must give up their breasts in order to survive breast cancer. None of this is necessary, and when a friend of mine survived breast cancer in 2024 due to my work she also kept her breasts and simply had a successful lumpectomy after previously malignant tumors converted to benign. It is far past time for more restorative approaches for cancer treatment. If an alternative approach of healing cancer is taken, instead of destroying it, suddenly cancer recovery is less painful, easier, and actually successful. Since cancer is already trying to heal itself, assisting the effort is more effective than trying to search and destroy every diseased cell, as is obvious by the rates of recurrence in cancer treatment. Another person who used my work still had cancer in her bones after chemotherapy and her family was preparing for her death, but months after following my example as laid out in the earliest version of this book before I had even discovered the solution to the Warburg Effect received a surprise "no evidence of disease" and was officially in remission.

While my descent into ill-health was terrible, and something I do wish to have never endured, my body became a walking laboratory. On the precipice between health and death, even little changes became more obvious than they would in a completely healthy person. Small improvements in body temperature or energy from certain foods or substances wrought obvious causations and correlations, allowing me to experiment, reason, and evolve the various interworking of the human body, aided by scientific research interpreted through correct physiological context and helping me deduce the path back to health without the help of contemporary medicine, which at best would have left me without a thyroid and thus dependent on thyroid medication for the rest of my life (which by the way does not successfully replicate thyroid function and will lead to yet more debilitating health issues down the road).

The specific juncture where cancer fails to heal itself is in inflammation. When cells die in their natural course of living they fall apart and leave behind chemicals signals which stimulate new cell growth. This new growth is in turn accomplished by swelling. Just like an embryo growing in a womb, new cells swell large so they can split into new cells, and the process repeats until all the new cells have matured, and once finished growing the mature cells put out new signals which tell the surrounding tissue that healing is complete, or rather the signals which stimulated the healing response are no longer expressed, and so no more new growth is necessary. Cancer cells swell and divide but aren't able to stop beyond that point. They continue to grow and divide because the chemical signals which stimulate the healing response continue to persist and never turn off. This is generally caused by a lack of energy in that area of the body, especially due to interference by opportunistic pathogens, and basically the cells are suffocating as they grow, unable to oxidize sugar in a normal manner because the hormones which stimulate growth also inhibit normal oxidative metabolism in order to facilitate growth. So the growth stimulus continues unchecked, stimulating more and more cells until a tumor mass forms. And though the tumor is the focus of the cancer treatment it is not the thing which actually kills us. There are countless cases of humans living for many, many years with tumors. In fact, all people over the age of 50 usually have tumors in many places in their bodies. Tumors are a natural part of aging. The part about cancer which kills a person are the *hormones* which the tumor and the cancerous area of the body continue to express. They are stress hormones meant to briefly facilitate growth and healing but a constant stream of them from a cancerous area eventually overwhelms entire systems, and as the tumor grows it produces more and more of these hormones which interfere with other body systems and eventually results in the death of vital organs and thus the body.

There is a delusion I suffered most of my life, indeed it is one which most of humanity suffers also, one that causes more pain, heartache, and broken bonds than that of any other to which we are susceptible. That delusion is the erroneous expectation that result is entwined with action. *Unreasonable expectations* is the phrase often used to describe the failure of outcomes to match what we expected, but it is more than that—whatever we undertake in life, whether making friends, taking tests, applying for jobs, entering into relationships and marriage, raising children, and even fighting cancer, it is never our job nor is it within our capacity to determine the outcome. That is far beyond our ability, and expecting ourselves to bend the course of life to what we think it should or what others may want leads not only to bitter disappointment and an ineffectual approach to life but to a misguided idea that outcomes make our experience. It is not our job to make people love us, to make children turn out, to get an employer to hire us. It's not even our job to not get cancer. Our only requirement is to show up for life and opportunity and to do our best. Beyond that it is entirely up to life, and fate, or whatever it is which determines if we live or die.

One of the greatest liabilities for cancer survival is fear. Many people suffering from cancer end up doing insane things because we believe it is our job to control mortality and not die, and actually end up hastening our own demise or instead bury our heads in the proverbial sand and do nothing because of fear. We only can strive, and knowing that our responsibility stops before the outcome not only helps relieve us of unreasonable pressure it also helps to improve the likely outcome because once we turn those things over to the forces which actually make them it frees us to be better at showing up, to meting our actual responsibilities, the ones which we actually can effect. In dealing with cancer especially we are required to come to terms with what it means to have no control over life, what it means to suffer, to live, and to love. If this is difficult to do you must address your trauma and control behaviors through inventory therapy and my other books, or it will only increase your suffering, frustration, and ineffectiveness. The further I get from my cancer the more convinced I am of the value of such difficulties. My life is endlessly more rich and satisfying because of these struggles which I would never otherwise have experienced. My view of life is both satisfied and deep. Fear of death is just a fear of dying with yet unamended wrongs, and being up against such realities changed me in ways I would never have otherwise. If we or others around us have cancer we can trust that we are intended to learn deep and meaningful truths about reality that not everyone gets to learn. It's hard, of course, and sometimes sad, but to us is given the chance to peer beyond the shallow surface of normal life.

There are quite a few biologists like Otto Warburg who have understood the basic nature of cancer for a very long time, and some medical professionals like Dr. Stephen Paget who first proposed the "seed and soil" characterization of cancer *all the way back in the year 1889*, stating that for cancer to grow the environment of the tissues must be right to accept it. Their careers have been spent studying cancers, hormones, and degenerative illnesses in clinical environments. But because they are not part of medical boards or institutions their ideas aren't spread throughout the medical community, even though Dr. Warburg is so important in biology that he has a Nobel prize and The Warburg Effect named after him. Dr. Peat understood the fundamental relationship between cellular energy production and cellular morphology, and the approach I took to healing my own cancer symptoms I learned from reading their work and applying the science to my own situation. It was one in which I got to heal rapidly and successfully, without great expense nor having to suffer horrible, radical treatments. Sometimes it might be necessary to remove a tumor through surgery if it has reached appreciable size, but radiation and chemotherapy, which damage and destroy other cells and promote destruction of the body should not be the primary treatment, but instead the instructions in this chapter and book. DO NOT confuse other 'alternative' approaches to healing cancer as equal to this book, however, as they are as poorly informed about the actual biology behind the etiology of cancer as mainstream treatment and while they may avoid the very harmful effects of chemotherapy or radiation they will not ultimately improve survival outcomes.

This whole book is essentially the cure for cancer, where this chapter only focuses on the specific factors, and this chapter will do nothing to help recovery from cancer if the diet and behaviors are not changed as discussed in other chapters and to adhere to principles of cellular respiration, human diet, pathogenic microbes, and metabolic health, and treatment using these strategies should also continue long after recovery is made, as reverting back to old dietary patterns will results in recolonization by opportunistic pathogens and thus also relapse of cancer. The effect of these approaches can and should be felt rapidly, such as one person who had stage four lymphoma and could barely swallow food due to the large, protruding tumors in their neck lymph nodes and the swelling it caused, but was able to eat again after just two weeks using these strategies (tumors do not shrink rapidly, though, and if very large should be surgically removed). They did not listen to my advice about taking it easy and avoiding stress, however, and spent their time obsessively day-trading in stocks and crypto which drove up their stress hormones and promoted self-destructive behavior. Just as necessary as nutrition and physical health when dealing with problems like cancer is the resolution of mental stress as this will not only lower stress but help promote better decision making and empower more effective life skills to more effectively deal with the stress of recovering from cancer.

In the mid 1900s the famous scientist, Otto Warburg, famously discovered one of the primary metabolic dysfunctions behind cancer which is now termed *the Warburg Effect*, where cancer cells are shown to lack oxidative respiration even when there is sufficient available oxygen (oxidative respiration is the oxidation of carbohydrate to produce the energy molecule adenosine triphosphate). Instead, cancer cells use backup pathways of energy production such as glycolysis or the oxidation of fats (which also involves converting sugars into fats first rather than oxidizing sugar). This shift in metabolism by cancer cells is often used by ignorant nutritionists and medical professionals to recommend a low sugar or low carbohydrate diet for those who have cancer, but because the problem in cancer is failure for cells to respirate properly and not a problem with sugar this never succeeds in treating or preventing cancer, and in many cases can actually contribute to cancer due to the chronic stress of low carbohydrate diets which chronically elevates hormones of stress and torpor which slow the metabolic rate. Cellular respiration occurs in mitochondrion organelles through the *electron transport chain* in which electrons taken from substrate like carbohydrate (which is first converted into pyruvate through the citric acid cycle) are passed through a series of proteins which then produce ATP, and oxygen then accepts those electrons at the terminal end of the transport chain and forms CO_2 as the end product. Since mitochondrial respiration is the major energy production route for human physiology, cancer cells are seen consuming a great deal of fuel but outputting very little ATP, since non-mitochondrial metabolism is so inefficient at producing energy, so cells do not have sufficient energy to heal themselves or the tissue which they inhabit and cancer cells become stuck in a state of excess consumption and deficient production. Fuel sources for energy production include the amino acid *glutamine* which, like carbohydrate, is metabolized through the citric acid cycle and can be converted into pyruvate for oxidation and run the electron transport chain. In fact, glutamine is a comparable energy substrate to sugar and the deficit in energy production is even more problematic for cancer because failure to produce energy leads to exponentially higher fuel consumption as cells attempt to restore energy deficits which then creates a growing negative feedback loop that more rapidly consumes fuel, eventually catabolizing tissues into useable sugar and amino acids (especially glutamine, methionine, and cysteine) which then causes wasting (cachexia) band eventually death.

It is not well known that mitochondria concentrate *silicon,* and silicon is shown in studies to increase mitochondrial consumption of oxygen (in opposition to the Warburg Effect), and although silicon does not receive much attention at all in medicine, biology, or even nutrition it is in nearly every food we consume (even meat) and is proven by a few studies to be necessary for some aspects of human health like bone and cartilage, which is why cartilage and silicon utensils have similar physical properties because silicon possesses useful polymerization characteristics for pliable durability in both biology and industry. While silicon's importance in plant physiology has also long been established silicon is also a *semiconductor,* which is an element that directs elections in a specific direction, which is the reason silicon is used in the manufacture of computer chips. When reading in research papers that mitochondria concentrate silicon I immediately understood that it would be involved in the function of the electron transport chain, because silicon would still have this semiconducting property in mito-chondria as it does in electronics, to direct electron flow and insulate the electron transport chain from leaking electrons to the surrounding environment. Leakage of electrons from the mitochondria would not only cause harm to cells and prevent the production of energy, since electrons leak from the transport chain without reaching the terminal end, but would also cause the premature reduction of oxygen meant for the terminal end which would thus further interrupt mitochon-drial energy synthesis. Not only this, but the premature reduction of oxygen would also form the harmful *superoxide* ion also highly present in states of cancer which damages cells and causes significant oxidative stress. Therefore, loss of mitochon-drial silicon is the cause of the Warburg Effect and thus the primary mechanism underlying most cancer.

This problem is also not isolated to cancer nor relevant only for those with very serious disease, and in fact affects all metabolic stress, aging, and illness contain some degree of silicon loss from mitochondria because this problem originates in digestion of food and silicon absorption and integration into mitochondria. Silicon dioxide is a widespread mineral found in nature, industry, and supplements but silicon's incorporation into plants and our own tissues comes instead from the form of *silicic acid* which makes silicon bioavailable. Silicon spontaneously forms polymers which prevent its absorption into the body, and uptake into the body is entirely dependent on acidification by stomach acid and short chain fatty acids produced by commensal microbes in the intestinal system to prevent polymerization and maintain silicon bioavailability, otherwise silicon can and does contribute to harmful conditions of *silicosis* such as during industrial exposure breathing in silica particles. To demonstrate this point the toxic compounds of asbestos are silicate minerals which, when breathed into the lungs, are nearly impossible for the body to remove and act like glass constantly cutting the delicate mucosal tissues and eventually causing cancer due to constant abrasion of tissues, and when I first started using supplements their added silicon dioxide or silica caused eczema as the silicon particles became lodged in cellular pathways.

Silicon also has an apparent relationship with water, which may be a primary reason for its incorporation into cells where it can help manage water (and why silicon is used as moisture packets in product packaging), and studies show that *aquaporin* channels which transport water also transport silicon, but aquaporin channels also function *better* when cells are replete with silicon, which may be from silicon's support of ATP production since ATP is required in ATPases which transport electrolytes that help manage water. Because ammonia is structurally identical to water, aquaporin channels also transport ammonia into cells for metabolic processing. But ammonia is also highly alkaline and strongly neutralizes acids, which is why microbes use it to raise the pH of the gut, and this gives ammonia direct opportunity to neutralize imported silicic acid to then cause deficiency of mitochondrial silicon, and indeed those with cancer always present with excess ammonia which is thus a primary driver of the cancer state through its neutralization of silicic acid.

For this reason, resolution of problems with ammonia and microbial ammonia producers is one of the most important steps in recovering from cancer (or preventing it too), such as is discussed in the chapter on parasitism and restoring the normal metabolism of dietary arginine through restoration of gut acetogens and dietary citrulline. Ammonia producers in the gastroinestinal system produce ammonia to compete with our commensal microbiome, not only inhibiting producers of short chain fatty acids required to dismantle foods and acidify dietary silicon but also causing ammonia excess to neutralize acids and acidified silicon, and production of streptavidin which also inhibit commensal biotin producers in our gut to promote continued biotin deficiency that is required to sequester ammonia into glutamine can entirely prevent normalization of ammonia metabolism if not addressed.

Factors like radiation cause cancer for similar reasons, for instance radiation adds energy to molecules which then causes them to release electrons for long periods of time which then mimics electron leakage from mitochondria to also cause the Warburg Effect, but loss of silicon and resultant mitochondrial dysfunction are primarily a consequence of colonization by ammonia producing pathogens like parasites, *Streptomyces*, *H. pylori*, and yeasts like *Candida* which disturb the normal acidification of dietary silicon, which is why even dinosaur fossils present with tumors, because cancer has been around as long as there have been opportunistic microbes which alter host physiology for their own benefit, which then impairs both uptake of silicon into cells and its required incorporation into mitochondria, both from ammonia in the gut as well as in local tissues like the breast, throat, gut, prostate, cervix, etc. Because even poor diets are high in silicon it is taken for granted that this nutrient should even be at the root cause of cancer, because even a diet high in silicon or use of a daily silicon supplement *will not reverse this deficiency* since the primary problem is the acidification of silicon which makes it bioavailable, not its absence, which is mediated by factors disturbed by opportunistic microbes like stomach acid and microbial short chain fatty acids.

When searching for studies which might contain relevant information to further elucidate or support this discovery I found one study which showed that acetylated silicon *adsorbs* to fats (meaning it adheres to their bulk phase rather than being absorbed into them), and mitochondria are encased in two phospholipid layers, the inner and outer membranes bilayer, which explains how silicon is physically incorporated into mitochondria. One very old study on rats which investigated the uptake of silicic acid into mitochondria identified that the silicon is located on inner membrane, confirming that silicon adheres to the membrane layer, which implies that it does function as a semiconducting insulator.

Since cancer cells are in fact already trying to heal themselves, cancer is actually one of the easiest metabolic disease to treat, since restoring these pathways enables cells to once again produce sufficient energy so they can properly reorganize and restore their normal function. But the reason I became so confident in having solved the Warburg Effect and thus the underlying cause of cancer is because this also happens to be the cause of *migraines* and headaches, because loss of silicon in *sphenoid* sinus cavity tissue due to colonization by parasites or other ammonia producing pathogens causes massive local electron leakage and inflammation of the very cramped recesses of the sinus cavities, which the body then cannot resolve due to impaired ATP production required to manage water distribution through the function of ATPases. To demonstrate how this works, the migraine I got which led to this discovery originated from eating a large helping of homemade macaroni and cheese, as although a thickened sauce might not seem very watery a white sauce for macaroni is just milk and cheese thickened with a roux and contains an abundance of both water and protein as potential substrate for microbial production of both ammonia and hydrogen sulfide (since microbes use water as a cofactor to produce ammonia from dietary arginine). That night I only experienced a slight headache but the migraine really began after breakfast the next day after a large carbohydrate breakfast since sugar (especially fructose) most strongly stimulates mitochondrial respiration, and since my mitochondria were depleted of silicon due to microbial ammonia production from my dinner the night before this resulted in massive electron leakage from highly active but silicon-depleted mitochondria to then cause massive water influx (inflammation). The migraine was so bad I could do nothing but turn off all the lights and sit quietly (even laying down made it worse), but it was an opportunity to contemplate migraines and the realization of they were also caused by the Warburg Effect, which I had been studying, popped into my mind. I immediately took some tea and carrots to suppress ammonia and hydrogen sulfide, and then mixed a plant-derived silicon supplement in a little tea with added citric acid powder to the acidity of lemon juice, then followed that with several apricots, an apple, and a small slice of cake (for sugar) and the migraine immediately began to fade and was completely gone within forty-five minutes and I was back at my computer working and listening to music with curtains open and sun shining in as if it had *never* happened, when a migraine that bad would normally take a day or more to resolve.

Specifically, a dose of about 500 mg of plant-derived silicon (such as from bamboo) in about 3 tbsp of vinegar or lemon juice, or citric acid in water or juice, followed by the generous consumption of sugar such as from abundant fruit, fruit juice, or sugar added to juices once a day is sufficient for treating cancer and migraines (children should use 1/2 the dose). While silicic acid is available as a supplement which can be used instead of this preparation the entire problem is disturbance of normal stomach acid and microbial populations, so the cure for cancer is not this acidified silicon but also in restoring the ability of the gut and commensal microbes to also acidify dietary silicon, and this step of using manually acidified silicon simply seeks to rapidly rescue mitochondrial silicon deficiency, to relieve symptoms and support recovery, but on its own without resolving patho-genesis and restoring immunity and digestion will not cure cancer in the long term.

It is also more effective to actually boil these acids and silicon in a little water similar to methods used for other supplementation, because hydration by hydro-gen molecules is what makes the silicon silicic acid and thus more bioavailable. Especially for recovery from migraine attacks, sugar is not optional and must be consumed immediately after a large dose acidified silicon since the resumed production of ATP is required to restart ATPase pathways and resolve inflamma-tion. Because vinegar can be quite unpleasant to choke down it can be slightly diluted with some tea or acidic juice like purple grape juice, especially to help children, but citric acid such as occurs in lemon is nearly as effective and far more pleasant to use which can be especially helpful for children. If symptoms of eczema emerge after use of silicon stop using supplemental silicon until it resolves, then reduce the dose afterward to prevent excess. As discussed in earlier chapters, our body produces citric acid from carbohydrate under the influence of vitamin D and zinc, and deficiency of endogenously produced citric acid is a primary liability in cancer which increases mitochondrial vulnerability to alka-line factors like ammonia, and a primary reason why dieting promotes cancer, by impairing citric acid production, so steps to resolve vitamin D deficiency and stay replete with carbohydrate also promotes these interventions.

The mechanism of electrons escaping mitochondria which causes migraines is also why light aggravates migraines, because light stimulates mitochondrial respiration as photons of light change to electrons when they strike the mitochon-drial electron transport chain which, missing its silicon, then add to the quantity of escaping electrons and resultant inflammation. It is also important to know that *silica* and *silicone* are not interchangeable terms for the element *silicon*—they are different silicon-based chemicals and will have the opposite effect of silicic acid and can actually promote oxidative stress and cancer and conditions of silicosis (predatory purveyors will try to cheat consumers with products when my work becomes well known, and much care will be required to avoid falling prey to cheats and opportunists). Many foods like spinach, dates, green beans, oats, bamboo shoots, etc., are also high in silicon and should be eaten daily to support normal mitochondrial function. In support of this discovery there are also surprising studies which show no association between breast cancer and breast implants, even though breast implants do cause other harmful complications, since silicone leakage from breast implants would actually provide some silicon that could be converted to silicic acid in the body. But there are also other toxic forms of chemi-cal silicon used in industry and manufacturing and even personal lubricants made from silicon which actually dull sexual sensitivity that do cause cancer because of the other elements and chemical structure of those silicon molecules, so all silicon is *NOT* universally protective or safe. Only plant-sourced silicon should be used supplementally. Horsetail is also a potent source but grasses like horsetail and bamboo also contain toxic *thiaminase* which causes thiamine deficiency, and if they are the whole plant must be treated to remove thiaminase to be safe. Even when using a supplement of silicic acid or bamboo silicon it can and does form insoluble silicon polymers in the gut if there is excess ammonia or deficiency of stomach acid—this is not harmful, it only prevents silicon absorption. I've also often heard that collagen peptides or gelatin can give people migraines and this occurs because collagen is especially high in arginine which is the primary substrate used by parasites and enzymes arginase and arginine deiminase, and since water is used as a cofactor for production of ammonia from arginine the act of taking gelatin or collagen in some water is one of the fastest ways to promote migraine and cancer when suffering metabolic illness (although many of us do this simply by taking tannin-free beverages with meals anyway). *Streptomyces* which cause autism and diabetes by inhibiting B vitamins as described in that chapter also produce ammonia by respirating on nitrate which they convert directly into ammonia, so consuming high nitrate leafy greens without immersing in water to remove their nitrate can also lead to migraines when stomach acid production is insufficient, although acids normally reduce nitrate into nitrite, which is why salads also often don't result in migraines because a vinaigrette is acidic, so only those with low stomach acid production will experience this (which is also a good diagnostic for it!).

Interestingly, there are many studies which have explored the relationship of migraine with cancer and there has been an established association of cancers of the head and neck with migraine, and of childhood cancer with migraine, but an inverse association of breast cancer with migraine. The connection with childhood cancer and migraine is especially interesting because pathogenic colonization as the primary explanation for most cancer, including childhood cancer, demonstrates how childhood cancer can be mostly prevented by a diet high in fruit because of its tannin, sugar, carotene, and silicon which children should be having anyway, which protects them more effectively from pathogenic colonization if they also get plenty of sunshine for vitamin D since childhood physiology is designed specifically to be more resistant to pathogens. One of my nephews developed a brain tumor before he was three-years old and while his parents fed him a supposedly healthy diet free of refined and processed foods it was mostly high in grains and legumes and were discouraged from eating sugary fruits and getting sun as his mother had the typical, harmful, misguided attitude that sugar and sunlight are bad which she took so far as to feed him foods like avocado in preference to grapes, apples, and oranges where avocado is very high in polyunsaturated fats which impair mitochondrial function through lipid peroxidation. As a toddler he began presenting with frequent headaches, which is not normal in children and can indicate such problems. Luckily his tumor, the size of a small apple, was not cancerous and the surgery to remove it and his subsequent recovery was entirely successful, and I was eventually able to convince my sister that fruit is not only safe for children but required for their health and development as not only is fruit high in silicon but also pectin, tannin, carotene, to promote microbial short chain fatty acid synthesis which further helps to acidify silicon in the gut from commensal microbes (avocados are great just don't feed them in excess to children). Even fruit juice can strongly promote resistance to childhood cancer unless you go and dilute it with water which not only increases the cofactor for ammonia synthesis (water) but dilutes the protective polyphenols, anthocyanin, tannin, citric acid, and sugar that would otherwise promote a protective healthy microbiome and healthy mitochondria.

The great scientist Louis Pasteur suspected silicon would be useful for curing disease, but not yet understanding the role of acidification and digestion in silicon assimilation, attempts at leveraging its benefits have not been realized, since, again, this is entirely a problem of pathogenic alkalization of silicon which prevents its bioavailability, since silicon is omnipresent in every diet but especially high in plants. I am glad to have proved Pasteur more right than even I could have imaged, but plant foods which are excellent sources of silicon are also very difficult (impossible, really) for the body to break down, because we do not natively possess the enzyme *cellulase* for digesting cellulose which is instead the job of our microbiome as discussed in other chapters, which in turn requires *cobalamin* (vitamin B12) to overcome the polarity of plant cells to adhere to their surfaces for digestion. When there is B12 our microbes not only thoroughly digest plant foods to liberate nutrients like silicon but also produce more short chain fatty acids like acetic acid to directly acidify silicon in the gut and promote its absorption directly to mitochondria, as well as the production of vitamin K2 and liberation and increased absorption nutrients, so the genesis of cancer, migraines, and specifically the Warburg Effect is also a function of vitamin D deficiency and loss of cobalamin producing *Thaumarchaeota* which then impairs the ability of our commensal microbiome to effectively digest and acidify dietary silicon.

In addition to having thyroid cancer and leukemia, a large skin lesion characteristic of carcinoma also appeared on my back around the age of thirty from a sunburn I got at the age of sixteen when when my father forced me to lay sod in the middle of a hot summer day after already having a severe sunburn from laying sod the day before, instead of doing it at hours which were safer for my wellbeing. The sunburn was the most severe I ever had, with my skin blistering and painful to even the slightest touch, and I remember thinking this was probably going to lead to skin cancer in the future, which it did, but even as my other symptoms of the other cancers resolved (like leukoplakia, fatigue, wasting, insomnia) the skin lesion did not heal. This is because skin metabolism is entirely independent from the rest of the body, because circulation to the skin is greatly limited during the stress response and the skin is designed to endure that stress, but when stress is especially high and chronic the skin's access to nutrition can also be chronically limited. Prior to solving the Warburg Effect (and an experience which would later lead to that), around the time I discovered that B12 could be used to assist the commensal microbiome to better digest foods, especially those like leafy greens which are harder to break down, the lesion healed over (carcinomas resemble scabs that never heal) for the first time in eleven years after a single, large salad with a large dose of supplemental B12 mixed into the vinaigrette dressing (there was still a small mass, discoloring, and scar tissue but no longer a scab). At first I thought it might have been increased liberation of vitamin K or some other nutrient, and during a later winter in which I did not get much sunshine and did not use B12 regularly the lesion reappeared, and I finally began to suspect silicon as being the primary factor, and only a couple more large salads inoculated with B12 and several doses of silicon in lemon juice to once again healed it and kept it healed, reliably reproducing these principles and demonstrating not only their validity but simplicity. Mixing a supplement of B12 into very healthy plant foods (such as a salad) high in silicon once a day is also requisite for healing, since local B12 production by *Thaumarchaeota* is likely absent in states of cancer, until such time that a recovery is made and endogenous vitamin D fully restored (remember that reduced gas and cravings for vegetables instead of meat are primary diagnostic symptoms for vitamin D repletion due to *Thaumarchaeota* cobalamin).

A particularly easy way to accomplish increased silicon acetylation favorable for the treatment of children with cancer (anyone with cancer, really), since they don't like strong acids is through the use of low-dose supplement of *pectin* mixed into high polyphenol fruit juice used to also dilute a small dose of the lemon juice/silicon mixture. As discussed in the chapter on gut health, pectins can only be metabolized to acetic acid, which not only supports microbial producers of short chain fatty acids but naturally acetylates nutrients like silicon in the gut microbial consumption of pectin. Since vinegar is difficult to consume it is entirely possible and useful to leverage this function of supplemental pectin to acetylate silicon in the gut from the action of microbes as not only a more pleasant than mixing with vinegar but also more effective since it also occurs immediately at digestion. Tea and coffee are also extremely high in potent prebiotics and robustly promote gut microbes (which is why any oxygen in their water can also promote aerobic, opportunistic microbes), and for adults the addition of some silicon to the water used to make tea or coffee is also an excellent method for both supporting cancer recovery as well as migraines and as a prophylactic against migraines for those whom it is a regular occurrence.

I personally found the addition of silicon in water for tea (added before boiling in order to hydrate it) to be very effective at preventing migraines. But the problem with these strategies *not* using acids directly is they will *only* work if the gut microbiome is at least marginally functional and would, for instance, not work while undergoing chemotherapy or using antibiotics since those kill off the microbiome (only use lower doses of silicon, about 100 mg per liter, to prevent undissolved silicon). But if there are some commensal microbes this works even better than manually acidifying silicon, and works so well to support recovery that complacency quickly takes root and neglecting treatment then occurs, which would be a significant mistake, and consistency is extremely important, even when feeling well, to make a full recovery. Two years after incidentally causing the carcinoma to heal over using B12 in foods, the daily use of a low dose of silicon in the water used to make tea or coffee caused the carcinoma scar to soften and lighten more to the normal color of skin, literally in a period of just two weeks, and continued, daily use of hydrated silicon through this strategy caused it to nearly disappear after several months. Whether these less aggressive treatments are working is also not vague or nebulous and would be immediately obvious from even a single administration in the increase in feeling energetic and well from the increased production of ATP which should occur, which has a near immediate effect (within hours) of increasing energy.

Yet while silicon plays this extremely important role in mitochondrial function it is also a crucial factor in the synthesis of healthy connective tissue such as ligaments, cartilage, and the extracellular matrix which actually holds cells in place. Even bone requires a substantial amount of silicon, and if the diet is too low in silicon or the gut has lost its ability to properly digest, acidify, and absorb dietary silicon then far more problems can and do occur to the human body than cancer, which is simply the most extreme manifestation of silicon deficiency, and it is not only helpful nor necessary to acutely treat migraine and cancer with silicon but to also raise the entire general intake of dietary silicon in order to reverse the deficiency which has led to these conditions, to rehabilitate the entirety health which, without adequate silicon, is not possible, since even the most basic cellular function is dependent on both mitochondria and support structures which hold cells in place and allow them to function properly. When I was in my mid-forties and experienced a surprise period of insomnia the use of spring water caused me to become exceptionally sleepy during the day, which I thought to be a function of chlorine and fluorine in municipal water, but spring water is often extremely high in dissolved silicon, and since silicon is taken up by aquaporin channels which transport water the solubilization of silicon in water is also one of the most ideal and effective methods of increasing its supply in the body. While spring water can certainly be used it can also expensive, and when I tried boiling a supplement of silicon (100 mg per liter of water) in tap water it caused the very same pronounced sleepiness and resolution of insomnia as had occurred with the spring water, demonstrating it was dissolved (hydrated) silicon in the water which was causal, and this method can eventually supplant the need for acute dosage of silicon once sufficient recovery has been made, should also be used alongside recovery without exception, and can rehabilitate many other conditions simply due to systemic repletion of mitochondria and structural tissues with silicon.

Even adding a little silicon regularly to meals which contain water like stews and soups would be effective, in addition to the increased used of high-silicon foods like green beans, spinach, snap peas, bamboo shoots, dates, whole grains, bananas, apricots, and other fruits (including things like cucumber), while promoting digestion as discussed in other chapters to leverage acetylation of silicon by commensal microbes. And, yes, also means that diseases like cancer are the result of a diets low in silicon such as commonly occurs in an industrial food system, but also due to municipal water supplies which are often not only low in silicon but to which the addition of chlorine and fluorine would also cause polymerization of what little silicon it does contain and thus entirely prevent if from being a source of silicon (which is another reason why boiling the water can help, since this also causes off-gassing of the chlorine, but not the fluorine, which instead simply must be avoided by ceasing fluoridation practices), and municipal water supplies could be inoculated with diatomaceous earth or other high silicon source to naturally increase the levels of dissolved silicon in drinking water, which could help improve the general health of the public and resistance to metabolic disease.

The next most important thing anyone with cancer should do is begin taking *aspirin*. It is the most effective, easily accessible medicinal therapy for cancer and studies have confirmed that aspirin used with traditional cancer treatment improved the survival and remission rates by an astounding margin, though of course the study authors concluded that chemo or radiation was the primary treatment even though patients without aspirin did not fare well at all and had dramatically increased rates of mortality. Generally a dose of one or two aspirin once or twice a day should be more than sufficient (325 mg each), where the *lowest effective dose* is best since aspirin does have side effects, but it can be used in higher doses if cancer is very severe if care is also taken to prevent its potential side effects. Due to the work of Ray Peat I used aspirin for my own recovery long before I discovered the cause of the Warburg Effect, because aspirin was shown in studies to promote mitochondrial respiration and inhibit glycolysis, which is opposite to the state of cancer. Discovering the role of mitochondrial silicon in the Warburg Effect makes it obvious that this benefit of aspirin was because it acidifies mitochondria to thus stabilize mitochondrial silicon and prevent its alkalization to thus support mitochondrial integrity, so aspirin works synergistically with restoration of silicon and promotion of normal mitochondrial respiration. It is important to use a brand of aspirin without toxic coatings, ingredients, or titanium (read labels!). Plain, normal aspirin is important, as the other substances added to inferior brands can contribute to metabolic issues and worsen cancer, although the use of aspirin is more important if finding better products is not possible. It has lately proved more difficult to find good aspirin products since companies try to dress up aspirin with coatings and ingredients so they can justify higher prices for something which should be cheap and widely available. One brand unfortunately called *GeriCare* comes as aspirin should be priced, 1000 tablets for $10. Aspirin is *not* expensive, and store brands with coatings and other crap are designed to make it look expensive rather than having any improved benefit. The best relief I got from aspirin was from the feeling of suffocation which enveloped my whole body, as by acidifying mitochondria which increases their rate of oxidative respiration aspirin helps oxygenate and invigorate cells and relieve some discomfort, and it does have some analgesic properties. But it is important to remember that *ibuprofen* and *paracetamol (Acetaminophen) are not aspirin.* Aspirin is aspirin, and other NSAIDs do not, at all, have the same benefit to physiology and can even promote cancer by oppositely suppressing mitochondrial respiration, and the use of all other such medications or even other "alternative therapies" should cease entirely because they can easily inhibit respiration and healthy forms of inflammation which are needed to recover from cancer.

Aspirin side effects include stomach irritation which occurs because aspirin stimulates the increased use of the amino acid *glycine* in metabolic pathways. This irritation is easily resolved or prevented by supplementing glycine (be sure to avoid brands which contain toxic and allergenic additives) or eating foods high in glycine (if using gelatin or broths care must be taken to include tannins to prevent more microbial ammonia production). Aspirin also depletes *vitamin K* more rapidly than would occur normally, so if using high doses of aspiring daily, especially if you are older or very ill, it will be necessary to consume foods high in vitamin K daily and to also use a supplement of vitamin K and K2. *Do not rely on supplements only* since vitamin K is extremely important for our gut microbiome, which is deranged during states of cancer. Without either of these safeguards aspirin can cause gastrointestinal bleeding, the risk of which is increased in people with severely compromised health or advanced aging. Children should never be given high doses of aspirin either, but the daily use of one baby aspirin could probably benefit childhood cancer, where the other nutritional and environmental approaches will be more beneficial. Very young children (neonates) do not have well developed carbohydrate oxidation pathways and their cells mostly run on glycolysis which is inhibited by aspirin, so it can actually be dangerous for the very young, and breastfeeding mothers of very young children should have diets high in silicon in order to transfer that nutrition to their newborns, which also helps prevent other childhood illnesses as discussed in the upcoming chapter on immunity. There is also some evidence that high doses of aspirin could interfere with white blood cell count in those with very advanced leukemia or lymphoma, so while aspirin will still be beneficial in those cancers careful monitoring of white blood cell count will important to prevent immune emergencies, and the aforementioned nutritional therapy will be more effective (echinacea is a good immune supporting supplement which can help those with immune-system related cancers like leukemia, but don't use other herbal treatments as those can interfere in recovery). Any significant fever during cancer likely indicates poor immune function and should be treated at an emergency room. This effect of aspirin on inhibiting the immune system in immune related cancers will diminish as therapy progresses.

The hormone *progesterone* also directly competes with some of the more cancer promoting hormones like estrogen, which is a hormone of growth, cortisol which catabolizes lean tissue, or serotonin, which slows the metabolic rate and results from ineffective healing pathways triggered by the cancer state, and can rather quickly raise the body temperature and metabolic rate by promoting thyroid function which is usually quite depressed in those with cancer. I used natural progesterone (avoid synthetics) intermittently throughout my cancer treatment and found it to be equal or better than thyroid medication for improving thyroid function and relief from cancer symptoms (because thyroid problems are not actually healed by taking thyroid). Progesterone is more of a female hormone, but all humans normally have it in abundance and it has the effect of invigorating tissues just like thyroid and aspirin. Using enough progesterone will help raise the body temperature and metabolic rate significantly, sometimes it can even produce fever-level temperatures of 100 F (37.7 C) or more, and this is a good sign if suffering from cancer as it would indicate the immune and thyroid system coming back (if it exceeds 102 though you probably have a true fever and should seek medical care). Women, especially those suffering breast cancer will benefit amazingly from progesterone use, and progesterone is being used in study after study to support cancer treatment. As discussed in the upcoming chapter on hormones, progesterone is actually antiparasitic, and since most cancer is a consequence of parasitism, such as by *Trichomonas* colonization of the breast, prostate, testicles, cervix, uterus, and ovaries (which are all mucosal organs) progesterone helps by suppressing parasites, which can and should then also be supported by the steps in the upcoming chapter on immunity.

Some women complain that progesterone makes their breasts too large (in those who are already well endowed) as progesterone can stimulate breast enlargement, in which case the use of *pregnenolone* may be an acceptable alternative. In men progesterone will lower testosterone while taking it, which has some significant effects but nothing long term or harmful. Progesterone does help maintain muscle mass, however, so what losses in libido occur during use can be offset by increases in youthfulness, energy, and strength. Especially if facing death, in my opinion, I chose rather to have the benefit of progesterone and put my libido on a temporary pause, finding that the libido reduction was not too severe anyway, and it returns within days of stopping progesterone. I would describe natural progesterone as an essential, emergency, life-saving therapy for cancer treatment, and anyone with severe cases should seriously consider taking progesterone. If the product does not state the source of origin, it likely contains soy derivatives and it is best to avoid those with soy. Studies which show negative effects of progesterone are usually done with the synthetic forms like progestin, where studies showing a positive effect were done with natural progesterone. Natural is less expensive anyway. Progesterone is also non-toxic, so overdosing is not a worry (overdosing produces symptoms of sleepiness and relaxation, and sometimes nausea in high doses because it softens internal organs such as occurs during pregnancy and morning sickness). Like aspirin, progesterone increases the metabolic rate and it is important to be well-fed when using it, especially with carbohydrate, and can help stimulate and support the citric acid cycle and energy production. Progesterone can also promote improvements in sleep, which will be comforting since most cancer patients also suffer insomnia. One of the most consequential side effects of progesterone is that it is also the hormone of *empathy*, so be prepared for a flood of emotions and take proper care of your emotional wellbeing and have compassion for your feelings and experiences, recognizing the role of progesterone in emotions and not to take them too seriously during this time.

Insufficient steroids are a bigger problem than excess since they rescue metabolic deficits, and most cancer will be accompanied by dysregulated cholesterol and steroid production (steroids are made from cholesterol) due to saponification of dietary fats as discussed in the chapter on hormones, and restoration of normal, endogenous steroidogenesis as discussed in the upcoming chapter on hormones can help promote long term recovery and resistance to cancer relapse once recovery is made.

Since estrogen is a hormone of growth it is directly involved in tumor growth and cancer progression, and progesterone also helps recovery from cancer because it protects tissues against many of estrogens growth-stimulation effects, for the same reason that progesterone protects a mother's body from the high estrogen required to grow a fetus. My body temperatures and pulse rose within days of beginning progesterone, which relieved me of the stiffness, lethargy, and histamine induced irritation from low metabolic rate and cancer almost immediately, years before I discovered the role of silicon in the Warburg effect and didn't have the benefit of using silicic acid. Because progesterone is generally safe it can also be used in the treatment of childhood cancer, especially to counteract the effects of soy exposure (which is a potent phytoestrogen), but this role of water in growth of tissues is another reason why silicon is likely useful in controlling cancer, because silicon is strongly involved in the movement, metabolism, and balancing of water in the body, and it is very common to feel dry mouth or other symptoms of increased thirst when beginning silicon repletion, especially since pathways which move electrolytes required for the normal metabolism of water are dependent on ATP which is increased by mitochondrial silicon repletion.

Natural *vitamin E is* another powerful tool to support recovery from cancer and other metabolic illnesses because vitamin E is a powerful antioxidant that synergizes with progesterone, vitamin C, and carotene to inhibit aromatization and lipid peroxidation. In fact, many natural progesterone products are formulated with vitamin E. Most problematic, ammonia producing pathogens like *Candida* and dermatophytes, which are fungi that colonize skin, achieve pathogenesis by producing oxidized lipid products like oxylipin as discussed in the chapter on pathogens. But vitamin E is a lipid-soluble, chain-breaking antioxidant, which means it stops the domino-effect of reactive oxygen species and thus the damage to our metabolism which otherwise promotes uncontrolled growth. Oxidative stress is a hallmark of cancer, and needn't even be very intense, just widespread, which keeps tissues in a constant state of stress, hypoxia, and excessive aromatization, but since vitamin E stops this chain reaction and returns cells to their normal state while also inhibiting pathogenic yeasts it is actually a very effective tool for resolving many cancers.

Because cancer cells produce large amounts of lipid-associated reactive oxygen species due to impairment of carbohydrate metabolism (because lipid metabolism is a backup) vitamin E deficiency can be one of the most significant but elusive causative factors in the etiology of general metabolic disease and thus the pathogenesis of cancer, especially because these oxidized lipid products impair the transport of chloride as discussed in the chapter on metabolic disease. There is a ridiculous term used in oncology—castration resistant prostate cancer—and yes that is exactly what it sounds like, the removal of testicles for the treatment of prostate cancer, because testicles can become the highest site of androgen aromatization into estrogen due to long-term colonization by *Trichomonas* parasites, and the aged prostate can become cancerous if metabolic health is sufficiently deteriorated because testicles continue to produce testosterone even if there is a high rate of aromatization and unresolved parasitism. But researchers and doctors think that androgens promote prostate cancer simply because they know men have high androgens rather than its aromatization into estrogen in poorly respiring and vitamin E deficient tissue, and are entirely ignorant to *Trichomonas* or other parasites being etiological mechanisms in cancer and other metabolic disease. If it were true that androgens caused prostate cancer every man in the world, regardless of age, would have prostate cancer. But they don't, because it is the aromatization of androgens caused by systemic ammonification from parasites and yeasts which causes prostate cancer in a metabolically fatigued prostate, and this same principle applies to all cancers regardless of their location, with *Trichomonas* distribution to breasts, cervix, lungs, gut, testicles, and even the head being achieved through casual and sexual exposure *Trichomonas* in the environment when the immune system and epithelial defenses have failed.

Anyone with cancer should use a supplement of natural vitamin E as discussed in the chapter on pathogens and metabolic disease. Dietary vitamin E is more important than supplemental vitamin E, and since we must eat food it's convenient and less expensive to get vitamin E from high vitamin E foods like nuts and leafy greens, but vitamin E can be destroyed by oxidation or saponification of fats and fat soluble nutrients in the gut as discussed in the chapters on calcium, immunity, and hormones also effectively blocks the absorption and distribution of vitamin E to cause deficiency which then also impairs chloride channels and thus our normal immune and metabolic function. Before the advent of agriculture our supply of dietary vitamin E came mostly from foods like nuts, seeds, wild grains, leafy greens, and fruit but, after we started hunting, animal fats and organs like the liver became an optional source, but liver tastes revolting because of its extremely high iron content which the tongue warns against as being potentially toxic, and plant sources of vitamin E are far more effective due to their generally protective phytochemicals like oxalate which help prevent saponification which animal products lack entirely. Grains like wheat, barley, or spelt began to replace nuts and seeds as they were more widely cultivated, since they were more convenient and available, but now that grains are most commonly refined, even bleached, their vitamin E content is minimal, and nuts tend to be very expensive, so our dietary traditions have in many cases shifted entirely away from high-vitamin E foods which then contributes to high rates of metabolic disease, oxidative stress, allergies, and cancer.

Soaking or sprouting nuts, whole grains, and seeds increases their vitamin E content, which is already considerable, by as much as 600%, turning these foods into literal vitamin E supplements (don't discard the soaking water, which will be high in tannin, and incorporate it into dishes like soups or sauces), although nuts do not always need to be soaked or sprouted to benefit from their vitamin E content it can be helpful to do when recovering or when in need of significant metabolic aid, and making bread from safe, sprouted whole grains as discussed in the upcoming chapter on bread can also be a delicious and satisfying solution to vitamin E deficiency and required silicon while also providing general calories and satiation and other nutrients (because of their high phytate content, whole grain products should *always* be soaked, sprouted, or fermented, so products like whole grain pasta should be avoided if they are not sprouted and choose refined option from safe grains like spelt instead). Hazelnuts, macadamias, and chufa (tiger nuts) are some especially convenient sources of vitamin E and are high in healthy fats like palmitic, stearic, and oleic acids. But these foods are also useful because of their high tannin content, which helps protect vitamin E from oxidation and saponification, and for those with cancer a low-dose of vitamin E in strongly brewed tea (yes, you can have it with milk or cream), is the most effective method for vitamin E repletion (do not overdose on vitamin E, just take one dose once or twice a day of whatever supplement you purchase). Following a vitamin E supplement with a supplemental dose of salt is so effective at restoring chloride channels it can immediately start promoting relief of tension and discomfort (though there may be some immune effects as well) within literal minutes of dosage. Remember that the only way to tell if a vitamin E supplement is natural is on the ingredient label and whether it identifies d-tocopherol or dl-tocopherol, though most natural forms will also indicate where it came from, such as sunflower. Also, there is something wrong with soy derived vitamin E. I have no idea what it is, but it does not act the same as sources derived from sunflower seeds, wheat, and other sources, so avoid soy products altogether.

While the lesion on my skin and thyroid tumors were my only confirmed oncological growths because of limited access to medical care, I suspect leukemia to have been the primary cancer which caused the majority of my symptoms. An obvious sign of leukemia is a markedly high white blood cell level and symptoms like the leukoplakia on my tongue and chronic gum disease, accompanied by easy and profound bruising because of the disruption to blood cell functions (I once bumped into a doorknob which left an enormous and strangely dark and patterned bruise on my thigh for weeks), and is often accompanied by significant gum disease. In the period immediately before my use of progesterone I also briefly presented with *petechiae*, which is an odd rash of small, round spots from subsurface bleeding and is a common symptom of cancers like leukemia, and progesterone and other strategies in this chapter should be used immediately if presenting with such symptoms as well as addressing the immune system. Those with cystic fibrosis are at high risk for developing both diabetes and leukemia or lymphoma, which makes a great deal of sense in retrospect considering all my health struggles, and those with cystic fibrosis will need to address that as discussed in the upcoming chapter on immunity otherwise the risk of cancer greatly increases. Leukemia is very likely caused by retroviruses or human T-lymphotrophic virus and cause cancer by replacing our DNA in the cells they infect with RNA which changes the function of those cells (that's how viruses work), and discuss these viruses in the upcoming chapter as thriving in oxygen-poor (hypoxic) environments, as retroviruses are not especially virulent, which is reversed by restoring boron and oxidative respiration, to oxygenize the tissues and restore the immune system in addition to the steps in this chapter, and leukemia, lymphoma, and other cancers of immune organs may directly benefit from supplemental thyroid hormone (T3) which, as discussed in the chapter on immunity, acts as a highly bioavailable iodine supplement.

It is described generally that cancer cells spread like a seed in the wind, coming loose and traveling to other parts of the body only to infect new areas of the body, but this is in fact entirely incorrect. The hormones produced by the environment of a body with cancer are what stimulate and promote its development in other organs, by suppressing the metabolism of all tissues, and systemic hyperammonemia and other problems of continued parasitism or other opportunistic microbes which impair metabolic health and make tissues prone to cancer. Stem cells which migrate are transformed into cancer cells by their environment, not by mutations, so if the environment is toxic then stem cells can become cancerous, but cancerous stem cells cannot spread in healthy tissue because those tissues support the normal metabolic function of cells that may migrate there. In a previous version of this book before I solved the Warburg Effect I recommended the use of supplemental lysine, glycine, and taurine to help further suppress the stress hormones and conditions which both result from and contribute to cancer, as these amino acids have potent regulatory effects in suppressing excessive nitric oxide stress, restoring cellular respiration, and protecting against excessive cellular excitation (respectively), and they can be used if desired but are likely to be unnecessary if enough progress is made quickly in the restoration of a healthy gut, immune system, silicon homeostasis, and normalization of cholesterol. A lysine-rich protein called 'leukemia protein' also helps suppress tumor growth, and because opportunistic pathogens (including those which cause oral disease) not only catabolize lysine but convert it to the toxic cadaverine, lysine deficiency cause by microbial dysbiosis is a likely driver of some cancers like leukemia and could be supplemented for some time, protected by tannins, until the gut microbiome is restored (since the gut microbiome is a primary source of lysine).

A particular issue at the core of cancer is that mitochondria, the site of the electron transport chain and production of energy, proliferate under the influence of vitamin A and thus dietary carotene, copper, and zinc as discussed in earlier chapters. In terms of metabolic health this is one of the best and most effective ways to get well since mitochondria are the source of most of our energy production, but in states of cancer and metabolic disease it also can and will result in more leaking electrons from silicon deficient mitochondria due to an increase in mitochondrial which can and will then result in an increase in oxidative stress and associated symptoms such as insomnia, irritation, or worsening of cancer states (although since carotene and vitamin A are also antioxidants they help restrain some of the damage). Restoration of carotene is not optional, however, because carotenoids suppress microbial hydrogen sulfide, promote vitamin D synthesis from sun exposure, and help power the immune system and thyroid function which are also required to recover from cancer. Vitamin A (and thus carotene) also strongly regulates tissue morphology, and is shown in studies to actually *suppress* tumor growth and regulate angiogenesis (growth of capillaries), a function which is likely dependent on mitochondria, and it is especially important for recovery of gastrointestinal cancers (where there is an abundance of hydrogen sulfide producing microbes) to use carotene frequently (with all meals) to suppress microbial hydrogen sulfide and tumors, and gut, rectal, and anal cancer are very likely a specific consequence of too infrequent consumption of dietary carotene even if those cancers can also be catalyzed by other pathogens like HPV (remember that copper is also required to absorb and distribute carotene), and the leakage of electrons from the increased mitochondria instead being a function of silicon repletion.

As amino acids are vital for recovery from cancer, to support tissue regrowth, immune dysfunction, and to relieve stress I used *casein protein* to great effect in the treatment of my cancer after learning of casein's superior protein quality. I ordered some to assist in meeting protein requirements since I was having a hard time doing so with a normal diet (and because whey protein is less nutritious) but also noticed that it helped prevent nightly muscle catabolism by supplying a continuous stream of amino acids (casein is slow digesting). Cachexia (wasting) is a common symptom of cancer due to protein wasting and excessive catabolism of amino acids by cancerous tissue. I began taking it several months after my tumors were discovered and within three days of taking it the places on my body which had been in constant, excruciating pain (my left ribcage, groin, and left tibia) for the last year or more of my life suddenly vanished. It wasn't even intermittent relief, but complete abatement. I didn't plan right and ran out of that first bucket of casein before its replacement arrived, and three days after not having casein the pain came back to those areas just as hard and bad as it had ever been. I was so relieved to get my new bucket of it and in another three or four days the pain went away again completely. It's now been years since that day and now that I am healthy I never really use casein anymore and there has been no return of pain to those areas. Considering that pathogens like parasites, fungi, and bacteria catabolize our amino acids for their own use and produce toxic ammonia, hydrogen sulfide, and amines which destroy our health, the primary issue underlying cachexia and other protein wasting problems is also that of opportunistic microbes, so using tannins, carotene, anthocyanin, and other polyphenols with all sources of protein also help to increase our benefit from that nutrition while inhibiting the pathogens which interfere, to not only help resolve the pathogens which cause cancer but increase the rate of recovery, and in my early recovery I often took that casein in smoothies made with an enormous quantity of frozen fruit and juice which inadvertently supplied those necessary polyphenols which probably had a great deal more influence on my recovery than I ever could have known at the time.

Because oncologists consider cancer an invasive disease and are prejudiced toward the destruction of cancer cells they consider high quantities of methionine and glutathione in tumors to be inhibitors of chemotherapy drugs, which are poisons, rather than this being evidence of cancer cells attempting to heal. But when patients die during chemotherapy treatment they die because the body becomes completely exhausted of its *sulfate* (methionine, cysteine, glutathione, etc.) because sulfate is also required to detoxify chemotherapy drugs from the body, and when sulfates becomes completely exhausted then chemo drugs, hormones, and other products normally detoxified from the body recirculate endlessly back into the body until it is poisoned to death, and people who die during chemotherapy treatment or naturally from cancer die due to complete exhaustion of important amino acids like glutamine, glutamate, methionine, cysteine, sulfate, etc. So consuming plenty of protein and sulfur while also protecting them with tannins and carotene is absolutely requisite to surviving cancer, especially chemotherapy treatment if that is chosen. Chemotherapy also completely eradicates the microbiome, so throughout the entire duration of chemotherapy there is no microbiome to produce the abundance of B vitamins, short chain fatty acids, vitamin K2, and other nutrients we require for our health which then leads to even more rapid deterioration including the loss of hair, energy, sleep, etc., and one person who died from gastrointestinal cancer likely did so because chemotherapy eradicated the commensal microbiome in his gut which was protecting him from the causative pathogens like *C. difficile* and *H. pylori* which had been protecting him, as he began critically bleeding shortly after chemotherapy (he was not someone using my work). Sometimes chemotherapy and radiation can help promote recovery from cancer, but when this occurs it is only because these toxic treatments can potentially also kill the invasive pathogens responsible for the cancer in the first place, but this is also why relapse then happens later because contemporary treatment does nothing to prevent reinfection by these opportunistic pathogens, often even carried by family members and lovers, and why it is so important to address the root causes of cancer, even when we don't have cancer, and especially to prevent its return, and there is no future for anyone with cancer, even if they survive, that does not require constant care of the body and meeting these requisites, and returning to past behaviors of neglecting the diet and self-care will absolute result in a return of cancer, since the causative agents like parasites and *H. pylori* and the requirement of our physiology on silicon (silicic acid) are universal.

One of the worst symptoms I had which anyone with cancer will be familiar was an insane, body-wide irritation which seemed to be located under the skin, deep within my nerves as if they were dissolving in acid. It worsened at night, when the sensation seemed to concentrate along my spine and was the primary driver of my debilitating insomnia. Even if you have cancer but don't have this symptom you perhaps have some kind of general feeling of restlessness and agitation. This is caused by overproduction of *histamine* and other amines in the gut by toxic microbial amine producers which thrive on salt and fructose malabsorption as described in chapter on pathogens and metabolic disease. This problem occurs because the parasympathetic nervous system is overstimulated by the excess histamine and the body overtaxed by adrenaline analogs like tyramine and phenylethylamine, and because histamine is highly activating and a mediator of growth it is in fact thought to be a primary driver of cancer due to its activation of the nervous system which then excessively excites cells and drives them to fatigue. This likely occurred to me due to the intake of A1 dairy combined with dieting habits like avoiding sugar which promoted amine producing microbes, so in addition to avoiding A1 dairy and consuming plenty of fruit, sugar, and high polyphenol foods a low-dose, nightly *antihistamine* can also be used to inhibit the stressful effects of histamine on the body and nervous system. Histamine also likely contributes to tumor growth, so the use of an antihistamine can help arrest tumor growth more effectively, so long as the other steps are also taken, until such time as excess histamine is resolved through these dietary strategies and resolution of amine producing gut microbes as discussed in chapter on pathogens and metabolic disease. Taking the right antihistamine is important, however, as some medications which pose as antihistamines are actually steroids or other non-antihistamine product with antihistamine-like actions but are not true antihistamines. The ones which are are safe and most effective for cancer treatment are referred to as *first-generation* antihistamines. Some are available as prescriptions, but many are also available over-the-counter (which I prefer anyway). *Diphenhydramine* and *doxylamine succinate* are two such forms available from many brands. These antihistamines also function as sleep aids (and are sold as such) and can also help cancer sufferers get some much needed sleep. I haven't, however, been able to find any products that don't contain at least some toxic additives, though some of the generic brands are safer with less ingredients and dyes. I would avoid types which have titanium, dyes, and other metals if possible but if you have these symptoms taking it for a short period of time to address them will be fine. Addressing histamine excess by histamine producing bacteria as discussed in the chapter on calcium is extremely important for long term resolution of this problem.

Niacinamide (vitamin B3) is also a useful tool with which to fight cancer because the cancer state in those who are no longer very young the metabolism is compromised such that the body can no longer produce adequate amounts of nicotinamide adenine dinucleotide (NAD) as discussed in the chapter on niacin therapy. Just like oxygen intended for the terminal end of the electron transport chain, the Warburg Effect causes NAD to be excessively reduced which then prevents its normal electron transport function in support of the citric acid cycle and the mitochondrial electron transport chain, and in response to this deficit cells increase their production of lactic acid from pyruvate normally intended for the citric acid cycle in order to maintain oxidized NAD but which significantly causes metabolic acidosis to further worsen metabolic respiration. Because NAD is an electron transport chain participant it can, however, increase the leakage of electrons from mitochondria if they are absent of silicon, so during cancer it is best not to use niacinamide until after silicon repletion has been achieved, and restoring mitochondrial silicon through this strategy thus also stops the inappropriate reduction of NAD to thus restore NAD function, meaning that supporting the NAD pathway through the steps in the chapter on niacin therapy or a low dose supplement of niacinamide will then further hasten recovery (a supplement really is not necessary if supporting NAD function through diet as described in that chapter, but if using a supplement no more than 250-500 mg per dose for adults and 50 mg for children once a day is required, and do not confuse niacinamide for niacin as while they are very similar their dosages are not the same and this high a dose of niacin will result in significant discomfort).

Lastly, because cancer is primarily caused by colonization with pathogens, the information in the chapter on immunity is not optional for cancer recovery. As will be discussed, halides like chloride, iodine, and the pseudohalide cyanide are primary factors in immune function, and iodine deficiency is specifically shown by studies to promote cancer of glandular organs like the breast and prostate because the peroxidase system uses halides like iodine to protect tissues from infection by pathogens which cause problems like internal production of ammonia or hydrogen sulfide. Most cancer is caused by colonization with pathogenic organisms, and restoring immune function as discussed in that chapter is absolutely required to make a full and complete recovery from cancer (as well as to prevent it in the first place), otherwise continued colonization with opportunistic parasites, yeasts, and other microbes will simply continue causing cancer and tumor growth. Cyanide is often marketed as a way to kill cancer cells, but this misunderstands its role in biology and instead supports the eradication of cancer-causing pathogens by the immune system and does nothing if the immune system is not working but can and does cause poisoning if taken in excess such as from supplemental amygdalin, laetrile, or so-called vitamin B17 (there is no such thing), and cyanide instead should only come from safe, dietary cyanogenic foods like brassicas (arugula, broccoli, kale, etc.) almonds, apricot kernels, yuca, or a few apple seeds, etc. Organs like the prostate, cervix, breasts, and lungs are primary sites of parasitic *Trichomonas* infection, and it has been shown in studies that *Trichomonas*, which is the most common non-viral sexually transmitted disease, can and does cause prostate cancer and should also be immediately treated with lithium light therapy as also discussed in the upcoming chapter on immunity.

Removing or destroying organs like the thyroid as a means to treat cancer is extremely misguided and is most definitely a case of the cure being worse than the treatment, especially since the thyroid and parathyroid together help to manage calcium homeostasis which is so crucial to so many metabolic pathways in the body. My friend who died of liver cancer after having this thyroid removed likely died in part because of the absence of normal thyroid function, but a friend who survived breast cancer in 2024 using these strategies did not even need a mastectomy and simply went through a lumpectomy and still has her breasts. Additionally, most people who die from cancer treatment die when treatment keeps going and going, as doctors who treat cancer often treat the patient's body as if it can resist such insane abuse but which in truth is eventually depleted of sulfate sources required to detoxify chemotherapy drugs the same as the cancer cells it is meant to attack. The young man I tried to help who had an extreme and aggressive form of lymphoma said his doctors had thought he was doing unusually well and so gave him a higher dose of chemotherapy than usual and it nearly killed him. Before he came to me for help he could not even swallow food his cancer was so advanced, and within about two weeks he had regained the ability to swallow and was progressing very well until his family pressured him to get traditional treatment and give up every single other strategy discussed in this book. A little bit of chemo treatment can theoretically be useful to destroy tumors and disinfect the body of carcinogenic pathogens, but the body cannot handle significant chemo-therapy stress and will eventually die from excessive treatment due to depletion of glutamine and sulfate. Even people with very advanced cancers find near immediate improvement through these strategies, and within days see noticeable increases in metabolic rate (as measured by the pulse and temperature diagnostic discussed in the chapter on self therapy), heat production, and feeling well because the body is designed to promote cellular respiration and this should be the primary approach with other strategies as supplemental therapy, not the other way around.

Emotional stress can also be a significant factor in survival and the reaction I have seen of family members to those with cancer is quite alarming as those without cancer pile all their fears of death, disease, control, and mortality onto the cancer patient and thereby hasten their departure from this life. The young man with lymphoma was so stressed by his situation and family pressure to subvert death he distracted himself with the drama of day-trading and crypto investing rather than focus on his recovery and self-care required to get well. Those with cancer are not your martyr sent to conquer death and must be given space and support, not pressure or stress, if they are to get well, and should cease working and physical strain and engage in much rest, relaxation, sleep, eating, and enjoyment. If this is difficult for the patient to do it is caused by stress both endo-crinological and psychological, the former treated by these nutritional and dietary strategies and the latter treated through trauma therapy outlined in the upcoming chapter on spirituality (or my other book, *The Perfect Child*).

When suffering cancer diet is paramount to survival, and eating common wheat or lots of meat is like pouring gasoline on a fire and will only cause more cancer and reduced chance of survival. Cancer sufferers *must* stop eating common wheat forever and ever, not only for its gluten but also the fortification by harmful additives like iron and nitrates, and maintain a diet high in fruits and vegetables for the protective effects of phytonutrients like tannin, carotene, anthocyanins, etc. Lactic acid such as occurs in yogurt and fermented foods strongly promotes cancer growth by directly lowering the metabolic rate and body temperature. Fish oil, seed oils, corn oil, and canola oils all exacerbate cancer because these fats are unstable in the high heat, high oxygen environment of the human body and produce metabolic byproducts such as abundant lipid peroxides, malondialdehyde, oxylipins, eicosanoids, etc., which interrupt the high-respiratory pathways that promote healing (such as a functioning kynurenine pathway). Sadly, most restau-rants use these inferior oils to cook their chips, omelettes, and French fries and if you have cancer your only choices are to entirely avoid all sources of these oils or stick to home cooking to make your own version of these foods without those oils (store-bought salad dressings, mayonnaise, and other fat and oil based products are major offenders too, so always read food labels).

Keeping blood sugar elevated at all times is also important for suppressing the stress hormones that drive cancer. Eat regularly—no less than every two or three hours. Some theories on sugar's connection to cancer claim that cancer runs on sugar and while this is technically correct EVERY CELL IN THE BODY RUNS ON SUGAR YOU FUCKING PSYCHOS, and cancer cells convert sugar into lactic acid and fatty acids for energy rather than oxidation in mitochondria due to the Warburg Effect which will be restored by restoring mitochondrial silicon. It does no good to remove sugars and carbohydrates when healing cancer because the other body systems which are needed to heal and prevent the cancer from worsening need carbohydrates and sugar to function properly, to fuel normal cellular respiration restored by reversing mitochondrial silicon loss which heals cancer.

When suffering from cancer it is silly to expect healing while drowning tissues in alcohol, but alcohol also suppresses many opportunistic microbes which cause us disease and can treat the condition which underlies alcoholism, and if you have cancer and continue to drink, well, you'd be exactly like me. Many people also smoke cigarettes and think it's what causes cancer, but tobacco is very high in cyanide which supports the immune system in suppressing cancer-causing pathogens and smoking is often a self-medication for disease in those who have a low cyanide diet. Certain drugs like cocaine are also antiparasitic, and those who abuse such drugs are also self-medicating undiagnosed parasitism. While it's fine to consume a little alcohol while recovering from cancer, even moderate consumption will prevent recovery, and the chapter on curing alcoholism and addiction provides information about what causes alcoholism and addiction and how to heal those underlying conditions and thus relieve ourselves of the burden of substance abuse.

It is also important for anyone with cancer to avoid estrogen products like birth control, estrogen prescriptions, and herbal supplements (as plants are often high in phytoestrogens) as estrogen stimulates growth and helps worsen the expansion and migration of tumors since estrogens are hormones of growth. As discussed in the chapter on hormones, high progesterone is a primary mediator of femaleness, not estrogen, and those who are on hormone replacement therapy or transgender and using hormones can still maintain their desired gender attributes through the use of progesterone rather than estrogen, which also helps to treat cancer by raising the metabolic rate, promoting thyroid function, and suppressing parasitism, and once a full recovery is made lower doses of estrogen can be resumed if needed. Oppositely, healthy estrogen levels are required for normal metabolic function (even in men) so using estrogen inhibitors for too long as is common to much conventional treatment can still cause harmful side effects and should be stopped as soon as the metabolic rate improves and remission is achieved, as continued practice of these dietary, metabolic, hormonal, and immune strategies will continue promoting remission even with normal levels of estrogen as the problem is not estrogen but the pathogens which dysregulate our metabolic and hormonal function for their own benefit. Other pharmaceuticals can directly contribute to cancer as well, for instance one person I helped had been using melatonin for years to combat their insomnia caused by dieting and unresolved trauma because they believed the lie that melatonin is safe because it is natural, but there is absolutely nothing safe about taking a hormone of torpor which functions in part by suppressing cellular respiration and lowering sex hormones. As discussed in the upcoming chapter on oral disease, essential oils can also disturb the polarity of cells and induce neurological dysfunction which can also impact cancer recovery. Unless it is specifically recommended in this book, pretty much all pharmaceuticals and alternative treatments will actively contribute to cancer and should be avoided and their relevant conditions instead treated as recommended by relevant chapters herein.

A person using these therapies should notice at least small positive improvements within days, especially reflected in the measurement of pulse and temperature, and without using this metabolic diagnostic tool as discussed in the chapter on self therapy you will be guessing your progress which will leave you uncertain, uniformed, and guessing. Measuring the temperature and pulse constantly as described in that chapter can empower you to visualize and directly measure your progress (or lack thereof), which can help you make adjustments or lean on especially useful strategies more strategically. Positive changes such as increases in body temperature, feeling more relaxed, lessened pain, better sleep, improved energy, etc., are signs that healing has begun, and prognosis thereafter is linked with alleviation of symptoms. This is not something that we wait for months to see, wondering if you're doing it right. It should begin happening right away and continue to improve linearly, continuously and consistently. If you don't see positive changes you are probably not adhering to one or more of the concepts, such as dieting or eating wheat or bad fats or continuing to use herbs not recommended in this book or pharmaceuticals and need to evaluate diet and behavior or reconsider supplement strategy.

The great temptation when improving is to begin taking health for granted once it starts to return, and to resume old habits and be less regimented in treatment. This is a mistake because symptoms will disappear even while the potential for recurrence is still high, as tumors may in fact never actually heal (it is not the tumors which kill but the hormones they secrete), and treatment should continue for several years after symptoms abate. Daily peak temperature and pulse should eventually reach 99° F and 85 bpm. While getting close to those numbers is great, if they are not reaching those or exceeding them more work is required.

Most people with cancer present with gum disease because those pathogens readily access the bloodstream and thus very strongly contribute to cancer, so gum disease should be immediately treated as discussed in that chapter, in those who are very ill a shot of *ceftriaxone* can be more rapid if it can be acquired, to wipe out gingival pathogens as quickly as possible, but this will not prevent reinfection and all sexual activity should be avoided until a complete recovery is made and resistance to colonization established as discussed in the chapters on immunity and oral health. The oxidized form of *vitamin C* is also is the active agent which shrinks tumors, but while this has been established in studies researchers don't know how it works, which is explained in the chapter on immunity and thyroid, to effectively restore vitamin C status, further eradicate pathogens, shrink tumors, and achieve full and permanent resolution of cancer, but not by injection of vitamin C as is commonly and errantly practiced by some physicians, which instead will promote cancer through excessive chemical reduction, and that physiology should be understood and practiced only as described in this book.

Cancer is not the frightening condition it is usually considered. While cancer is often catalyzed by pathogens it is also just the body trying to get well, so you can help it along with a little care and planning and it is easier to heal from cancer than other diseases like diabetes or cystic fibrosis since cancer only occurs from the most fundamental failures of human biology which are very easy to reverse since the body itself is inclined already to do so.

CHAPTER 16
IMMUNITY, VIRUSES, AND ALLERGIES

When I was twenty-one, shortly before my suicide attempt, I one day came down with debilitating fatigue and a slight fever. I had no heath insurance at the time and it was not serious enough to warrant a hospital visit on my low income, but my fears of contracting HIV fueled by the shaming from conservative communities as well as the alarmist leaders in the queer community itself led me to believe, without evidence, that I had contracted the virus. Months later my suicide attempt was motivated in part believing I would never again be accepted back into my family if I became HIV positive. That I thought I was HIV positive was ridiculous. I had not had any unprotected sex except with my boyfriend, whom I had broken up with almost a year before. There was no way for me to have actually contracted the virus, but so malicious was the hatred and rhetoric toward homosexuals I just assumed I had contracted it. Of course when I finally got checked a few weeks after my suicide attempt the test came back negative. But even after having unprotected sex far more regularly than I should over the next twenty years of my life I still never contracted HIV. What I did contract during that two weeks of infection in my youth was the *Epstein-Barr virus*, known colloquially as *Mono*. Epstein Barr is a herpes virus often responsible for *mononucleosis*, sometimes called 'glandular fever' in other parts of the world, which is got through the act of kissing. Most people get Epstein Barr while they are yet children, and never know they actually have it as it is much safer for children to contract than grown adults. Getting it as a child might cause a short, mild fever, but getting it as an adult, such as in a person like myself who never even kissed another person until he was nineteen-years old because of the psychotic sex abuse that occurs in religious communities is devastating and can produce life-long fatigue and inflammation and make a person more susceptible to other diseases (especially if they have preexisting conditions like cystic fibrosis). Years later out of curiosity, and after learning what Epstein Barr was, I got tested for the Epstein Barr virus with a positive result.

Every single person who lives will at some point contract at least one herpes virus, if not many more. There are nine known forms which cause chickenpox, shingles, so-called "cold sores," as well as those which infect the genitals. If you think you don't have herpes you are completely wrong. Most people don't even know about types such as *Cytomegalovirus*, which is a herpes virus the majority of people catch also while young and which infects more than half of all humans (probably more). Epstein Barr is transmitted through the lips just like the more visual *Herpes virus 1*, but its lesions are impossibly tiny and impossible to see around the very outer ridges. It has been known for a relatively short while now that herpes viruses permanently alter functions in the body, and I believe that Epstein-Barr (or another such virus) is the root cause of *Hashimoto's* thyroid disease, and no one really has any idea what *Cytomegalovirus* really does or why it even exists, let alone the implications on our long-term health, although disturbances in beta oxidation of fatty acids and the production of energy as well as association with diabetes has been established, and it generally inhabits the salivary glands which gives it ready access to distribution among the population. With more and more people succumbing to mysterious cases of chronic fatigue and other diseases which seem to present without obvious causation more researchers are investigating the possibility of microbial origins. But it is quite obvious that most disease is caused by microorganisms because if we lived in a vacuum from such pathogens the human body would not have mechanisms to self-destruct or become ill after so many millions of years of evolution. The general absence of obvious signs of infection by so-called "latent" viruses has caused the belief that most herpes are generally harmless, but it is obvious to those of us who suffer chronic metabolic conditions that such viruses cause chronic-low grade changes in metabolic function and fidelity and are anything but benign or inactive. I personally believe most chronic diseases are caused by infection with such viruses, where initial infection is enabled by dietary and environmental stress, and then the virus perpetuates decline in metabolic rate thereafter to sustain its own survival, and that 'non-latent' phases are simply for communication and not reflective of any difference in 'latency.'

When a virus infects a cell it hijacks our cell's DNA and reprograms the cell to make copies of the virus. Viruses do this because they cannot reproduce on their own, and have no obvious metabolism. Some viruses like Influenza or Ebola are quite virulent while others like the Herpes strains are chronic and inconspicuous. This is because there are two ways that viruses replicate in cells—The way in which viruses like the Flu reproduce is to hijack a cell and quickly multiply, then cause the cell to burst and spread more infectious viral agents through the disintegration of the cell (called lysis). These viruses are easily detected by the body and once the symptoms clear the virus has been destroyed. In the case of chronic viral infections like the Herpes types or those which cause hepatitis, which infect us for a lifetime, they have evolved ways to commandeer our own cells in a clandestine fashion, masking their presence to our own biological programming using things like fatty acids to conceal themselves from the monitoring immune system. These viruses cause more harm in the long run because they permanently alter the functioning of entire systems, such as what happens in the case of chronic fatigue or even cancer, reducing the quality of life and preventing the ability to rebound after infection, even with a generally good diet and healthy behaviors.

Normally when a cell's integrity becomes compromised as it does in infection (or even just worn out) the cell automatically destructs in a process called *apoptosis* in order to recycle the contents of the cell or to expose infectious agents which allows immune cells like macrophages to come and clean up all the debris, pathogens, and foreign or damaged particulate. This process also signals to other cells the presence of pathogenic organisms through release of *interferon* that stimulates surrounding cells to seal themselves up against possible infection which slows spread of disease. Chronic-type viruses achieve their inconspicuous ends by turning off the process of apoptosis as well as the signals which would normally be sent by a cell to indicate infection. It is a hostage situation (or an invasion of the body-snatchers situation) where the surrounding cells have no idea that their buddy has been hijacked, murdered, and zombified. By creating their own signaling molecules from our cells the virus is able to stay put in perpetuity, and thus cause chronic illness to set in. Not only that, but their emergence from infected cells to other cells also goes unnoticed, allowing long term viral infections like Herpes, HIV, and Hepatitis to continue unchecked.

The consequence of associating HIV with gay men even though HIV was also raging in the heterosexual population eventually led to the disease being extremely widespread because, as the COVID-19 pandemic deftly illuminated, we often want to believe that disease is associated with groups of people or behaviors we can control and blame instead of employing the intelligence and compassion required to effectively manage infectious microbes we cannot see with the naked eye. Indeed human history is riddled with many instances of bigotry surrounding disease, majorities laying blame on minorities or invoking religious mythology which only serves to further endanger even those who espouse such bigoted beliefs since disease does not, in fact, discriminate against any humans and will still infect those who employ prejudice and fear for control and power. During the coronavirus pandemic the President of the United States purposefully withheld effective containment because they stupidly thought the virus was mostly contained to cities dominated by his political opposition. Later his own brother (and nearly himself) became a casualty before it ended, along with significant populations of his supporters which also ironically had the effect of removing votes from his reelection campaign. Many people, especially those who professed to believe in God, celebrated AIDS for taking the lives of us gay men, even most of our own mothers would not visit us while dying alone in the hospital during the AIDS crisis, a responsibility instead taken up by many of our lesbian sisters who stood beside their gay brothers in our time of need, and this hatred met no introspection even after God and medicine saved us because the persecution by hatemongers never has anything to do with God or faith but fear and the desire to control that fear. Hubris condemns us and our loved ones to suffer as a lesson of prejudice and ignorance as the immutable laws of cause and consequence do not care about beliefs, demographics, or even intelligence or lack of it, and the very generation who persecuted, ignored, and rejected victims of the AIDS crisis and taught their children to hate and discriminate against those with illness were, in their old age, those most vulnerable to COVID-19 who were in turn abandoned mercilessly to die alone in retirement homes and hospitals by the very people they raised to behave that way in the face of illness and death.

Karma really is the ultimate bitch, but Karma does not actually do these things out of malice or even vengeance—those are human traits we anthropomorphically attribute to reality. Karma simply exists that we may experience the full breadth of life, where life without consequences would not be meaningful or fulfilling (nor actually life), and the reason that COVID raged unchecked and took those who abandoned people with HIV is because they did not take the time during other pandemics to assimilate wisdom, establish responsible and equitable systems and institutions, or set up our government and society to care for those in need. We all become ill and die because we all must experience the fullest depths of mortality, to fully understand what it means to be alive, which is the entire purpose of our existence in the first place, death being the ultimate subversion of the ego and experience of surrender. At some point we all must come to terms with mortality and if we don't do this willingly life will force upon us experience after experience which does. It is understandably difficult to do, because fear at times can be over-whelming, and in terror we grasp at denial, religion, conspiracy theories, or bigotry and xenophobia to protect our fragile minds from fears we have not strength to endure, but in the end become a victim of our own willful ignorance, fear, and hatred because none of us can control reality. Nobody who died of HIV deserved to die, and nobody who has HIV, or COVID, or cancer, or who otherwise experience the limitations of mortality deserve it either. We are simply creatures living for a limited amount of time in this incredible world and there are diseases and limita-tions on our potential as a mortal creature, of which many of us are afraid only because we do not yet understand why it is we are here nor the purpose of life, even and especially when we selfishly subscribe to powerful theocratic institutions and authoritarianism which exploit our fear of disease, death, the unknown, and desire for control.

HIV is a retrovirus, and retroviruses are not usually very difficult for the body to resist, which makes its spread in the human population very perplex-ing. I first began to be suspicious of the origins of the Human Immunodeficiency Virus infection observing those who used an inhalant drug colloquially referred to as '*poppers,*' which have a strongly chemical smell, and boys who used them very often showed side effects such as to lose erections entirely. This seemed to indicate that poppers had a very powerful effect on vasodilation so great as to reduce blood pressure sufficiently for erections to fail. While popper abuse is common today among the gay community for the sensation of euphoria and relaxation they bring, poppers were for nearly a hundred years in the 19th and 20th Centuries a drug most common among all the general population as a form of inhalable *nitrite,* and the etymology of the word 'poppers' came from the form in which they were first manufactured way back in the Victorian era, beginning in 1867 as small glass spheres which were "popped" by crushing in a rag or hand-kerchief and then inhaling the released fumes. Inhalable nitrites were used for cardiovascular problems such as angina which is a painful condition in the chest in which arteries constrict tightly and can be mistaken for a heart attack. By dilating the cardiovascular system poppers helped relieve sufferers of the symptoms of angina and anxiety, but their high nitrite content also produced strong feelings of relaxation bordering on euphoria. Because drugs were not highly regulated until the mid and latter half of the twentieth century during the advent of the unfortu-nate and poorly conceived "War on Drugs," poppers were as much a recreational drug of convenience as tobacco, cocaine, and even heroin which could all be purchased from convenience stores and sold as common consumer products (such as early Coca Cola which was originally formulated from the coca plant and thus contained cocaine). Even though most drugs eventually came under regulation, in 1960 the FDA eliminated the requirement for prescription for poppers, and the reason that poppers even came into prevalence in the club scenes of the 70s and

80s was because it was already in use recreationally in high schoolers in the 60s and 70s who had unfettered access to inhalable nitrites because of their deregulation, with one study reporting eleven percent of high schoolers in 1979 as having used poppers. When access to inhalable nitrites was finally recognized as a health hazard and access began to again be restricted it was deceptively repurposed as household and cleaning instruments which failed to inhibit access entirely until their specific chemicals were outright outlawed in 1988 and 1990, and use of nitrites among high schoolers dropped to 1.5% by 1992. Today the most toxic forms are illegal but others are still widely available and legal and sold duplicitously as chemical cleaning agents, and while our heterosexual counterparts from the 70's and 80's moved on to more hardcore drugs like cocaine and heroin poppers remained in use in the gay community for its ease of access and ignorance to potential harm.

Nitrates and *nitrites* are also a component of artificial fertilizer, and nitrates and nitrites do occur in nature although in much smaller amounts, and are even made in our own bodies from the oxidation of nitric oxide which is important for cardiovascular health and immune function. In fact the mechanism of vascular dilation caused by endothelial nitric oxide does so in part by forming nitrite, which is then recycled back into nitric oxide but exposure to high exogenous sources exhaust those enzymes and are toxic to many systems in the human body including the immune system. During the advent of the AIDS crisis intelligent medical professionals and those who were also members of the gay community rightly recognized the potential for inhalable nitrite from poppers as a cause of the disease. By this time nitrite and nitrates from artificial fertilizer had been recognized as toxic chemicals with the potential to cause poisoning and death from high nitrate runoff from agricultural fields, and it just made sense that the potentially toxic nature of nitrites could impair the immune system when used recreationally. A few studies began to explore its role in the etiology of the mysterious illness affecting gay men, finding for instance that it might alter human lymphocyte viability. But as soon as the HIV virus was identified interest in nitrite as a causative factor of HIV infection evaporated and efforts instead fixated on preventing infection, without further seeking to understand the disease. Renewed interest in the nitrite origination of HIV infection began in the late nineties and continues today, but because of very common mistaken beliefs about HIV, AIDS, and the nature of the immune system it has failed to gain much attention.

There have been several attempts to develop a vaccine for HIV, all of which have failed because even most virologists do not understand how the immune system actually works. While many vaccines have successfully controlled or eradicated diseases like polio, measles, mumps, etc., there is nothing inherently immunologically special about vaccines—the only thing that vaccines do, even the most complex mRNA vaccines, is to trigger our own immune system. If, such as in the case of human immunodeficiency virus, the immune system is not working correctly in the first place (due to inhibition by factors like nitrites and nitrates) there is nothing for vaccines to actually stimulate, so there can never actually be a vaccine for HIV. When the coronavirus vaccine started being propagandized as the promised solution to the coronavirus pandemic I was extremely frustrated understanding that coronavirus are highly adaptable and since an individual can be infected numerous times and resistance lasts only several months it would not be possible for one vaccine to resolve the pandemic, and the prospect of vaccinating even the majority of people several times a year until the pandemic finally reached its natural end was impossible, and so dialogue by the government and pharmaceutical companies promising a vaccine solution was incompetent at best and purposefully dishonest at worst, and while the vaccine did marginally help end the pandemic the entire discourse and official decision-making surrounding the virus demonstrated just how little authorities on viruses and infectious diseases actually know about the immune system and communicable disease.

Nitrate and nitrite have been found specifically to have suppressive effects on the immune system, which is not something we would desire in the first place while suffering an immune disorder such as what is caused by HIV, even if it weren't participating in pathogenesis, though it is. At the very least, using poppers while having HIV is like refusing to pull the parachute cord while skydiving. My experience studying nitrates, nitrites, reactive nitrogen species, and nitric oxide in relation to other biological purposes like erectile dysfunction, insomnia, aging, immunity, and oral disease has made it apparent that excessive nitrites and endogenous dysregulation of nitrite is the primary etiology of HIV infection, not the virus itself, whose presence is facilitated instead through the inhibition of our natural immune function by nitrite dysregulation and excess whether through drugs, agriculture, oxidative stress, or microbiome dysbiosis. For instance, the stomach normally secretes ascorbic acid (vitamin C) in gastric juice during digestion because ascorbic acid neutralizes nitrates and nitrites, but even stomach acid can neutralize nitrites and nitrates, converting them into safer nitric or nitrous oxide which also inhibits nitrate reducing microbes. Because pathogens like *H. pylori* and parasites inhibit stomach acid and cause vitamin C deficiency, chronic colonization by opportunistic microbes is the primary factor which makes us vulnerable to nitrite and nitrate toxicity, especially from industrial agriculture, and thus infection by other opportunistic pathogens like HIV. Use of poppers must unequivocally cease as a recreational drug and rates of HIV in populations which use them would plummet.

Of course, the use of such drugs serve as a cheap and valuable treatment for the conditions of depression and drug and alcohol dependence as discussed in the chapter on alcoholism and addiction, and general avoidance of artificial sources of nitrate, nitrate, and promoting antioxidant systems as discussed in this book and chapter can resolve immune inhibition to promote recovery and resistance to HIV. For instance, HIV infection is shown to correlate with reduced NAD production, so restoring the kynurenine pathway as discussed in the chapter on niacin therapy and supplying niacin can be useful, and in fact one study showed that the use of niacinamide was effective in inhibiting HIV-1 in vitro. Incidentally, a lot of people use lysine to suppress outbreaks of Herpes viruses, and indeed lysine inhibits the growth of herpes viruses because lysine competes with arginine into cells and thus robs herpes viruses of amino acids required for its replication, but in another study researchers sought to uncover if lysine would have a similar effect on HIV and instead found that lysine caused an *increase* in the spread of the virus. This probably occurred because nitric oxide derived from arginine (and citrulline) is a primary component of the immune reaction which not only kills viruses but also stimulates migration of immune cells to areas of infection to help suppress viruses, and in contrast to herpes arginine oppositely suppressed HIV. But arginine does not normally circulate in the body because it is otherwise metabolized to ammonia by opportunistic pathogens to alter the body's pH and inhibit the immune reaction. Instead, dietary arginine and proline are catabolized in the intestines to citrulline, glutamate, glutamine, creatine, and nitric oxide, then arginine is resynthesized at sites when needed and, as discussed in the chapters on gut health and parasitism, the domination of the gut by lactic acid producing microbes such as occurs from dieting behaviors and deficiency of sunlight, vitamin D, and microbial cobalamin (B12) required by commensal gut microbes to produce short chain fatty acids inactivates normal arginine catabolism to then promote ammonia producing pathogens, inhibit the immune system, and cause arginine deficiency.

Being that LGBTQI+ children are often traumatized in our childhood by hateful and homophobic parents and communities we suffer higher rates of trauma motivated behaviors like body dysmorphia, obsessive dieting and exercise, or workaholics that fail to get sufficient sunshine, which then destroys the commensal microbiome, immune system, and increases vulnerability to health problems like HIV or other infectious pathogens, not to mention higher rates of drug and alcohol addiction. Under no circumstances should anyone with HIV engage in dieting behaviors or excessive, strenuous exercise, and instead focus on sustaining a healthy microbiome through the ubiquitous consumption of fruit, use of supplemental pectin, supplemental B12 (or Swiss cheese for its B12-producing *Propionibacterium*), and restoration of vitamin D. Respiration which is driven by carbohydrate, vitamin C, and sunlight is also the primary catabolic pathway for nitrate and nitrite which reduces them back to nitric oxide, so recovery from HIV can never be accomplished while dieting, but the immune system is also comprised of a great many micronutrients like zinc, molybdenum, copper, glycans, arginine, etc., and is directly supported by the gut microbiome which are all casualties of dieting behaviors which must be restored through a generous and consistent diet high in fruits and vegetables. Resolution of psychological trauma which motivates such behavior and obsession with rejection is resolved through inventory therapy as discussed in the upcoming chapter on spirituality and my other book on psychology.

While much immunology focuses on immune cells such as T-cells and other leukocytes the immune reaction itself is primarily facilitated by enzymes which participate in the *Peroxidase System*, in which peroxidase enzymes consume the oxidant *hydrogen peroxide* and use it to in turn oxidize *halides*—fluorine, iodine, chlorine, and bromine, and the pseudohalide cyanide—into hypohalous acids which are exceptionally potent antimicrobials. This system is employed by immune cells during the immune reaction to kill invasive microbes including bacteria, fungi, parasites, archaea, and viruses. The role of peroxidases in consuming hydrogen peroxide is often considered their only important function when in fact their primary function is to use hydrogen peroxide to kill pathogenic microorganisms, and some of the peroxidases relevant to our immune response are *lactoperoxidase*, *myeloperoxidase*, *eosinophil peroxidase*, and even *thyroid peroxidase* which is the enzyme that also makes thyroid hormone. Like many enzymes in our body peroxidases are based on *heme*, which is iron-dependent and thus also on vitamin A and D which regulate release of iron from tissue storage (while supplemental or preformed vitamin A might seem like good options to reverse this problem it can be quite toxic when supplemented, and is instead derived from generous consumption of dietary carotene). Consuming meat, which is high in heme iron, can actually mask impaired endogenous synthesis of heme as discussed in the chapter on iron, which is itself caused by depletion of sulfur by opportunistic pathogens consuming our sulfate which then also results in iron over-saturation of cells and tissues, so while dietary heme can support the immune system it can also disguise and inability to produce sufficient quantities for effective immune function, and the immune peroxidases are most strongly promoted then by repletion with sulfur through consumption of non-proteinous dietary sulfur (kale, brussels sprouts, broccoli, collards, onions, garlic, etc.) while also protecting that sulfur with dietary carotene to prevent microbial production of hydrogen sulfide.

Nitrite, nitrate, and hydrogen sulfide are also powerful inhibitors of heme and heme based enzymes, by binding to the iron in heme, which is how products of nitrosative stress and pathogenic bacteria inhibit the immune system as seen in HIV and other chronic illness, and nitrate poisoning causes illness and sometimes death by directly inhibiting heme dependent proteins like the peroxidases or cytochrome oxidase, so because industrially grown produce usually contains far higher quantities of nitrate due to the use of artificial fertilizer industrial diets actively and directly promotes immune dysregulation. Processed meats, wheat flour, rice, and other foods also commonly contain added nitrate like *sodium nitrate* or *thiamine mononitrate* and consumption of industrially grown greens, grains, commercial sausage, pepperoni, and baked goods like bread and pasta and other common wheat or grain products can and do impair heme function and promote opportunistic nitrate reducers like *Streptomyces* which also block biotin. All metabolic conditions are in fact also immune conditions because the immune system would normally easily evict those pathogens which cause these illnesses, but especially in severe conditions like HIV, diabetes, cancer, autism, cystic fibrosis, etc., it is absolutely critical to avoid any and all sources of excess nitrite and nitrate by avoiding these products and eating organic food as is possible (regeneratively grown is best). The reason we find the odor of hydrogen sulfide instinctually offensive (such as halitosis or smelly feces) is because our biology has long evolved to recognize and avoid potential colonization with harmful sulfate reducers which not only causes immune dysfunction but also chelates molybdenum and copper and poisons copper enzymes. Because we can now mask hydrogen sulfide malodor (and related compounds like methyl mercaptan) with minty toothpastes or mouthwashes it's even easier to become infected or infect others with these pathogens or remain willfully ignorant to their presence, and carotene absolutely must be employed frequently to keep hydrogen sulfide suppressed, even using carrots or other carotene sources to keep breath fresh as discussed in the chapters on vitamin D and oral health, rather than oral care products, and feces free of malodor (remember that sodium deficiency prevents necessary sulfur absorption).

Peroxidase enzymes are themselves composed of *calcium*, so adequate intake of calcium as well as normalization of calcium metabolism as discussed in the chapter on calcium is absolutely required for adequate immunity (the use of calcium citrate can be especially useful if dietary calcium is not adequate). The calcium in the peroxidase enzymes attracts the halides, which allows them to be oxidized into the hypohalous acids. Fluorine, which is considered the most reactive of all the elements, has such a high affinity for calcium that it can in high doses such as what is added to municipal water and oral care products actually destroy the peroxidase enzymes and interfere with other calcium channels. Natural fluoride in the environment occurs mostly as calcium fluoride which then prevents that fluoride from reacting to the calcium already in our body, but fluoridation of water, milk, salt, and oral care products is typically done through the addition of sodium fluoride or fluorosilicates which then promote fluoride reactivity to tissue calcium which can and does disrupt sensitive calcium pathways. Fluoride's reaction to calcium is the justification for its use in dental care, because fluoride attaches to hydroxyapatite of which enamel is made, but fluoride ingestion in excess is in fact a toxic mechanism that also can and does disturb other calcium pathways and thus contribute to metabolic disease rather than prevent it. Studies also show fluoride accumulates in the cells of people with cystic fibrosis to inhibit endocytosis, which is a process by which cells subsume extracellular content such as the process of phagocytosis by which immune cells engulf and destroy microorganisms, and during any metabolic disease associated with reduce calcium metabolism such as aging, osteoporosis, cystic fibrosis, etc., the reduced ability to absorb and manage calcium properly very likely increases the harmful potential of fluoridation on the immune system and other pathways, as the immune system is also directly connected to bone mineralization, and avoidance of artificially fluoridated water or foods is likely requisite to help restore a normal immune response so the less reactive halides chloride, iodine, bromide, and cyanide have better support of the immune response (fluoride toothpaste can be used occasionally if needed, since toothpaste is spat out). Fluoride is extremely difficult to remove from water, so campaigning to have water fluoridation removed from municipal water supplies will be very helpful to general wellbeing, where natural food sources like tea and fruit are far preferable (if required for dental health, fluoridated toothpaste can be used occasionally, since that is not swallowed).

Chloride is the most abundant halide in the body and regulates many pathways including cellular metabolism, the production of stomach acid, and tone of the cardiovascular system, but chloride's most important role is being the primary substrate for oxidation by the peroxidase enzymes in the immune reaction. But this chloride oxidation produces *hypochlorous acid*, which is *bleach*, and as such is the most oxidizing and damaging of all the hypohalous acids, but it is also the most effective and generalized immune strategy and chloride deficiency or malabsorption is the most common cause of metabolic and infectious disease. Although chloride is the most oxidizing halide, a deficiency of chloride leads to even worse oxidative stress as the peroxidase enzymes instead oxidize proteins, amino acids, and hormones during chloride deficiency, to prevent pathogenic ingress further into the body, so chloride repletion is one of the most important parts of the functioning immune system.

Some insane people take chlorine dioxide as a "supplement" or alternative medical treatment and is just as dumb as drinking bleach because in high doses it causes the same type of poisoning and oxidative stress. Just because chloride participates in biological functions does not mean that all forms of chloride or chlorine are safe, and hypochlorous acid production by immune cells occurs locally and within immune cells which protects the rest of the body from oxidative damage as much as possible, where engaging in dumb behaviors like taking chloride dioxide instead oxidize our tissues generally and can even risk death. Perchlorate is a chlorine molecule but is so toxic than even small quantities can cause serious illness because the effects of the halogens on pathogens are the same on our own cells, and it is only that we have specific immune strategies which pointedly direct their toxicity when immune cells target pathogens, a function that is not at all replicated by taking things like chlorine dioxide.

While low dietary salt intake (dietary salt is typically sodium chloride) is a common cause of low chloride status, it is primarily caused by factors which impair or disrupt normal chloride uptake into the body such as antacid use or colonization by pathogens like parasites, *Candida*, and *H. pylori* which disturb chloride homeostasis through the production of substances like ammonia and oxylipin as discussed in the chapter on pathogens and metabolic disease. Chloride must be acidified by stomach acid for entry into chloride absorption channels, but because stomach acid is primarily composed of hydrogen atoms derived from carbohydrate the practice of dieting behaviors is one of the fastest ways to impair the immune system through stomach acid deficiency which then prevents the uptake of chloride, and colonization by pathogens often occurs during periods of dieting, fasting, and starvation for those reasons. Many people have what is called "salt hunger" which is a marked craving for salt due to malabsorption of chloride, and the increased desire for salt is not easily sated because even though large quantities might be consumed the pathways which absorb chloride are impaired. Simply increasing the quantity of dietary salt can sometimes work for people who are not too ill, and too much salt intake can make a person vomit, so no more than about 1 tsp should ever be used in one sitting or dose, and because salt malabsorption also increases amine producing bacteria in the gut it is not a good idea to only increase the salting of food, but to restore stomach acid production as discussed in the chapter on parasitism and metabolic disease using the strongest of bioavailable tannins such as from astringent fruit like chokecherries, aronia (chokeberries), gooseberry, persimmon, currants, lingonberry, sloe berries, etc. If deficient in chloride this will result in acid reflux, however, as the restoration of hydrogen secretion into the stomach will leach chloride from surrounding tissue to cause failure of the esophageal sphincter muscles (which allows acid into the esophagus). If and when this occurs it is an excellent time to supplement chloride such as from a small dose of extra salt (never dose more than 1/2 tsp at a time, as excess will cause vomiting) in juice or tea as this will acidify chloride in opposition to the alkalizing effect of ammonia to promote greater absorption of chloride and sodium to restore the esophageal sphincter contraction, chloride immune pathways, and other roles of chloride.

As also discussed in the chapter on metabolic disease, yeasts impair chloride transport through the production of oxylipins which is directly and only inhibited by vitamin E, which is a potent, fat-soluble antioxidant, and oxylipin is so powerful at inhibiting chloride transport that a person can become dangerously low in chloride even when the diet contains excess. As discussed in the chapter on oral health, halides keep the mouth free of infection and teeth white and bright, so one easy symptom through which to diagnose chloride deficiency, even if plenty of chloride occurs in the diet, is the staining of teeth, which should be naturally close to white without the use of commercial whiteners and cleaning, and any chronic metabolic disease will always be accompanied by chloride deficiency due to oxylipin production by opportunistic pathogens which can be reversed rapidly by dosing some supplemental salt (no more than 1/2-1 tsp per dose, depending on size) in juice or water after using vitamin E in tea or other high tannin solution. This can be done up to three times daily but should be felt in near immediate effects and result in rapid improvement in many symptoms if at least some production of stomach acid has been restored.

Though chloride is the most important halide, *iodine* is a comparable antimicrobial and has been known as an effective universal disinfectant for many decades, and can be used to address many diseases when used with restraint and skill as discussed in this chapter. Unlike antibiotics, iodine does not permanently kill all bacteria but in the capacity of the peroxidase system primarily kills those which are harmful to our health, including parasites and some fungus and viruses as well. This happens because pathogenic organisms have physical structures such as exposed tyrosine residues which are necessary for them to infect us but which are also vulnerable to iodination (or other halogenation) and thus oxidation by hypohalous acids like hypoiodous acid made by the peroxidase enzymes. Iodine has been denigrated over the last few decades where it once enjoyed a place of esteem in the medical profession, treating everything from gout to bronchitis to syphilis. It was also common to administer it in very large doses, although iodine is very caustic and should never be given in excess (doses more than 20 mg are needlessly excessive and not very helpful anyway), which demonstrates a misunderstanding of how iodine is employed in our immune system since large doses of any halide can result in significant oxidative damage but will not necessarily work to remove pathogens if the immune system is not working properly as discussed in this chapter, and excess iodine can suppress our own commensal microbes as well and should never be used in high doses for long periods of time.

To demonstrate the purpose and strategy for iodine I was one day called by my sister in a panic as her children had come down with an alarmingly painful stomach condition. Her doctor diagnosed it as *gastroenteritis* which means the doctor had absolutely no idea what the fuck was going on as the term simply means inflammation of the gut lining, and is used as a catchall diagnosis for mysterious gut ailments doctors don't understand. My nieces and nephews had clearly contracted some kind of bacterial infection as each child lost the desire to eat which is a natural defensive reaction by our body toward most invasive pathogens, to starve them of nutrients, but the doctor sent them home untreated and in much pain. I suggested my sister give each of them one drop of 2% potassium iodide in a small amount of water and it was so effective that each of my nieces' and nephews' pain stopped within about thirty-minutes and all were totally well and back to their normal, boisterous selves within little more than a day. One took too much water and threw up the solution, but even the small quantity of iodine which entered her gut was still sufficient to resolve her infection, which demonstrates just how powerful iodine actually is and why high doses are *not* necessary to achieve these effects.

Another woman I once helped who did not have health insurance had a tooth infection which moved down into her chest and was alarmed at the pain, especially considering her lack of healthcare since we live in the United States which, unlike other developed nations on the planet, does not provide healthcare to its citizens. At my advice she took iodine diluted in liquid every day for several days and the infection in her chest completely disappeared (though not the tooth decay as that is more complex as discussed in the chapter on oral health). As discussed at the end of the chapter on gut health, the far majority of lower back pain is also caused by pathogenic bacteria eating our tissues and producing toxic metabolites in the gut which cause stiffening of the psoas muscles which are then easily injured and struggle to heal and regenerate to then cause chronic lower back pain. During the decade of my chronic back pain I would often get massages and use copious amounts of toxic NSAIDs, which very likely actually made it worse by depleting sulfate, and nothing worked to even alleviate the pain until I found out how to properly use iodine which completely cured my back pain in a single day (also because of my improved diet that supported the commensal microbiome). Occasionally over the years I have sometimes had a slightly sensitive back on waking in the morning (about four or five times), and a dose of iodine would immediately knock out that discomfort by midday. Iodine deficiency during fetal development or childhood can and does also result in severe developmental deformities, and because the immune system can also be chronically activated during chronic infection with parasites or opportunistic bacteria iodine can also become easily exhausted, since many of these pathogens are also communicated through intimate contact, causing iodine deficiency which impairs our immune system or developing fetuses or during breast feeding.

Iodine deficiency has long been a problem, and in the contiguous United States the Northern regions were long identified as *The Goiter Belt*, goiter being a condition where the thyroid enlarges due to chronic iodine deficiency, because such a significant number of the population presented with severe endemic goiter (it's literally a huge mass of growth in the neck and unmistakable). This phenomenon has been incorrectly attributed to a reduced quantity of iodine across the whole of North America due to the melting of ice age glaciers, which is total horseshit as indigenous Americans who lived in North America for tens of thousands of years before the genocide perpetrated by European colonialists had no such epidemic of goiter whatsoever. Instead, iodine is actually highly volatile and when exposed to air evaporates to the atmosphere, and traditional farming practices like ploughing the soil instead causes iodine to evaporate from soil and thus deficient quantities in the plants we grow. This is even more damning considering there is an iodine cycle in which atmospheric iodine falls in rainwater, so if soil is left intact it will, over time, accumulate iodine unless of course practices like ploughing soil continues. Indigenous Americans did not plough the soil so it retained its iodine content and thus their produce contained a far higher quantity of iodine which prevented goiter.

After the genocide of indigenous Americans their remaining populations were not only forced onto reservations by genocidal racists in the U.S. government but also forced to practice Western monoculture and ploughing (as their children were also forcibly abducted or made to attend Western education to eliminate language and cultural traditions) which then lead to the same kind of malnutrition and metabolic illness which to this day still plagues all populations who reside here. Goiter was a common problem also in Europe because tilling soil has been a practice for several millennia after agriculture technology developed in the Middle East which used to be called The Fertile Crescent but now is a dry, barren desert due to the destruction of non-regenerative farming practices on the environment, and many places which lack iodination of salt still present with goiter regardless of their geographical location or cultural traditions as modern food production continues to degrade soils and produce poorly nutritive food. Although salt was famously iodized as a comprehensive strategy to treat endemic goiter it is far less than what is required to promote adequate metabolic and immune health, and contemporary herbicides and agrochemicals can also bind iodine and cause thyroid disease even if there is sufficient amounts in the diet. Besides the immune system, iodine is also required by glandular tissue such as the breast and prostate as well as the brain, liver, and many other important organs, and deficiency in those organs is a strong promoter of cancer due to local immune failure which then facilitates ingress of pathogens.

Although it is no real solution to the problem of soil iodine deficiency, iodination of salt was incidentally a very effective treatment to iodine deficiency because iodine is taken up into cells through a sodium importer (the iodine-sodium symporter). It is very likely my health problems worsened in my early thirties after switching to non-iodized sea salt as became so readily available in markets since, because of our poor food systems, is often the only source of iodine for most people where my partner, who often experienced salt hunger, would consume far more iodized salt at restaurants or from movie theater popcorn and so did not experience as severe an iodine deficiency as I did. Lactoperoxidase which prefers iodine and cyanide as substrates is primarily located in glandular secretions like saliva, tears, and breast milk, and the reason it is located in saliva is not to convert iodine secreted by mucosal tissues to hypoiodous acid but to convert all dietary iodine to it, utilizing that which is supposed to occur in the diet to help constantly protect our gut and mucosal tissues from opportunistic pathogens. For this reason, dietary iodine is best, especially for children, but in order to reverse deficiency in those with chronic metabolic illness or poor immune function extra iodine should be taken such as from the frequent consumption of seaweed or iodine supplement derived from seaweed, which should be chewed in the mouth or swished with a tiny bit of water in order to activate it to hypoiodous acid via salivary lactoperoxidase, as while swallowing iodine can help it won't do much for those already colonized by opportunistic gut pathogens which disturb digestion and impair absorption of nutrients like iodine as well as the immune system.

One major problem is that the primary uptake pathway for iodine is the sodium-iodide symporter which is in turn entirely dependent on the presence of *butyric acid*, which is a short chain fatty acid produced by our commensal microbiome from substrate such as indigestible carbohydrate. Root vegetables are in turn the most reliable food for butyrate production (where fruit is instead best for acetate), so failure to eat root vegetables sufficiently frequent to support butyrate producers results in failure to uptake iodine and thus persistence of immune dysfunction even when supported by iodine supplementation. For those who are very ill such as with diabetes, cancer, cystic fibrosis, etc., starting every day with root vegetable such as sweet potatoes, potatoes, turnips, yuca, carrots, or other roots (I find sweet potato most effective) will help supply butyrate required for the rest of the day. After this, the supplemental use of iodide such as is available from *Lugol's solution* (*not* povidone iodine though, which is only for topical disinfection) and *potassium iodide* will be required due to the poor quantity inherent to industrial food systems. Iodine is caustic, however, and should never be used in very high doses. About 1-5mg per dose, depending on size (children won't need more than 1/2 mg), mixed into tea, juice, milk, or water for several days, reducing the amount and frequency of dose as progress occurs. The sudden introduction of iodine after long periods of deficiency as are common in those with metabolic disease can potentially trigger a temporary *hyperthyroid* state as described in the chapter on thyroid, so doses should not be high or frequent for several days to slowly introduce iodine back to the body, or stopping completely if hyperthyroid symptoms occur and are unpleasant until they subside. Incidentally, the iodine skin patch test which is so prevalent an anecdote is total bullshit as iodine simply evaporates into the air, so the rate at which iodine disappears when painted on the skin is determined by air temperature and humidity, not body iodine stores (about 12% of iodine applied to the skin is absorbed into the body). A leaky bottle of iodine once turned all the walls of my cupboard yellow, which demonstrates this volatile, evaporative nature of iodine.

Both chloride and bromine are also used in the synthesis of collagen (which also requires vitamin C) through the peroxidase *peroxidasin*, and halide deficiency or chemicals which interfere with normal halide peroxidasin function (like bromine fire retardants or fluoride in toothpaste or municipal water) is the likely factor in *Ehlers-Danlos syndrome* which can likely be addressed by consuming more dietary chloride and bromine such as from seaweed and avoiding fluoridated water and other halide base chemicals as much as possible. Bromine was also formerly used in the treatment of epilepsy, which is very likely also caused by pathogenic colonization (and discussed in the chapter on calcium since calcium dysregulation also underlies seizure), but bromine has an extremely long half-life so bromine medications or supplements often resulted in serious side effects because researchers and medical professionals did not realize bromine's participation in the immune reaction, and it was not fully effective because of factors inhibiting the immune reaction as discussed in this chapter also prevent the potential usefulness of bromine and high doses easily caused toxicity from chronic administration. Immune cells called *eosinophils* are specifically designed to fight parasites, and *eosinophil peroxidase* specifically prefers bromine rather than the other halides for their immune reaction. Some conditions like *muscular dystrophy* present with deficiency or dysregulation of eosinophils which probably demonstrates zinc deficiency since zinc is required to synthesize proteins used in the production, growth, and function of immune cells, but there are also conditions of eosinophilia characterized by excess production of eosinophils which likely demonstrates ineffective eosinophils to which the body responds by trying to produce more. Zinc also has an interesting function in that during an immune reaction it helps shrink the size of normal human cells at sites of infection which then increases the extracellular space which then allows passage of immune cells like eosinophils, to better congregate at sites of infection.

Thiocyanate from dietary cyanide is the most effective and least oxidizing immune substrate and is especially important for immunity in body fluids like saliva, semen, breastmilk, and the mucosal fluids which line the lungs, sinuses, and digestive tract because cyanide also scavenges hydrogen sulfide so dietary cyanogenic foods are absolutely required to restore good immune function and resist the influence of harmful hydrogen sulfide producers. To further support the fact that *Prunus* fruit are an original dietary staple for our pre-human ancestors the kernels of *Prunus* fruit like almonds are a potent dietary source of cyanide. The taste of almonds is actually the taste of cyanide which, when not taken in excess, is sweet to our sense of taste for this very reason. Other foods high in cyanide are brassicas like broccoli, kale, mustard greens, cabbage, etc., bamboo shoots, yuca, sorghum, and apple seeds. There is even a little cyanide carrots, corn, and other common foods (though not enough for this purpose). But cyanide is released from foods like almonds, apricot kernels, and brassicas by enzymatic activation on exposure to water and acids, and cooking can and does also ironically prevent cyanide release from plant foods. Many animals such as ourselves seem to have evolved to exploit dietary cyanide in the immune defense which in turn requires chewing fresh plant food sources of cyanide in order to activate the enzymes which in turn release cyanide. Being elements this is not the case for the halides such as iodine, chloride, bromide, and fluoride, which are converted to their hypohalous acid forms by salivary lactoperoxidase regardless of the state of food, but in order to benefit from dietary cyanide it must be chewed from fresh, uncooked food sources like almonds, apricot kernels, brassicas, bamboo shoots, etc., as cooking can and does otherwise reduce the cyanide content up to about 98%. This does not mean that all cyanide sources must be uncooked—only that when attempting to recover from metabolic disease fresh sources must be used medicinally, and for maintenance of immunity afterward the regular consumption of fresh sources can also be very useful. For instance it has long been recognized that dietary cyanide benefits cancer, but which is erroneously misunderstood to kill cancer cells when in reality it helps the immune system eradicate parasites and other pathogens which cause the cancer. While cooking certainly advantaged our species and provides an increase in nutrient bioavailability it did also disadvantage us such as through reduced exposure to dietary cyanide which normally empowers the immune system.

Cyanide is certainly poisonous in excess, especially when we are deficient in dietary sulfur which detoxifies cyanide to thiocyanate which means the functions of dietary cyanide are also dependent on sulfation factors inhibited by hydrogen sulfide producers, and there are many instances of illness and death from the overzealous and wishfully naive use of cyanogenic foods. Many products are also sold which concentrate cyanide or even fraudulently try to advertise it as a vitamin, which it is not, and cyanide's function in the immune system is never, ever a function of potency but of biochemistry and the conversion of cyanide to thiocyanate to hypothiocyanous acid, so consuming large quantities of any source of cyanide will *not* restore immune function better but *will* cause poisoning, where its efficacy is instead dependent on a functioning immune system and consistent intake. For instance in the early eighties a religious group in California poisoned eight of its members after preparing fresh elderberry juice in which they included the leaves of the plant which contain far more cyanide than the fruit, nearly killing its members, and in the nineties a professor who should have known better was also poisoned from preparing a tincture of elderberry as tinctures strongly concentrate cyanide in very high quantities. But this also illustrates most people's myopic fixation on killing microbes rather than promoting immunocompetency, which are two entirely different things and only the latter is effective at restoring health. Our ingenuity and technology can often have unintended consequences and the proper way to restore cyanide sufficiency is simply through the normal and rational consumption of cyanogenic foods and restoring the body's ability to use cyanide in the first place, not desperately trying to poison microbes, which will only instead poison us.

With regularity the trend of juicing fresh cabbage gets discovered and rediscovered all the time, with its health benefits errantly and ignorantly attributed to its low calorie or nutrient content rather than being a perfect example of how fresh, enzymatically liberated sources of dietary cyanide provides cyanide and supports the eradication of opportunistic microbes via the immune system. Other fresh preparations of brassicas like coleslaw (a traditional Dutch food) can also effectively achieve this, but ferments of brassicas like sauerkraut or kimchi have much less due to microbial inactivation of the cyanogenic glycosides and degradation of cyanide over time, and simply taking time to chew fresh shredded cabbage, brussels sprouts, arugula (rocket), broccoli, cauliflower, etc., daily can easily provide plenty of dietary cyanide. Brassicas are especially useful because they also contain plenty of sulfur which supports conversion of cyanide to thiocyanate, and health problems in regions of the world which rely excessively on yuca or lima bean for nutrition and can develop neurological disorders after many years of consumption due to varieties which are ridiculously high in cyanide due to protein and sulfur deficiency which impairs detoxification of cyanide to thiocyanate, and cyanide itself is not quite as toxic as its famous reputation. In fact, while illness often results from cyanide intoxication instances of actual death from food sources is extremely rare. No one in the above cited examples of cyanide poisoning actually died and unlike many other toxic substances does not make us sick at all unless consumed in excessive quantities or in forms which amplify its toxicity. Synthetic cyanide and concentrated cyanide from *Prunus* pits, specifically bitter apricot seeds, were promoted as a misguided and ineffective alternative treatment for cancer which resulted in the unfortunate deaths of several children who accidentally ingested those preparations, and there is also an account of death from cyanide poisoning in children fed a dessert normally made with almonds that instead used apricot kernels. Regular consumption of dietary sources like brassicas (broccoli, brussels sprouts, watercress, arugula, kale), almonds or other *Prunus* kernels, bamboo shoots, or apple seeds are all safe for adults and effective when eaten as food and not as prepared concentrates. The effect of cyanide can even be felt as a numbing sensation on the tongue when chewing high cyanide sources like apple seeds or non-almond *Prunus* kernels, which can be a useful barometer for avoiding excess.

Thiocyanate also spontaneously scavenges hypochlorous acid, converting to hypothiocyanate without requiring enzymatic production while also converting hypochlorite back to less oxidizing chloride, and because hypothiocyanite is minimally oxidizing to our tissues the consumption of dietary cyanide can and should result in an obvious and dramatic sense of relaxation as oxidative stress is suddenly lessened (for instance this occurs by thoroughly chewing cyanogenic foods but not by rapidly swallowing them). This function of cyanide scavenging hypochlorite is acutely experienced by smokers of tobacco, which is very high in cyanide, and the primary reason for the relaxing effects of a cigarette and thus its 'addictive' nature is not from nicotine at all but from its cyanide which scavenges hypochlorous acid throughout the body to instead promote (temporary) relaxation as well as suppression of the pathogenic organisms which trigger the immune reaction. Smoking is often associated with gingival disease which researchers and medical professionals assume is caused by smoking which is instead the instinctual self-medication for treatment of pathogenic colonization, not a behavior of addiction, for the effect of cyanide in both scavenging hypochlorite and eradicating pathogens. This is why those trying to give up smoking never find nicotine gums or patches an effective replacement nor cure for the 'addiction,' because although nicotine is a stimulant like caffeine which can help us cope with stress (or cause withdrawal symptoms when abstaining) it does not have the antioxidant and immune functions of cyanide, so smokers continue to crave smoking. Because smoking is harmful, and those who smoke also don't usually have healthy dietary habits, the daily consumption (chewing) of dietary cyanide sources will resolve addiction to smoking. During recovery in alcoholics anonymous I tried to become a smoker, in part because I had never smoked but I also wanted to experiment with nicotine and see if it had any useful properties, but to my surprise not only did I not become addicted, I would outright forget my cigarettes or vape at home in their drawer for days and weeks at a time because at that point my diet had finally included many dietary cyanide sources. To prove this further, most cyanide in canned bamboo shoots will actually be located in the packing water, not the shoots, because cyanide is water soluble, and drinking bamboo shoot packing water will produce the very same profound sense of relaxation as smoking a cigarette. Providing daily, rational amounts of dietary cyanide is thus also the cure to 'nicotine addiction' which also then supports immunocompetence.

Much like nitric oxide, cyanide and thiocyanate inhibit mitochondria as a regulatory mechanism, and I believe that the increase in nitric oxide seen in metabolic illness is a backup for the primary function of thiocyanate in keeping cells clear of invasive pathogens. Though there is no science which yet explores this I believe that, similarly to nitric oxide, thiocyanate is also removed from mitochondria by exposure to sunlight, which then reduces the molecule and makes it available for acceptance by peroxidase enzymes or to further scavenge hypochlorous acid and other reactive oxygen species, because following consumption of dietary cyanide with sun exposure results in far more profound sense of relaxation and improved immunity than without, and conversely exposure to sunshine without having chewed up some dietary source of cyanide like arugula, yuca, or almonds is a missed opportunity. This also simply makes sense in terms of human evolution, browsing cyanogenic foods under the light of the Sun, but because cyanide is lost to cooking or soaking and only occurs in specific foods the increase in metabolic illness which accompanies industrial diets as reflected in the work of Weston A. Price is in large part a consequence of cyanide loss or absence from the diet, replaced almost entirely by refined grains and animal products and yet another factor which affects health which has nothing to do with calories, fat, lack of exercise, discipline, etc. Likewise many relatively healthy young people find easy resolution of bloated guts, weight gain, and slow metabolisms simply through the increased consumption of brassicas, almonds, yuca, and other dietary sources of cyanide, which will be more obvious if these foods are eaten for breakfast or preceding any sun exposure, because their still competent immune systems and microbiomes easily leverage dietary cyanide for the production of powerful hypothiocyanous acid to resolve opportunistic microbial colonization. The nature of cyanide in the immune reaction is also not at all subtle and ineffective immune reactions during chronic illness cause chronic, significant feelings of agitation, irritation, and restlessness as peroxidase enzymes oxidize proteins, hormones, and other nutrients during deficiency of dietary cyanide. In fact this is a symptom and cause of alcoholism and addiction as discussed in that upcoming chapter as alcohol or other drugs help to suppress opportunistic microbes and thus the discomfort caused by chronic immune activation. The emotional state of consuming cyanogenic foods (without overdose) immediately before generous exposure to sunlight is so profound as to make this relationship between dietary cyanide, immunity, and sun exposure an easy and effective means to address metabolic illnesses of all types.

The condition of *cystic fibrosis* is also one in which the pseudohalide cyanide has received some attention because the pathway at issue, the *cystic fibrosis transmembrane conductance regulator* (or CFTR), exchanges thiocyanate, chloride, glutathione, and bicarbonate (and probably others), directly linking CFTR dysfunction to immune function. Cystic fibrosis is often discussed as a disease of genetic inheritance and indeed a far higher concentration of the illness exists among those of European descent, but mutations do not so easily get passed down when they cause highly mortal conditions like cystic fibrosis, and genes can actually improve or degrade across generations simply from the quality of diet, which is in direct conflict with ideas of immutable genetics. Most heritable diseases are also inherited not by DNA but by food traditions and dietary behaviors, and especially the sharing of microbes between family members which one could argue are more easily passed in families than DNA since there is a maximum limit of genes we can receive but none such limitation for pathogens. DNA also appears to be self-healing, and cells recognize when DNA is dysfunctional and will either repair it or undergo apoptosis) to eliminate damaged DNA from the body's gene pool, making such illnesses very unlikely to be genetic in origin. Men with cystic fibrosis are also infertile because the epididymis and prostate are also mucosal tissue like the lung and pancreas which, because of CFTR dysfunction, impairs sperm maturation and migration to the prostate and thus also related functions like fertility, which is another reason I was never diagnosed since, being gay, I never had opportunity to fail trying to impregnate anyone. Another symptom of cystic fibrosis is that young men and women with the condition never have *wet dreams* which, because of my hateful, religious upbringing I mistakenly thought was some kind of divine punishment for jacking off or being gay and thus never even told anyone. The inability for men to genetically pass down cystic fibrosis is entirely counterintuitive to it being a genetic disease, as such reduced odds and high rate of mortality would have caused such "mutations," if they existed, to die out long ago. But existing science on cystic fibrosis already proves it is not a genetic disease, with only about two-thirds of those with the condition even having the supposed mutations attributed, a fact not readily apparent from even professional characterization of the condition. There is also a whopping two-thousand other supposed "mutations" now associated with the illness which is a ridiculous number that serves only to impugn the research and medical establishment as entirely unserious.

Places like Japan which have an exceedingly rare rate of cystic fibrosis also have the highest consumption of iodide and bromide as seafoods are very high in halides which, like cyanide, would be oxidized by salivary lactoperoxidase during the act of chewing to better inhibit oral and gastroinestinal pathogens like *H. pylori*. Fruit and tea such as is more commonly consumed in many regions also with low rates of cystic fibrosis are high in natural fluorine and iodine as well as oxalate which helps sequester calcium away from pathogens. If scientists cannot see the forest for the trees, geneticists cannot see it for the leaves. Blaming DNA, inheritance, heredity, etc., for health problems is also not a novel function of genetic science or medicine but actually continues a long practiced tradition of blaming people for their disease when insecure and egotistical doctors and researchers are not able to cure or understand it. Not that they should—science and medicine are very hard and the behavior of saying 'it's the patient's fault' rather than 'I don't know how to cure that' is entirely a voluntary defense mechanism which originates from experiences of trauma and insecurity (as is discussed in my book on childhood trauma) desiring control over mortality, because if it's the patient's genetic fault that means we both don't have to do anything about it and can avoid it by not interbreeding with them, which is not at all how life works. Before 'genetics' was even invented the word 'heredity' was used in exactly the same context, irrespective of evidence with absolutely no idea that genes even existed. This tradition is most harmful not because it hurts patients, which it does, but because it actively prevents researchers and the establishment from finding actual cures to existing diseases when conditions such as with HIV or cystic fibrosis are finally "understood" and the entire machine either stops research or moves myopically in a single direction due to sunk-cost fallacy no matter how many failures evidence the folly. The insistence that only doctors can cure disease even while those with suicidal depression, diabetes, and cancer continue to die in vast numbers is nothing but complete and delusional submission to systems of authoritarianism and desires for control entirely in opposition to how realty and disease functions which does not care one bit about your fucking credentials.

Not only is cystic fibrosis not a disease of genetics, it is also more widespread than is commonly understood because only those with the most serious symptoms are even suspected, let alone diagnosed. In reality, cystic fibrosis is caused by parasites, most likely *Trichomonas* (or possibly *Cryptosporidium*) which specialize in colonizing mucosal tissue and, to further emphasize the degree of incompetence of our medical systems, unless you've had it you have never even heard of the misogynistically named *Trichomonas vaginalis* though it is the most common non-viral sexually transmitted disease and not only infects vaginas but also the prostate and urethra of penises, and this institutional misogyny causes it to be more widespread as vulnerable populations remain ignorant to it even existing let alone the ability to identify and address infection. Studies show that *Trichomonas* downregulates the cystic fibrosis transmembrane conductance regulator but even though this is confirmed by studies it has never been factored into cystic fibrosis research. Other mucosal tissue include the lungs, nasal passages, oral cavity, pancreas, and gut which are also the organs affected by cystic fibrosis, and studies show that colonization by *Trichomonas* also increases risk of infection by HIV, because of course it fucking does. There are also many *Trichomonas* species which can colonize all mucosal tissues, and they spread like any other parasite or pathogen from all sorts of vectors like shaking hands, sneezing, coughing, spitting, sex, food, bathrooms, dentistry, water, and even childcare.

Healthy, well fed people are highly resistant to infection, as one study showed when zinc-replete or sodium-replete seminal fluid rapidly killed *Trichomonas* in the prostate (which is not a function of zinc but simply reflective of working immune pathways). So while *Trichomonas* are very widespread they are not extremely virulent and, like those microbes which cause autism, all humans at some point do contract *Trichomonas,* which is why many of the symptoms of cystic fibrosis like chronic lung infection and impaired immune function are also those seen frequently in aged persons, and cystic fibrosis is also essentially a condition of premature aging caused by premature immune dysfunction caused by *Trichomonas* colonization. Besides producing ammonia, parasites also inhibit the immune system by catabolizing purines which results in an excess of uric acid which competes with thiocyanate for lactoperoxidase and myeloperoxidase (so gout is also a symptom of parasitism), and theft of purines like adenosine in turn also causes ATP deficiency and promotes insomnia as discussed in the upcoming chapter on sleep, and those with metabolic conditions like cystic fibrosis present with high uric acid which can also cause gout conditions and promote other secondary infections.

But the immune system, or immune defenses, are not only active, chemical strategies as these, and there are many environmental, structural, and innate factors which also help to protect us from colonization by pathogens, such as the production of immunoglobulins or the relatively dry barrier of the skin since microbes generally require moisture to grow and proliferate. In the chapter on cancer I discuss how silicon becomes polymerized when exposed to an alkaline pH, and it just so happens that skin, connective tissue, and the cellular matrix are normally very high in silicon, which not only provides structural support to our own body but also an inherent defensive barrier to microbes like parasites and *H. pylori* which produce highly alkaline substances like ammonia, sulfides, etc., the liberated silicon then polymerizes, and since those pathogens do not like acidic environments and do not produce acids to dissolve the polymer the silicon then forms an impenetrable barrier through which they cannot ingress. This means that one of the primary defensive mechanisms inherent to our health and wellness is silicon repletion, but which is a far more complex problem than simply taking a silicon supplement since we cannot absorb or use normal silicon and it is the acidification of silicon as discussed in the chapter on cancer which allows silicon to be incorporated into the body. After discovering the usefulness of loading drinking water with silicon (only so much as can be dissolved by boiling, which is about 100 mg/L), this began to strongly promote even more recovery from symptoms of cystic fibrosis than what I was able to achieve from earlier research and restoration of the immune system. But, unsurprisingly, immune cells like macrophages and eosinophils which are so important for actually attacking and destroying invasive pathogens are also dependent on bioavailable silicon, not only having mitochondria but also producing reactive oxygen species which actively harm pathogens but which process could also similarly result in massive leakage of electrons if those cells are also deficient in silicon as what occurs in states of cancer and metabolic disease as discussed in the chapter on cancer.

Cystic fibrosis then specifically occurs when parents harbor *Trichomonas* parasites, then pass to their children not only *Trichomonas* but also dietary behaviors which perpetuate silicon deficiency which then prevents spontaneous recovery by children which can and will otherwise recover if this deficiency is reversed, since children are naturally better resistant to *Trichomonas*. Like many parasites, *Trichomonas* does not obviously cause symptoms of disease but merely downregulates the immune system, and disease is instead revealed by secondary infections such as those which cause yeast infections, urinary tract infections, prostate inflammation, premature ejaculation, HIV, prostate cancer, cervical cancer, chronic post nasal drip, chronic sinusitis, gum disease, and chronic cough from chronic pulmonary (lung) infections such as by *Pseudomonas aeruginosa*. As *Trichomonas* readily colonizes the prostate, loss of robust erectile arousal as discussed in the chapter on erections is a primary symptom of *Trichomonas* colonization, because the arginase enzyme produced by parasites consumes arginine that is otherwise used for endothelial nitric oxide which mediates vasodilation and erectile tumescence (and the immune response also results in greater inducible nitric oxide production to combat pathogens which also then chronically depletes arginine and suppresses mitochondrial respiration), and colonization is not limited also to areas like the prostate and urethra but will also include the oral cavity, sinuses, lungs, pancreas, cervix, breast ducts, nasal passages, the gut lining, and any other mucosal tissue. Because of this, *Trichomonas* are a major catalyst of cancers in mucosal organs like the breast, prostate, etc., and since sex partners can and do also harbor *Trichomonas* but may remain asymptomatic they can also remain a vector for repeated infection or exposure. Because collagen synthesis utilizes peroxidase enzymes and halides, the fibrosis also seen in fibrotic conditions like cystic fibrosis, uterine fibroids, pulmonary fibrosis, etc., are caused by chronic and ineffective immune reaction in response to the presence of pathogens which then results in the spontaneous and cumulative synthesis of collagen fibers to cause fibrosis, but since those fibers are also generally low in silicon they then fail to protect tissues from increased colonization that would otherwise occur if silicon was generously present. During the worst of my cystic fibrosis my coughing was constant and so severe it directly contributed to my inability to sleep, and looking back on how severe it actually was I'm even more amazed nobody in my life was very concerned or helpful (as discussed in my book on psychology trauma is often handled through dissociation and avoidance), and though restoration of the immune system generally and dramatically improved my cough, it was after finally discovering the role of silicon in cancer and immunity and the repeated, daily, consistent repletion with silicon (especially by dissolving it in drinking water, since silicon is taken up by aquaporin channels) finally resolved the feeling of chronic fibroses, tightness, and irritation in my lungs that associated with the coughing.

Early in my recovery even as many of my other symptoms and conditions improved I would still be woken nightly by a coughing fit that would last several minutes, and every morning started with a coughing fit (or two or three or four). Even the chlorine off-gassing from a hot shower would trigger coughing, and after using a vitamin C water filter so I could shower without having my lungs spasm I had the idea to start supplementing vitamin C and eat high vitamin C foods daily for the first time in my life. Suddenly my cough began to improve so I kept making sure to sustain my vitamin C. Years later during my research I found studies that showed the CFTR pathway is restored by vitamin C and citric acid. As discussed in the chapters on parasites and calcium, both endogenous oxalate produced from vitamin C (and other substrate) and dietary oxalate from specific plant foods also helps sequester calcium away from mucosal tissue specifically, which is the primary site of colonization by *Trichomonas,* but diets high in grain and animal products such as is so common to industrialized food systems are low in vitamin C which in turn promotes microbial colonization of mucosa such as by *Tricho-*

monas, and indeed those with cystic fibrosis are found to present with deficiency of vitamin C and higher circulating oxalate, indicating active parasitism. Studies show CFTR regulates oxalate secretion to mucosal tissue, so CFTR impairment by parasites likely prevents oxalate secretion out of the mucosa that would otherwise inhibit them. For this reason sun exposure for endogenous production of citric acid (which also requires carbohydrate and zinc), and high dietary vitamin C is even more important for recovery from any immune disorder, to help restore normal mucosal oxalate secretion, and especially important for recovery from any microbial related conditions such as cystic fibrosis, diabetes, autism, etc., in order to restore normal metabolism of calcium to prevent its acquisition by pathogens.

Even as I was investigating and writing about cystic fibrosis, since its symptoms were similar to the ones I presented because I fucking had cystic fibrosis, I never actually considered it and not cancer was the reason for my chronic cough, profuse sweating, poor digestion, libido problems, insomnia, pain, premature aging, and cancer. Cystic fibrosis increases the risk of both diabetes and leukemia or lymphoma, which explains why my health fell apart so rapidly and at such a young age, and the average lifespan for those with cystic fibrosis is sadly no greater than early thirties. The CFTR channel at issue in cystic fibrosis is thus primarily an immune channel, but it is also mischaracterized even by specialists and is not merely a transporter of thiocyanate and chloride but an *exchanger* which imports chloride and secretes thiocyanate simultaneously, to preserve chloride and help sustain hydration of cells while using thiocyanate as the primary immune substrate, if it is available in the diet, as cyanide is widespread in plants. This discrepancy is illustrated best by conflicting characterization of CFTR function of sweat glands compared to other mucosal organs, where chloride is secreted by non CFTR channels but is *reabsorbed* by CFTR, to prevent loss of chloride, not secreted which, when dysfunctional, then causes increased chloride loss to then impair not only immunity but also the metabolism of water and synthesis of collagen and other connective tissue. As in all other organs this function occurs in sweat to disinfect epithelial (outer) layers, but when the body is low in thiocyanate chloride is not resorbed, to replace missing thiocyanate as a less effective backup to the immune reaction. This is also why those with cystic fibrosis lose so much chloride and sodium in sweat but also present with immune dysfunction and dry mucous since deficiency of thiocyanate then promotes deficiency of chloride and then also of sodium and water. Increasing dietary cyanide from the daily intake of brassicas (broccoli, cabbage, watercress, brussels sprouts, mustard, etc.), yuca, apple seeds, almonds, etc., followed by generous sun exposure (at times and duration that does not risk sunburn) enhances chloride retention and is required for recovery from any metabolic illness, since all metabolic illness is underpinned by parasitism, but this also has implications for other body functions like blood volume, cardiovascular health, and erectile function since everyone has the CFTR channels which help metabolize water and electrolytes. While CFTR is activated by vitamin C (and citrate, probably any acid) and thus benefits from a diet high in vitamin C (more on vitamin C is discussed in the upcoming chapter on thyroid), vitamin C becomes unstable from reaction to alkaline factors like ammonia (vitamin C is an acid, after all) and vitamin C deficiency in turn is mostly facilitated not by dietary deficiency (even potatoes contain a lot of vitamin C), but by chemical neutralization of vitamin C such as when the gut is colonized by high-ammonia producing microbes like parasites and *H. pylori,* which is why eating high tannin, astringent fruits as recommended in chapter on pathogens and metabolic disease can be so therapeutic.

Studies also show that CFTR is also regulated by *cholesterol*, and most people do not know that all cells in the human body also contain a sulfated cholesterol lattice throughout the membrane, as fats and cholesterol are not only required for things such as hormones and bile but also the very structural makeup and biomechanical function of living tissue, and without an abundance of high-quality and well-functioning cholesterol cells become weakened and more vulnerable to stress and invasion by opportunistic microbes. When I discuss the human evolutionary niche this does not only include *Prunus* species of fruit trees or a semi-aquatic habitat on the shores of ancient lake Mega Chad, but also the microbiological niche wherein the makeup and construction of human cells occupies a separate biological niche than those microbes with which we compete, such as the fact that much of our physiology is dependent on silicon, and this also includes the composition of physiological fats which are used in such structures as cholesterol which are different than those used by parasites, bacteria, and fungi, which then give our cells greater resistance to competition and thus also increases the integrity of cellular structures in turn such as the CFTR channel required of normal immune function. As might then be expected, those with cystic fibrosis and other metabolic illnesses like diabetes, autism, cancer, depression, etc., also present with dysregulated cholesterol, though because of the bias against cholesterol this has never received appropriate attention and research, but if the integrity of every CFTR channel in the body is in turn entirely dependent on the cholesterol composition of those cells then this means that restoration of abundant and normal cholesterol function is the key not only to reversing cystic fibrosis but every other metabolic disease as well, which in turn then helps restore both normal immune function and the metabolism of water which supports immune and defensive barriers.

As mentioned also in chapter on pathogens and metabolic disease, *lithium* also paralyzes parasites, which does not kill them outright but helps the body to better mount an immune response to eradicate them, and a low dose supplement of lithium daily (2-5 mg, depending on size) can help also to suppress symptoms and improve the rate of recovery. Foods like leafy greens, peas and beans, nuts, tea, and fruit are also generally good sources of lithium which are sufficient for those whom are already healthy, but bioavailability of nutrients like lithium is greatly misunderstood and for those that are very ill even high doses as commonly occur in pharmaceutical lithium will not provide this benefit without correct administration. Bioavailability is often measured by how much gets excreted in urine, the fact it was absorbed and secreted being used as evidence of bioavailability. But rapidly urinating out nutrients like lithium shows its bioavailability is actually quite low, which is why those on pharmacological lithium therapy are often given such absurdly high doses, which are required to overcome its otherwise low bioavailability, doses which are in fact potentially very toxic and often to result in complications and hospitalization. Tannin (and anthocyanins, which are tannin) actually complexes with lithium and makes it highly bioavailable, and cinnamic acids most strongly promote lithium uptake, likely by inhibiting the production of the hydroxyl radical which otherwise reacts to lithium, and using lithium along with sources of tannin such as fruit juice or tea increases its bioavailability so effectively that if high doses typical of pharmacological lithium prescriptions were mixed with tannin it could very well send someone to the hospital, so only low doses are necessary and useful. Lithium is atomically related to sodium, and in those with cystic fibrosis who present with sodium deficiency lithium can also temporarily reduce the volume of air exchange in the lungs if care is not taken to first restore sodium sufficiency, using tannin to block ammonia which will promote the uptake of sodium, otherwise lithium, being similar to sodium, will insert itself excessively in sodium dependent pathways and produce an outsized effect. Otherwise, lithium stays in the extracellular space where it helps paralyze parasites to promote better recovery from illness.

Lithium itself also binds ammonia, to directly mitigate some of the harm of ammonia excess and mechanisms by which parasites inhibit immune channels, but this also means that ammonia is also a primary causative factor in lithium deficiency, so the general absence of tannin from diets is also a major cause of lithium deficiency, and using tannin to suppress gastroinestinal ammonia and cucurbits to promote renal ammonia detoxification also potentiates the effect of lithium treatment (which is most strong when accompanied by cinnamic acid sources). Lithium is highly water soluble so the natural occurrence of both lithium and tannin in sources of drinking water during our evolutionary history was probably a major health resource which became lost once we started drinking water low in tannin such as from wells or reservoirs, but leaves and nuts are also often high in lithium. Studies which show an increased rate of violent crime associated with areas deficient in lithium and nutritive diets, which is likely a consequence of psychological illness due to widespread parasitism and the effects of ammonia on the brain and endocrine system as a consequence of lithium deficiency (in combination with trauma and other factors like economic stress which prevents healthy diets and healthy dietary behaviors).

One incredible property of lithium which has been heretofore unknown, however, is that its emission spectrum (the wavelength it emits when exposed to light) is also the very same wavelength of 670 nanometers which is attributed to the therapeutic effects of red light exposure therapy. I have not discussed red light much yet in this book as it is widely known as a therapeutic tool, but for some reason nobody has yet recognized that lithium is the only element which has this emission spectrum and thus that many of lithium's healthful benefits actually come from exposure to light and in fact mediates many of the the beneficial effects seen from light exposure. What's even more useful is that since lithium is shown to negatively affect parasites it likely does so through production of the 670 nm wavelength which likely causes irradiation stress in parasites to outright kill them. Early in my recovery I took supplemental lithium twice daily and it turns out that much of my early recovery came from sun exposure while replete with lithium which in turn eradicated the parasites which cause cystic fibrosis and otherwise impaired my immune system. When I made this discovery ten years later and purposefully preceded light exposure with a dose of 5-10 mg of supplemental lithium its antiparasitic effects on my lung and immune function were so profound that it entirely alleviated symptoms of cystic fibrosis for the first time in my entire life. Because these parasites colonize all mucosal tissue including the breast, prostate, cervix, lungs, pancreas, and even the oral cavity which can and does also cause cancer, anyone with any kind of metabolic illness will require a low dose supplement of lithium aspartate or lithium carbonate to suppress *Trichomonas* and other parasites, which can be added to the boiling water used to make coffee or tea (with some added cinnamon), or to undiluted fruit juices, lemonade, soup, etc., after which the body will once again resume the absorption of nutrients like sodium, chloride, and dietary fats and fat soluble nutrients, and will benefit more rapidly from a healthy diet in the restoration of health and wellness. Although the effects of this therapy are quite rapid, it should be continued for anyone with cystic fibrosis even well after symptoms have resolved, since *Trichomonas* is very common in our environment.

The peroxidases which oxidize halides to produce the hypohalous acids which attack pathogens also first require an oxygen donor, and as such are supplied with *hydrogen peroxide* made from the powerful oxidative radical *superoxide* by another family of enzymes called *oxidases* which use *water* as a cofactor, so dysfunctional aquaporin channels caused by deficiencies of silicon and vitamin C also impairs the immune reaction by literally causing water deficiency. This is the reason why water helps mitigate hangovers after a night of excessive drinking of alcohol because *aldehyde oxidase* processes alcohol to acetic acid, and the more alcohol drunk the more water is required for aldehyde oxidase to process it. This is the same reason lots of water is often required during acute infectious illness, but superoxide is also produced as a byproduct of normal cellular metabolism when electrons leak from mitochondria as discussed in the chapter on cancer, and when not converted to hydrogen peroxide is one of the most destructive and stressful reactive oxygen species produced in the body. For this reason, superoxide is converted (*dismuted*) to hydrogen peroxide by the enzyme *manganese superoxide dismutase* which is obviously dependent on *manganese,* which you will remember is also stolen by opportunistic pathogens which use manganese to produce ammonia that causes ammonia toxicity which inhibits uptake of sodium, chloride, vitamin C, silicon, etc. The immune myeloperoxidase is capable of using superoxide directly when hydrogen peroxide is not produced due to dismutase deficiency, but when this occurs myeloperoxidase indiscriminately oxidizes important nutrients and amino acids like tryptophan and tyrosine as a massive immune overreaction to prevent pathogenic ingress into the body but which in turn causes literal deficiencies of important nutrients like tryptophan and tyrosine. As discussed in the chapter on niacin, tryptophan is required for niacin, NAD, serotonin, and melatonin production, and tyrosine is required for dopamine and adrenaline (and the immune system itself), and immune system oxidation of amino acids causes their deficiency and is one of the primary reasons for wasting and atrophy that are associated with long term chronic illness and even the condition of aging in general, which is in turn a specific consequence of manganese deficiency and thus the increase in superoxide and myeloperoxidase mediated oxidative stress, so the body cannot even make NAD and sometimes even serotonin and melatonin without resolving dismutase and manganese deficiency.

Manganese is also required for a pathway called *cGAS-STING* which is how the body locates pathogens in the first place. Most people understand that viruses live inside our actual cells but even parasites and bacteria can and do as well as human cells are comparatively enormous but which then makes it more difficult for the immune system to hunt down and destroy them. This detection system uses the chemical *interferon* which alerts surrounding cells and the immune system to the presence of DNA in the cytosol of a cell because DNA is normally contained to the nucleus and mitochondria so any DNA in the cytosol is a way to identify either damaged cells or the presence of pathogens, a function entirely dependent on manganese in cGAS-STING. One murine study on *Cryptosporidium* parasites which are commonly associated with HIV infection found that manganese helped inhibit and in some specimens resolve colonization entirely. Because manganese is also a cofactor in the enzymes *pyruvate carboxylase,* required to produce insulin, and *glutamine synthetase* which sequesters ammonia into glutamine, restoration of manganese though an occasional, low-dose supplement can greatly help restore normal immune function but in anyone that is diabetic the use of a manganese supplement can cause dangerous insulin spikes which should be prevented by careful monitoring of blood sugar and eating accordingly.

While a supplement of manganese might be useful, any healthy diet will contain plenty of manganese, and instead deficiency is mostly caused by pathogens like parasites stealing our manganese, not lacking in the diet. Those with cystic fibrosis, for instance, present with less manganese in sputum which would otherwise prevent the biofilm formation of *Pseudomonas aeruginosa*, the primary pathogen which causes chronic coughing and fibrosis, so after resolution of *Trichomonas* with lithium and light therapy the restoration of nutrients like manganese will be far more easy to accomplish, even without the use of a supplement. However, there is also a protective immune protein called *calprotectin* which binds manganese (as well as zinc, iron, copper, and nickel) to sequester away from sites of infection and colonization. Many diseases like diabetes, cystic fibrosis, IBS, Crohn's, and ulcerative colitis present with up to ten times the amount of detectable calprotectin in feces indicating rapid loss of calprotectin and ineffective nutritional immunity, so manganese deficiency is primarily due to dysfunctional calprotectin which allows its theft by opportunistic microbes. Part of the nomenclature of calprotectin is that its binding strength is entirely dependent on calcium, where it cannot bind manganese without calcium and only weakly binds zinc, meaning this too is also a casualty of disturbed calcium homeostasis and regulation. Calprotectin is abundantly produced in the body and neutrophils, which carry the most, with studies showing white blood cells carry as much calprotectin as red blood cells carry hemoglobin, with up to sixty percent of their cytosolic protein being calprotectin. During an immune reaction calprotectin is secreted as a net or web across tissues, digesting food, and microbial colonies, and while the primary effect of calprotectin is thought to function by sequestering away nutrients I suspect that calprotectin may also turn these ions directly into antimicrobial factors that may actively destroy pathogens.

But studies which show high calprotectin activity alone do not also show high antimicrobial function, only in the presence of elements like calcium, zinc, or manganese, where plain calprotectin actually does not itself necessarily present with broad antimicrobial effects. Corroborating calcium dysregulation as a cause of calprotectin dysfunction are studies showing that high calprotectin loss in feces also correlates with high rates of inactive matrix glutamate proteins (vitamin K dependent proteins) which can be reversed by the daily consumption dietary vitamin K, even or also with additional sources of calcium such as the preparation of tea in milk, creamed spinach, cheese in a high vitamin K salad, pesto, etc. Experimenting once with zinc citrate I discovered the necessity for calprotectin, because significant uptake of zinc in such a bioavailable form led also to a significant coughing fit I had not experienced in several years, since *P. aeruginosa* which accompanies cystic fibrosis exploits zinc for its own purposes. After regular consumption of tea brewed in milk (during vitamin D repletion) this not only never occurred again but also made the use of zinc exceptionally effective in suppression of parasitism and restoration of immunocompetence such that even considering my large size a supplement of zinc is only required about once or twice a month. Libido is the easiest and most reliable metric to diagnose zinc deficiency—if you have one, you're fine on zinc, if not there is zinc deficiency even if zinc occurs in the diet or a supplement for reasons like calprotectin dysfunction. Manganese is thus also similarly dependent on calcium homeostasis and should not require a supplement, and while a supplement could be used to more quickly reverse deficiency a supplement will not help long term until calprotectin function is restored, through the restoration of calcium metabolism, after which the consumption of foods high in manganese like mussels, germ of cereal grains, pine nuts, hazelnuts, pumpkin seeds, etc., will be more than sufficient.

The role of zinc in mediating extraction of citrate from the citric acid cycle under the influence of vitamin D is another reason zinc is required for immune function and why calprotectin is required for immune function. Although vitamin D is primarily thought to be activated only by the liver and kidneys, studies prove that T-cells, macrophages, and even periodontal tissue (the gums) directly activate vitamin D, which means local production of citric acid from carbohydrate is a primary immune defense mechanism, which likely functions by actively depriving pathogens of the calcium they require to buffer our immune response. Since vitamin D binding protein and cholesterol (from which vitamin D is made) are dependent on sulfur and selenium, microbial reducers of sulfate and selenate which result in the offensive malodors of breath, feces, and flatulence also indirectly impair immunity by directly interfering with vitamin D homeostasis. The misunderstanding of deficiency of sunshine and vitamin D as a major etiological factor in disease is a major fallacy behind common convalescence procedures in hospitals which usually imprison patients away from sunlight and vitamin D required for healthy immune function and activation of mitochondrial respiration. This is done out of caution for exposure to cold temperature, as cold does impair the immune system by impairing, though unaware of the mechanism, where cold impairs the migration of immune cells and saturated fats, which are highly dependent on heat, since polyunsaturated fats synthesized in the body when exposed to cold (or what are eaten in the diet) competes with vitamin D for vitamin D binding protein, but this role of fatty acids and temperature in the immune response is also why we get fever when sick because heat increases the body's ability to transport saturated fatty acids to sites of infection to thus support robust immune function and tissue regeneration. Interestingly, during the years of my experimentation with oral infectious bacteria I never got a fever, even from coronavirus during the pandemic, and I believe that certain pathogens like those which cause gum disease can and do inhibit the pyrogenic fever response which not only helps them persist in the human body but promotes other persistent pathogenic colonization. Using gentle, safe supplemental heat as well with saunas, spas, heat lamps, and blankets by *slowly* bringing up the body temperature without causing heat stress can help to raise heat and engage the transit of our most useful saturated fatty acids which stabilize vitamin D and promote immune function. Making sunlight exposure safe and effective through dietary carotenoids and restoration of cholesterol, sulfate, selenium, vitamin C, and dietary cyanide can also help during convalescence through the increase in heat and vitamin D and thus citrate, careful not to cause sunburn or overheating which will instead increase illness and discomfort.

Lymphoma and leukemia such as what I likely had are also caused by retroviruses, which are some of the oldest viruses in nature and which are shown in studies to normally be easily destroyed by the immune system, even unable to exist in healthy cells that are properly saturated with oxygen (normoxia, as opposed to hypoxia which is low oxygen) even without direct immune defense, and it is very likely that retroviruses originate from when most biology was not oxygen-dependent and when our ancient, ancient ancestors evolved oxygen respiration it also then greatly diminished vulnerability to retrovirus colonization, since retroviruses are shown to associate with states of hypoxia. HIV is a retrovirus and has been befuddling for its widespread distribution since retroviruses are normally so easy for the body to resist. Boron is also required for activation of vitamin D, by inhibiting excessive hydroxylation and chaperoning oxygen to mitochondria as described in the chapter on vitamin D, and boron has also been shown in studies to inhibit HIV protease, an important enzyme required in its replication, and heme also facilitates oxygen delivery to cells I believe any disease caused by a retrovirus such as leukemia, lymphoma, or HIV/AIDS to be a function of hypoxia induced by anemia, boron deficiency, iron excess, sulfur deficiency, and oleic acid (which stabilizes the respiratory cytochrome oxidase). Studies confirm already that 40% of children with HIV present with anemia, while adults with HIV present with 50%, and since anemia is driven by factors like iron excess, impaired heme synthesis, and boron status it is very easy to see how HIV and cancers like leukemia are driven by dieting, diabetes, industrialized foods supply, malnutrition, and colonization by hydrogen sulfide and hydrogen selenide producing opportunistic microbes.

The entire cardiovascular system is also lined with sulfated cholesterol and is a target for sulfate and selenate reducing oral pathogens once they gain access to the cardiovascular system, and since this cholesterol barrier is meant to prevent water escaping from the bloodstream many with HIV then also present with edema of the face, arms, legs, etc., as their cholesterol and sulfate are depleted and which impairs the CFTR channels and synthesis of heme (which is dependent on sulfur) and promotes boron dysfunction due to excess accumulation of iron. Since heme is required not only in hemoglobin but also the immune peroxidases themselves, HIV and other retroviruses then directly benefit from reduced immune activity. This means the cure to HIV is likely from the reversal of iron overload by protecting dietary sulfur with dietary carotene, which will also help reverse boron deficiency (since boron status is impaired by iron overload), and restoring heme synthesis through greatly increasing dietary sulfur intake protected by dietary carotene, for which the use of a low-dose boron supplement will be helpful (but only useful inasmuch as iron excess is resolved) and since cyanide also spontaneously scavenges hydrogen sulfide the dietary intake of cyanide through brassicas, almonds, yuca, etc., can help further scavenge hydrogen sulfide in the body. This might also seem difficult to resolve but boron status directly regulates the rate of respiration (which is why those with severe HIV present with reduced breathing rate), so an increase in respiration rate and volume of gas moved through the lungs is an excellent way to evaluate progress (too little means no progress while increased volume and rate means it's working).

The oxidases which support the immune reaction itself are in turn dependent on both *molybdenum* and *riboflavin* (vitamin B2), the latter being a prolific generator of reactive oxygen species and used in nature primarily for the purposeful production of reactive oxygen. For instance, when oxygen disturbs the gastroinestinal microbiome it does so by reacting to flavins which spontaneously form hydrogen peroxide which then kills our commensal microbes, and the body uses this property of flavin in pathways such as oxidase enzymes to purposefully oxidize pathogens or other foreign particulate. Just as there is nicotinamide adenine dinucleotide (NAD) there is also *flavin adenine dinucleotide* (FAD), and dependency on riboflavin means FAD is also inhibited by *roseoflavin* producing *Streptomyces* (which you will remember also inhibit biotin) respiring on dietary nitrates as discussed in the chapters on pathogens and metabolic disease. Since all humans are eventually colonized by *Streptomyces,* roseoflavin produced by opportunistic microbes which competes with riboflavin producers is one of the etiological factors which underlies many conditions of immunoincompetence and aging, because this predisposes us not only to immune dysfunction but also poor oxygen transport as *hemoglobin,* our primary oxygen transport in blood, is also highly dependent on riboflavin, and when the COVID-19 pandemic started I researched and wrote an article about riboflavin being a primary tool used by the immune system to fight viruses and even very aged people with poor health using riboflavin easily fought off the virus (i.e. my seventy-year-old parents who instead gave credit to their superior constitution and religious beliefs). Because riboflavin is also required for the transportation of oxygen I believe mortality from coronavirus during the pandemic (and other pandemics) most commonly occurs from total depletion of riboflavin by the massive immune response in those already deficient in riboflavin due to opportunistic roseoflavin producers. I caught COVID-19 two times (possibly three) in spite of my strict efforts to avoid it, because cystic fibrosis made me highly susceptible to infection, but even with severe symptoms and active cystic fibrosis which directly impairs lung and immune function the use of riboflavin and aspirin helped me recover fully each time in about thirty-six hours compared to the few weeks common to much healthier people, and without any symptoms of long covid.

Unlike streptavidin which binds to biotin, roseoflavin merely mimics riboflavin, so taking extra riboflavin as a supplement for the treatment or prevention of infectious illness can be very, very effective. During the coronavirus pandemic in 2020 many patients presented with hypoxemia (low blood oxygen) and were put on ventilators, which is kind of ridiculous because there is plenty of oxygen in the atmosphere and hypoxemia is clearly a problem of biochemistry that was very likely caused by severe depletion of riboflavin due to colonization with roseoflavin producers, and if those with hypoxemia (or everyone, preventatively) had been put on a supplement of riboflavin the rate of mortality would have likely been far less than it was. Because riboflavin also promotes the storage of glucose in glycogen, obesity is almost always a reliable diagnostic for riboflavin deficiency, but because riboflavin is also a requisite for the kynurenine pathway as discussed in the chapters on niacin therapy and hair loss those factors can also be used to establish the presence of roseoflavin producers and need to supplement (otherwise it's not necessary) until the gut microbiome can be restored. Supplements of riboflavin tend to be far too high in dose (not harmful, just unnecessary), so opening up a capsule and using smaller doses like 10-20 mg once a day is very economical and more than enough for efficacy, and elimination of *Streptomyces* through restoration of gut health and immune function will restore natural riboflavin synthesis by the commensal microbiome.

A diet high in molybdenum from foods like peas, nuts, and cucurbits with care taken to suppress hydrogen sulfide (since hydrogen sulfide forms toxic thiomolybdate when reacting to molybdenum) will supply necessary molybdenum better than supplementation. But exposure to toxic agrochemicals like glyphosate also strongly causes molybdenum deficiency, so it may also be required to take a low-dose supplement occasionally (like once a week) in order to restore oxidase activity. This should also be taken with high anthocyanin foods like cherries, plums, purple grapes, blueberries, etc., because anthocyanin forms a high bioavailable complex with molybdenum which will make the supplement more effective. Studies show that the immune oxidase-peroxidase system easily destroys HIV and other retroviruses, and it is possible that molybdenum depletion by toxic agrochemicals combined with anemia (low B12) and low boron are the hypoxic conditions that allow retroviruses ingress to the body which can possibly be cured by restoring B12, boron, molybdenum, and riboflavin (and riboflavin producers in the gut by restoring the gut microbiome).

Another primary purpose of oxidase enzymes related to the immune reaction is the oxidation of any foreign matter in the body to prevent interference with our metabolic pathways. All proteins, peptides, and amino acids have direct effects on our physiology and foreign particulate be it pollen, toxic chemicals, microbes, dust, animal dandruff or saliva, or the enzymes of infectious microbes and must be neutralized. During insult by foreign particulate the body thusly increases oxidases to oxidize and neutralize foreign particulate so it can be detoxified before triggering or interfering in our own metabolic pathways. Without oxidases even pollen proteins from plants interfere with our biological pathways (pollen is plant sperm, after all), which is why allergies to things seemingly as benign as pollen or peanuts can induce severe allergic responses and is in fact due to the oxidative stress caused by our own oxidases which in turn causes a chain reaction of oxidative stress to our own tissues and resultant inflammation and other symptoms which accompany allergies. Cytochrome oxidase, our primary respiratory enzyme, also uses this same exact function to facilitate respiration to oxidize carbohydrate (pyruvate) for energy, and thus the principle mechanism underlying our entire biology, and without oxidases many systems in our body cannot actually function.

But this problem with oxidases is also the cause for *autoimmunity*, since the immune reaction creates reactive oxygen species to attack not only pathogens but any foreign material. This problem is usually treated by suppressing the immune system with pharmaceuticals, such as by blocking oxidase activity, but this only makes us more susceptible to disease and infection, not less, as pathogens are then able to further colonize tissues and spread throughout the body due to a pharmacologically inhibited immune system. One person I know with severe, chronic autoimmune issues used more than twenty different medications and only barely got by due to their massive health problems and overreliance on the medical system. In fact there is actually no such thing as autoimmunity, and what is mistaken as autoimmunity is the immune system instead doing exactly what it is supposed to, which is to seek and destroy foreign material, and all antibodies do is clean up foreign particulate or damaged cells, and pathogens like viruses which can and do invade nearly every type of tissue in the body. Many autoimmune conditions involve the skin and are in fact ingress by pathogenic fungi due to the absence of commensal skin microbes as discussed in the chapter on diabetes which can be resolved by recruiting skin microbes from the environment by exposure to healthy soil and plants such as in the act of gardening (which is dependent also on skin carotene). But the way autoimmune conditions are usually characterized and managed is as if the body is wrong, mistaken, or dysfunctional, so treatment is also ineffective, never mind the fact that viruses, parasites, bacteria, yeasts, and other pathogens often live even inside human cells and there is absolutely *no* reason to believe actual pathogens aren't located at sites of supposed autoimmune conditions anyway.

Instead, the real problem occurring in autoimmunity and allergies is the uncontrolled oxidative chain reaction first catalyzed by oxidase and peroxidase in response to colonization, which is instead a symptom of *vitamin E* deficiency. Vitamin E is not a generous consumer of reactive oxygen species but is instead a powerful chain-breaking antioxidant, which means it can and does easily stop the chain reaction of reactive oxygen species created by the immune reaction, which then prevents the oxidative cascade that triggers the inflammation, swelling, redness, etc., which accompany allergic reactions and autoimmune conditions. During an allergic or immune reaction even a small amount of oxidation can trigger a massive chain reaction cascade which can, in severe cases, even become life-threatening *anaphylaxis* as an oxidation chain reaction can and will continue until it is interrupted by vitamin E. Thus, allergies or autoimmunity are mostly just a symptom of vitamin E deficiency, either through low dietary intake or impaired absorption, and all oxidases also require and deplete vitamin E. This includes non-immune oxidases like *sulfite oxidase* which produces sulfate from dietary sulfur, so consuming dietary sulfur can also result in negative reactions and supposed sulfur intolerance because of the role of sulfite oxidase in oxidizing sulfur into useable sulfate. But vitamin E is also regenerated by glutathione which, also being a product of sulfite oxidase and casualty of hydrogen sulfide, is a primary factor in vitamin E recycling, and when this recycling pathway is not functioning correctly even large quantities of vitamin E will fail to sustain sufficiency, and thus the function of vitamin E is also extended by resolution of hydrogen sulfide and repletion with vitamin C and other factors in this chapter, and every time I have worked with people presenting with so-called autoimmune antibodies the antibodies eventually fall after weeks or months addressing these problems.

While a supplement can be very helpful or even necessary for people with severe disease like cancer, a nephew of mine who had regular airway constriction from allergic reaction to grass began consuming soaked and roasted hazelnuts, with enthusiasm and since has not had an allergic reaction though he was not also told about this reason for being given them but suspiciously craved them where his other siblings who did not present with allergies did not care much for nuts. As nuts are also a source of molybdenum, zinc, manganese, lithium, and boron they can easily cover requirements for proper immune function which helps prevent allergic reactions, and those who are allergic to nuts should instead use sprouted whole grains like brown rice or oats, or sunflower seeds or pumpkin seeds. But because vitamin E is fat soluble its absorption is also inhibited by saponification as discussed in the chapters on calcium and hormones, and resolution of gastroinestinal saponification of fats must be achieved to benefit from dietary and oral supplemental vitamin E, and dermal application of vitamin E can not only help circumvent that problem but is also required to suppress pathogenic skin fungi as discussed in the chapters on erections and skin health.

The sprouting of nuts, seeds, and grains also increases their vitamin E content up to a whopping 600%, making them even more potent sources than some supplements—to be clear, sprouting only occurs in live nuts, seeds, and grains and not after roasting, grinding, refining, cutting, etc., although sources like nuts or sunflower seeds are so high in vitamin E that soaking is not always even necessary, but can greatly help those with severe symptoms while also improving digestibility. The toxicity of polyunsaturated fats is in large part a function of lipid peroxidation, and the entire purpose of vitamin E in plants is to prevent the oxidation of fats, so even seeds high in polyunsaturated fats like pumpkin or sunflower can be safe when consumed whole (avoiding oxidation which occurs from oil refining) because of the presence of the vitamin E. In fact, many inflammatory mediators which trigger the immune response and allergies like the prostaglandins are actually derived from polyunsaturated fats, so use of dietary vitamin E also helps to reduce the toxicity of polyunsaturated fats on the body, though preferable to consume from sources high in saturated fats like almonds, hazelnuts, macadamias, pistachios, etc., and as sources of other nutrients like lithium required for suppression of parasites are most effective when consumed alongside roots and fruit rather than apart. Though chufa (tiger nuts) are rather tough they also contain a lot of vitamin E (they are not actually nuts so sprouting is not necessary), and its flour can be used in baked goods, smoothies, or made into delicious traditional horchata for even more options, and regular intake of vitamin E sources will help to mitigate or resolve allergies and autoimmune conditions when also supported by all the other factors herein required of a good immune system. But because vitamin E is fat soluble its absorption is also inhibited by saponification as discussed in the chapters on calcium and hormones, and use of a natural supplement of vitamin E (without causing overdose) in tea or other high tannin medium can be extremely useful to more rapidly resolve symptoms than dietary sources alone in those who are very ill.

Asthma is also similar to these conditions except that asthma also presents with elevated *eosinophils* which are the largest immune cells which attack parasites and fungi, and asthma likely represents chronic colonization of the lungs by fungi or parasites which is also why asthma attacks occur during physical exertion and emotional excitement since adrenaline releases sugar from glycogens storage which then reaches those opportunists in the lungs. Eosinophils also require silicon, and the condition of asthma is likely just a silicon deficiency which can be reversed by a high silicon diet, use of silicon drinking water, and good digestion, but *not* a supplement of silicon alone which otherwise causes silicosis and immune cell dysfunction, since silicon must be acidified and bioavailable for proper integration into physiological pathways to help control the transport of elections used in metabolism.

Xanthine oxidase is another very important oxidase which controls levels of the purine *xanthine* which is otherwise exploited by parasites because parasites cannot produce their own purines. Many people get migraines during caffeine withdrawal because caffeine downregulates xanthine and thus also xanthine oxidase, and then giving up caffeine causes a rebound in xanthine levels which, if there are parasites, will then promote parasite activity to induce migraine (as discussed in the chapter on cancer, which is then also a good diagnostic for parasitism). Since water is the oxygen donor for xanthine oxidase headaches can and do also occur from dehydration, so caffeine withdrawal headaches or headaches resulting from dehydration are also symptoms of parasitism which indicates impaired immune function and likely deficiency of vitamin C. Sickle cell traits are also shown by studies to provide greater resistance to parasitism by red blood cells such as occurs from parasites like *Plasmodium* and *Babeisa,* and characterization of sickle-cell as a disease is a great example of institutional racism since this condition is often presented as a genetic condition rather than evolutionary adaptation which requires resolution of parasitism, not therapy for sickle-cell, and studies show that xanthine oxidase induces sickle cell anemia due to oxidative stress from the enzyme, which is thus likely also a symptom of vitamin E deficiency.

Oxidases also possess *nitrite reductase* activity, meaning they can reduce nitrite back into nitric oxide, which not only helps sustain the nitric oxide pool but prevents nitrite and nitrate excess which otherwise impairs the immune system and conditions like HIV, with studies specifically showing enzymes sulfite oxidase and xanthine oxidases generating nitric oxide from nitrite (which is the oxidized form of nitric oxide), thus helping to prevent the nitrite and nitrate inhibition of peroxidases. Important also for the immune reaction is also riboflavin's relationship with light, as when exposed to light, especially ultraviolet, riboflavin becomes irradiated and directly participates in oxidative reactions which help kill pathogens. For this reason our skin mostly protects blood and inner body parts from ultraviolet light which would destroy all of our light sensitive nutrients like riboflavin, folate, vitamin K, etc., and if the skin is properly supplied with carotene ultraviolet light only only penetrates a few millimeters into the skin (melanin which makes skin dark also protects from UV damage), but as discussed in the chapter on vitamin D sun exposure to the skin also stimulates an increase in local endothelial nitric oxide (if sufficient in citrulline) to increase blood flow to the surface, which then also increases the production of small amounts of riboflavin photoproducts like *lumichrome* and *lumiflavin* which are highly antiviral and antifungal and very likely assist in the disinfection of skin and blood by colonizing pathogens, so regular sun exposure is also helpful for immunocompetency for more reasons than vitamin D status alone. One study for instance found that rats kept in the dark during riboflavin supplementation did not present with circulating lumichrome, where those exposed to light did, and restoring riboflavin or taking a dose of riboflavin and getting generous light exposure can and does result in some light oxidative stress and inflammation in areas of chronic infection but which can be helpful for those suffering long term, chronic immune dysfunction.

One of the most important immune factors is copper which is used by the immune system to intoxicate microbes and increase their susceptibility to oxidation since, like iron, copper so rapidly switches redox states (is oxidized or reduced rapidly), and without copper the immune system is actually quite ineffective in actually killing pathogens it targets. Copper was used to sterilize water and treat wounds even in ancient times, and workers in nineteenth-century copper smelting plants were actually spared from cholera epidemics due to incidental copper exposure. *Metallothionein* is an immune copper chaperone which spontaneously releases copper into the environment during pathogenesis to cause copper intoxication of pathogens, especially those which accumulate or produce hydrogen sulfide which has a high affinity for copper, which then forces their oxidation by immune cells. But for this same reason copper is never purposefully liberated from chaperone proteins except in the presence of pathogens, because copper can and does also oxidize our own cells and free copper can also spontaneously activate copper dependent enzymes such as the copper dependent oxidase, *tyrosinase* that oxidizes tyrosine to make melanin, and it is free copper like this which causes skin hyperpigmentation like *acanthosis nigricans, dermopathy,* or *liver spots* that so frequently accompany diabetes and conditions of aging. *Ceruloplasmin* is a particularly important copper dependent protein in health and disease because it is also a molybdenum dependent ferroxidase which oxidizes iron to attach it to transferrin which protects iron from pathogens during transit, so dysregulation of copper also directly results in dysregulation of iron which then means more free iron is released into circulation and targeted by pathogens.

Copper is also required for synthesis of connective tissue, in lysyl oxidase, and disorders of tissue synthesis like stretchy skin and joints (Ehlers-Danlos) involve copper dysregulation, but resistance to pathogenic ingress by the basement membrane is also impaired in conditions like cystic fibrosis due to poor copper status that affects immunity and morphology, manifesting also as posture and alignment problems, and even early greying due to loss of copper dependent tyrosinase (children as young as six with cystic fibrosis will present with greying hair). But becauset of the potential dangers copper can cause, simply taking a supplement has potentially harmful consequences, and if very ill the use of copper will do nothing but promote disease. For example, one study presented the case of a sixty-year-old man taking 8 mg of copper daily for several years at the instruction of his doctors for the condition of neuropathy (which it didn't appear to help) but which then destroyed his liver and required a transplant, which he did not survive. Unlike many other kinds of proteins the function of metallothionein in releasing or binding copper (and zinc) is not dependent on enzymes but instead by environmental pH, so it's function cannot be inhibited by pathogens and is instead activated any time that pathogenic activity disturbs the normal pH of human organs. But because of this copper homeostasis which determines our ability to effectively clear pathogens is also disturbed by any factors which imbalance normal pH, such the production of ammonia by pathogens which also disturbs silicon homeostasis, or dysregulation of calcium as discussed in the chapter on calcium. Since calcium metabolism is highly dependent on vitamin D for the endogenous production of citric acid from dietary carbohydrate, one of the fastest ways to cause long-term illness and increased susceptibility to pathogenic colonization is thus low-carb dieting which destabilizes calcium metabolism and then also copper homeostasis required to combat infectious and opportunistic microorganisms. The body also does not normally store very much at all, and at any one time there is no more than about 100 mg of copper in an adult body, depending on size, because copper is normally also so commonly available in the diet. But because copper sensitizes pathogens to oxidation, copper status is actually more important for effective immunocompetence than most other factors discussed in this chapter and since copper status is not a function of dietary copper or supplementation, the safe repletion of copper first requires the normalization of pH disrupting factors like ammonia dysregulation and calcium metabolism, including the restoration of vitamin D, endogenous citrate production, vitamin K, and dietary oxalate. Specifically, having oxalate such as from foods like plantains, spinach, almonds, dates, etc., along with a low-dose of copper or high copper food like shellfish very effectively promotes copper absorption by temporarily binding free calcium in the digestive tract and pathogenic biofilms.

Over the years of my research I often used supplemental cocoa powder to address problems like insomnia, and cocoa is high in both copper and oxalate. Shellfish, nuts, and leafy greens are also excellent sources of copper, so supplementation is often not actually required, but for copper the citric acid cycle is also extremely specific because another metabolite of the citric acid cycle, *malic acid*, is upregulated by the presence of copper which inhibits the *malic enzyme* just as zinc upregulates citric acid by inhibiting aconitase. There is no science currently which explores this, but just as zinc uptake for regulation of citrate is regulated by vitamin D, this copper mechanism which promotes malic acid is also likely mediated by vitamin D and thus also is copper dysregulation rooted in deficiencies of vitamin D and dietary carbohydrate. Those with Wilson's disease, which is a condition of severe excess of copper, present with symptoms like insomnia and deficiency of vitamin D, demonstrating how it is not merely absorption into the body of nutrients like copper which mediate their function, since this conditions presents with a harmful excess, but of properly working biological pathways which in this case requires malic acid which is in turn mediated by vitamin D status. Those with Wilson's disease, cystic fibrosis, and other metabolic illness will benefit from a diet high in malic acid such as from lots of sweet fruits intake (purslane and sumac are also high malic acid sources), while also working to restore vitamin D function and never avoiding carbohydrate. A low dose of copper (about 2 mg) had very promising effects on my coughing and mucous production (causing mucus to be more wet and runny), but sometimes the copper would also cause nausea even at very low doses, which is caused also by silicon deficiency and leakage of electrons which produce reactive oxygens species like superoxide, and after restoration of silicon and calcium homeostasis this no longer occurred. Tannins in tea and fruit also complex with copper, and studies in animals show that copper-tannin complex is strongly antibiotic and results in elevation in copper status, so taking a dose of copper with tea a few times could help if needed (never put copper in boiling water though as it will rapidly oxidize).

Cellular secretory pathways which release bound copper into circulation for use in immunity and iron transport are also *ATPase* channels which require ATP to transport elements and maintain their regular and normal flux through cellular pathways, which is also why restoration of silicon also helped restore copper homeostasis, but since ATPases are actively inhibited by the hydroxyl radical produced from hydrogen peroxide by pathogens (as discussed in the chapter on iron) the hydroxyl radical also inhibits copper homeostasis and is also relieved by the cinnamic acids which consume the hydroxyl radical. Cinnamic acids are also shown to regenerate the peroxidase enzymes and, as might then be expected, communities which use spices regularly in their cuisine and have a high intake of fruits and vegetables like some Latin American, Caribbean, North Africa, and Middle East countries also have some of the lowest rates of HIV transmission even though they do not have robust health systems or sex education awareness. Bangladesh is one of the most densely populated countries on the planet, because of high rates of sex, by which babies are made, and plagued with abysmal rates of corruption, human rights violations, economic instability, and an abysmal health system (at the time of this writing, which hopefully improves after their recent revolution!), but actually has one of the lowest rates of HIV transmissions and coronavirus mortalities among countries with poor health systems because of their high consumption of fruit and spices in Bangladeshi cuisine which helps normalize copper status and thus also carotenoids which then directly supports robust immune function. Oppositely, countries with the highest rates of HIV transmission like Eswatini, Botswana, and South Africa colonized and subjugated by white Europeans during the previous two centuries have diets which greatly resemble Western attitudes about food dominated by grains, protein, and animal products very low in spices, fruit, or other sources of cinnamic acids (remember I use this term to describe cinnamic acid as well as its many dietary derivatives which include ferulic acid, gallic acid, caffeic acid, curcumin in turmeric, compounds in ginger, etc.). Copper directly inactivates the HIV protease and is shown in studies to directly inactivate the virus, so promoting transport of copper through a high cinnamic acid diet is pivotal for resistance to such illness.

Peroxidase enzymes have two or three charges each before they must be regenerated, otherwise they irreversibly accumulate hydrogen peroxide and become inactivated, and so are more potent and persistent if supported by a diet high in fruit and spices or supplemental dose of cinnamon or other high cinnamic acid source like turmeric, ginger, Indian bay leaf, sassafras, etc., especially preceding or accompanying high copper and high carotene foods. After consistent use of tannin sources to also suppress ammonia producers this effect is quite profound and can help resolve many metabolic illnesses in a short period of time when supported by other requisites (such as vitamin D repletion). The effect of cinnamic acids in the body are also quite persistent, and hydroxyl radical stress is very strongly and easily suppressed by the purposeful addition of cinnamic acid sources for several weeks (or always if suffering severe conditions like HIV or cancer). There is more than enough cinnamic acids in fruit and vegetables for those who are already healthy, especially children, and the daily supplemental use of cinnamon or other potent sources of cinnamic acid is only necessary for those with severe or chronic metabolic disease. Especially for those with cystic fibrosis and related conditions the use of supplemental cinnamon with dietary carotene, copper, and daily sun exposure should rapidly result the normalization of mucous and rapid improvement in lung function, reduction in coughing, improved energy, etc.

Stress has also long been known to impair immune function, and this occurs also in large part because the amino acid *tyrosine* which is the precursor to catecholamines like dopamine and adrenaline is also vital for immunocompetency, because many proteins designed to support immune function like transferrin and ceruloplasmin which bind and transport iron and copper are made from tyrosine, so depletion of tyrosine by excessive stress, dieting, and resulting high adrenaline then depletes available tyrosine required by the immune system. Specifically tyrosine acts as a buffer to protect iron and copper from reacting with hydrogen peroxide to produce the hydroxyl radical, which then otherwise impairs ATPases among other very harmful side effects. Copper is also a factor in *nitrate reductase* which also reduces nitrate back into nitrite to prevent nitrosative stress, and those with cystic fibrosis are found to present with about four times as much nitrosylated tyrosine (a product of nitrosative stress) than healthy persons as well as elevated hydroxyl radical stress. The peroxidase system also actively halogenates tyrosine during immune reactions which, I believe, is meant to protect tyrosine from acquisition by pathogens which can and do also convert it to harmful tyramine which acts like adrenaline and promotes excessive release of glucose and sodium flux through cells during fructose deficiency of malabsorption (remember that fructose prevents hyperglycemia triggered by adrenaline and its analogs). Thyroid hormone is iodinated tyrosine (iodotyrosine) made by thyroid peroxidase which, I believe, functions to protect both iodine and tyrosine on their transit to cells. Interestingly, *Toxoplasma* parasites cause excessive dopamine production, which likely also depletes tyrosine, and it is well known that rodents infected with *Toxoplasma* lose their inhibition toward predators like cats, which are required to complete the *Toxoplasma* lifecycle, as it intoxicates mice with excessive happiness and lowers their inhibition, demonstrating exactly the role of dopamine, not serotonin, in happiness, but also the parasitological depletion of tyrosine which would otherwise support the immune system. Some humans are occasionally insufferably happy, with an almost pathological optimism and giddiness and are unfortunately probably colonized by *Toxoplasma* if they have other metabolic disease, likely contracted from cats or rodents, and other conditions associated with dopamine dysregulation like Parkinson's or bipolar disorder are direct consequences of dysregulation of tyrosine and catecholamine by parasites in the gut and brain which are resolved through the immune strategies in this chapter.

Supplementing tyrosine does nothing to reverse this problem, however, as the problem is excessive conversion of tyrosine to adrenaline (or microbial adrenaline analogs like tyramine), so stress reduction *is not optional* for restoration of a healthy immune system, by resolving factors discussed in the chapter on depression and finding empowerment and resolution of trauma as discussed in the upcoming chapter on spirituality and my other book on psychology. Because of tyrosine's role in catecholamine production its catastrophic depletion due to the immune response during the pandemic is likely responsible for conditions of 'long-covid' which appear to have affected people with preexisting eating disorders or other severe catecholamine dysregulation. In the early nineteen-hundreds a disease called "sleeping sickness" or *encephalitis lethargica* would cause people to experience extreme fatigue so bad they would often even lose awareness of their surroundings and be unable to move or respond to their environment. While the disease was rightfully considered likely viral in origin it was, decades later, treated somewhat successfully with the administration of dopamine but which only had a limited effect that eventually wore off, demonstrating the interconnected role of tyrosine, dopamine, adrenaline, and stress in the etiology of traumatic immune dysfunction. Reversing this chronic depletion of tyrosine by addressing parasites and emotional stress and then consuming plenty of protein protected by the use of tannins, carotene, etc., can help normalize tyrosine levels to restore dopamine and immune function.

Lastly, the most important immune organ in the body is the *thymus*, a gland you have probably never heard of which sits just behind the sternum in the chest cavity below the suprasternal notch. It is a two-lobed gland similar to the thyroid and is the seat of our immune system and thus also that our longevity, as there is a direct correlation between the health of the thymus and that of our entire metabolism. The thymus specifically matures and programs immune cells and is shown to require nutrients like vitamin K2 made by our commensal microbiome from dietary vitamin K for this process. But the thymus is alternatively larger during childhood and begins to involute (shrink) during early adulthood, and by the time we are very aged the thymus is only about a tenth the size it once was and most of it is converted into nothing but fat, rendering our immune function wholly dependent on already circulating immune cells which can actually multiply and propagate indefinitely so long as they are also supported with good nutrition and low stress. While the thymus is an immune organ it also secretes hormones which circulate throughout the body and thus is also an endocrine organ which regulates and stimulates other systems not only limited to our immune function. Deficiency of vitamin K2 also promotes calcification of the thymus, and the loss of hormones produced by the thymus eventually prevent the immune system from functioning robustly, and as the supply of T-cells diminishes and those which already exist fall to the stresses of aging our body begins to succumb to the stresses of chronic infection.

Treatment for a disease called *myasthenia gravis* which affects the nervous system and is characterized by a droopy eyelid and reduced muscular strength during aging was commonly *thymectomy* (removal of the thymus) because researchers noticed a so-called autoimmune component to this condition and, misunderstanding so-called autoimmune diseases, thought simply taking out a very important organ as an acceptable solution. But recent studies showed that thymectomy fails to improve the prognosis of Myasthenia Gravis, with one showing a higher incidence of Lupus in those with thymectomy as well as an ironically higher autoantibody count. Myasthenia Gravis is caused by viral infection of the nervous system by herpes viruses (such as cause chickenpox) and the so-called autoimmune component is the immune system fighting the virus as it progresses through tissues, not aberrant immune function. There is in fact no such thing as autoimmunity, and all so-called autoimmune conditions are not the immune system errantly attacking our own cells but instead the immune system attacking cells infected with viruses, parasites, fungi, or bacteria, and impaired effectiveness of the immune system in controlling that infection. Removal of the thymus only makes Myasthenia Gravis worse because it impairs the production of new immune cells as well as the endocrinological role of the thymus, and is another case of limited powers of human observation misunderstanding how biology actually works. Many people in fact present with myasthenia gravis, only very subtly, where one eyelid will droop lower than the other, and supporting the immune system, especially the factors which control oxidative stress, will oppositely improve so-called autoimmune conditions like myasthenia gravis.

While restoration of other immune system factors should occur first, it is possible, after chronic infections are resolved or suppressed and requisite nutrients restored, to regenerate the thymus and restore its support to the immune system. A study on mice suggests this to be the case, when supplemented with the thymus hormone *fibroblast growth factor 21* (FGF21) their lifespan extended by a whopping forty percent. But the thymus cannot regenerate unless vital dietary and environmental factors are also restored, for instance being highly sensitive to levels of vitamin C, copper, zinc, boron, pregnenolone, iodine, vitamin E, glutathione and, most especially, light. Adequate thiocyanate status is likely the most causal factor in thymic health, involution, and regeneration and it should not be expected to regenerate the thymus without functioning CFTR, thiocyanate repletion, and restoration of copper homeostasis. Mostly, the thymus is highly sensitive to light deprivation and dietary starvation, and regenerates and degenerates more rapidly than any other organ, increasing or decreasing in size in direct proportion to light and nutritional stress. It can entirely disappear altogether during prolonged fasting and extended light deficiency, which is a primary reason why those with eating disorders or perpetually indoors become very susceptible to chronic infection, cancer, and other metabolic disease. Even when it has totally disappeared due to stress the thymus can still regenerate by generous exposure to light and repletion with calories and nutrients on which it is dependent.

I accidentally discovered this therapy while trying to use light therapy to regenerate my thyroid and at first attributed the benefits to thyroid health rather than thymic. As earlier discussed, the warm colored wavelengths of light provide free energy to cells which in turn facilitate regeneration pathways, and bright light inhibits hormones of torpor which inhibit regeneration and promote catabolic stress hormones like cortisol responsible for thymic involution. But light therapy is especially effective for restoring the thymus because red wavelengths of light specifically liberate mitochondria from the inhibitory effects of nitric oxide to restore the production of ATP. As I discovered recently after a decade of research, this effect of red light is mediated by the element lithium, and studies show various effects of lithium on thymus function and immune cell activity, typically dose dependent, meaning that both deficiency and excess of lithium is harmful while adequacy is beneficial, which is another reason that a low-dose supplement rather than high doses is most effective. Most red-light devices are too weak and ineffective or ridiculously expensive (or both), and what is most important in leveraging the regenerative effects of light is that it be *bright*, and must only be merely in the warm spectrum (warm meaning its color spectrum, not heat) and should be 3000k or less in color temperature, not specifically red as warm white light contains plenty of red wavelength.

Sunlight is the best and most effective light source which absolutely cannot be replicated by any artificial sources, not to mention being free, but an artificial light can augment sunlight exposure if exposed to the thymus (behind the suprasternal notch). LED lights work well if they are very bright and on the warm or red spectrum, but many LEDs are actually in the cold spectrum (as are all compact fluorescents or CFL), and those will negatively stimulate tissue by promoting ATP consumption, not production. Red and near-infrared light is the most effective as long as they are also bright, while infrared only supplements heat and does nothing for this purpose. Using light directly on the lungs (from the back, especially), and other organs at issue for those with cystic fibrosis and or other diseases of mucosal and glandular tissues can also enhance recovery with lithium. As with all therapies, do not push this past your feelings of comfort. One person was using light therapy on their head for so long it gave them headaches due to heat stress because they were also using a hot lamp in spite of my advice not to (infrared saunas and other infrared devices do nothing but add heat). Reason and common sense must always prevail and if you feel uncomfortable you are probably doing something incorrect or acting too hastily or in excess. A full course of successful thymus regeneration will last quite a while—a year or more if sources of stress are avoided, chronic infections resolved, the endocrine system balanced, with no interruptions to light exposure—and should occur daily for as many weeks as you are decades in age, in addition to regular, outdoor sun exposure. Calcification is one of the primary catalysts of thymic involution, so this therapy absolutely will do nothing to improve health unless previous steps are taken to reverse dysregulation of calcium, oxalate, and vitamin D as well.

Finally, aspirin is also highly effective in directly suppressing other viral infections, with studies showing profound inhibition against pathogens like cytomegalovirus and other herpes species, and aspirin can be used to inhibit viral replication, the outbreak of coldsores, shingles, coronavirus exposure, and other chronic viral problems, but should never be given to children in high doses and none at all to very young children since aspirin inhibits glycolysis (which neonates and toddlers highly rely for energy production). Viruses like HIV, COVID, and Herpes hide from the immune system and do not activate interferon, but aspirin increases the synthesis of interferon in the cGAS-STING pathway which is partly how it also helps inhibit the spread of viruses in the body. Aspirin is antiviral because of its ability to inhibit glycolysis which viruses promote when coloniz-ing cells (babies primarily run on glycolysis, which is why they should not have aspirin), as well as blocking fatty acid synthesis needed for viral replication. Many therapies in this book promote exposure to sunlight, which can trigger outbreaks of herpes viruses due to restoration of factors like vitamin A, D, etc., which is also a symptom of insufficient arginine catabolism by the gut as discussed in the chapter on parasitism, but topical coconut oil also strongly treats herpes outbreaks (including cold sores) through stimulation of local pregnenolone production by lauric acid, and immediately and repeatedly applying coconut oil during an outbreak can often even prevent it from erupting from the skin, or at least mini-mize it.

While this chapter helps to restore the immune system, upcoming chapters on oral disease, thyroid, and even hormones are required to make a full recovery. Appendicitis can also specifically be prevented by these immune strategies, espe-cially the regular consumption of cyanogenic foods like yuca and brassicas, a short course of iodine, and resolution of calcification and excess ammonia. A primary symptom of appendicitis not commonly recognized is dark, malodorous urine, especially when accompanied by pain or chronic discomfort in the lower torso or low back, and being aware of this and using these strategies can help people avoid appendicitis attacks and surgery (the appendix is a reservoir for bacteria to help maintain a healthy gut, but it's fine to have it removed if necessary). Many other diseases such as Multiple Sclerosis, ALS, Alzheimer's, etc., are all also associated with chronic viral infections such as Epstein-Barr or other herpetic varieties, and can also be improved by adhering to these principles of immunological compe-tency since, even though the viruses cannot be eliminated, they can be very easily controlled. Neurological conditions like multiple sclerosis also present with high citrullination which indicates the presence of arginase producing pathogens such as parasites, and can likely be treated also through the steps in this chapter and book.

Restoration of the immune system can promote more than just good immune function—energy, happiness, and feelings of satisfaction are a direct reflection of pathogenic colonization and our ability to eradicate them. Because vitamin D and the health of the thymus is so inextricably connected to light, we require generous, daily sunshine exposure if we wish to restore and maintain a working immune system and resistance to disease. Not all lifestyles accommodate this, but nature does not care. If the choice is a cushy desk job and being ill or being financially poor but physically and mentally healthy I would choose the later and abscond away to more affordable places to grow a garden or work in farming or other outdoor occupation. Many windows produced nowadays block lots of beneficial sunlight that would otherwise help, and glass which is tinted green or blue in contemporary residential and commercial construction is a huge problem for our metabolic health and requires even more exposure to the outdoors to compensate. Take up lifestyles and jobs which get you out of the house and doing things to care for your body, not just your bank account. Start a garden and build your environment to be walkable, accessible, and outdoors as much as possible. At least get supplemental lights and big, clear windows, and access to the outdoors to reverse the stress of an unnatural environment on our modern lives and generous use of traditional foods like fruit, nuts, tea, and spices which directly promote and sustain a healthy immune system.

CHAPTER 17
THYROID DISEASE AND VITAMIN C

I come from good stock. Part of the reason I was the favorite grandchild, apart from being the patriarchal heir, was an obvious good score in the genetic mash-up, reassuring both sets of grandparents that their genes were truly a success and would persist long after they pass (though it kind of threw a wrench into things later, my bubbly, gay personality probably charmed them as well). I found a clip of my mother from the mid 1970's in her role on an episode of the television show *CHiPs*. Her scene was one in which Eric Estrada and Larry Wilcox chase down two bikers and are surprised when my mother and the other actress remove their helmets and shake out their feathered, Farah Fawcett hair like models in an expensive shampoo commercial. My mother is a beautiful woman, inside and out, but it was her physical health and beauty which enabled her brief career as model and beauty queen. My father too has always had a washboard stomach and broad construction-worker shoulders and a head of hair that never quit. They are the kind of couple everyone gawks at and remarks about how beautiful their children are, and I was constantly praised for my appearance when growing up.

In fact, a great deal of our family's energy was spent on appearance, and we were 'handsome' or 'pretty' when we were happy, but 'ugly' when sad or angry. Physical appearance was used as a weapon to cajole and coerce, but I also understood it as a tool for manipulation and control and as I began to grow into manhood the heads which turned when I entered a room gave me a great sense of power over others and thus a better feeling of safety that was so fleeing in my tormented young life. So you can perhaps see my frustration when around the age of eighteen, instead of growing into an impressive specimen of a man I found myself riddled with acne, depressed, and spilling out of my jeans. Other young men were developing muscles, maturing, and going out into the world with an excess of infectious virility where I could barely get myself out of bed in the morning, let alone develop an impressive set of abdominals. Having been a promising athlete I tried to muster myself into disciplined exercise routines, keeping gym schedules faithfully or engaging in the sports I so loved, as well as structured dietary practices, until eventually fatigue would return and sabotage my efforts. Muscle-building was frustrating, slow, and quick to disappear, and staying lean became a herculean task never mind my awful skin and constantly tired appearance, and struggling to find happiness in a homophobic and hateful world.

Sadly, many young people are sent into adulthood with a misplaced sense of responsibility, ill prepared to deal with life on life's terms we are instructed to forge it instead, even to control biology and manipulate humanity to make our success. My dad often crowed over his genetics, how rarely he got sick, or his talent for putting away a bowl of ice cream every night without getting fat while he criticized my mother's persistent weight gain or my failure to thrive as if we merely lacked the willpower to bend life to our desires, completely ignoring his indulgent lifestyle and her herculean dieting efforts. The reality is we wield very little control over life, and absolutely none over biology though we strive to do so with astounding effort. Sometimes we appear to have success, but more often reality is merely that of delayed consequences of the abuse and desecration of the human body which eventually catches up with everyone sooner or later.

Most of us are actually dealt great cards when it comes to genetics—Two arms, two legs, ten fingers and toes, a nose, a mouth and lungs, a heart and brain. That we are alive at all despite eons of natural disaster, predation, and competition is testament to superior genetics, not whether skin is this color or that, or hair, eyes, stature, intellect, or any other superficial attribute which become fodder for prejudice and presupposition of insecure narcissists. People with no understanding of even simple biology hail genes as the end-all to life's lottery, because they've heard it in the news or saw it on social media and consider themselves "smart," and then proceed to destroy their body and relationships because of contempt for our physical body and subjugation to mortality or prejudice for our fellow humans, blaming everyone else for problems which in truth we all suffer as a condition of life.

In the early nineteen-hundreds the disease tuberculosis killed one in seven of every person living. It was a massive plague of a disease which had been haunting humans since before the time of the Greeks, but since the concept of germs and microorganisms were not known tuberculosis was commonly attributed (without evidence mind you) to one of inheritance. The bigoted doctrines of race, class, of divinely anointed inheritance infected even medical institutions which were supposed to be objective and scientific, and because of this prejudice and stupidity no one decided to investigate why some people get this disease and others not. If they had, someone like Dr. Robert Koch who discovered that tuberculosis is caused by *Mycobacterium* might have occurred centuries or even millennia earlier and saved many millions of people from an unfortunate death. But even after Koch's discovery no one ever thought to ask why the disease doesn't effect everyone, because most people, now as then, continue to believe in the false doctrine of genetic superiority, in one form or another, because we delusionally want to believe each of us is somehow exempt from laws of mortality and fate and thus the grief caused by suffering and death. We push our bodies until it breaks because we want to be immortal, yet we know we are not and so wonder in disbelief why he could have had a heart attack when he was so fit, or how she could have gotten cancer when she ate so healthy. It must be genetics. No more fretting needed.

Our biology is *not* mistaken about the parameters for health. You are. We don't want to be sick, and we don't want those we love to be sick, but reality doesn't care about what we want so instead we condemn others for their suffering, disease, and blame character, choices, or genetic inheritance or the unfathomable mysteries of God. But just like the billions of other people and creatures that have come before us, we also will not live forever, and relying on hope or prejudice is never a strategy to deal with illness, but rather acceptance and knowledge, and because enough brave men and women fought for those with HIV and stood against those who wished to ignore it that epidemic only destroyed a generation of lives, instead of hundreds.

Biology can create morals, but morals do not create biology. Neither discipline, nor deprivation, nor self flagellation will synthesize testosterone or promote the mitochondrial electron transport chain, nor defend against the microbes which cause cancer. Unfortunately neither will kindness, patience, nor long-suffering or even prayer because biology runs on laws of chemistry, the laws of which are finite and absolute, immutable and indiscriminate. Every time citric acid encounters sodium bicarbonate there will be a chemical reaction that can be mathematically measured—That is how precise chemistry is. The formation of fat cells, cancer, or infections from natural-born viruses such as the flu and herpes and ebola are not the fault of promiscuity, laziness, or even gluttony. Your ex did not invent the herpes virus nor are they the reason you caught it. You caught herpes because of biochemistry and because herpes viruses exist. You are fat or have cancer because of biochemistry. You lost your attractiveness because of biochemistry. Biology has no morals. It does not care if we are born in the United States to Christian parents or in Iran to Muslims or in Poland to Atheists. That's why all demographics of humans suffer the same diseases, the same maladies, and why you were devastated by the loss of your wife to ovarian cancer even though she did everything she was supposed to, loved God, and ate a 'healthy diet.' It is why metabolic disease ravages the citizens of the United States because biology does not care about faith and good intentions and especially not wealth, but it does care about herbicides, dioxins, and the microbiome. Genes guide the function of an organism much the way blueprints guide the construction of a home, but blueprints do not dictate the quality of the lumber nor what to do if the plumbing subcontractor doesn't show up again for the fourth fucking time. Genes can only work inasmuch as they have the expected and appropriate materials to work with. That anyone should expect genes to function exactly the same in an absence of sugar or an excess of iron is a travesty of arrogance.

Basic medical textbooks point out the necessity for certain conditions to be true for life to survive. But how to *thrive*? Luckily our progenitors have lived for billions of years and our biology has inherited many abilities to deal with many uncertainties. We torment our physiology with starvation, deprivation, insufficiency, toxins and poisons and purposefully inflict stress and yet we stay alive, in spite of our best efforts, for long stretches of abuse. The fact that I am still alive after the events of the past twenty years is not a testament to the cost of disease but the resilience of our biological engineering already passed down unwittingly through countless generations and the robustness of living organisms. Our bodies do not trend toward death and decay, they trend toward life, or did you not notice the seven-billion other people on this planet? The ease with which health can be restored constantly astounds me. Most cells in the body turn over very quickly. Skin heals in a matter of days. Bones repair in weeks. Nerve cells heal in months. Of course, the conditions need to be favorable for this to happen, but all that requires is accurate knowledge of how and why, not what I want and wish, and certainly not dogma either secular or religious.

When I first recovered from cancer and general metabolic illness I woke up for the first time in my adult life with my fingertips nice and rosy-colored and my feet warm and toasty and not wanting to get out of bed. When I woke in the morning for the first five years of my thirties my fingers and toes were white and pale, void of meaningful circulation, and my body felt stiff and achy and took many hours to get it revved up again. I would later find this was caused by thyroid disease and cancer. But this isn't an aesthetic issue. The color of fingertips as described in the chapter on self therapy directly corresponds with metabolic rate. Even in Palm Springs, California I would shiver in ninety-degree weather until I got into a hot, hot shower or steam room. As we get older, or suffer disease, our fingers and toes turn white as the circulation to our extremities is dampened by stress hormones redirecting blood flow to the core to support more important organs, and our ability to maintain constant body temperature becomes compromised and difficult. It is a sign that things are not going well for our internal machinery. In older people doctors call the whitening of fingers and toes Raynaud's disease but in younger people they just call it being a baby, because doctors are taught that what is likely is also fact and it *used* to be likely that a thirty-two-year old white male walking into their office did not have cancer. Now it is not so unlikely for young people to develop severe metabolic illness while yet young but the medical system is more interested in tests and numbers to turn a profit than symptoms and quality of life, leaving many young people to suffer needlessly, or abandoning older people to their fate simply because they're old. It turns out if you don't feel well, there probably is something amiss. Though it is probably not cancer, most people can tell when their health takes a downturn and it can be upsetting, not only because we know something is wrong but because it seems as though no one can help us.

Discovering how to cure hypothyroid disease was a serious turning point, before then all my efforts seemed merely to be plugging a leaky dam, managing symptoms day to day without any permanent healing, and any lapses causing major setbacks. I have read countless medical studies and articles and papers on biology from a wide range of authors, piecing together disparate biological information that fit within my understanding of human physiology. One article done years ago might suggest how certain types of cholesterol influences adipose tissue, and then another recent study talks about how vitamin C influences the composition of cholesterol, and suddenly I understand how steroidogenesis, interrupted by a deficiency of vitamin C, results in hypothyroid disease, which no doctors are currently aware.

When I first began my recovery from cancer I excitedly told my fiancé how these nutritional factors could restrain the progression of my illness and that I could possibly overcome it. The anger on his face as I explained the mechanisms of why saturated fats could protect my thyroid function made me realize not many people possessed the ability to understand science the way I did. I am also struck by how easy it is to find solutions when looking in the right place. A lot of notable scientists like Linus Pauling and Otto Warburg knew that the majority of medical philosophy is not actually representative of real physiology. But these kinds of distractions are why so many diseases have gone so long uncured, and seem to not have any real hope of a cure even though we can smash together subatomic particles or peer billions of years into the past with a telescope positioned one million miles from Earth—you are not going to find grandma's house lost in the woods. Those leading efforts to cure persistent diseases lack nothing in talent or intellect, they are merely pointed in the wrong direction. My elucidations on human health have been easy to come by because of the available research of others, because the biologist Ray Peat pointed me in the right direction, and it's easy to find what you're looking for when actually looking in the right place.

In addition, I also asked what conditions our evolutionary ancestors might have experienced which promoted or harmed their health. Unlike popular dieting trends which ignore realities of our past ancestors such as the fact that they ate bugs, it turned up more answers than many like to believe (and certainly has nothing to do with "paleo" diets). We also don't need to find a "receptor" for vitamin C to know that levels of vitamin C directly govern the function of the endocrine system. Such variability in thyroid function is another reason I advocate using the temperature and pulse diagnostic to evaluate thyroid function and not test results for thyroid hormone or TSH, because it is the functional metabolic rate which determines health, not test results, and TSH and thyroid hormone measurements can be mismatched to symptoms. My thyroid tests came back 'in range' while I had three types of cancer and was dying of alcoholism and cystic fibrosis likely because my body could not even produce adequate amounts of TSH that would normally appear in severe illness.

Though some organs might have a specialized function they are exposed to and exert influence on and from every other organ in the body. Discussing organs like the thyroid and their functions without considering others runs the risk of missing how each is reliant upon and influences the whole. In fact, the entire function of thyroid and thyroid hormone has been generally misunderstood by science and medicine which has led to ineffective treatment of all thyroid diseases. Generally thyroid hormone regulates the rate of metabolism of human cells, controlling the rate both of energy production and consumption, and the thyroid gland which produces thyroid hormone directly communicates with with the brain, the pituitary, the parathyroid, the liver, and the adrenal glands but is also influenced by the intestinal system, the pancreas, the immune system, the blood, and even the microbiome. The condition of *hypothyroidism* is defined as insufficient thyroid hormones which in turn downregulates the rate of metabolism, and hyperthyroidism is when the body has too much thyroid hormone, upregulating the metabolic rate. These conditions, however, are often diagnosed by tests that not even doctors really understand, and practical hypothyroidism, meaning the experience of illness felt by the individual and not test results, is not always obvious nor measurable by laboratory tests, which only measure total hormone and do not actually determine the effects of those hormones on individual metabolic wellbeing. Nor is the condition of hypothyroidism ever cured by thyroid medication since medication only functions to supplement hormones which does nothing to heal the thyroid gland or restore normal, healthy production by the body. Hypothyroid states, regardless of hormone levels, develop when the body either won't or cannot produce enough normal oxidative energy from carbohydrate, because some conditions can cause high levels of thyroid hormone but which do not actually affect cells and thus result effectively in a hypothyroid state that is more accurately measured by factors like pulse and temperature and gas exchange in the lungs. I say won't because most systems in the body also have rate-limiting fail-safes to prevent the exhaustion of other limited resources and respond to such deficiencies by downregulating metabolic pathways to slow or stop its function in order to protect us and keep us alive as long as possible.

Thyroid production is also cyclical and rises and falls with the time of day and the time of year, not because our body wants us to suffer but because certain conditions like winter (in evolutionary terms) make the production of thyroid hormone dangerous to the long-term survival of the individual since thyroid hormone drives a higher metabolic rate. Thyroid rises when there is enough carbohydrate, vitamins, and sunlight to risk the oxidation of sugar which then results in enormous amounts of biological energy as ATP if mitochondrial respiration is working properly. Thyroid drops in the wintertime to prevent the overuse of nutrients traditionally scarcer during the wintertime, like vitamins D, E, C, K, A, carotene, and sugar, not because we are human but because we descend from ancestors which possessed these survival adaptations, as all vertebrate animals have a thyroid gland. Because of this, hypothyroidism usually first develops during the wintertime when thyroid is low, and most people don't initially recognize their doldrums or lethargy as a hypothyroid state and probably assume they just have low-energy or a temporary lull in health but then adopt harmful behaviors like more frequent workouts and dieting which then increase stress and harm to the body less able to respond to such stresses in a hypothyroid states. Light regulation of thyroid function can and is also affected by increased sequestration indoors away from natural light which artificially mimics conditions of wintertime, and one of the first and primary requisites to good thyroid function is daily, generous exposure to bright, natural light.

Thyroid hormone itself is also made by the same peroxidase system which runs the immune system, where *thyroid peroxidase* oxidizes the halide iodine to hypohalous acid which attaches iodine to thyroglobulin resulting in thyroid hormone. As discussed in the chapter on immunity the effect of industrial farming practices and tilling and disturbing of soil also promotes the volatilization of iodine to the atmosphere, thus causing deficient iodine in our food supply for which iodized salt is used to treat deficiency. Anyone living in any industrialized food system where food originates in tilled soil, especially those who present with metabolic disease, will require extra added iodine for normal thyroid function, which can come easily from sources like seaweed or other seafoods or an occasional, low dose of iodine product like *potassium iodide* such as one drop (1 mg) added to a large carton of juice from which can be drunk regularly to achieve several hundred micrograms in dosage per day (for adults, about half as much for children). As discussed in the previous chapter, iodine uptake is inhibited by the hydroxyl radical in those whom are metabolically ill, due the presence of opportunistic microbial colonization and chronic immune reaction, and in the case of anyone who is ill must be protected and promoted by cinnamic acids which are abundant in the most delicious tasting fruits and most potently in cinnamon, turmeric, ginger, and other spices).

But restoration of iodine alone almost never reverses thyroid disease, and I first suspected my hypothyroidism was a disease primarily of *vitamin C* deficiency after first using vitamin C daily in the form of a naturally sourced supplement, which I had never done before in my life, which immediately caused changes in my mood, energy, and physical wellness expected from proper thyroid function. As I researched thyroid function and metabolic respiration it became clear that vitamin C was the primary mediator of healthy thyroid function which occurs for several reasons, but mostly because vitamin C is also highly misunderstood in that our body does not actually absorb vitamin C at all, but instead cells *only* take up the *oxidized* form of vitamin C, called *dehydroascorbate*. It is well known that application of heat to vitamin C leads to formation of dehydroascorbate, which leads people to think dietary vitamin C is destroyed by heating since dehydroascorbate is technically *not* ascorbic acid, but since our cells *only* absorb dehydroascorbate, heat and cooking of vitamin C actually *increases* its bioavailability (as long as it's not cooked so much as to also destroy dehydroascorbate), and dietary vitamin C is actually oxidized as it reduces elements during digestion such as in the case of iron which then promotes iron uptake while also oxidizing vitamin C to dehydroascorbate which is then absorbed.

Hydrogen sulfide as discussed in so many previous chapters which inhibits the immune system and causes much illness is also directly detoxified in the body by *glutathione*, which is also our primary storage site for sulfate, and though glutathione is often considered our primary antioxidant hydrogen sulfide is also a powerful antioxidant but which is highly toxic to our wellbeing, and the oxidized form of glutathione actually serves to *oxidize* hydrogen sulfide into harmless polysulfides which not only keeps hydrogen sulfide from inhibiting the peroxidase enzymes and cytochrome oxidase but transforms hydrogen sulfide into a form which can be metabolized back into sulfate and thus also makes it a source of sulfur nutrition instead of immune inhibitor. This role of glutathione is entirely regulated by and dependent on dehydroascorbate which oxidizes glutathione which in turn sustains glutathione's ability to oxidize hydrogen sulfide. Vitamin C is most often considered an antioxidant, but the primary role of vitamin C is actually *not* as an antioxidant but a *pro-oxidant* to oxidize glutathione, because hydrogen sulfide inhibits mitochondrial respiration, so vitamin C increases the metabolic rate by oxidizing glutathione which in turn oxidizes hydrogen sulfide to liberate mitochondria *and* the immune system (heme based enzymes).

This well-known pathway between vitamin C and glutathione includes NADP+, but is usually characterized as NADP+ reducing glutathione reducing ascorbate which in reality it is the reverse direction where oxidized vitamin C oxidizes glutathione which oxidizes NADP+, because oxidized NADP+ is also required for transporting electrons in the mitochondrial transport chain and a molecule cannot accept more electrons when it is perpetually reduced. Most animals produce their own vitamin C endogenously from dietary carbohydrate but primates (including ourselves) and a few other animals like guinea pigs and fruit bats do not, which has always been a bit of a perplexing mystery in biology since it would logically seem advantageous to produce vitamin C. But the oxidation of glutathione by dehydroascorbate explains our lack of endogenous vitamin C production as an evolutionary survival adaptation, since deficiency of vitamin C during times of food scarcity or pathogenic colonization will naturally downregulate the metabolic rate by allowing hydrogen sulfide to inhibit respiration and thus prolong survival by sparing nutrients. Our tissues also produce hydrogen sulfide during protein deficiency and unfortunately this adaptation also makes our bodies very resistant to dieting and starvation which then leads us to believe that dieting is not as harmful as it really is due to this valuable survival adaptation which, if we did produce our own vitamin C like other animals, would more rapidly demonstrate wasting during dieting behaviors.

The oxidized form of vitamin C, dehydroascorbate, thus enters cells to oxidize glutathione to liberate the respiratory chain from hydrogen sulfide, which is then oxidized to polysulfides and eventually converted back to sulfate. Vitamin C is one of the only nutrients shown in studies to be directly antiparasitic, which occurs similarly to oxidize the thiols of parasites (glutathione is a thiol) but which they do not have compensatory reduction pathways and thus which leads to their oxidation. A study on Plasmodium parasites which cause malaria, however, showed that parasitized cells accumulate vitamin C, not dehydroascorbate, demonstrating how parasites can hijack reducing pathways for their own benefit to subvert this otherwise useful defensive mechanism of vitamin C. Similarly, studies on *Schistosomes* show higher vitamin C status *increases* parasite burden, while iron repletion *decreases* parasite burden, which occurs because oxidized iron kills parasites but vitamin C reduces iron to its reduced state, and because science and medicine does not yet recognize the importance of dehydroascorbate in maintaining redox balance and preventing problems caused by excessive vitamin C to dehydroascorbate ratio the use of vitamin C as a supplement rather than dehydroascorbate can actually be a problem and is one reason why dietary vitamin C is far safer and more effective than a supplement. Immune cells also accumulate large quantities of both cholesterol and dehydroascorbate, and those with cystic fibrosis are unsurprisingly found to present with about 90% reduced glutathione content in the lungs where healthy controls only present with 50% reduced lung glutathione. If the function of glutathione and vitamin C were their antioxidant properties, this would be reversed, but it's not, because oxidation is more important in these pathways than reduction.

Both redox states of vitamin C are also shown to chelate copper, and thyroid dysfunction (especially nodules) has been shown to be associated with increased blood copper, which occurs during chronic colonization with opportunistic pathogens as discussed in the chapter on immunity, because copper is spontaneously released from metallothioneins when the environmental pH of the body changes unexpectedly such as what occurs from infection. Free copper also causes other problems, and the copper binding-properties of vitamin C is likely the primary mechanism through which it improved my thyroid function. Free copper also oxidizes cholesterol which contributes to atherosclerosis (heart disease caused by buildup of cholesterol), and many hormones are also synthesized from cholesterol, so impaired vitamin C absorption due to ammonification of the gut, calcium dysregulation, or low dietary intake directly promotes metabolic disease, heart disease, hyposteroidogenesis, and other metabolic illness by impairing the normal metabolism of cholesterol even if cholesterol production is sufficient, which isn't usually the case since vitamin C is also required for cholesterol synthesis in the first place.

Vitamin C is also required for synthesis of collagen and the epithelial layer, and when the body has no vitamin C it begins to actually disintegrate in scorbutic disease (scurvy) such as was characteristic in sailors of previous centuries due to reduced availability of fresh fruits and vegetables on long sea voyages. Vitamin C can last up to three months in those who are healthy but vitamin C is also destroyed more rapidly in alkaline pH such as is caused by hyperammonemia (because vitamin C is an acid), so states of gut dysbiosis and parasitism also more rapidly destroy vitamin C stores which then directly causes thyroid disease and other metabolic disorders. Vitamin C is also a primary substrate for endogenous production of oxalate as discussed in the chapter on calcium which serves to help decalcify mucosal tissues in order to rob parasites of calcium they otherwise use to neutralize the immune system. Vitamin C declines rapidly in wintertime, not only from reduced consumption of vitamin C foods but because the decline of endogenous citric acid production which is dependent on vitamin D requires the body to in turn rely more on endogenous oxalate made from vitamin C to maintain calcium homeostasis and resist parasitism. Because vitamin C is also required to make cholesterol from which vitamin D is made during sun exposure, dietary vitamin C is also required to restore immune function through restoration of membrane cholesterol in support of CFTR, CFTR directly, and vitamin D synthesis for the restoration of endogenous citric acid production (which is a reason citrus fruits high in vitamin C like lemon are so helpful).

The adrenal glands also concentrate more vitamin C than any other organ in the body since adrenaline synthesis also requires vitamin C, and when they are exhausted of vitamin C we lose the ability even to make adrenaline (and dopamine) to release glucose from glycogen storage to fuel the metabolism which then increases catabolic cortisol that tears down tissue to release glucose. Many people present with symptoms of high cortisol such as agitation and anxiety, weight gain, and stretch marks in spite of diets with adequate carbohydrate, which normally lowers cortisol. Especially if accompanied by depression since dopamine synthesis also requires vitamin C, these symptoms indicate chronic vitamin C deficiency (even if has occurred in the diet!), which is even more likely during dieting behaviors since they make the body over-reliant on adrenaline and thus more rapidly deplete vitamin C than in those who do not engage in dieting behavior.

Vitamin C is also shown in studies to help reverse some damage of fluoridation and exposure to fluoride as caused by common fluoridation of municipal water sources, but this also causes vitamin C deficiency since fluoride is highly reactive, and studies show that exposure to fluoride raises TSH in children, pregnant women, and those with active thyroid disease, and fluoride causes harmful effects in cells by strongly raising the internal pH while factors like vitamin C are acidic, and the reason vitamin C helps reverse illness is in part likely by helping to restore intracellular pH in opposition to factors like fluoride, ammonia, hydrogen sulfide, etc. Interestingly, the testes require high throughput of calcium to make sufficient testosterone, and are also a highly mucosal organ and target of *Trichomonas* species, but studies also show that vitamin C repletion promotes an increase in testosterone production and sperm quality, so impaired calcium metabolism and impaired vitamin C status is also a reason for muted secondary male characteristics which may occur in conditions like childhood cystic fibrosis, autism, diabetes, etc., because the ingress of Trichomonas due to deficiency of cholesterol and vitamin C also alters sex hormone production and maturation, and resolving these problems led me to experience an increase in secondary masculine characteristics such as more sinewy muscles and greater thickness of body hair in more masculine distribution patterns even at the age of forty-five than what I had in the entirety of my young adulthood.

During some research into cancer and immunity I one day realized that vitamin C may have some affinity for silicon, since vitamin C is an acid and might help form silicic acid (technically in this case it would be silicon ascorbate), and if true would then be transported primarily through aquaporin channels which absorb silicon and water (and ammonia since ammonia is structurally similar to water which in so doing also neutralizes vitamin C and silicic acid which is the whole problem underlying cancer). I experimented by boiling ascorbate in a little water with plant-sourced silicon and took a dose. Unlike even dietary sources of vitamin C this caused near immediate symptoms of vitamin C repletion, and because silicon has a high affinity for water which increases the absorption of water by aquaporin channels it very quickly made me very thirsty, and my mucosal tissues temporarily dried out even more than they already were as water was sucked back to the bloodstream (when mucus membranes dry out and is not accompanied by urination it means water is being pulled back to the bloodstream, or being used by oxidase enzymes). This effect confirmed my suspicion that the primary problem in cystic fibrosis is *Trichomonas* parasites which produce ammonia that neutralize vitamin C, but also that dry mucous as seen in cystic fibrosis is not failure to secrete water (excessive sweating refutes this idea) but in fact prevents the *reabsorption* of water, and that healthy mucosal tissues very likely reabsorb water after secretion, which both hydrates mucus but also prevents excessive water loss and dehydration, and after taking vitamin C I began to experience some of the most regularly normal mucus production for the first time in my adult life, which was then fluid and wet rather than thick and dry. Mucosal protein made in goblet cells lining mucosal tissue is also held in place by a calcium pin which is removed on mucous release, which causes the mucosal protein lattice to expand a thousand times is original volume and give mucous its gel-like viscosity, which also serves to literally push microbes off the epithelial surface as well as to distribute immune factors, and though bicarbonate is often cited as the factor which pulls the calcium pin this could also be a role of oxalate made from vitamin C or dietary vitamin C and oxalate since they are also acids and thus would also react with that calcium pin, and thus help restore normal mucous.

Studies already confirm that aquaporin channels take up vitamin C, but why this hasn't been identified as a vitamin C transporter is befuddling, but it can be restored by consuming fruit daily (which is naturally high in vitamin C and silicon), suppressing microbial ammonia production (though daily use of tannins), restoration of calcium homeostasis, and preparing silicon ascorbate by adding vitamin C and silicon to boiling water (the use of silicon ascorbate will at first cause an increase in thirst, which should be heeded, as the body sucks up more water to restore blood volume first). Taking too high of doses of silicon ascorbate can overly oxidize our own glutathione, however, and at first might often cause a slight headache due to the increase in mitochondrial respiration (but because of the silicon will resolve over time). Because in the state of cystic fibrosis our glutathione is excessively reduced this is very useful, but it should be used with caution, such as only once a week at first, and never in extremely high doses. However, I also believe this is the mechanism by which our body kills cancer cells, and it has long been established in studies that vitamin C causes tumor cell death, without researchers knowing why, which occurs because tumors have very little glutathione which is then rapidly depleted by dehydroascorbate to cause cell death from oxidative stress, but which could also theoretically occur in other healthy cells if excessively high doses are consumed. Many health professionals have tried intravenous vitamin C for treatment of cancer, but that would introduce an excess reducing environment to actually *promote* cancer growth by protecting tumor cells from its oxidized form (over time the vitamin C would get oxidized, however), but the idea also to use intravenous dehydroascorbate is just as stupid as that would massively oxidize many nutrients in the bloodstream, and vitamin C should *ONLY* ever be taken orally through the use of natural food sources or silicon ascorbate as through the heating of ascorbic acid with a silicon supplement in water. The dose an adult should use are about 500 mg of ascorbic acid with about 100-200 mg of plant-sourced silicon (such as from bamboo), in about 1 cup of water boiled for about 1-2 minutes (there should not be so much silicon that it remains undissolved after boiling, however). Allow this to cool and do not dilute when taking, using half this dose or less for children if required such as to help recover from cancer, and only continuing to dose if side effects from previous doses have fully resolved.As mentioned in the chapter on calcium, thyroid and parathyroid also strongly regulate calcium homeostasis because thyroid synthesis also requires *calcium*, and when thyroid levels are sufficient the thyroid releases *calcitonin* to limit calcium circulation but when thyroid is low the parathyroid instead releases *parathyroid hormone* to increase calcium mobilization, either from the bones or increased absorption from the diet. This has long been thought as a regulatory role of calcium in thyroid production but halides like fluoride and iodide strongly react to calcium and I believe the increase in calcium flux through the thyroid are attempts to scavenge calcium iodide and draw iodine into the thyroid using its affinity for calcium, as the thyroid gland also lies immediately adjacent to the carotid arteries and grow in size to filter more blood when iodine levels decline. In fact, the reason calcium is utilized by pathogens to buffer themselves from the immune system is for calcium's reactivity with halides to neutralize the hypohalous acids produced in the immune reaction, so calcium dysregulation caused by poor intake of vitamin C, oxalate, insufficient vitamin D, and dieting behaviors also impair thyroid hormone production by excessively binding iodine. In my opinion, the purpose of thyroid hormone is primarily a vehicle to protect iodine from reacting to other elements like calcium as it is distributed throughout the body, and thus excessive calcium dysregulation and calcification can and does impair thyroid function and reversing calcium dysregulation through the restoration of vitamin D, K, oxalate, and vitamin C as discussed in the chapter on calcium is required to restore normal metabolism of iodine in production of thyroid hormone.

Taking thyroid hormone as medication thus works to improve health by functioning as a iodine supplement that is more bioavailable and potent than simply taking iodine on its own, which then also increases immunity to defend against pathogens. But thyroid function must restored endogenously to achieve long term recovery, and while taking thyroid hormone can be very helpful for overcoming the symptoms it never heals thyroid disease on its own because the underlying problems which cause thyroid disease are never addressed. Restoring thyroid function is one of the easiest things to do and should be done as soon as possible instead of taking thyroid unless it is absolutely needed (such as after thyroidectomy) because taking thyroid hormone also downregulates our own production which causes its own problems.

I was also first able to stop using thyroid medications when I changed my diet to include copious amounts of butter and other good fats like coconut oil, cocoa butter, and nuts high in saturated fats like hazelnuts, almonds, and macadamias because fats are required for production of cholesterol required for vitamin D which is required to reverse calcium dysregulation for restoration of thyroid production and immunity. But iodine required for synthesis of thyroid hormone also readily reacts with and saturates the unsaturated bonds of unsaturated fatty acids, meaning that highly polyunsaturated fatty acids also cause thyroid disease in part by also diluting and chelating iodine required to make thyroid hormone, and because saturated fats have no shared bonds (and monounsaturated which have only one) a diet low in polyunsaturated fats but high in saturated and monounsaturated also helps spare iodine. As organs like the hypothalamus and pituitary which regulate the thyroid gland also require iodine and cycle through about 2 mg each day this problem of iodine status can and does affect more than just the thyroid and includes the immune system, liver, breasts, and prostate too and cancers of those glandular organs are specifically associated with iodine deficiency, which I recognize as being a consequence of poor immune function and greater colonization of mucosal surfaces by Trichomonas parasites. For the same reasons iodine is oxidized to produce thyroid hormone many studies also show iodine to be an antioxidant which also protects glands of the body such as the breasts or prostate from oxidative stress (caused by the immune system in reaction to those pathogens). As studies show vitamin C and citric acid to upregulate the CFTR channel which coordinates halide transport to the immune reaction, thyroid function and iodine homeostasis can thus never be restored without also that of vitamin C.

Albert Szent-Györgyi, an important Nobel Prize winning scientist, first discovered vitamin C and its consequent importance to general human health. Most importantly he also recognized that vitamin C uptake was accompanied by flavonoids required for the normal metabolism of vitamin C, which is why synthetic supplements of vitamin C are not always reliable and why natural sources are so important (a synthetic can be used when added to juices, tea, or heated with citric acid). Linus Pauling, a giant of biology awarded both the Nobel Prize for chemistry and peace, further elucidated the role of vitamin C as a cornerstone of human health, though most of the public is only familiar with a reductionist version of his work showing vitamin C could even prevent the common cold. This was a valuable insight, but the reason is not because vitamin C fights cold bugs but the role of vitamin C in maintaining thyroid function and distribution of iodine throughout the body as established by my work here. Although I had many health problems in the last decade of my research in that time I only ever had one cold because of my regular and substantial vitamin C intake supported by the regular intake of iodine, carotene, and exposure to sunlight. Even bile which protects the microbiome from the inhibiting effects of dietary fat requires vitamin C through the synthesis of cholesterol, so to say that vitamin C is not so crucial or useful for our health is to betray serious ignorance of human physiology, and reversing deficiency is required for recovery from thyroid disease, diabetes, cancer, and improving overall human health including the reduction of unwanted adipose tissue and promoting the youthfulness of skin, hair, and libido because of its role as a distribution system for needed iodine. Incidentally, dry-eye conditions which are commonly suffered by small breeds of dog is similarly caused by excessive chlorine exposure from tap water, which destroys vitamin C, of which small dogs produce only a small amount, and providing filtered drinking water from our refrigerator permanently cured my little dog, Brahms, of his chronic and painful dry eye which had otherwise required eye drops five times daily. A veterinarian even proposed a surgery to reroute his salivary gland into his eye which would have required changing his diet to prevent the saliva from dissolving the eye (how the fuck do doctors come up with this shit?). Removal of chlorine from his drinking water allowed his body to restore synthesis of its own vitamin C and cured his dry eye in a matter of weeks, never requiring eye drops again, but somehow not even veterinarians are aware of this role of vitamin C (and harm of chlorinated water on the health of pets and people alike).

As Linus Pauling advanced in age he continued to advocate higher and higher doses of vitamin C, but like many scientists incorrectly adulated synthetic molecules while ignoring the complex biological dynamics of natural food sources and lacking knowledge about other roles and factors that affect vitamin C such as my work has elucidated. Our primate relatives are reported to consume upwards of 900 mg of vitamin C a day, yet our recommend dose is a measly 100 mg, and most people consume even less than that. As discussed in the chapter on immunity, our inability to synthesize vitamin C is an adaptive survival trait which allows hydrogen sulfide to inhibit mitochondrial respiration to help us better survive famine and other nutritional stress, and most studies on vitamin C have been done on rats and other animals which actually synthesize their own vitamin C whom do not always respond to it the same way we do, so those studies can be highly misleading and irrelevant. Because ammonia producing pathogens and ammonia dysregulation also strongly interferes with vitamin C homeostasis, vitamin C deficiency is primarily caused by pathogens such as parasites and H. pylori which produce ammonia. Most people are not aware that vitamin C (ascorbic acid) is actually secreted into the gut during digestion, which the body does to scavenge nitrates, oxygen, and to reduce elements like iron, copper, and manganese which must be in their reduced states for absorption, which also oxidizes the ascorbate to dehydroascorbate, but since the stomach is a primary site of ammonia production by pathogens this ends up destroying a great deal of vitamin C and causing systemic deficiency even when the diet is high in vitamin C. Because so many systems like immunity, oxalate, vitamin D, steroidogenesis, bile, collagen synthesis, immunity, and redox homeostasis are based on vitamin C, it is one of the most important nutrients required for our health and thus on which most of our biology is based, and thus this strategy of resolving ammonia and making dehydroascorbate can help improve health more than most therapies in this book, and it is common for people to see many profound symptom improvements even after a single dose (which, again, should *not* be taken frequently).

Other factors required for property thyroid function include *vitamin A* derived from dietary carotene, because vitamin A promotes iron release from tissue storage required for the production of heme which is a cofactor in thyroid peroxidase. Vitamin A and carotene also act as antioxidants which helps protect heme from excessive oxidation that can and does destroy heme and impair peroxidase enzymes required to produce thyroid, but since the absorption of dietary carotene is impaired by copper deficiency or copper dysregulation as discussed in the chapter on immunity the problem which impair copper homeostasis also impair thyroid function through disruption of carotene absorption regardless of how much carotene might be in the diet, and taking steps to restore normal copper metabolism while increasing dietary carotene sources that are also high in copper can rapidly help restore thyroid function and thus many other biological functions.

It has also long been known that *selenium* is protective not only of the thyroid gland but is also a cofactor in *deiodinase* enzymes which release iodine from thyroid hormone once thyroid has reached its destination. While nobody really understands the fate of iodine once it reaches cells it is clear that iodine has both regulatory and immune effects when reaching cells, for instance channels called *pendrin* exchange iodine and chloride and the delivery of iodine to cells by thyroid hormone, released by deiodinase, then promotes an increase in chloride channel activation to increase the metabolic rate by drawing in sodium which then drives calcium flux to run mitochondria, the endoplasmic reticulum, etc. Severe thyroid disease is also often accompanied by hair loss probably because iodine is actually deposited in hair follicles to inhibit hair-eating mites (which likely also cause conditions of alopecia). This oppositely means that selenium sufficiency is required to even benefit from iodine and thyroid hormone, and while selenium is quite abundant in the diet selenium is also a casualty of oxidative stress and is thus also a function of manganese and calprotectin dysfunction and thus increased superoxide stress as discussed in the chapter on immunity, but consumption of foods high in selenium like Brazil nuts, brewer's yeast, or even a low-dose selenium supplement first boiled in water taken only once or twice a week can help reverse acute deficiency, but healthy diets usually contain plenty of selenium and its deficiency is instead a function of manganese dysregulation and selenium reducing microbes which reduce selenium the same as others reduce sulfur which, after addressing those factors, will easily sustain selenium repletion from a healthy, normal diet and occasional supplementation.

Many conditions of thyroid disease like Hashimoto's thyroiditis are also considered autoimmune conditions, and studies often show that populations deficient in iodine have lower rates of thyroid autoimmunity then used to postulate that iodine itself promotes thyroid autoimmunity as if goiter and hypothyroidism are acceptable alternatives. As discussed in the chapter on immunity iodine is a crucial substrate for the immune reaction and its participation in autoimmune conditions is instead evidence of immune response to pathogens and not any harmful nature of iodine itself, and what is mistaken as autoimmunity is in fact the immune system attacking and destroying cells colonized by pathogens like viruses, parasites, yeasts, and bacteria which can and do live inside human cells. Of course the thyroid is also susceptible to oxidative damage from oxidases and peroxidases that make thyroid and participate in the immune reaction which requires vitamin E to prevent the inflammation and oxidative stress which accompany so-called autoimmune conditions (and being so reactive polyunsaturated fats increase allergic reactions), but many pathogens such as the herpes viruses and parasites specialize in colonizing human cells and it is not well known that Epstein-Barr virus, which causes the colloquially termed disease *mono* (mononucleosis, also known as 'glandular fever,' which I caught in my early twenties and mistook for HIV), can and does preferentially colonize the thyroid gland. Herpes viruses cannot be entirely eradicated from the body, they are just too well adapted to evade the immune system, but most people get Epstein-Barr when they are little children which produces hardly any symptoms, and a healthy person's immune system is well designed to suppress herpes viruses quite effectively most of the time until we age or become very ill. Disruptions to immunity (including immune suppressant pharmaceuticals) then causes infection to spread to more tissue causing the appearance of autoimmunity as the immune system inelegantly tries to control their spread by destroying more and more tissue.

It is commonly recommended that those with thyroid disorders avoid *cyano-genic* (cyanide) foods like brassicas and almonds which are mistakenly called "goitrogenic," meaning it can cause goiter, because *thiocyanate* can and does also compete with iodine for entry into the thyroid gland. Cyanide also competes with iodine for thyroid peroxidase, but it has slightly less affinity than iodine, and other truly harmful halides like perchlorate do not react with thyroid peroxidase demonstrating its narrow and specialized function. In fact, studies which adminis-ter thiocyanate fail to to produce any harmful changes to thyroid if iodine supply is adequate, so any potential interference of cyanide with thyroid is a function of iodine deficiency, not cyanide. Thiocyanate also competes with iodine for deio-dinase, and thiocyanate, like iodine, also participates in the immune reaction but where thiocyanate preferred by immune peroxidases and is even more antibiot-ic than iodine while also less oxidizing to our own cells. Cyanide's entry into the thyroid is thus a purposeful design of our biology, and likely helps to keep the thyroid free pathogens like Epstein-Barr virus, *Streptococcus*, or *Neisseria*. If cyanide did truly cause thyroid disease smokers would present with higher rates of auto-immune thyroiditis, because cigarette smoke is extremely high in cyanide, but smokers oppositely have acutely reduced risk of Hashimoto's and thyroid peroxidase antibodies. What's more interesting is that studies also show seemingly contradic-tory results in that acute cyanide toxicity can and does cause *hyperthyroid* states as measured by thyroid hormone, not hypothyroid as would be expected if cyanide were harmful. It is well known that, like hydrogen sulfide, cyanide actively inhibits respiration, which is how cyanide poisoning kills, but our body is clearly adapted to utilize cyanide in functions like the immune system and thyroid, so why isn't cyanide also transported to every cell in the body for use as a mitochondrial brake to iodine's gas? Indeed my observation is that there exists cyanogenic thyroid hormone which also serves to distribute thiocyanate throughout the body just as iodinated thyroid which also helps to *regulate* the metabolism by inhibiting mitochondrial respiration opposite to iodine's promotion.

Conditions like Hashimoto's as well as addiction to smoking or other tobacco use are thus *caused* by insufficient intake of cyanogenic foods because thiocyanate is required for a functioning immune system and properly working CFTR chan-nels to exchange for chloride, which otherwise replaces thiocyanate and causes an increase in oxidative damage as discussed in the chapter on immunity. Anecdotally, I have always seen those who refuse to increase their consumption of brassicas find worsening of Hashimoto's, while those who do eat more see improvement, espe-cially when supported by the other factors in this chapter and that on immunity, even one case of a fifty-five-year-old woman whose thyroid antibodies complete-ly vanished after a year of using these strategies, and entirely cure addiction in smokers simply through consumption of dietary cyanide sources daily. As discussed in the chapter on immunity it is dangerous to use distilled, refined, or concentrated sources of cyanide, and this therapy is achieved only through the consumption of safe dietary foods high in cyanide like brassicas, almonds, kernels of other *Prunus* fruit, yuca, apple seeds, bamboo shoots, etc. Even excess apricot kernels can be toxic, and this therapy is not achieved by poisoning pathogens which will also poison us, but instead by restoring thyroid, vitamin C, deiodinase, calprotectin, manganese, selenium, iodine, etc., and the normal immune and thyroid response. After doing so, however, the surge in deiodinase from a single dose of selenium and consumption of dietary sources of cyanide (more potent ones like apple seeds or *Prunus* kernels will be required in those who are very ill) can cause a temporary feeling of euphoria exactly like smoking a cigarette as the production of reactive oxygen species is resolved. In fact, this is the easiest and most reliable way to diagnose healthy thyroid function, including cyanogenic thyroid, is whether intake of selenium or dietary cyanide results in feelings of relaxation and reduced tension. If dietary cyanide from ample sources like several apple seeds, *Prunus* kernels, or bamboo shoots does not result in obvious feelings of relaxation this indicates calcium dysregulation which disturbs vitamin C and thyroid function.

Interestingly, iodine supplementation also had the benefit of improving skin hydration, which I have seen repeated in others who are iodine deficient, since hydration is mediated by sodium which is mediated by chloride which is mediated by thyroid hormone. Too much iodine (or use of iodine after severe deficiency) can cause temporary hyperthyroidism, however, because of the body's countermeasures to raise thyroid during iodine deficiency, so iodine should be slowly introduced to the body, and those who are severely hypothyroid will often rebound strongly into hyperthyroidism regardless, until TSH function normalizes, so its dose should be gauged to manage this, taking breaks if symptoms of hyperthyroidism occur, and since iodine can suppress our own gut microbiome not to use it in high doses chronically. No more than a few hundred micrograms per day are required for thyroid function, which can be easily achieved by adding just a single drop of supplemental iodine to a large carton of juice or milk. Around the age of forty-five I experienced a return of some thyroid problems which had otherwise been resolved long before which no amount of iodine or cyanide could resolve, which turned out to be copper deficiency causing impaired carotene and vitamin A status, and after resolving that problem the use of iodine and dietary cyanide resumed their normally profound benefit, so if the use of dietary or supplemental iodine and cyanide, even in low doses, along with sufficient dietary carotene does not produce obvious improvements that is likely a useful diagnostic for deficiency or dysregulation of copper which must first be restored.

Thyroid hormone itself is also made from the amino acid *tyrosine*, which is another reason stress causes illness since adrenaline excess depletes tyrosine, and both phenylalanine and tyrosine are also targets of biogenic amine producers which use tyrosine to produce the adrenaline analog tyramine, so resolution of gut dysbiosis and restoration of a healthy microbiome is absolutely required for good thyroid function. Thyroid is even secreted into the gut where it reacts with acetic acid, if it is present, which helps activate and regulate thyroid.

Since fructose so strongly turns on the metabolism, consuming fruit or sugar first thing in the morning with breakfast (or invert sugar for those with diabetes) can promote longer regeneration time each day for organs like the thyroid and adrenals, but waiting until later in the day to eat food prolongs catabolic stress, and waiting until we are hungry to eat is far too late when recovering from metabolic disease because the hunger impulse indicates release of stress hormones that impair regeneration, and maintaining instead a high metabolic rate through consistent intake of carbohydrate and other healthy foods is required to recover from any thyroid disease. Make sure to use the pulse and temperature diagnostic to measure thyroid activity, not subjective symptoms like weight, feeling cold or warm, or energy as those can be highly misleading. Hot flashes, for instance, is the loss of heat from the core as discussed in the upcoming chapter on sleep, not being too warm, so many people with declining metabolic rates don't understand they have thyroid disease and their body temperature is dropping, not rising.

A deficiency of sunlight will *always* downregulate thyroid function, and a full recovery absolutely cannot be expected during light deficiency. A *minimum* of two hours of unobstructed, direct sunlight exposure to skin each day is necessary for the full functioning of the hypothalamus-pituitary-thyroid axis (sitting behind a window is fine if light directly contacts the body but ambient light exposure absolutely will not serve this purpose). If this is not possible it will be necessary to supplement extra light by using a bright artificial light as explained in the chapter on depression, to stimulate the thyroid and parts of the brain which would otherwise downregulate the metabolic rate. Infrared light can also be used on the body in the wintertime to supplement extra heat and is particularly pleasant when it's cold outside, but infrared is only heat and alone will not improve or reverse thyroid disease and can even cause heat stress, but it does make the body more comfortable when it's cold out and picks up some of the effort required to maintain body temperature if more supplemental heat is required.

Though thyroid medication can often help and may even be necessary sometimes such as in those who are very aged or missing their thyroid, misuse or abuse of thyroid hormone such as to lose weight, which it does not do, will result in symptoms such as strong nighttime elevation of adrenaline, so it's not always useful to use thyroid, and first and foremost should be the restoration of our own natural thyroid function. The heretofore ignorance of cyanogenic thyroid hormone is probably the main reason why those with thyroidectomy eventually experience worsening health over many years, and production of synthetic cyanogenic thyroid hormone could greatly prolong their survival (if you're missing your thyroid or any other organ it might be prudent to explore organ transplant). Thyroid illness has long seemed impossible and persistent, but that is only because we tend to overcomplicate or anthropomorphize biology and take for granted the basic and commonplace nutrients which are actually more important than is typically assumed. Being so widely available, the use of dietary vitamin C can quickly restore thyroid function in even the most severely diseased, so long as it is supported by the other factors discussed in this chapter.

CHAPTER 18
ORAL HEALTH

Several years into my thirties when my health really began to decline further and earlier than I ever thought possible my gums started bleeding profusely whenever I brushed my teeth. My partner at the time was neurotic about his own oral care, spending no less than ten minutes each morning and night brushing, flossing, and swishing copious amounts of mouthwash. The only time I ever flossed was when food got stuck between my teeth because they were (are) very tightly packed and very difficult to floss without breaking the gum line. Brushing just once or twice a day had always been more than effective in keeping my teeth very healthy—The only time I have ever been to a dentist at the age of 18 showed not a single cavity (the dentist, though, said I had "deep groves" in my teeth that should be filled so he could make money, and a return visit three months later for that procedure also conveniently revealed what he said were "two genetic cavities," whatever the fuck that means, which also had to be treated). Embarrassed by what I thought to be poor oral hygiene I started brushing my teeth apart from by boyfriend to avoid spitting the red tinted effluence in his presence, and increased my brushing and even began using mouthwash, but no matter how much I cleaned my teeth or how many products I used the bleeding did not stop until my relationship with him finally ended when a course of (injected) antibiotics for exposure to sexually transmitted illness also entirely eradicated my gum disease which then stopped, without any other oral care or dentist visit, in a matter of days.

It was no coincidence that the rapid decline in my health occurred in correlation with this development of periodontal disease because many oral pathogens are extremely virulent, and once they reach the bloodstream have access to the interior of the entire body to catalyze cancer, cardiovascular disease, hypogonadism, insomnia, and even diseases of the brain like Alzheimer's and Parkinson's. Oral pathogens are so virulent because they skillfully inhibit the immune system, which is also why dentists and dental products can't and won't cure gum disease. I did not know during this time of my own involuntary motor and vocal tics, as instead of helping me my fiancé also withdrew and abandoned me even though it was his disloyal and risky sexual behavior which had caused me to be infected in the first place, which is why he was so neurotic about his own dental care because he had the same problem but was able to better control it because he didn't have cystic fibrosis. It was not until filming my first social media content a few years later taken completely by surprise seeing myself twitching and smacking and clicking my tongue and lips on camera. Oral disease is extremely serious and can lead to a myriad of other complications, but its treatment by medical professionals usually consists of doctors telling patients to see their dentists and dentists telling their patients to buy more oral care products which does shit all to resolve these virulent microbes that have evolved for millions and millions of years to colonize teeth and gingival tissue.

The resolution of many of my symptoms including periodontal disease from an injected antibiotic (ceftriaxone) was very interesting because no dentists or other medical professionals are willing to treat oral disease like this, even when it is life threatening and clearly caused by highly infectious microorganisms, choosing instead to blame patients and their oral care routine which has absolutely nothing to do with it. After putting my life back together and returning to dating I eventually found myself again catching the same symptoms I experienced with my ex, since I did not yet know I had cystic fibrosis which impairs the immune system. During the AIDS crisis when government refused to help those being infected, hundreds of leaders in the LGBTQI+ community like Morris Kight, Don Kilhefner, and Larry Kramer (who were also anti-war activists) helped establish free clinics and services to provide sexual health education and care for those who didn't have coverage. These clinics still exist and being very poor myself regularly got free testing. But each time I came down with symptoms the tests came back negative for common sexually transmitted diseases, so I lied to the clinicians and claimed to have been knowingly exposed to gonorrhea or chlamydia so as to get treatment with the antibiotics I knew worked but otherwise had no access. Because of my success discovering the cures for alcoholism and addiction, depression, hair loss, thyroid disease, and recovery from cancer I was a bit overconfident and the last time I got infected I resolved to remain untreated as to find out what exactly was happening and how it could be treated without third-party intervention, thinking at most it would take six-months, maybe a year, but the other conditions I solved are generally failures of human biology which, while affected by pathogens, is naturally designed to achieve health, and pathogenic microbes possess their own, separate biology entirely designed to destroy ours so it instead took more than six years and serious, debilitating effects on my body (and self-imposed celibacy to avoid infecting others) before I was finally able to understand and resolve them too.

Oral pathogens are in fact some of the most virulent of all those which affect human health, and individuals can and do harbor infection for decades and decades, especially in monogamous relationships, passing organisms back and forth betwixt family members but never having reason to suspect intimately transmitted disease or occasion for incidental eradication such as when single, sexually active persons like myself contract and treat other commonly known illnesses. All oral disease is in fact a sexually transmitted illness because we typically catch it through salivary exchange with intimate partners, and any gum disease which includes redness, bleeding, or recession of the gums indicates the presence of these opportunistic gingival pathogens which cause and contribute to all meta-bolic illness. Dentists also cannot treat these conditions because oral pathogens like *Porphyromonas gingivalis* live inside the actual cells of our gums, not only on the surface, which is why an injection of antibiotic like ceftriaxone was required to eradicate it where oral antibiotics like penicillin, tetracycline, and clindamycin had absolutely no effect.

Researching oral disease was also very difficult in part because every single study of the literal thousands which addresses oral pathogens show *in vitro* efficacy of every single herb, nutrient, product, and pharmaceutical tested but which have absolutely no effect in the actual human body (*in vivo*), and required instead the metaphorical search for needles in an immense haystack of information (in which that information also had to be inferred from other studies combined with my intuition and practical experience). As a result, I also know now that *all* common treatments claiming to resolve oral illness whether conventional or natural utterly do not work.

Oral disease and tooth decay are most commonly attributed to sugar, but sugars like sucrose (common sugar) generally show broadly therapeutic and antibacterial properties, especially in wound healing and tissue regeneration. Although the reason for this is not clear to researchers it is plainly because of its promotion of energy production in human cells through the citric acid cycle and other sugar dependent pathways which promote immunity, cellular function, production of citric acid, etc. Fructose is also actually toxic to many microbes, even to *Streptococcus mutans*, the very bacteria which causes tooth decay, and *S. mutans* produces an abundance of biofilm in the presence of sugar not to colonize the mouth, which it has already done, but to buffer itself against fructose exposure (it does use glucose contained within sucrose, however). The virulence factor or toxin of another problematic oral pathogen and potent hydrogen sulfide producer, *Aggregatibacter actinomycetemcomitans*, is also shown in studies to be inhibited by fructose. Listening to common anecdotes on sugar and oral health one might think that sugar itself dissolves teeth, but sugar has no properties which are harmful to human health and instead tooth destruction comes from acids made by bacteria from metabolism of all carbohydrate, a fact lost even on the hundreds and hundreds of scientists writing studies which state sugar causes tooth decay, which it absolutely fucking does not, rather than the pathogens which do. Some studies even state that tooth decay is non-communicable but, seriously, how do we obtain tooth decay microorganisms? Spontaneous generation? Fuck me.

When considering things like sugar in a moral sense rather than one of biology important facts are often overlooked and questions not asked like, what is point of fructose in sucrose anyway? Many studies and articles on sugar, especially in relation to tooth health, are notorious for using inferences in their conclusions which, if we are supposed to be acting scientifically, is not allowed, yet many authors discuss the contribution of sugar to tooth decay as if it is a foregone conclusion even when their studies do not directly design controls for it or result in data which opposes those biases. If other studies are to be believed, which are better designed and lack bias against sugar, it is actually shown to be highly antibacterial as study after study show that fructose inhibits aspects of pathogenic bacterial growth and virulence factors and assists in wound healing, recuperation, and food preservation. Remembering that the majority of glucose taken up by cells is also actively converted to fructose, even when it is synthesized back into glucose, fructose and sugar did not just appear on the recent dietary stage as is so often suggested but we and our ancestors evolved on fructose alongside those plants which produce it in cooperative evolution against pathogenic organisms. Fructose and sucrose account for our long evolutionary relationship with fruit, which has been used by plants as an enticement for distribution of their seeds along with the various other nutrients which come from them like tannin, anthocyanins, cinnamic acids, vitamin C, carotene, mannose, malic and citric acids, iodide, fluoride, boron, etc. Indeed, studies show time and time again that higher fruit consumption, though high in sugar, is associated with far lower incidences of oral disease, tooth decay, and cardiovascular illness which is in complete opposition to accepted ideas on sugar promoting oral disease as fruit is some of the highest possible sources of dietary sugar.

Sugar is also much maligned because of religious desecration of the human condition and there are many, many articles and studies which assume sugar's evils because of its reward stimulation which in reality is the evolutionary survival instincts of human biology trying to get us to consume a potent energy source to fuel life and survival since sugar so strongly promotes mitochondrial respiration. Much unsupported science also attributes the advent of dental problems to the rise of agriculture and thus increased access to sugar and carbohydrate, but this is absolutely not supported by fossil and anthropological records nor critical thinking or the scientific method since human organisms have often had access to high quantities of sugar even before the advent of agriculture, or likewise severe tooth decay long before man ever even thought to cultivate plant life. A population of hunter-gatherer humans who lived in Morocco around 15,000 years ago, for instance, in a cave called the Grotte Des Pigeons showed some of the absolute worst dental conditions of any sample of humans from any population record ever studied, with severe dental issues on up to 90% of all their teeth, besting even the worst industrial age dental health such as what occurred during Victorian Era England. This population of humans had a diet very low in sucrose and fructose and high in foods like acorns which are extremely high in phytic acid which strongly promotes calcium deficiency (especially in low calcium diets) which then can and does disrupt salivary pH to strongly promote tooth decay. French adolescent populations have the highest rate of good periodontal health in the world and the French also have a custom called goûter in which it is customary for children to indulge daily in an after-school meal of intensely sugary foods like chocolate, sweet croissants and other pastry, fruit, and other treats. These are not cheap, crappy, industrially produced candy with chemicals and other shit common to industrial food production but real, well-made, and traditional confectionary and patisserie but still loaded with sugar. If sugar was the cause of oral disease French children should have the worst oral health in the world, not the best. French adults stop participating in goûter, however, and because adults more widely contract oral pathogens through sexual activity French adults display similar rates of periodontal disease as the rest of the world.

Pathogens like *Porphyromonas gingivalis* which cause periodontal disease express protease enzymes (those which digest protein) which prematurely activate our own proteolytic enzymes to dissolve our cells from the inside out and feed on the released nutrition. *P. gingivalis* is especially interested in amino acids like glycine which is a primary component of connective tissue, and has been shown by studies to directly cause other disease by increasing calcification of cardiovascular tissue, a feature which is also common to cancerous tumors and cardiovascular disease. Many oral pathogens cause hydrogen sulfide malodor as they consume our sulfated amino acids, and as they colonize the cardiovascular system they strip the sulfated lining that prevents water leakage, and pathogens of periodontal disease directly cause cardiovascular illness and cancer as they access the bloodstream and distribute throughout the body. *P. gingivalis* is even found in the brains of those with Alzheimer's and to cause spontaneous abortion (miscarriage), causing many couples frustration and confusion as they try to conceive, and not only lives in calculus and biofilm on the surface of the gums and teeth but also inside the cells of our mucosal tissue. *P. gingivalis* is even shown in studies to actually farm other microbes for its own benefit and coordinates and exploits hydrogen sulfide produced by other microbes to directly inactivate the immune system and prevent resolution of pathogenic colonization.

Hernia is also a condition entirely without explanation in the medical industry but is in fact also caused by these same pathogens due to destructive proteolytic enzymes which degrade and weaken connective tissue. Surgery, sometimes with implanted mesh, is the only method by which hernia can be addressed by medical treatment, a procedure which comes with a high rate of complications (because our body always tries to remove foreign material implanted into the body). The human body should be able to repair and heal such simple damage as hernia, but hernia conditions present with a high degree of circulating proteases which is not a normal state of the body but exactly what is caused by oral pathogens. Forms of collagen which are associated with youth are easily destroyed and consumed by oral pathogenic organisms as they target glycine and arginine, which is also why supplements of gelatin or collagen can often exacerbate symptoms like migraine since it can also feed such opportunistic pathogens and parasites. This problem then requires the body to produce inferior forms of collagen which are stiffer and less elastic but better resists pathogens, and once these organisms access the cardiovascular system they circulate throughout the entire body to also cause arthritis, hernia, and problems with posture.

Snoring and sleep apnea are also direct consequences of colonization by these oral pathogens due to degradation of the structural integrity of the nasopharynx, which causes it to collapse and airway passages to deform and constrict, which is why snoring is also associated with cardiovascular disease as they are caused by the same infectious agents (seriously how the fuck does nobody know any of this shit???). I was alarmed at just how loudly my partner snored, which also contributed to my insomnia, as he had probably long been infected by these oral pathogens to cause significant collapse of his nasopharynx tissue, and as my own condition progressed resulted also in sleep apnea. One of the reasons radiation and chemotherapy has an apparent benefit on cancer treatment, when it doesn't kill the patient, is simply because it eradicates these pathogens and the parasites which impair the immune system to enabled secondary infections which cause oral and cardiovascular disease and thus then cancer, but which usually return afterward due to reinfection by untreated family, friends, and lovers, and thus then cancer, since cancer treatment does not prevent reinfection and the role of infectious microbes in cancer etiology is almost entirely ignored by the medical and scientific establishment. But this also highlights how breast cancer occurs which is through sex and the transfer of oral parasites and gingival pathogens to the nipple which then invade the mucosal breast tissues, as does cunnilignus transferring them to the urethra, cervix, ovaries, and uterus to result in cancers of those organs, and fellatio which does the same to the urethra of the penis, prostate, and testicles. Whenever I help someone with cancer who is not very old and still retain their gum tissue they always have red, inflamed, or bleeding gums and I advise them to immediately get a shot of injected antibiotic such as ceftriaxone to immediately wipe out these virulent pathogens and afterward avoid all intimate contact with any person until their immune system and symptoms are recovered. This results in the rapid resolution of some of the most excruciating symptoms of cancer and helps promote sleep and catalyzes the beginning of recovery. The young man who came to me with stage four lymphoma so severe the large tumors on the sides of his neck caused him difficulty swallowing regained the ability to swallow in a matter of days after starting the practices outlined in my chapter on cancer (in the version of this book before solving the Warburg Effect) and began to improve even more dramatically after getting a shot of ceftriaxone.

Most people think of oral disease as a problem of bleeding but in fact blood supply to the gums is impaired during periodontal disease as there exists massive clotting beneath the surface of gingival tissue which directly contributes to gingival hypoxia (low oxygen). As discussed in the chapter on calcium, citric acid is the body's primary anticoagulant which increases blood flow, but citric acid also helps to keep periodontal tissue free of calcium to prevent its availability to pathogens. Studies also prove that periodontal tissue activates vitamin D so periodontal disease is likely first initialized during transient deficiencies of zinc, sunshine, and low-carbohydrate diets which impair endogenous production of citric acid. Calcium is also the primary factor which sustains normal salivary pH to inhibit acid which otherwise dissolves enamel, so restoration of normal calcium metabolism and regular consumption of dietary calcium is the first and primary requirement to reverse tooth decay. Dieting is often a behavior ostensibly used to increase sexual attraction, but since dieting also reduces endogenous production of citric acid the behaviors of dieting and then dating, kissing, and having sex is the absolute best way to contract oral disease and initialize metabolic illness as this directly exposes us to pathogens during times when periodontal production of citrate is inadequate to protect us against infection. Often when I was younger and experiencing mild symptoms of illness like tiredness or an expanding waistline they would disappear after jogging down San Vicente boulevard in Los Angeles, leading to the incorrect belief that exercise and not simply exposure to sun and thus increase in vitamin D and citric acid was the causal remedy. Cystic fibrosis is also associated with elevated risk of oral disease, diabetes, and leukemia or lymphoma because immune dysfunction caused by *Trichomonas* also prevents the body from mounting an effective defense against communicable pathogens which use calcium to buffer themselves against the immune system, and leukemia is always accompanied by severe oral disease although oncologists consider it an effect of leukemia rather than a cause, which is ridiculous considering that oral pathogens are extremely virulent, suppress immune function, circulate in the body to other organs, and literally eat our tissues for their own nutritional benefit, which is why my only consistent test results year after year were elevation of white blood cells, which all but the doctor who imaged my thyroid routinely dismissed as inconsequential but which is in fact a common symptom of cancer because the medical profession has yet to recognize the role of communicable pathogens in cancer.

Calcium is also secreted in saliva in the form of *hydroxyapatite* for the maintenance of tooth health, but the dysregulation of calcium metabolism as we age facilitates pathogenic colonization and formation of biofilm like plaque and calculus and promotes loss of vitamin C (which is an acid neutralized by alkaline factors like calcium and ammonia). Fluoride helps prevent cavities by hardening hydroxyapatite, but this has led to the use of fluoride fortification of water, milk, and other foods which leads to toxic fluorosis of the nervous system and skeleton, and fluoride should never come from fortified, ingested products but only natural sources (sometimes natural sources can even be excessive), while the occasional use of fluoridated toothpaste (like once a month) can be used if necessary. Bu as discussed in the chapters on parasites, mucosal tissue also actively secretes oxalic acid derived either from plant foods or produced in the body which, along with citric acid and vitamin K carboxylation of calcium proteins, serves to deprive pathogens of free calcium they use to infect our oral tissues. Oxalate secretion by mucosa is the primary mechanism by which buildup of calculus (calcium phosphate) is prevented or resolved, and calculus buildup on teeth is always a sign of calcium dysregulation and poor vitamin C status (remembering also that high oxalate intake can cause oxalate toxicity and kidney stones if deficient in vitamin D). Higher salivary calcium has long been established as a primary factor protective against tooth decay since calcium reacts to acids, so when salivary hydroxyapatite is adequate the acids produced by microbes in the mouth react with salivary calcium rather than calcium in teeth, and hydroxyapatite can and does help repair cavities if they are not too large, so restoring calcium homeostasis is required to sustain tooth health and prevent tooth decay. Popular commercial beverages formulated with phosphoric acid, especially in a low calcium diet, strongly promote tooth decay because excess phosphorus in ratio to calcium strongly antagonizes calcium, and one of the fastest ways to cause tooth decay is to drink sodas without taking enough calcium which gets blamed on the sugar content of soda which instead is a function of the phosphorus to calcium ratio, so tooth decay must also be treated by resolving calcium dysregulation and calcium deficiency.

In the course of my recovery, however, I also noticed that my teeth felt harder after several months of reversing silicon deficiency as frequently discussed throughout this book (especially the chapters on cancer and immunity), and in my research then found the existence silicon hydroxyapatite, which suggests the possibility that silicon is also necessary for tooth health and preventing loss of enamel. It is well known that silicon participates in bone and connective tissue, and decay of non-enamel tooth structures is certainly a function of silicon deficiency, for instance the fact that silicon polymerizes when exposed to alkaline pH such as is caused by most infections microorganisms which, when liberated from tissues, then forms a barrier of polymerized silicon that mechanically prevents further ingress into tissues. Obviously this defensive mechanism requires repletion with silicon in the first place, which is unfortunately disturbed by alkalizing pathogens and loss of good digestion, but reversing silicon deficiency even as a forty-five-year-old with a long history of oral health problems still resulted in obvious increase in the hardness of my teeth and integrity of oral tissues in a matter of months, with no signs of carries or other active decay.

But calcium is *not* the only primary protective factor against tooth decay, and studies also show that when oral microbes have access to the amino acid *proline* secreted in our saliva they produce almost none of the acids which dissolve tooth enamel, and while proline (and arginine which can be converted to proline) can and do come from dietary protein they are primarily synthesized in the body from dietary citrulline most commonly found in the cucurbit fruits like cucumbers, watermelon, squash, pumpkin, and other melons. As discussed in earlier chapters our body does not readily use or metabolize arginine unless there is a generous dietary supply of citrulline (called the arginine paradox), and domination of the gut by lactic acid producers which inhibits arginine catabolism (as discussed in chapter on pathogens and metabolic disease) prevents catabolism of arginine to citrulline. During oral disease there is a high rate of citrullination of gingival tissues, meaning that arginine in tissue proteins is converted to ammonia by pathogens when commensal microbes no longer have access to salivary proline they require in order to help fight against opportunistic infection.

After discovering this role of the citrulline pathway in the maintenance of oral microbes an informal survey of parents I knew confirmed that children with the least amount of cavities (i.e. none) regularly consumed cucurbits (*Cucurbitaceae*) such as cucumber while those with cavities did not. Even within one family a child who hated cucumber (but we raised all our children the same!) had extensive cavities and required significant dental care while their sibling who loved and ate cucumber regularly did not have any cavities at all. Dietary citrulline is thus the strongest predictor of our ability to resist cavities, especially in children and young adults, and since watermelon is a cucurbit most enjoyed by children and the highest source of dietary citrulline it should be used as much as possible when available and cucumber is always an excellent backup, with squashes and melons like chayote, pumpkin, cantaloupe, etc., also very acceptable options which should be consumed daily as a regular part of the human diet to prevent oral disease, and any persons or children with tooth decay or other oral disease should consume cucurbits every single day to rapidly arrest decay and restore salivary proline to cultivate commensal oral microbes. Oral disease is thus also a consequence of watermelon deficiency, since watermelon and other cucurbits were a primary food source responsible for the evolution of humans, and indeed the only aspect of my health growing up that was always excellent was my teeth, with watermelon, other melon, and cucumber some of the only healthy foods consistently present in our diet.

Besides redness, bleeding, and gum recession the most obvious and easy symptom for diagnosis of oral pathogens is *halitosis* (offensively bad breath) due hydrogen sulfide producing pathogens which also interfere with sulfur metabolism required for normal sulfation pathways. The mouth and breath should never smell malodorous *even when not brushing your teeth or doing any oral care whatsoever,* and any bad breath is evidence of colonization by these microbes and potential for disease. Because carotene inhibits sulfate reduction by pathogens any and all symptoms of halitosis or other oral disease should be immediately and consistently treated through increased frequency of carotene consumption such as from carrots, peaches, watermelon, dates, red and orange bell peppers, etc., which can and will entirely suppress halitosis if used sufficiently frequent, even without the use of other oral care products. Accompanying all meals with carotene is often sufficient for those with insignificant disease, but these pathogens also consume our mucin proteins and gum and connective tissue so in those with established oral disease it is usually required to more frequently use carotene such as every two or three hours, for which the absence of fresh breath is an excellent diagnostic, and high carotene foods should also be the first and last things eaten every day until oral disease is resolved.

Unfortunately these warning odors can be easily masked with toothpastes, mouthwashes, gum, and other breath fresheners which not only fail to protect us from these pathogens but readily disguise their communication to other persons or enable self-delusional thinking like they aren't a problem. But it's even much worse as oral care products actively increase risk of infection—One day when using a shampoo formulated with peppermint oil, which can feel uncomfortably cold on the skin even though I diluted it to reduce this effect, the small remaining amount of peppermint still felt so uncomfortable the sensation made me wonder if it was actually safe to use mint compounds on the skin or body (I had been contemplating oral disease nearly every day for the last five years so this was normal for me). Toothpastes and oral care products usually contain mint or its constituent chemical *menthol* which is, wrongly, thought to be inert to the human body, with stupid people explaining the effects of peppermint and menthol as interacting with "cold receptors" in the skin and membranes as if cold isn't one of the most harmful insults to human cells. Like carotene, menthol is a terpenoid and rapidly penetrates into biofilm and tissues but menthol functions in nature as a pesticide which kills microbes and insects by *depolarizing* their cells and, as discussed in the chapter on gut health in terms of vitamin B12 and digestion, polarity is a very important biological principle which facilitates the directional travel of energy and elements for the function of living tissue which is also used in defense against microorganisms which literally electromagnetically repels them from our epithelial surfaces. The human body is no exception and this means that depolarizing chemicals like menthol in oral care products, even those which are 'natural,' have a depolarizing effect on our tissues which then allows pathogens to adhere to our mucosal surfaces, and the pain comes from the impairment of our cellular depolarization and the cessation of energy production they require to remain alive. In smaller lifeforms with low body mass like microbes and insects the terpenoids in mint and other plant 'essential oils' are easily fatal, and while we are a much larger organism these chemicals don't kill us but do directly impair our defensive epithelial polarization, so while oral care products can kill some microbes they also destroy the very defensive mechanism against those microbes and oppositely *promote* colonization by opportunistic pathogens. Because salivary exchange with others is always preceded by the behavior of brushing teeth and freshening breath with menthol products the use of mentholated toothpastes, gums, mouthwashes, etc., ironically increases risk of pathogenic infection.

Unlike menthol, our biology is designed to expect and use dietary carotene in our biological function, and because carotene is also a terpenoid and rapidly penetrates mucosal layers it serves to also freshen breath, especially through the inhibition of sulfate and selenate reducing microbes, and because carotene is converted to vitamin A which stimulates mitochondrial biogenesis and the creation of energy for ATPase channels which transport electrolytes the consumption of carotene also helps reestablish polarity, and studies do show that vitamin A helps to restore polarity of cells which means that consumption of dietary carotene is also one of the primary methods to reverse gingival disease, to not only reverse halitosis but to promote regeneration of gingival tissue and repel opportunistic pathogens. This property of carotene can be easily felt by chewing a carrot or other high carotene food as carotene feels like menthol as it penetrates mucosal tissue and leaves mucosal tissues feeling fresh, and the best way to protect against both infection and bad breath before romantic encounters is not to brush your teeth with toothpaste, ever, but to chew on a carrot or other high carotene food which will help maintain cellular polarity to repel pathogens (especially if chewing is slow to allow saturation of all mucosa). Carotene is so effective in promoting this function it has breath-freshening properties that last even longer than oral care products anyway, and teeth will stay cleaner for longer periods of time between brushing.

Studies also show that gingival disease is associated with increased copper in tissues, which occurs since copper chaperones automatically release their copper during environmental changes in pH such as what are caused by opportunistic pathogens, since copper intoxication increases susceptibility of pathogens to oxidation by the immune response as discussed in the chapter on immunity. But since carotene uptake by cells is also dependent on copper this means that chronic gum disease is a symptom of copper dysregulation or deficiency which then prevents carotene uptake that would otherwise restore and repolarize gingival tissue through mitochondrial biogenesis. Studies also confirm that menthol causes proteins which chaperone copper and iron to release them, which in turn contributes to oxidative damage and depletes gingival tissue of the copper required for an effective immune response and uptake of carotene and vitamin A, so using any oral care products further exposes gingiva to opportunistic pathogenic colonization by literally impairing copper homeostasis and the very defense mechanism required to resist infection.

This problem of cellular depolarization is also not only relevant to oral health as all parts of body utilize polarity for their function, and losing polarity causes cells to leak their potassium and water. Because it is highly dependent on polarization for its function the nervous system is particularly susceptible to depolarization by menthol and other 'essential oils,' and many people who practice aromatherapy or use copious amounts of essential oils in or on their person often develop severe neurological disorders because of the depolarization caused by terpenoids and related chemicals even when they are natural. Some studies do outright confirm this harmful effect of oral care products by showing increased risk of oral disease from mouthwash, but which obviously have not seen much attention in the general public since it is antithetic to the capitalist exploitation of disease for profit. Other chemicals in oral care products like sodium laureth sulfate act as detergents and surfactants which literally strip the epithelial layer of fats and proteins and expose the underlying tissue to infection by pathogens, and canker sores are in fact a common manifestation of the damage that oral care products cause to oral tissues and defensive barriers which are then infected by opportunistic pathogens including viral causes of canker sores, and in the two years since I stopped using any oral care products I have not had a single canker sore even though my gingival health was not even fully restored. Considering how destructive oral care products actually are for oral health, and that infectious oral bacteria cause or contribute to a wide range of diseases from cancer to arthritis to cardiovascular disease to schizophrenia, and that heart disease which is catalyzed by infectious oral pathogens is the number one cause of death in most countries, oral care products appear to be the number one contributing factor to all death and disease, even more than alcoholism and smoking (which in truth are also self-medication for treatment of these pathogens). There is nothing wrong with consuming herbs culinarily, and I will never avoid mint ice cream, but oral care products are often highly potent quantities applied directly to gingival tissues for extended periods of time every single day, but other charged molecules such as sodium bicarbonate can still also strongly depolarize mucosal tissue, so even 'natural' commercial oral care products are all actually harmful to use in the oral cavity and should not be used at all, instead relying on dietary carotene as the primary oral care strategy and for keeping breath fresh.

As might be expected, I believe that oral disease is also an effect of mucosal colonization by *Trichomonas* parasites which inhibit the immune system and then allows for secondary opportunistic colonizers like *P. gingivalis*. Since light activation causes lithium to be strongly antiparasitic a very useful treatment for all oral disease is to hold a solution of water and lithium (1-5 mg) in the mouth during exposure to bright sunshine or supplemental, warm-spectrum light as discussed in the chapter on immunity. This works so well it can help lesson pain even from a single treatment, which makes it tempting also in turn not to do it frequently, but this therapy should be repeated daily until the full resolution of all symptoms of oral disease. Within days of using lithium and light exposure it caused the small deposition of calculus behind my front, lower teeth to completely break up which, when it happened, I first mistook for a piece of tooth, since calculus is extremely hard. Taking a mouthful and swishing it while on a walk or sitting in the sunshine for ten minutes or so is quite simple to do, but generally taking a dose of lithium and getting light exposure will also still assist in the resolution of oral disease and resistance to colonization without swishing it every time, and swishing should only be required for a short period of time as indicated by the resolution of calculus buildup.

Saliva also naturally contains lactoperoxidase, the immune enzyme which produces hypohalous acids from dietary cyanide, iodine, chloride, fluoride, and bromide as discussed in the chapter on immunity, and after resolution of oral parasitism through lithium the efficacy of halides in the resolution of oral disease should be more obvious. Lactoperoxidase shows preference for cyanide, iodine, and chloride, but immune dysregulation as discussed in the chapter on immunity due to dysregulation of cholesterol and the CFTR pathway prevents the effectiveness of halides in the resolution of oral disease. Teeth are also kept white by the hypohalous acids, especially chloride, so discoloration of teeth is a useful symptom to diagnose impaired chloride status caused by factors like excessive ammonification or production of oxylipins by pathogens due to vitamin E deficiency which can and does occur regardless of chloride intake. Commercial teeth whiteners do use hypochlorous acid (bleach) to whiten teeth, but the amounts are so high as to cause significant oxidative damage and risk harming the tooth and gums, but they also mask symptoms of impaired chloride transport like discoloration which then makes it more difficult to establish causal diagnoses, and normal dietary salt should be enough to keep teeth mostly white even while consuming things like tea or coffee daily. Any oral disease represents immune dysfunction, but restoring chloride homeostasis is the most important which can be achieved in turn by restoring vitamin E as discussed in the chapter on immunity. Never use more than 1 tsp of salt per supplemental dose juice, tea, or water otherwise it will induce vomiting (1/2 tsp for children, if needed), and should result in brightening of teeth within as little as 24-48 hours, which will also provide immune support for the rest of the body and gingival tissues too. Other halide channels like CFTR and pendrin which also transport cyanide and iodine require chloride to function as discussed in the chapter on immunity, so restoration of chloride will also then cause iodine and cyanide to be more effective in resolution of oral disease too, and afterward the active chewing of dietary sources of cyanide such as arugula, cabbage, almonds, etc., and low-dose supplement of iodine will help resolve gingival disease. Because oral pathogens are communicated most commonly through salivary exposure, the active use of supplemental salt (with natural vitamin E), iodine, and chewing dietary sources of cyanide can and should be used to both prevent and treat disease in anyone who is sexually active, even if monogamous, to prolong and maintain oral health. Pregnancy is highly affected by oral disease, and miscarriage or infertility are frequently caused by oral pathogens communicated by romantic partners or sexual predators of children, their victims not knowing they have been exposed and suffer illness due to the assault. Those in high-risk occupations for oral pathogen exposure like dentistry, nursing, sex work, etc., should also use these strategies prophylactically to better resist colonization.

The physical act of brushing which manually debrides teeth of plaque, biofilm, and food detritus is the only real benefit of brushing, not the use of chemicals, as this also stimulates salivary secretion from oral tissues which then increases the quantity of saliva, salivary antimicrobial peptides, and peroxidase enzymes to better promote oral health, and a high quality, soft toothbrush can be very useful in keeping teeth clear of biofilm and buildup, while being consistently replete with dietary citrulline and vitamin C confers resistance to pathogenic colonization. In fact, the act of brushing should result in an abundance of salivary stimulation which assists the process far better than any commercial product since saliva contains active immune factors designed to keep the mouth naturally free of disease. The coconut oil swish as discussed in the chapter on self-therapy can also help stop tooth decay, as the fatty acids like lauric acid released from the action of salivary lipase on coconut oil triglycerides are not only highly antibiotic and effectively disinfect cavities but also directly promote our own tissues through the increased production of pregnenolone and stabilization of cells by saturated fat. Tooth pain should thus be treated by a thrice daily coconut oil swish for a prolonged period (at least fifteen minutes) until the pain is resolved (which should occur in no more than two days otherwise the problem is very severe and should be treated by a medical professional). A visit to the dentist for a thorough cleaning and removal of calculus can also springboard your recovery since buildup acts as a reservoir for pathogens, and to treat any severely decayed teeth beyond saving. But do not get x-rays since radiation is very harmful to human cells and directly disrupts ATP production (you can refuse dentists if they insist), and since many dentists in capitalist economies are outright dishonest always get a second opinion for any major dental work. Metal implants, even titanium, also usually cause toxicity in the body since the body will always try to dissolve foreign material, and high-tech, ceramic implants are likely the safest if needed. Implants made from silicon would be ideal, but none are yet developed as I can tell.

As this chapter has demonstrated, most traditional or alternative therapy or products not only do not work to cure oral disease they can often actually promote it, and oral care should be limited to gentle brushing with metabolically complimentary ingredients. Tannin has also been shown in studies to bind iron and form a lattice over cavities and dentin to facilitate remineralization, so the inclusion of tannin in the diet such as from tea and nuts (with their skins) also naturally inhibits tooth decay. Oral disease can be devastating to our overall metabolic health, as many other metabolic diseases such as cancer, diabetes, autism, cystic fibrosis, arthritis, cardiovascular disease, multiple sclerosis, etc., also involve oral disease, and this therapy is required for full recovery of all chronic illness since many pathogens take up permanent residence in the oral cavity, and understanding the principles of oral disease and immunity is required of all humans regardless of metabolic status, as we all eventually contract oral disease which contributes to later metabolic decline and mortality and spread pathogens to others when our bodies and diets lack these nutrients and self-care strategies.

Fragile Things

Porcelain doll,
Pane of glass,
Cup from Ikea,
not meant to last.
Bubble of soap,
A new downy chick,
Tired balloon,
Flower, fresh picked.
The curl on a cupcake,
A butterfly's wing,
Young man's voice,
on a high note sings.
A wet piece of tissue,
Resolve at the start,
The first day of spring,
My lover's heart.

CHAPTER 19

CURING ERECTILE DYSFUNCTION

When I was almost fourteen my upcoming birthday brought with it the promise of drawing nearer to manhood. In a few short years I would get to drive a car, date, and perhaps even get to have sex. Birthdays happen regularly in a house of eight people, and every few weeks there is some kind of celebration be it a holiday or a special day for one of our family members. My mother is one of those women who takes great joy in piling on as many gifts and decorations as she can assemble, and as the week progressed a pile of perfectly wrapped gifts began to climb higher and higher on the dining room table. We were not that well off, and the appearance of each new present filled me with surprise and gratitude for my loving family. But the night before my birthday my parents took me out to dinner at an expensive restaurant they usually reserved for their own special date nights. I had never been alone with them in a setting like this, and our lack of conversation quickly turned awkward. "We have an early present for you," they said during a moment of uncomfortable silence, then crassly slid a fifty-dollar bill across the table. Not in a card or anything, just the plain bill.

"Oh," I said, taken aback by the vulgarity of cash. *Why this, when all those presents are on the table?* I thought, almost handing it back to them. I didn't want money. The evening alone with them was enough, even though my growing awareness of my different interest in other boys, such as the handsome waiter who constantly passed our table, had begun to make me feel separated from them, unable to talk about who I really was for fear of betraying myself to danger.

"Happy Birthday," said my mother the next morning when she came into my room. "Thanks," I said, suppressing that childish overexcitement for birthdays which, it turns out, no one ever really grows out of no matter how much they may protest. Because it happened to be the weekend, by lunch my mother had gathered everyone at the table and we went right to opening presents. But a strange hesitation seemed to hang on the family, as if no one but my mother had really been aware of the day or what was actually in any of the gifts. My first present was presented as from my first sister, but of course it was not from her at all—she was only a year younger than me and had no money of her own and nobody had accompanied my mother on trips to shop for these. We all knew full well that birthdays were done in complete and total orchestration by our mother, assigned gifts already wrapped and set out for the event. I suppose my mom had grown so used to doing this when we were toddlers that she never thought to change the process, and she always desired that celebrations be as perfect as possible, and opening the first gift I was immediately confused, perplexed. "A fish?" I said, peeling the wrapping from a small wooden knick-knack of a river trout painted in muted earth colors atop a dowel on a square wood base. "For your desk," said my mother. "Oh," I said, trying not to sound like a disappointed brat. Maybe there was something about it I didn't get. Maybe she wanted me to take up fishing. I certainly had never expressed a like for trout, or fishing. I'd figure it out later. "Thanks!" I said with a smile so fake any perceptive parent would easily have seen through it.

The next present was from another sister who was only ten and had even less means to shop for a birthday present. It was a rug. "It's a prayer rug," she said with extra, forced enthusiasm because no kid in the entire world ever wants to give their sibling an earth-tone, woven, "prayer" rug. My mom must have seen the look of confusion on my face, "So you can remember to say your prayers in the morning when you get out of bed," she said. *But it doesn't say 'prayer' on the rug,* I thought. *It's just a normal, dull, coarse, oval rug. I also didn't have a problem remembering my prayers. Did they think I did? And my bedroom is carpeted—*"Thanks," I said instead. Suddenly, on the day of my fourteenth birthday, it began to dawn on me for the first time just how truly alone I was in my own family, a stranger to the very people who gave me birth, viewed with indifference by my own siblings—and I still had to make it through several more presents.

The next was from my brother. The package was large, light, and plush to the touch. "It's a blanket," said my mom before I even got the wrapping open. *I already have a blanket!* I thought angrily. "It's like the one we have," she said unctuously. "It's so soft, open it up and feel it." The fabric was coarse, rough. Maybe I was feeling the wrong part. I pushed my hand down farther. "Is it supposed to feel like this?" I said. My mother took the blanket. Her face fell in disappointment. "Oh, I got the wrong one," she said. "We can go exchange it," and set the package down next to her.

Suddenly I felt guilty. Her perfect birthday was not going well. How could I tell her that none of this was necessary? That while it was terrible I would have been overjoyed by a package of nice colored pencils and drawing paper, or a few comic books which were only a couple dollars each, which I could also use as a reference when drawing superheroes with oversized bulges. I didn't understand how my interests were apparently so nebulous. Was I a mystery to them? Was I really so uninteresting? "Thanks mom," I said instead, feeling my throat starting to catch. The blanket alone had taken up a great bulk of the pile. Without it, the volume of gifts now seemed much less than it had appeared, and the reason for the fifty-dollar bill was becoming apparent. Every present seemed like one to give a mom or grandmother, to appoint a home in my mother's particular taste, not a single one appropriate for fourteen-year old boy, even if he was a fairy. Maybe the last one, a thin, brick-shaped box, was some markers. *Please be markers.*

Picking it up I realized it was a book. Maybe it was a fantasy novel, since I loved to read. One of the *Dragonlance* books of which I had become obsessed. At last, one thing to confirm their interest in me as a person.

'*How to train your dog,*' read the title of the book. My heart jumped for joy. This is why my birthday sucks! I thought. At my tenth birthday they had got me a doughnut-colored cocker spaniel whom I promptly fell in love with, but whom my father later gave away while we were gone visiting our cousins because Dudley had bit my little sister after going crazy being forced to live in the backyard alone in the harsh Northern Utah weather. Losing Dudley was the first time my heart ever broke, but the present which teased his arrival was a wrapped collar and leash. I had been asking for a new dog for years, so the book and crappy birthday presents were all because they got me another dog! Finally they decided to make amends for breaking my heart all those years ago. But looking through the glass sliding door to the backyard for the sight of a little muzzle, big eyes, or a wagging tail I saw only faded grass and the scattered red and yellow leaves of autumn. Confused, I looked to my dad for answers. "Oh," he said, realizing far too late the mistake they had made, "there's no dog this time."

My throat tightened quick. Tears immediately threatened to expose my heart-break. Instead of the dawning of manhood my teenage years seemed to portend ignominy and grandmotherly accouterment. "Thanks for the birthday!" I said, then quickly gathered my gifts and rushed to my room before the tears had a chance to escape.

My "room" was actually the den in the basement which I shared with my twelve-year-old brother, which had only three walls and adjoined the basement family room. Privacy was a rare thing for our family anyway, but which made this prudish environment all the more perplexing and frustrating, and I could not hide and cried quietly at my desk. "What's wrong?" said my brother. I looked up in surprise and wiped my eyes in embarrassment. He was genuinely concerned. "I don't like my presents," I said, sadly, grateful at least for someone to share my feelings but sounding exactly like the spoiled brat I was trying hard not to be. How could I find the words to explain that I felt invisible in a house with eight people, except when I disappointed them, about the violent storm of emotions which whipped my insides, fearing for my safety if anyone should ever discover that I looked at boys or masturbated into my old teddybear pretending it was a cute boy, a fear which separated me from everyone I loved now compounded by the reali-zation that my parents didn't even know I liked comic books or thought I would enjoy a goddamned *prayer rug*. Was that really the person they thought I was? Was *I* really that person?

My brother left me alone and a few minutes later my mother came storming downstairs. "You ungrateful brat!" she screamed. My face flushed red with fear and embarrassment. My brother had told her what I said, though he had meant to help and later apologized it would make no difference. "Where's the money we gave you last night?" she demanded. I pointed to a small box on my dresser. She opened it and took the fifty-dollars, then stormed out of the room. I began to cry again, and was later commanded by my father to apologize to my mother for being ungrateful for receiving a fish knickknack, a brown rug, and a book on training dogs when I had no dog, for my fourteenth birthday. They never replaced the blanket, or the fifty-dollars.

I retreated further into my own world, taking solace in the very small spaces of my own—my desk, my art, showers, and the endless world of my imagination. Being able to draw brought me attention and was a source of pride, but I could also retreat from this volatile environment into my fantasies and draw powerful dragons, silly cartoon characters, or ripped, muscular, nearly naked men with huge bulging packages and enjoy a clandestine outlet for my pent up sexuality as long as they had a line across the neck, the wrists, and ankles to indicate skin-tight spandex of a superhero outfit (and while writing this I suddenly realized why they probably didn't encourage my superhero obsession). Of course, more risqué drawings had to be hidden carefully. Only a few days before I had gathered the courage to draw my first penis. It was beautiful and made me feel like less of a freak for having one and wanting to use it. It was too precious to throw away, so I placed it within a large stack of drawings. Later when I was alone I sifted through my art to find the image. It had been vandalized.

Gross!!!

The word was written in blue ink, in fine handwriting underlined many times and with three exclamation marks as if to avoid any mistake of intention. I was mortified. The penis wasn't even very big, or veiny or hairy. It was just a nice penis. My one small space of privacy, my artwork, had been invaded, defaced, and used as a tool to humiliate me. I crumpled the paper and threw it in the trash.

Sharing a room also without a wall meant finding time to beat off in secret. A good strategy was to pile the covers up enough to create a wall, and since my brother's bed was lower than mine and on the other side of the room it was impossible to get caught unless he woke up and turned on the lights. One morning, however, I woke very early and, overcome by hormones, did what any normal teenage boy likes to do. I must have been fully entranced by the fantasy I was having because suddenly I heard a noise across the open end of the den which looked out onto the basement living room. The covers of my "wall" had sunk away entirely and my erection, firmly in the grip of both hands, was in clear view of one of my sisters who, groggily wondering what she was staring at, stood near the bottom of the stairs which means she had passed across the entirety of the open wall of our bedroom while I had been fast at work. We both realized at once what was happening. I yanked the covers up and she darted up the stairs, and we never discussed it.

I had a very active libido which had begun somewhat younger than what is usually considered typical. Gay boys actually enter puberty on the same timeline as girls, at an earlier age, and I had my first orgasm just before turning twelve. It happened under the sheets late one night while quarantined in a room with all five of my younger siblings because my father was yet again remodeling the house we lived in, one-half entombed in a wall of plastic to keep the construction dust from contaminating what spare livable space remained. For a few years we lived like this, moving from house to house while tearing them apart and trying to eat, clean, and cook amongst the constant interruptions of electricians, plumbers, and drywall dust. My siblings hadn't had as much trouble sleeping as I did, still tucked naively in the comfort of pre-adolescence, and not realizing I was even touching it suddenly found myself in the alarming throes of what I would later learn to be an orgasm. It was exhilarating, like nothing I had ever experienced. I felt there should be more to it as eleven is usually too young an age to ejaculate, and sure enough it became a very different experience a few months later.

It would be something with much importance and consequence on my life, jerking off, one of the only tools with which I could bring myself rare comfort during the fast approaching tumult of my religion-addled adolescence and destabilizing family life. But that I discovered my sexuality so early is also no coincidence—religious groups are often obsessed with sex. Sex and genitals are spoken of with much frequency, even with those who are very, very young though usually in the context of not touching them or not sharing them with others. Every Sunday there were lessons in which church leaders described sex and variations on it, in detail, under the pretense of religious instruction, then demeaned and shamed it and those considering its engagement who probably weren't even thinking of it until you brought it up in church but thanks now that's all I can think about. I could not get away from discussion of sex even if I wanted to, and I often very much wanted to. Now that I am a grown man I recognize many of those adults as sexual predators, their fetish for exposing young people to eroticism veiled as religious instruction, enabled by a culture comfortable with shame, secrets, impunity, and authoritarian patriarchy. One creepy religious leader who often took to discussing sex behavior when leading our young men's group was later arrested for criminal sexual conduct at his place of work, assaulting a female colleague and hiding cameras in the women's locker room. I first learned of anal sex from my own father at the age of thirteen during our first sex talk in which he described anal sex between men with graphic and familiar detail, but refrained to inform me about gay people and the ability to love and be loved by someone of the same gender, betraying an obsession with sex but ignorance to love and affection. By that time I had already found myself attracted to other boys and I think he suspected and meant to warn me against acting on it, but with the newfound knowledge that I could put my penis in another boy I was struck not by the possibility of penetrating one but in finding comfort from drawing so near, to think another boy's smile could be meant for me, the touch of our skin during a warm embrace, a passionate kiss.

At the beginning of my adolescence I got caught humping the wet porcelain surface of an empty tub after a bath in the bathroom known to everyone not to have a lock by my mother who entered accidentally on purpose. Caught other times while in bed, being walked in on by my parents who knew full well they should knock on the closed door of a teenager, even as an older teenager while working out in my underwear on our home weight-lifting set when my imagination got the better of me and stupidly thinking I was alone in the house. I heard later from a psychologist that stressed children instinctively self-pleasure as means to cope with stress, and my childhood (like many others) was anything but stress-free. I found it impossible to suppress the overwhelming urge to ejaculate sometimes even two or three times a day, especially when being by myself was the only peace I could ever find. This same demanding compulsion carried far into my adulthood even when I began to experience erectile dysfunction and could not actually have sex, even with myself, and sex was such an overwhelming, depressing, and shameful experience from even my early childhood and yet I was unable to resolve my compulsions and find satisfaction in desire, which made my pain, frustration, and loneliness utterly unbearable.

It turns out that an overactive sex drive is rooted in biology and is not, as it is so callously and sadly regarded, a defect of moral character or something which can be controlled (the impulse, not acting on the impulse, which can be controlled). Sexual compulsion is also incorrectly regarded as an addiction, with many people suffering "sex addiction" finding it disruptive to their personal lives and even 12-step recovery programs for it. But an overactive sex drive is actually mediated by high *nitric oxide* stress, as nitric oxide stimulates sexual arousal by upregulating such factors as *gonadotropins* and *luteinizing hormone*, and dilates the muscles which prevent blood flow to the corpus cavernosum which facilitates engorgement of the penis (or clitoris), and because nitric oxide stress and excess also occurs from metabolic disease in response to metabolic illness sexual compulsion is actually not an addiction at all (which is why recovery programs for it do not work) but a biological response to potential expiration of an organism intended by nature to promote an increase in mating and thus increased chance of insemination and creation of offspring before death. In animals and our ancestors the kind of stress which causes nitric oxide dysfunction usually only came from famine, infectious disease, and competition, and such stress was *always* associated with significantly heightened chance of mortality, so sexual compulsion is actually our biology's attempt to promote our species, at our individual expense, by trying to force the increased chance of mating.

But because of contemporary medicine, food supply, and sanitation it is now possible for ill adults to live many, many years through stresses that would otherwise have easily caused death in our ancestors, and so persist for years and years with compulsory sex drive that frustrates and imperils personal wellbeing, especially since this problem is also usually addressed through ideology and shame which don't do anything except perpetuate the problem because the underlying problem is entirely biological. Conditions that stimulate sexual compulsion are also accompanied by high adrenaline and cortisol and colonization by parasites and other pathogens which further increase discomfort which then associates sexual compulsion with suffering rather than emotional fulfillment as occurs in normal sexual experiences, so many millions of men and women find compulsive sexual behavior to be unpleasant and unceasing and sit at their computers reading forums on sexual 'health' which instead encourage abstinence which they cannot achieve anyway because abstinence is based in ideological moralizing, not biology. There is nothing wrong with an active libido except that in cases of compulsive sexual desire it is associated also with suffering other stress, and the vague burden upon a person's psyche which is only relieved by sexual activity, so sex also becomes unfulfilling and burdensome and merely medicates the discomfort caused by excess nitric oxide rather than a healing, fulfilling experience it can and should be.

One of the most common sources of exogenous nitric oxide which exacerbates sexual compulsion is *thiamine mononitrate* added to wheat flour to supply dietary thiamine but which, adding significant nitrate, spontaneously stimulates sexual arousal, and if I were inclined to believe in conspiracy theories I might think this was done on purpose in order to force populations to have more sex and increase procreation, but the people running these things are too ignorant of biology to know it even has that effect and if you are very perceptive you may have noticed that consuming pizza, pasta, or sandwiches can result in sexual arousal within as little as ten to thirty minutes after as its additive nitrate content is rapidly detoxified into nitric oxide if your body sill possesses that ability as described in the chapter on immunity (if it doesn't this nitrate instead inhibits mitochondrial respiration and immunity).

This effect of exogenous nitrates in the food supply is even more burdensome in children from abusive homes such as the religious hell in which I was raised because the food supply literally forces sexual compulsion which is then demonized, shamed, or ignored. Many young men driven insane by the forced stimulation of sexual arousal from added food nitrate and artificial fertilizer in religious homes which constantly talk about sex and shaming sex behavior end up becoming sexual predators, even of their own family members, because of a lack healthy skills to fulfill sexual desires and constant, unrelenting, forced stimulation of arousal. Because of this role of nitric oxide sex addiction is not a thing at all, but is instead the human body's programmed response to nitric oxide and environmental stress which is meant to promote the success of our species at the expense of the individual who then sacrifices relationships and personal wellbeing to relieve themselves of the burden caused by biological function, and children and adults burdened with sexual compulsion become tormented, insane, cause harm, and even become suicidal since they have no idea what is actually going on.

Because the sex response in humans is also social and bonding, even to oneself, it promotes some reduction in stress, but unless the underlying nitric oxide dysfunction which stimulates sexual compulsion is addressed this condition does not change which is why men and women persist for years, striving willfully to overcome sex compulsion, even failing with therapy or incarceration, because the condition is based in our endocrinological biology, not the psyche. To be clear, the idea that this needs to be changed at all has nothing to do with sexuality or morality but only because the increased stress of nitric oxide dysfunction also further destroys metabolic health and sexual function, including mental health, and causes a great burden on the lifespan and quality of life of an individual. A person is still responsible for their choices and behavior while suffering health problems, but many also do not possess healthy and effective mental and social coping skills to handle the kinds of stresses which illness causes, let alone the biological knowledge to fix it, with many people being raised with entitled worldviews in which they are allowed or encouraged to satisfy personal selfishness which the stressed human metabolic state triggers, and so also become burdensome to others and society, motivated by biology but enabled by poor parenting and the lack of effective life skills (my other book, *The Perfect Child*, is all about psychology and how to be a good parent).

Since nitrate and nitrite also come from industrial agriculture and synthetic fertilizer in addition to being naturally common among many plants it is extremely easy to have diets and lifestyles which actively cause excess of nitrate, nitrite, and dysfunctional nitric oxide and thus high sexual compulsion. *Sodium nitrate* is another source used as a preservative common in processed meat products like sausages and bacon, but even "healthier" options contain celery powder because celery is naturally very high in nitrate, and processed meat products should be pre-cooked if they are not immediately sold, which eliminates the need for any nitrate preservation, and healthier preservatives like ascorbic acid or citric acid would be healthful rather than harmful, and these kinds of meat products can also be purchased fresh from a butcher to avoid nitrate preservation (always ask because many grocery stores still use nitrates on meats sold by the butcher). Celery does not need to be avoided, but avoiding it can help if suffering from sexual compulsion, cancer, and other metabolic disease, and organic foods will always contain considerably less nitrate than their industrially grown counterpart.

Problems with sex also only get worse as we age, and in spite of my high libido as a young man I first experienced erectile dysfunction around the age of twenty, but it wasn't until the age of forty-one that I found I had cystic fibrosis which, in addition to inhibiting the immune system, also causes libido problems, especially in males, and entirely prevents sperm production and wet dreams. Suffering libido failure at such a young age confounded my struggle to be happy and healthy and played into the ridiculous reward-punishment ideology of my rearing, and I only enjoyed about two years of sexual activity with partners unencumbered by problems with sex, not to mention that my idea of it was mostly an activity of necessity rather than an expression of love, my emotional connection to others long severed by the dissociative personality developed in response to a lifetime of heartache, punishment, and derision at the hands of my family, friends, and community.

Early on my problem wasn't serious, occurring only if I was especially spent or anxious. It began while on my own, at times finding no energy to bring myself to orgasm even when I had not been active and in spite of an overpowering impulse for sexual encounters. This occurs in large part because colonization by arginase producing microbes also consumes arginine for production of ammonia, and because parasites like *Trichomonas* colonize mucosal tissue including the reproductive organs this directly results in endocrine disruption, hypogonadism, and other problems with the sex organs.

Medically, the absence of sleep orgasms is often explained as a problem of reduced sperm production, but young women get wet dreams too, and my reproductive organs definitely had no problem producing seminal fluid in the prostate. In my early twenties I also suffered from a strange sensation that could only be described as a debilitating need to urinate even when there was no urine to be discharged, which I tried to discuss with doctors who would literally pretend like I hadn't asked about it since they didn't know what I was talking about but which would leave me debilitated and confined to the bathroom for long periods of time. I finally realized when writing this book around the age of forty that this sensation was inflamed prostate due to secondary bacterial infection as a consequence of *Trichomonas* colonization and cystic fibrosis and was the same problem as urinary tract infection as occurs in the vaginal urethra also then affecting the prostate which causes it to spasm. Many men suffer quietly with similar conditions because patriarchy ironically also ignores or shames men with health conditions, and incompetent doctors are only interested when disease progresses to more obvious, serious conditions like prostate cancer. As nitrates, nitrites, and nitric oxide excess all cause sexual compulsion and rapidly interfere with sexual function through the inhibition of mitochondria the compulsion to get off during an inability to do so can be especially infuriating. Of course, the guilt and shame indoctrinated into me said I had arrived at this miserable situation precisely because of my overactive sex drive, use of pornography, and being gay so I abided my struggles, failing to recognize them as a defect in health and the society in which I lived rather than anything wrong with me as a person. By the age of twenty-eight I started to have truly alarming difficulties with libido and sexual health, easily winded during sex, sweating excessively, or losing erections from the simplest interruption or over-exertion. I tried to be strong and to be okay in spite of my increasing difficulties, which I now realize was actually just down-playing my own suffering and marginalizing my self-worth due in no small part for knowing no way out.

I also experienced testicular pain which I found out later was from *varicocele* which is a condition like varicose veins which prevents proper blood drainage from the testicles, and nearing my thirties and still suffering these problems I finally asked another doctor for help but he also didn't understand what I was asking and scheduled a testicular cancer screening. As had happened countless times the medical profession failed to assist in any helpful way and so I gave up, accepting with embarrassment the increasing inability of my still young body to function normally when excited partners found me instead unable to meet their expectations.

Later a partner had access to erectile dysfunction pills (and also put me on finasteride even though I wasn't yet losing hair because of his own controlling, superficial insecurity). Those drugs made sex fun again for a moment but taking them too often or at full dose left me with stuffy sinuses and a puffy face, especially under my eyes, and more prone to inexplicable exhaustion afterward which I now know is because of the inhibitory effect of nitric oxide on mitochondrial respiration. My health also began to decline severely, my waist line increasing while the hours I could sleep decreased, which compounded my emotional tumult and desperation for relief. Never did I consider these medications were unnatural and that someone my age should *not* be suffering erectile dysfunction let alone being given erectile aids by unconcerned partners or doctors who should have instead promoted healthy lifestyles and educating young men how to properly care for their sexual health and bodies. By the time I developed thyroid cancer it was impossible to have sex even with myself, and boner pills didn't help with erections at all but made my other symptoms even more excruciating. Sex was always accompanied by fatigue, sweating, and was generally an unpleasant experience for everyone involved, made worse by an unsupportive partner and overwhelming fear about my waning health and appearance. Eventually he left and my physical state suffered so much that sex with others wasn't really an option. Thankfully, along with my journey out of ill-health I was also able to discover what causes erectile dysfunction and how to cure it and after finally recovering the ability to bone someone I regained some of the confidence lost during youth. Being a male does not always mean having an erection but losing a body function is always demoralizing, and regaining it is a reason to be grateful.

My penis has no concept of morals (I mean this literally, not figuratively, as decisions I make with my penis are *always* moral) and should work whether or not the rational mind does. Unfortunately, erectile problems are now all too common among young men and made worse by the ubiquitous desecration of the human body by religionist bullies and self-loathing victims of shame-based rearing, and the absence of experienced or empathetic fathers, friends, and brothers (and prudish mothers) too pussy to share helpful and encouraging information and support. The truth is we usually don't or shouldn't have to deal with arousal issues until forty, fifty, or even sixty years of age if very healthy. While I have no sexual experience with women, sexual arousal is more or less the same in all humans regardless of gender because hormones have the same function regardless of what body they are in, and the information in this chapter, though focused on men since that is my experience, is not limited to the male experience since women also get boners (they're just much smaller).

Sexual health does not start with nor does it end with the reproductive organs, and focusing on them is demoralizing and distracting if you have issues. Sexual health is a mirror. Unhealthy bodies have deficiencies with sex. Healthy bodies do not. Unlike hair, which falls out or grays at even moderate stress the reproductive system will continue working even when health is very poor because reproduction is crucial for the survival of species it is one of the very last traits to succumb to ill health, so a working sex drive does not necessarily mean a person is healthy by any means. When erections finally fail it is because of serious metabolic decline, and should rightly be of concern, especially if it happens earlier than is expected as this is a sign of very serious health issues (or health issues to come).

Because all humans have sexuality (yes, my ace friends, even you) it becomes a convenient fulcrum for exploitation and control, and sexual health problems are viewed by self-pitying ideology which seeks control of life, people, and reality as evidence of wrongdoing or deficiency of moral resolve, many men and women experiencing shame for biological responses which are instead a part of our natural existence. In reality sex is intended to fulfill our moral obligations as social and reproductive creatures, and moralizing or idealizing sex only serves to further add to the stress causing health problems in the first place! To make this point, a pathogenic bacteria called *Mycoplasma* is commensal to *Trichomonas* parasites and specifically causes many of the symptoms associated with cystic fibrosis such as male infertility, pelvic inflammatory disease, or bacterial vaginosis, but can also be "asymptomatic" and *Mycoplasma* are the smallest known free-living organism and also cause pneumonia and other illnesses, and stress depletes tyrosine since it is the substrate for adrenaline but tyrosine is also required in the immune system and to transport iron, so stress makes the body less able to fight the very pathogens which contribute to illnesses manifest through symptoms like sexual dysfunction, demonstrating just how complex issues with human health can be which often don't have anything to do with behavior at all, apart from diet, and everything to do with nature, and absolutely nothing to do with ideology except the stress and suffering it causes.

The biological response to nitric oxide dysfunction which motivates compulsive sexual behavior is also why sex so often becomes the pivot point of relationships, where those with elevated nitric oxide and impaired ability to recycle nitrite and nitrate as discussed in the chapter on immunity and thus sexual compulsion find sex to become problematic in the fulfillment and maintenance of relationships, not because sex is the problem but for the unsettling and unful-filling nature of elevated nitric oxide and other stress hormones which inhibit the bonding response of true intimacy. Of course, sexual activity can also relieve stress by temporarily lowering stress and raising dopamine and oxytocin, and so we engage in this behavior just as we eat food when we are hungry or sleep when we are tired, because the nature of biology is immutable, but those with sexual compulsion in turn treat their partners as mere tools to satisfy needs rather than experiencing the true depths of a fulfilling sexual relationship. If the goal is to get well it is unhelpful to consider sexuality outside the context of biology, because it is the rules of biology, not ideology, which define its function, and focusing on behavior and ideology is an attempt instead to control nature and biology, which we absolutely cannot do. Resolving stresses physical, nutritional, environmental, and emotional reduces fixation on sex and helps normalize nitric oxide status to not only relieve sexual compulsion but restore the fun and fulfilling nature of sex which then becomes restorative instead of a necessity or associated with feelings of guilt, shame, or the inability to bond with a partner. Even self-sex can result in unpleasant and demoralizing experiences when excess stress hormones cause outsized deficits on metabolic function and depress the usual healthy hormones whereas resolution of this problem restores the healthful, moral function of sex which is to promote love, whether it is with oneself or with a partner.

Firstly, boners do not actually work the way we generally understand them (including that women also get boners) and certainly not what we hear from media and pharmaceutical companies looking to make money from our erectile dysfunc-tion by products or clicks. Because of nitric oxide's role in sex it is a primary target of erectile dysfunction medication, and while nitric oxide does help facil-itate arousal by dilating blood vessels and allowing blood flow to the sex organs nitric oxide also acts like a stress hormone, and its role is not actually to facilitate arousal but to *guarantee* it. Sexual function is one of the last metabolic processes to be lost because the body has many methods to keep sexual functions operating as long as possible, even at the expense of physical health, to ensure a greater chance of reproduction, even at the expense of the individual, and because nitric oxide can and does also inhibit mitochondria the elevation of nitric oxide such as is caused by erection aids also accelerates the aging process by inhibiting mitochondrial production of energy and most men who regularity use erectile aids or workout supplements to raise nitric oxide soon show premature and advanced aging, faster greying hair, severely thinning skin, and reduction in muscle mass. Like many metabolic processes nitric oxide has its rightful place but this does not mean it also lacks side effects, and the long histories of ancient and contemporary practices of abstaining from sex to improve health based on many stupid theories ranging from the retention of sperm to retention of metaphysical energy does not result from abstinence from sex but instead the abatement of some nitric oxide excess which then frees mitochondria to respire. Especially since it is entirely possible to limit excess nitric oxide excess while maintaining erectile function it is misguided to engage in such practices, even futile, as nitric oxide production is defined by the state of health, diet, and environment, and *not* sexual activity.

The natural molecule for erection facility is instead *carbon dioxide* (CO_2), which also relaxes blood vessels the same way nitric oxide does, although not in such an extreme manner, but also comes with health restorative effects rather than detrimental ones because carbon dioxide oppositely promotes an increase in mitochondrial activity and proliferation, where nitric oxide inhibits respiration. In cardiovascular function, nitric oxide fills in the difference between what is achieved by carbon dioxide and what is needed otherwise, but over time a decline in mitochondrial health and thus CO_2 production increases dependence on nitric oxide which then begins to worsen CO_2 deficiency by inhibiting mitochondria and which eventually entirely prevents nitric oxide's ability to relax blood vessels in the first place. Paying attention to breathing during sex will reveal an increasing shallowness of breath as the body grows nearer to orgasm because holding the breath instinctually retains carbon dioxide (and nitric oxide) and this is how the body manually increases CO_2 during sex, by preventing its ventilation, which then helps to facilitate even greater blood flow and oxygen exchange to sustain mitochondrial respiration required for physical exertion. Nearing orgasm men actually hold their breath, unconsciously, an instinct which helps complete sexual performance because for a moment it drives the level of both carbon dioxide and nitric oxide through the roof to achieve erection maximum.

The increasing and chronic elevation of nitric oxide through deterioration of the metabolism due to dieting, poor diets, and chronic colonization by opportunistic microbes eventually thus causes failure of the libido altogether since mitochondria eventually become chronically inactivated by nitric oxide, hypoxia, and other mitochondrial dysfunction and are then unable to produce enough CO_2 to maintain normal respiration and pH, and erectile dysfunction occurs when the metabolism is such that carbon dioxide production has declined sufficiently that arousal can no longer be achieved. Firstly, the resolution of parasites like *Trichomonas* as discussed in the chapter on immunity is required to restore reproductive function. The first time testing lithium (applied topically) in the restoration of sexual function caused an orgasm which shot ejaculate over my head, at the age of forty-five. Restoration of normal cellular respiration as discussed also in chapter on calcium and respiration such as through the use of dietary oleic acid which potentiates the cytochrome respiratory enzyme and results in greater production of CO_2 also increases reproductive function by improving mitochondrial respiration. In fact, one study on rats showed that tiger nuts, which are high in oleic acid and a traditional, ancient human food source, specifically improved sexual performance and activity as well as testosterone levels. Foods high in oleic acid should make an almost daily appearance in the diet, and restoration of robust CO_2 production results in an immediate increase of CO_2 output after consumption of carbohydrates which is so great it becomes very noticeable as an increase in the rate of breathing and gas exchange required to maintain normal O_2 and CO_2 saturation.

More than carbon dioxide the largest problem of erectile dysfunction is, obviously, a deficit of *testosterone* (regardless of gender), which occurs either from a deficit in synthesis of testosterone or excess conversion to estrogen in a process called aromatization which is also enhanced by parasitism since parasites like *Trichomonas* exploit our estrogen for their reproductive functions. In fact, estrogens are synthesized from androgens like testosterone, and conditions like polycystic ovary syndrome result in failure to produce sufficient estrogens and thus an increase in masculine features (due to parasitism). Before gay men won legal protections we were often forcefully treated with testosterone by stupid, hateful people who knew nothing about biology and surmised that homosexuality was caused by testosterone deficit, but this only had the effect of making gay men hornier and even more gay because hormones merely activate sexual arousal by acting on organs like the brain which already exist, and is instead a process that occurs during gestation and development. Young women with healthy arousal don't have high androgens but they do have a high cellular respiratory rate compared to those with libido problems, and testosterone is still the agent of arousal in women. Due to widespread mischaracterization of cholesterol by the food and medical industry many people also do not realize or know that sex hormones are made from *cholesterol*, and that without properly functioning cholesterol as discussed in the upcoming chapter on hormones it is impossible to make sex hormones required for healthy sexual function and arousal. The entire purpose of cholesterol is simply to transport dietary fats and fat soluble nutrients which are delivered to parts of the body via sulfated glycoproteins like chylomicrons and cholesterol, and while our body can synthesize fats a low fat diet is a great way to impair sex hormone production. Synthesis of hormones also requires *vitamin A* and thus carotene, without which the body cannot make them, and as such both dieting or carotene deficiency is often the first and primary cause of erectile dysfunction— Go eat two large carrots or a bunch of peaches right now and see if you can't get rock hard in fifteen minutes.

But vitamin A synthesis is also inhibited by microbial hydrogen sulfide production in the gut which binds to the enzymes that convert carotene to vitamin A, so if there are any symptoms of malodor like halitosis or smelly feces and flatulence that will be inhibiting normal sex hormone synthesis which must first be treated by using carotene sufficiently frequent to suppress all malodors (remember that ammonia, tannin, sodium, and molybdenum are also required to complete normal metabolism of dietary sulfur). Studies also show that dietary carotene (not supplemental) directly has a protective function for the gonads, but as discussed in previous chapters carotene also requires copper for uptake and transport and carrots are so deficient in copper that while they can be great sources of carotene for healthy people and to inhibit hydrogen sulfide producing microbes it will be required to consume other sources that are also high in copper or with other high copper foods (or a very low dose of supplemental copper) in order to absorb and use carotene. Studies also show that vitamin A lowers cholesterol, which makes sense because too much vitamin A can cause excessive steroidogenesis (and vitamin A toxicity), so the body regulates vitamin A delivery to cells by regulating cholesterol production, and high cholesterol is likely a symptom of poor vitamin A status either from insufficient intake of high carotene foods or microbial hydrogen sulfide production indicative of malodors of the mouth, breath, feces, etc., and oral care products should also not be used, not only because they disable our epithelial polarity defenses against microbes contracted from intimate contact with others as discussed in the chapter on oral health but also because they actively promote copper dysregulation and mask malodors of hydrogen sulfide which must instead be identified and resolved.

The reproductive organs are also designed to handle nitric oxide since it is one of the elements which facilitates arousal, but excess nitric oxide and its inhibition of mitochondrial respiration is also a significant inhibitor of genital regeneration, making the reproductive organs particularly susceptible to nitrogenous stress if the system of nitric oxide regulation is not working properly. The two primary factors which relieve mitochondria of nitric oxide inhibition are *thiols* and *sunlight*. Thiols are a sulfur analog of alcohol derived from dietary sulfur and related to glutathione which helps to protect the mitochondrial respiratory pathway, and red wavelengths of light interact with our primary respiratory enzyme, cytochrome oxidase, and in so doing dislodge nitric oxide through the donation of an electron (which chemically reduces it). Sunlight deficiency, even to the testicles themselves, is a primary cause of libido problems since direct sunlight exposure removes nitric oxide from mitochondria while chronic darkness allows nitric oxide inhibition. During light deficiency nitric oxide migrates to mitochondria to inhibit cytochrome oxidase on purpose to serve as a regulatory mechanism which downregulates the metabolism to preserve nutritional resources and lower oxidative stress. But inadequate sunlight also stimulates a chronic increase in the hormone *melatonin*, which directly inhibits sex hormone production. In fact, high melatonin is the factor by which children are biologically prevented from going through puberty until the appointed time, and the onset of adolescence lowers melatonin to enable the development of secondary sex characteristics which means that deficiency of daily sunlight also actively downregulates the production of sex hormones through chronic elevation of melatonin, but also that taking melatonin as a supplement or medicine also does the same. The role of sunlight liberating testicular mitochondria from inhibition by nitric oxide is why young men who do not go outdoors often enough develop debilitating and premature physical disease and overactive libido accompanied by ironic erectile problems because sunlight deficiency so strongly raises melatonin and nitric inhibition of mitochondria to inhibit healthy sex hormone steroidogenesis, combining to produce young men who are both chronically aroused but also sexually frustrated which then blame other people for not fulfilling their needs rather than neglect of their own health.

It is also this sensitivity to light and light's function on our mitochondria why human testicles are on the outside of the body and sheathed in such a thin layer of skin, not only for temperature regulation as is widely believed but more that the testicles are specifically stimulated and regulated by exposure to sunlight, and studies show that exposure to light actively stimulates testosterone production in the testes by three to five times than otherwise. Many species experience an increase in testicle size and function when exposed to certain qualities of light, and this action of sunlight on the testes is in part why the nature of nitric oxide in sexual health is poorly understood since there is no benefit to increasing nitric oxide for sexual health if there is not also generous sunlight exposure and normal sulfur homeostasis (meaning the absence of pathogenic hydrogen sulfide producers) otherwise an increase in nitric oxide simply serves to suffocate mitochondria and in turn lower testosterone. It is no coincidence that Americans and other highly prudish cultures which avoid being unclothed out of doors or excessively sequestered away from sunlight due to obsessive attitudes about work, career, and discomfort with the human body also suffer from increased metabolic disease such as systemic erectile dysfunction, as achieving generous exposure to sunlight is highly important for cardiovascular and sexual health, but direct sun exposure to the genitals becomes even more important as men age and the tendency of nitric oxide to inhibit mitochondrial respiration increases. Both breast cancer and gynecomastia (enlargement of the breast tissue in males) are caused by *Tricho-monas* colonization of the breast duct and mammary glands (yes, all males have mammary glands), and gynecomastia is an especially specific consequence of insufficient light exposure which would otherwise activate the antiparasitic effect of lithium, and which can be reversed by applying some lithium in water topically to the breast area and then exposing the chest to bright sunlight or strong artificial, warm-spectrum light while also generally treating the entire body with supplemental lithium and light exposure for elimination of parasites from the prostate, testes, etc.

Making matters more complex, there are actually three different types of nitric oxide—*endothelial, inducible*, and *neuronal,* although they are the same molecule and this distinction describes where they are made, and the role of nitric oxide in facilitating health or inhibiting metabolic respiration is actually a more complicated issue than simply total nitric oxide burden on the body. Endothelial nitric oxide is created in the lining of the cardiovascular system and promotes vasodilation which increases the flow of blood and in terms of sexual arousal facilitates engorgement of the reproductive organs. Inducible is that which is produced within cells and its location directly inhibits mitochondrial respiration but also helps protect cells against pathogenic colonization. Neuronal nitric oxide functions within the nervous system to help regulate the nervous system and may also play a role in the inhibition of viruses like herpes which colonize nervous tissue. Nitric oxide rapidly diffuses through cells and each can function like the others and its function depends on its location, not origination, and exogenous nitrates and nitrites like thiamine mononitrate directly contribute to all different types of nitric oxide so they can force arousal in those who are healthy and impair mitochondria and eventually promote erectile dysfunction. Even the use of poppers (inhalable nitrates often abused for recreation) raises nitric oxide stress but they can also even cause excess nitric oxide in partners who did not use them as nitrogen species diffuse so rapidly through all tissue and can enter a body of another person from intimate contact to then inhibit the sexual sensitivity of their sex organs and impair arousal and not only in the person using them. Raising endothelial nitric oxide in preference to inducible is the best way to achieve an active and healthy libido, but because of nitric oxide's effects on mitochondria this also restrains the aging process and resolves sexual compulsion since it is the general ability of mito-chondria to respirate which regulates aging and stress.

Several other nutrients also regulate the production of or balance of nitric oxide and studies have shown that vitamin C deficiency increases inducible nitric oxide but lowers endothelial nitric oxide, which helps downregulate mito-chondrial respiration to prevent oxidative damage during nutritional deficiency. *Anthocyanins* which are the pigments common to purple, blue, and dark red fruits and vegetables like plums, berries, cherries, purple cabbage, and purple potatoes which prevents loss of sugar in the urine as described in the chapter on diabetes also strongly shifts nitric oxide from inducible to endothelial. This occurs because vasodilation promotes increase blood flow to the skin which then risks heat loss, so the body uses the availability of anthocyanins to regulate seasonal adaptability by reducing blood-flow to peripheral tissue during times which may indicate colder weather or reduced food supply when retaining heat is so important. Anthocyanins are very potent and efficient so after repletion can be maintained with regular, small amounts if they prove expensive (and since many anthocyanin sources are converted into preserves, jams, frozen, or juiced this makes their use in the diet very accessible). Studies on animals show that one of the organs in the body which does accumulate anthocyanin are the gonads, and since reproduction activity is often upregulated during favorable seasonal conditions such as occurs when fruit comes into season anthocyanin may directly regulate sexual health and activity. Anthocyanins are thus one of the best ways to promote and enhance a healthy libido, by upregulating the function of endothelial nitric oxide synthase in preference to inducible (beets are colored by *betalain* and it's not certain if betalain has the same function as anthocyanin).

Without a supply of endothelial nitric oxide the libido will not work well and while the body can use nitrates and nitrites to synthesize nitric oxide it is primarily and most healthfully synthesized from the amino acid *citrulline* found in high amounts in *cucurbits* such as watermelon and cucumber, with watermelon being the highest source in nature. Citrulline is interconvertible with arginine, proline, ornithine, glutamine, and glutamate so these are often also discussed as sources of nitric oxide, but arginine is preferentially metabolized by arginase into *urea* and *ornithine* to participate in more important pathways like the urea cycle and the removal of waste ammonia, and if the body only receives arginine and *not* dietary citrulline then endothelial nitric oxide (boner nitric oxide) is actually downregulated in order to preserve arginine for use in urea. Citrulline is efficiently converted into arginine in the body and is actually twice as effective at raising arginine levels than arginine itself, so the body perceives citrulline availability as a marker of the seasonal availability of nutrients and as such also allows endothelial nitric oxide to rise sufficiently only when citrulline is available in the diet, specifically access to watermelon during the growing season in our environment as an evolutionary human animal, so cucurbits should be consumed daily to support reproductive health, the cardiovascular system, immunity, etc.

Nitric also oxide rapidly oxidizes into nitrite and nitrate which then increases the rate of nitric oxide synthesis and thus more rapidly depletes arginine and citrulline, and vitamin C also helps to reduce nitrite and nitrate back into nitric oxide which then both lowers the rate of nitric oxide synthesis and protects cells against the more harmful effects of nitrite and nitrate, which also oxidizes vitamin C to help maintain sufficient ratio of oxidized glutathione to neutralize hydrogen sulfide, and plenty of vitamin C can thus also help increase storage of arginine and citrulline while also protecting the body from the harmful effects of nitric oxide dysregulation. As cucurbits also contain high amounts of molybdenum required for oxidases such as sulfite oxidase which consume nitrite as an oxygen donor to produce usable sulfate from dietary sulfur and hydrogen sulfide cucurbits also directly help maintain and regulate nitric oxide.

One major problem when it comes to failure of libido and sexual function is the decline of physical sensation. This not only creates problems of satisfaction, anticipation, and self-esteem but also destroys the reinforcing physical stimulus of the sex act. When we are young our nervous systems function on pointe, conducting stimuli to the brain without any inhibition. This occurs because our cellular health is more or less running as it should, and cellular respiration is the norm rather than the exception and so electrical conductivity of cells is very high. Over time the nervous system begins to deteriorate from excess stress, a poor diet, pathogens, nitric oxide stress, and contaminants such as bad fats or even toxic metals and pesticides. Bad fats are a primary cause of neurodegeneration because they are unstable in the high heat, high oxygen environment of nerve cells and cause the formation of lipid peroxides, malondialdehyde, or oxylipins which in turn raise nitric oxide and other stress hormones which in turn suppress cellular metabolic rate. You can imagine the energy which is conducted along the nervous system which not only has its own metabolism but also the duty to move electricity from one cell to the next. Moving electricity generates heat too and the nervous system is subject to intense wear and tear if the components are not made of the most sufficient elements. When bad fats, inhibitory metals, or toxic chemicals contaminate nerve cells they impair a cell's ability to run properly. This decrease in metabolic rate causes the cell to swell with extra water as it tries to repair itself but which in turn lowers the conductivity of the cell (this is inflammation), thus slowing down electrical stimulation. This swelling and impairment of conductivity dampens the potent neurological impulses of physical sex, dulling the response to touch and turning the reproductive organs into barely-sensitive vestigial organs. In turn this may make us feel that our partner is no longer alluring or stimulating when in reality our inability to enjoy them because of the decline of the nervous system is at fault.

An especially problematic metal which interrupts the nervous system is *aluminum,* which is ubiquitous in our diets and environment and actually increased by agrochemicals like glyphosate. Aluminum directly impairs the conduction of physical stimulus along the nervous system for a number of reasons—It reduces the metabolic rate of cells and is a poor facilitator for the nervous impulse, which I don't entirely understand but is probably the same reason for aluminum's *specific heat* property, which is a measure of how much energy it takes to raise the temperature of a substance, which is quite different for aluminum when compared to other metals which promote health like zinc, iron, and copper. The presence of aluminum essentially muffles neurological conductivity (which is why it is also implicated in Alzheimer's disease). Aluminum uptake is increased by glyphosate, but it's also usually part of the formulation of glyphosate sprayed on crops, so excess aluminum is supplied along with the very chemical which promotes its absorption, both in the plants we eat and also in our own bodies. Avoiding aluminum exposure by eating organic food, avoiding preservatives, medicines, household products, electric kettles, and aluminum cookware is one necessity to restore the nervous system and sexual sensitivity (restaurants commonly use inexpensive aluminum pans which react with acidic foods). One sneaky source of aluminum is in baking powder, with most popular brands containing aluminum, which is completely unnecessary but contained within a large fraction of baked goods, and aluminum-free products are available.

Simply avoiding aluminum intoxication can allow the body to resolve excess easily but *silicic acid* which is the bioavailable form of silicon derived from plants as discussed in the chapter on cancer also helps the body detoxify aluminum, and mitochondrial respiration such as is facilitated by mitochondrial silicon directly supports neurological conductivity, so restoring silicon metabolism as discussed in that chapter also directly result in the increase of sexual sensitivity and stimulus. Aluminum also directly antagonizes the enzyme which makes endothelial nitric oxide, which means it impairs the mechanism of action for sexual arousal. It has also been shown to concentrate in the pineal gland of rats, which it likely does in us as well, and since the pineal gland is the center of melatonin production it would definitely seem to negatively affect many aspects of health, including sexual function, through this mechanism. So addressing aluminum toxicity by avoiding aluminum products like aluminum baking soda and aluminum cooking pans is one of the most important things a person with arousal dysfunction should do, since the nature of aluminum is so persistent and ambiguous.

Because our mind, which is also a sexual organ, does not so easily lose its ability for arousal since it is the very center of sexual arousal, not the genitals, poor neurological conductivity of physical sexual stimulation then leaves the mind as the only effective tool for eroticism in those with sexual dysfunction which in turn motivates an increased requirement for novel, mental stimulants such as pornography or infidelity for a person to feel sexually stimulated. Most people inexplicably seem to think the genitals are what control sex even though they would have absolutely no function without the brain, which is the primary sex organ, and the genitals are merely sensory organs which respond to but do not control the actual neurological stimulus for arousal. This is also why transgender people are the gender with which they identify, and not that of their genitalia, because it is the brain which controls and mediates sexual and gender function, not genitalia, which are instead merely the tools through which sex and intimacy are expressed, but then used to categorize people by those who are stupid and insecure who wish to feel more in control of life, fear, and anxiety. For those with declining sensitivity of the sex organs and robbed of emotionally satisfying experiences due to excess elevation of nitric oxide and deterioration of the nervous system, sufferers of libido problems can then only enjoy or even engage in sex if the mental capacity is engaged, which with a long-term partner physical satisfaction is then impossible, whereas in those with still-functioning genital sensitivity sex with the same partner can be just as exciting (or more) even after decades of familiarity. Additionally, the repetitious use of one hand position while whacking off accustoms the brain to expect this during sex in those whose neurological health is compromised, and many men mistake the lessened intensity of intercourse for effects of pornography when really the brain is just expecting the same death grip and technique used in masturbation required for those with reduced neurological health. If you have this issue but can still orgasm manually, the next time you watch porn jack off with a different hand using a different technique— You will find the very same difficulty to orgasm that you have during sex, which has nothing to do with pornography and everything to do with neurological health.

Circumcision also greatly compounds problems with sexual function because the removal of nerve endings and scarring of the penis (or removal of the clitoris in female circumcision) further impairs or even eliminates physical stimulation, accelerating the decline of nerve cells required to facilitate sexual health and the normal pair-bonding effect of sexual intercourse. Even in long term relationships physical satisfaction has an undeniable role in the support and maintenance of bonds between couples and when this tool is absent because of circumcision or poor health the sex act not only fails to support physical bonds but can actively undermine pair bonding due to feelings of failure, inadequacy, and frustration in one or both partners. Feeling ashamed of their inability to perform satisfactorily a partner may withdraw from the source of their shame which are encounters with their chosen partner, then the only solution for any type of satisfaction for the natural sex drive are those found in mental stimulation such as is enabled through pornography or novel sex partners and activities. Plenty of physically healthy individuals can engage both in pornography use and also partner sex without difficulty, as it is only when the physical capacity of the nervous system to conduct sexual stimulus fails that the sexual response becomes impaired and pornography or cheating become one of the only options for sexual arousal that it seems like a problem.

Thankfully sexually sensitivity can still be increased in spite of male circumcision, but circumcision and nitric oxide dysfunction can also cause *soft glans* where the glans of the penis fails to tumesce during arousal. The glans has a separate arterial system than the corpus cavernosum (shaft) of the penis which runs along the dorsal side of the male anatomy, and this artery and the glans itself can be damaged by circumcision or the inability of the glans to regenerate itself. A condition called *calciphylaxis*, which is a serious disorder of calcium deposition in skin and fat, proves that glans physiology is separate from the rest of the penis because it causes the glans to become necrotic without doing the same to the rest of the penis, and during even mild calcification the glans can become stiff and fibrotic which impairs tumescence, a trend only exacerbated by circumcision and the absent protection of foreskin, not caused by it. A working glans is a reproductive adaptation to regulate pregnancy by stimulating the vagina to orgasm which in turn causes semen to be siphoned up the vagina into the cervix, and it is much more difficult to achieve vaginal orgasm (sometimes impossible) without a properly tumesced glans. This is no accident of nature, however, as soft glans is a purposeful characteristic of human biology designed to reduce fertilization from metabolically ill males and potentially unhealthy sperm and exactly why the glans is on a separate arousal system than the rest of the penis which then prevents its function in those who are not healthy. The glans is supposed to be as wide or wider than than shaft of the penis and quite prominent when fully tumesced, which then causes greater stimulation of the vagina and, bringing a partner to orgasm, causes the cervix to convulse which then siphons up semen deposited in the vagina.

Glans sensitivity is primarily a function of chloride status, as chloride is fundamental to the function of the nervous system, so poor sensitivity in the glans can also be used as a diagnostic for chloride homeostasis, which is primarily an issue of colonization by pathogens which inhibit chloride absorption and transport as discussed in the chapters on metabolic disease and immunity. Vitamin A is required for tissue morphology and growth, so deficiency of dietary carotene also impairs cellular regeneration and renewal and thus also impairs soft glans regeneration, and because the glans is on a separate arterial channel than the shaft even very young men can suffer from soft glans without ever knowing what a properly working glans is actually like due to poor intake of dietary carotene or colonization by hydrogen sulfide producing microbes. While circumcision can damage the glans of the penis it is a very sensitive organ that also constantly regenerates to facilitate sensitivity to stimulus, and circumcision is not a significant barrier to reversing soft glans and it sis still possible to achieve full erections while having a soft glans which also prevents them from recognizing that anything is wrong, but stimulatory sensitivity is also reduced from soft glans which makes sex less enjoyable and orgasm more difficult to achieve, especially when accompanied by other metabolic issues, and since the glans is meant to stimulate the inside of a vagina a soft glans does not really do this and makes it more difficult for both partners in heterosexual coupling to reach orgasm.

The glans is also shaped like a shovel or scoop because we evolved as human beings in social groups with multiple sex partners (to be clear there is nothing wrong with either monogamy or polyamory) and the human penis evolved to be longer and more complex than our other primate relatives to compete with the sperm of other males by literally scooping out other sperm during intercourse. This is also why males instinctually stop thrusting after orgasm, because doing so would remove their own sperm, and is not a learned behavior but one of instinct. A healthy glans will tumesce significantly when aroused from its flaccid state and have a smooth, more moisturized appearance, where a soft glans does not tumesce much at all, lays flatter against the shaft of the penis, and may be keratinized, dry, and cracked in appearance and evolutionarily prevented a male with soft glans from removing the sperm of other males which were healthy. "Moisturizing" in skin is achieved through ionic channels and fat deposition, not water alone, and the keratinization which occurs in soft glans or from circumcision is specifically evidence of problems metabolizing chloride and other elements such as during thyroid disease or colonization by pathogens which interrupt ATPase channels, and regeneration of the glans and increased sensitivity should be rapid and obvious from successful intervention in pathogenic colonization.

I am convinced that rates of circumcision are *the* major driving factor besides childhood trauma in high rates of divorce, and there is a direct correlation in the aging of circumcised individuals (aging being a promoter of keratinization and fibrosis) and the prevalence of divorce and marital conflict versus other populations who are not circumcised (in countries which do not also prevent divorce). Do you even know *why* you are circumcised? What is the excuse for cutting off the body parts of children? This practice as popularized today was pushed on Western cultures by an insane, child-abusing seventh-day adventist after which a popular cereal company is also named who was convinced that masturbation was the cause of childhood misbehavior, and he engaged in punitive cutting of the foreskin and cauterizing of the clitoris in children without anesthesia whom he personally diagnosed as engaging in masturbation. He championed this to medical boards and institutions and today the practice is continued due to his lunatic, child-predation pseudoscience as if it has any medical justification which it absolutely fucking does not. *Circumcision serves absolutely no medical purpose*, but it does actively cause significant mental trauma which lasts into adulthood, creating men who are more easily frightened, stressed, volatile, and timid, and directly damages the penis which prevents the normal function of sex including the effect of sexual intimacy on pair bonding. Surgeries also on those who are born intersex to make their genitals conform to stereotypes of binary gender conformity can and usually does permanently destroy their genitalia and prevent sexual arousal as an adult, and parents who birth intersex individuals should refrain from this heinous and abusive mutilation of children's private parts which purpose is only to satisfy prejudiced gender ideology of adults without any foundation in medical necessity nor the welfare of the child who should be the one making decisions about their own body when they are older.

Genitals are not parameters of existence nor a leash for our self-conception but are tools through which we connect emotionally and intimately to each other and reproduce as a species, and the use of genitals as a litmus for indoctrination into cultural fraternities or stereotypical gender expectations are merely the machinations of emotionally traumatized adults and systems of control and authoritarianism who use the body as an anchor in a world which can be inconsistent, surprising, and sometimes even frightful but which only serve to inflame those problems, not solve them. Circumcision is a mutilation of God-given body parts, parts which have a *necessary* biological purpose to perform for our wellbeing and engender pair bonding or else they would not be there, and I cannot fathom how when asked to remove a piece of their infant child's body for no legitimate medical purpose any parent could possibly respond with *yes*. The only correct answer is *no*. The reproductive organs are not meant to be carved up, and any person who believes that circumcision is beneficial for anyone does not consider how the removal of the system which creates biological pair bonding can do anything but harm a person and prevent their ability to bond with their mate later in their lives. Males deprived of their full sexual functioning during the entirety of a relationship due to the harm of circumcision later find themselves impotent with a chosen partner after the novelty and mental arousal wanes, increasing shame and guilt associated with failure to fulfill and embody the sexual stereotype in which they find themselves. Then, not understanding their situation and emotionally dulled by excess nitric oxide and scarring and years of mental dissociation reach for the only salves which will assuage their sexual ego which are the stimulation of pornography or novelty of adultery as their only options to any kind of satisfying sex life, or their husbands and wives frustrated by the emotional wall which arises from this situation do the same.

Because the genitals are directly connected to the cardiovascular system their function and quality of tumescence is also a direct reflection of cardiovascular health, and the size and quality of arousal in both men and women can also be used as a diagnostic tool to evaluate health of the cardiovascular system in general since low blood volume prevents adequate tumescence of the sex organs. Because the protein albumin is the primary mediator of blood volume and dysfunction of the genitals is a warning sign the cardiovascular system is under stress and deficient in water this is mostly a function of albumin status as discussed in the chapter on vascular insufficiency. Cinnamic acids which help restrain the hydroxyl radical and promote ATPase channels that maintain electrolyte and water status are also a powerful inhibitor of inducible nitric oxide and nitrosative stress and can strongly help to reverse erectile dysfunction and sexual compulsion. In fact high, daily doses of cinnamon, turmeric, or ginger daily in addition to other steps to resolve nitric oxide dysfunction (especially adequate sun exposure) can completely resolve compulsive sexual arousal and lower libido to a normal level in a matter of days.

Consumption of nitrates has been historically used to increase nitric oxide for functions like arousal and while a healthy body can effectively convert low doses of nitrate into nitric oxide metabolic illness instead results in excess nitrate and nitrite which more strongly disrupt respiration and immunity through the binding of heme based proteins like cytochrome or peroxidases as is relevant to HIV and immune function. Acids reduce nitrate and nitrite so dietary sources of nitrate like leafy greens are safer to consume when treated with acids like lemon juice or vinegar before consumption, or pre-boiled and drained beforehand. Human nitrite reductase is dependent on heme and molybdenum, both of which are impaired by microbial hydrogen sulfide. Turmeric can also scavenge nitrate and reactive nitrogen species and can compliment efforts to resolve dysfunctional libido and lower sexual compulsion. A temporary and strict nitrate avoidance diet can even more strongly improve the health of the sex organs and result in rapid and obvious increases in the volume and force of ejaculate as well as endurance and stamina during sex since this doing so both liberates mitochondria to respirate and deprives harmful *Streptomyces* of their respiratory substrate and production of harmful antibiotics like avidin and roseoflavin. A low nitrate diet is very hard to accomplish so while this can be helpful it is not feasible in the long term and restoration of stomach acid, vitamin C, anthocyanin, oxidases, cucurbits, and sunlight which regulate normal metabolism of nitrate is more effective.

Sometimes during sex there is also a discrepancy between solo performance and that with a partner where erections are possible until there is another actual person involved. This is often termed *performance anxiety* but is not really about anxiety at all and a man may be perfectly confident going in to an encounter and still meet boner failure. Sexual arousal stimulates the release of adrenaline in order to raise the metabolic rate so that our body can meet the demands of physical exertion by increasing the influx of sodium and glucose to produce more energy, but because sodium also maintains blood volume the condition of performance anxiety is caused by excessive loss of blood volume as described in the chapter on vascular insufficiency wherein there is not enough sodium (or chloride) in the bloodstream to maintain normal water volume and thus erection once adrenaline activates the increase flux of sodium into tissues. The enzyme *renin* stimulates transfer of water from blood to surrounding tissues through the function of chloride and sodium for things like intracellular water needs or sweating, and is activated by the release of adrenaline, so higher adrenaline expression caused in the first place by low sodium or low carbohydrate (such as occurs from diabetes or dieting) causes even more loss of sodium and water. So an encounter with a sexual partner stimulates adrenaline release, either from simple anticipation and excitement or actual physical exertion, and this then stimulates water efflux from the bloodstream to the surrounding tissues which then lowers blood pressure and impairs tumescence.

Renin release is also inhibited by sodium, and sweating profusely during sex is an excellent warning sign of colonization by *Trichomonas* and other pathogens which produce ammonia and consume sugars required to activate sodium absorption and transport to thus promote excess water loss from sweating. Sex is a primary transmission factor for opportunistic microbes like *Trichomonas* but any close contact during immune deficiency can and does result in colonization. Reversal of blood volume loss by resolving parasites, calcium dysregulation, ammonia, oxylipin, vitamin E deficiency, and acidifying supplemental salt (sodium chloride) with tannin and dietary acids like lemon juice, tannin, etc., can rapidly help restore blood volume if other dietary and metabolic stress like dieting, excess exercise, and light deficiency are discontinued. Not much salt is required to reverse this problem, since the issue is impaired absorption and transport, and once absorbed the body retains sodium and chloride for quite a while but a low dose can be used two or three times a day until blood volume is restored which will be made obvious by the return of rock hard erections. Contraction of the muscles which prevent blood flow into the corpus cavernosum is also mediated through calcium channels (these muscles relax during stimulation which allows in blood), so dysregulation of calcium such as what promotes parasitism and aging also then prevents tumescence by keeping contraction sustained, and resolution of calcium dysregulation then not only helps to solve problems like parasitism and blood volume but also restores greater relaxation of the smooth muscle which facilitates arousal.

Not many foods pharmacologically upregulate testosterone but mushrooms and sorghum are two options. Sorghum also contains cyanide which strongly promotes reproductive health by promoting the immune system. Most herbs are actually estrogenic, even those which are promoted to improve virility (meaning medicinal herbs, not culinary herbs which are used in far lower amounts), so it is safer *not* to use herbs meant to "treat" any disease and to instead simply address diet and environmental strategies as discussed in this book. For instance while herbs like *saw palmetto* are claimed to increase arousal they do so by strongly promoting inducible nitric oxide which strongly impairs mitochondrial respiration and accelerates aging and lowers energy production and CO_2 output, so even if it helps you get some stronger erections now it will cause their elimination later, but promoting mitochondrial respiration instead as described in this book will both increase arousal quality now and in the future. Seminal fluid is also rich in fructose, and the *leydig cells* of the testicles which produce testosterone are shown to release more testosterone in the presence of fructose, so it would seem that a diet with adequate fructose is also important for semen function and testosterone production. As discussed in the chapter on cardiovascular disease, the epithelial sodium channels which take up sodium to promote expansion of blood volume on which erectile volume is dependent are also activated by fructose, so low sugar diets actually promote erectile dysfunction by lowering the amount of sodium which is absorbed into the body. This likely occurs as a regulatory mechanism to lower the metabolic rate when sugar is scarce in the environment since sodium drives cellular metabolism, but it also means that erectile quality cannot be restored without the frequent use of sugar, and supplementing some extra salt in something very sugary such as fruit juice, lemonade, or even some sugar water can help to more rapidly restore erectile quality. Those who are very ill whom present with hypertension will also need to address that, however, through increased dietary potassium and daily sun exposure to reverse calcium dysregulation and hormones of torpor which promote cardiovascular stress.

The loss of testosterone to estrogen through the process of *aromatization* is the second biggest factor for insufficient testosterone. This is a natural process in our bodies because estrogen is necessary for growth, tissue regeneration, and cellular division and thus aromatization of testosterone to estrogen is necessary for staying alive and healthy. Aromatization even participates in sexual function, for instance the inflammatory properties of estrogen help any organs which require water in the production of secretory, voluminous fluids such as seminal fluid or breast milk to acquire sufficient water for those purposes. But hormone balance also determines the appearance of the body and because all humans regardless of gender also have nipples and mammary glands excessive aromatization can cause cis-gendered men to grow breasts and develop soft feminine features even while being bigoted toward those who are transgender who chose to alter their appearance on purpose. By the way, transitioning is not what makes a transgender person transgender and they are transgender whether they transition or not, and if hormones and genitals were the determining factor in gender all cisgender, heterosexual men would transition to identifying as female or gay as they age and produce as much estrogen as women not on their cycle because of high rates of aromatization which soften their bodies and stimulate gynecomastia (enlargement of the breasts).

While aromatization plays an important role in endocrine homeostasis and tissue growth the aging process and metabolic disease increases the rate of aromatization and this problem is especially amplified in males during sexual arousal because arousal is achieved by the release of testosterone from its chaperone *sex hormone binding globulin* which allows testosterone into cells, but free testosterone is susceptible to aromatization so arousal and orgasm during states of metabolic disease such as is caused by colonization with microbial hydrogen sulfide producers and sunlight deficiency results in greater rates of testosterone aromatization to estrogen. Oppositely in healthy men with normal thiol status and daily sun exposure arousal and orgasm causes an increase in masculinization from free testosterone which is instead oppositely converted to more of the active form of testosterone, *dihydrotestosterone*. Specific sexual dimorphic characteristics of low aromatization and high dihydrotestosterone in males are larger, hairier, more vascular forearms as well as chest and body hair that appears to collect toward the center sagittal plane (the center dividing line of the body) rather than being evenly distributed across the torso, to advertise a healthier physical body and thus increase in sexual attraction. Interestingly, free copper oxidizes cholesterol from which steroids are synthesized (which then also causes atherosclerosis) but vitamin C in both its oxidized and reduced forms also scavenges copper, and studies show that free copper inhibits synthesis of dihydrotestosterone which indicates this is a purposeful biological change in response to vitamin C deficiency, and since vitamin C is also required to synthesize cholesterol the strongest promoter of high dihydrotestosterone and characteristic male dimorphic features is vitamin C status, though vitamin C metabolism is quite complex and is discussed in the chapter on thyroid. Unexpectedly, the far greater rate of aromatization of testosterone actually occurs in the testicles themselves, so males with metabolic illness can benefit a great deal by raising the metabolic rate and getting light exposure to the testicles (either from sunlight or bright, warm artificial light) to raise their metabolic rate while avoiding chronic sunlight deficiency which will oppositely promote aromatization.

Both aging cisgender women and transgender women usually receive only estrogen in hormone therapy and since estrogen is a hormone of growth which is accomplished through influx of water into cells and inhibition of mitochondria by nitric oxide they in turn see more rapid acceleration of aging, including loss of libido and hair, and should instead use *progesterone* as the primary female hormone, supported by lower doses of estrogen. Likewise, transgender men and aging cisgender men usually only receive testosterone in hormone therapy in part because it is wrongly believed that dihydrotestosterone (DHT), contributes to hair loss, but DHT does not easily aromatize the way testosterone does so cisgender and transgender men with any metabolic stress see very slow results from using testosterone only. *Dehydroepiandrosterone* (DHEA) can also be supplemented in transgender men or aging men to promote more masculine features along with testosterone and dihydrotestosterone since DHEA does not require a prescription but has fairly strong androgen properties. Progesterone can and does also improve libido and fertility in both men and women because an excess of estrogen to progesterone ratio regardless of gender can be caused by dieting, poor nutrition, lack of sunlight, consumption of legumes, parasitism, and exposure to endocrine disrupting chemicals. Because of problems with aromatization, taking exogenous steroids like testosterone for purposes of bodybuilding come with horrific side effects such as the enlargement of the skull, protruding navels, liver damage, and shrunken testicles as the body attempts to resolve the excess caused by abuse. The "need" to supplement hormones in the first place is often a way to cope with destructive dietary and behavioral habits like eating low-carb, fasting, or drug or alcohol abuse which lower the metabolic rate to increase aromatization and production of catabolic hormones like cortisol which make it difficult or even impossible to grow muscle naturally as discussed in the upcoming chapter on muscle which then also disrupts libido and sexual function, and hormones should only ever be taken when it is absolutely necessary.

A problem which very much mimics the aromatization of testosterone into estrogen are phytoestrogens called *isoflavones* from leguminous foods like beans and lentils, especially things like soy and flax but can even come from delicious pinto and black beans since all legumes are producers of strongly estrogenic isoflavones. Not all phytoestrogens have strong estrogenic properties but isoflavones can be a problem when eaten frequently (peas are an exception and quite low, however, but whether they are true legumes is apparently also a point of debate). In healthy women the effects of dietary phytoestrogens are almost imperceptible because high levels of progesterone block the growth effects of estrogen from inhibiting mitochondrial respiration, but anyone without significant quantities of progesterone such men, aging women, and transgender women the effects of phytoestrogens can be quite harmful and even contribute to problems like hair loss as described in that upcoming chapter. In healthy people the occasional consumption of legumes is not a problem because isoflavones can be easily detoxified through the liver, but since detoxification pathways can be disrupted by sulfate reducing microbes they and other harmful substances can be repeatedly recirculated into the body as if they were far greater quantities. Since all legumes are high in isoflavones they should not be dietary staples in anyone experiencing metabolic stress of any kind, especially the avoidance of soy products, and legumes should instead be replaced by low phytoestrogen foods like fruit, vegetables, and properly prepared grains. Because phytoestrogens stimulate inducible nitric oxide legumes can also contribute to sexual compulsion. For the same reasons an alternative to pharmaceutical estrogen for aging women or transgender women is the use of hibiscus tea or hibiscus root as they contain very high levels of phytoestrogens, but these too must also be complimented by generous use of progesterone to prevent negative effects. The root of hibiscus is so high in estrogen, in fact, it can also potentially cause miscarriage as estrogen causes the uterus to contract to shed the uterine lining and thus disrupt a pregnancy, and is shown in studies to be a potential abortifacient and should not be taken during pregnancy.

Because good fats are stable in the human body and do not result in lipid peroxidation or the inflammatory prostaglandins they are another of the reasons men have a long history of enjoying foods like beef as ruminants have bacteria in their gut which convert bad fats into good fats (ruminants are animals with multi-chambered stomachs like cows, sheep, goats, bison, deer, etc.). But beef is also high in iron and a potential target of ammonia producing parasites and pathogens so high meat intake is then also why high meat diets also results in rapid aging and severe metabolic disease, and these good fats can also be gotten from things like hazelnuts, almonds, macadamia nuts, olives and olive oil, butter and cream, coconut oil, shea butter, etc., and a diet based in plant foods which accomplish the same underlying principles is healthier due to higher amounts of important libido promoting nutrients like silicon, vitamin K, oxalate, tannin, carotene, potassium, magnesium, sugar, etc., if the gut microbiome is capable of breaking down plant foods as described in the chapter on gut health. Coconut oil being very high in lauric acid strongly stimulates the synthesis of pregnenolone, the master hormone of the body, which can in turn supply ample amounts of testosterone, progesterone, estrogen, and other sex hormones but which then also rapidly uses up vitamin A which then can give the appearance of hormone deficiency which in reality is a deficiency of dietary carotene (or inability to convert it to vitamin A). To stimulate extra production of all helpful hormones it is then as easy as using coconut oil regularly while taking care to get ample dietary carotene. In fact, the largest promoter of aromatization is itself a carotene and vitamin A deficiency since they also function as lipid-associated antioxidants, so if you want to restore your erectile function rapidly (and health in general), having orange and yellow fruits and vegetables every day can saturate the body with sufficient nutrients to inhibit aromatization and thus restore normal testosterone production (if eating too much results in *carotenemia* or discoloration of the skin take a break then cut back on quantity, but not frequency).

Endocrine disrupting chemicals like dioxins, flame retardants, non-stick chemicals, many plastic chemicals, chemical cosmetic products, and certain artificial food additives are also major impediments to reproductive health and wellness because they directly interfere with normal hormonal function. Dioxins originate from industrial pollutants, pesticides, and non-organic fertilizers and because dioxin is lipophilic it accumulates in fat, so chickens, cattle, and pigs which eat feed laden with fertilizer and pesticides concentrate dioxin in their own fat and then we consume this concentrated food in the form of non-organic meat and dairy products, although the same process happens to our own fats when consuming pesticide laden produce and processed foods, especially ones dense in vegetable fats like soy and canola oils which also concentrate the lipophilic dioxins. Dioxin also has an *extremely* long half-life (7-30 years depending on the type) so it does not degrade sufficiently once it is present in food or body tissues. People like Dr. Harvey Wiley fought so that we could have safe food but corrupt and dishonest manufacturers always try to adulterate products to increase profit margins at the expense of people and there are a great many more chemicals and adulterants in industry than ever and a great vigilance must be maintained if we are to avoid being poisoned and killed by the demons of capitalism which is best achieved by eating locally, organically, regeneratively, and getting personally involved in politics and running for office (or in party leadership which is often more influential) to help create and maintain regulations that protect farmers, the environment, and the food supply. One very sneaky way in which chemical toxins enter our bodies is through clothing, bedding, carpets, flooring, and furniture. Textiles and home decor products are increasingly manufactured with harmful plastics and chemicals which are unregulated and not disclosed to the consumers. Polyester and other synthetic fabrics are made from petroleum chemicals, but harmful chemicals are also sprayed onto clothing to impart marketable slogans like wrinkle-free or certain finishes, and coming in direct skin contact with these products causes endocrine disrupting and carcinogenic chemicals to diffuse into the skin and then into the body. I once owned a blanket gifted to me which made my skin felt sticky and tacky whenever my bare skin touched it (so it went in the trash). I used to shop at a famous clothing store because of their tall sizes but increasingly their shirts and tops began making my skin feel soapy and I now avoid all their products. Besides buying 100% natural or organic textiles, clothing, and bedding, there is an easy way to detect products that will cause these problems which is that if touching a product causes the skin to feel soapy, sticky, or otherwise changed from the way it was before this means there are harmful endocrine disrupting chemicals on or in the product and it and all other products made by that manufacturer should be avoided entirely.

Many medications such as *finasteride* strongly lower testosterone, which is the entire point of many hair-loss pharmaceuticals due to incorrect conception of testosterone in in the etiology of hair loss as discussed in that upcoming chapter. Most medications cannot be used without experiencing significant side effects, and the pharmaceutical industry exists not to cure illness but to make money, which is also why they torture of animals in the name of research, because the end purpose is also the exploitation of suffering people for their own financial benefit, and it is best to avoid all medications as is reasonably possible, especially if the reason for their use is one of vanity like hair loss, acne, weight loss, etc. The active form of testosterone, *dihydrotestosterone* (DHT) is necessary for the most masculine of male physical qualities and thus these medications are a type of chemical castration and stopping their use while addressing dietary, behavioral, pathogenic, and environmental factors which affect sex hormones will restore many normal biological pathways since all systems in the body are intertwined and dependent on each other.

Testosterone is also specifically made in accordance with a high rate of *calcium* flux through the gonads (testicles and ovaries) since calcium is an important factor in the function of the endoplasmic reticulum where products of cellular function are produced, which means that both calcium deficiency and calcification of the reproductive organs due to dysregulation of calcium metabolism in diets also low in oxalate, vitamin K, and deficiency of sunlight and vitamin D is a primary cause of hypogonadism and hyposteroidogenesis and thus libido problems and deterioration of the reproductive system and organs. Because calcium is needed to supply this function but can also cause problems with calcification the active consumption of high calcium foods like leafy greens, nuts, or dairy will help support robust testosterone synthesis and calcium should always, always be accompanied and maintained by dietary oxalate and vitamin K while supporting vitamin D synthesis in anyone who is experiencing health issues. Because dairy is a good source of calcium and can be made useful through its combination with dietary sources of vitamin K and oxalate such as brewing milk in tea or preparing many traditional green such as creamed spinach (a little calcium powder added to leafy greens could be an alternative for those who cannot have dairy) this is not too difficult to accomplish.

Some men suffer from the opposite of erectile dysfunction and instead exhibit what is called *premature ejaculation*, where a man ejaculates quickly at the onset of sexual intercourse. There is much speculation about the causes of this condition, especially ones of a psychological nature, which is ridiculous because the mind does not control nervous stimulation impulses (the brain can send signals but does not regulate what is received) and shows a total lack of understanding about the physical body and what role the psyche actually plays (or does not play) in the health of the body. I agree with the marginalized notion that premature ejaculation is caused by *prostatitis*, which is inflammation of the prostate, because this inflammation would make the prostate more susceptible to estrogen which in turn increases its sensitivity to contraction and thus it would go off with much less required stimulation than those without the condition. This same kind of problem occurs in those who have to urinate frequently, where the contraction of the bladder is sensitized under the influence of higher estrogen, or even miscarriage when there is insufficient production of progesterone and the uterus contracts prematurely. The cure for premature ejaculation is simply reducing inflammation through a diet such as what is recommended by this book, avoiding common inflammatory factors like common wheat and concentrated sources of polyunsaturated fats like vegetable oils and soy, and resolving colonization by opportunistic pathogens as premature ejaculation is primarily caused by microbial infection of the prostate and likely reflects colonization also by *Trichomonas* such as what also causes urinary tract infections and yeast infections since inflammation is often a response to infection. One study on premature ejaculation using antibiotics showed a near total resolution of the condition with no recurrence afterward. Many of those whom I coach found total resolution of premature ejaculation simply from dietary changes and the use of aspirin, which strongly opposes inflammation and slightly inhibits bacterial and viral infection, but restoration of vitamin A and other immune factors as discussed in that chapter will also help resolve this issue.

Much like melatonin, when it comes to both arousal and physical stimulus, lactic acid also plays a large role in the diminishing of the sex response because lactic acid also directly inhibits mitochondrial respiration as as response to environmental stresses such as excessive physical exertion or deficiency of thiamine. Most people are familiar with lactic acid as it relates to working out (*"Bro—I'm so sore after my sesh'.» "That's lactic acid, bro!"*). But lactic acid is also in a lot of food choices such as yogurt and sauerkraut, where as discussed in the chapter on gut health yogurt also supplants our healthy microbiome with one which excessively produces lactic acid, and bacterial lactic acid is even more potent than the type made by our own body, and prevents healthy levels of testosterone, erections, sleep, and many other desirable health benefits. In severe metabolic illness lactic acid is produced even when not working out, such as at night, or all the time as happens in diabetes, hypothyroidism, or cancer. It is imperative to remove foods which contain appreciable amounts of lactic acid from the diet, like yogurt, and to restore a healthy gut microbiome.

The element boron is also shown in many studies and observational experience to increase testosterone and arousal, and in fact a boron deficiency due to poor intake of *Prunus* fruits like apricots, peaches, nectarines, and plums is extremely detrimental to the effectiveness of the reproductive system, as well as the health of bones, teeth, and the immune system (grapes and raisins are also high boron, though). Boron achieves an increase in testosterone by liberating testosterone and other sex hormones from their chaperone protein, *sex hormone binding globulin* (SHBG). It likely does this by changing SHBG from a lipophilic state (fat) to one of hydrophilic (water), because boron has a high affinity for making hydrogen bonds. Sex hormone binding globulin is very important because it prevents hormones from prematurely interacting with cells and tissues they are not supposed to. For instance, estrogen is a hormone of growth so free estrogen unbound by SHBG can stimulate any cell in the body to induce growth responses. By binding hormones, SHBG prevents this from occurring except where it is supposed to. But since boron is required to liberate sex hormones a deficiency in boron ends up causing sex hormone binding globulin to never release its hormones, thus causing hormone deficiency in spite of an abundance of it. Boron also has a strong relationship with calcium regulation where during a boron deficiency parathyroid hormone activity is increased as calcium is lost from the body in higher rates and significantly more calcium is leached from the bones. Boron is shown to stop the loss of many elements likely because of its resistance to forming chemical bonds with most elements. When the body is deficient in boron it must then support the sex drive with stress hormones like luteinizing hormone which over time destroy metabolic health and reduce hormone circulation. Boron is part of the reason why we grow a skeleton during youth, which acts a reservoir for trace nutrients like boron which are needed in adulthood, and so poor childhood nutrition (especially deficient in fruit) can result in early-onset boron deficiency as an adult, since it's not abundantly available in the diet, which in turn results in premature libido dysfunction when boron is eventually depleted. But because boron is also needed for immune function and our commensal microbiome, problems like libido dysfunction due to poor boron intake always correlate with conditions like oral disease, fatigue, and gut dysbiosis.

Albumin binds more hormones than sex hormone binding globulin but less strongly (by about 4-fold), and a symptom of successful elevation of albumin as discussed in the chapter on vascular insufficiency can be a surprising and abrupt decline in libido since less free testosterone will be circulating in the body. Albumin also binds and carries boron which also liberates hormones from it as well so this side effect is a specific symptom of boron deficiency caused by albumin deficiency (which promotes boron loss) then sudden repletion (which then binds all circulating sex hormones). As discussed in the chapter on vitamin D, boron absorption is dependent on endogenous production of malic acid from the citric acid cycle and is likewise disrupted by problems like vitamin D deficiency, sunlight deprivation, or the presence of excess ammonia. Boron absorption is so sensitive and we require so little that ammonia excess is typically the primary causative factor in its deficiency, and if eating any raisins, prunes, plums, or other high boron foods or a low dose supplement does not result in the near immediate restoration of libido this is a definite sign of other problems like ammonia excess which requires dietary citrulline (also acidified as discussed in chapter on pathogens and metabolic disease) to resolve.

Some controversy exists around boron supplementation because some studies also show boron to increase estrogen in men, but others show significant decline in estrogen and increase in testosterone and this disparity occurs because the high rates of aromatization in sluggish metabolisms and low mitochondrial respiration is the etiological factor, so more liberated testosterone in high-aromatizing individuals means more estrogen while high-metabolism and low aromatizing means less estrogen and higher testosterone. Because of this, boron supplementation should be used only when first supported by changes to diet and behavior which strongly elevate the metabolic rate as measured by the pulse and temperature diagnostic, especially daily sunlight exposure, otherwise boron supplementation risks excess aromatization (in both men and women). When used in a high metabolic state and well fed body will instead promote greater testosterone and actually reduce aromatization, and should be avoided at times like winter when sunlight exposure is not possible. Because it does release sex hormones too much boron can also result in a general ache in and around the genitals because of excessive free testosterone aromatizing into estrogen and it should never be used in excess (no more than 6-9 mg per day, depending on size) and if this occurs take a break before resuming much lower doses taken less frequently since this indicates a high rate of aromatization.

Ironically, aromatization of testosterone to estrogen in men happens primarily in the testicles because of reduced mitochondrial respiration. But, unknown even to the research and medical professions, are that common fungal dermatophytes such as which cause jock rash are the primary cause of this problem, and that anyone who gets jock rash or other acute manifestations of dermatophytosis will also have chronic colonization with those fungi. These fungal pathogens like *Trichophyton* target keratin and keratinocytes, so their presence in the skin also destroys the skin's structure, but their location also prevents the immune system from eradicating them because the immune system cannot reach the corneum stratum (the furthest, outer layer of skin). Contrary to commonly accepted, stupid characterizations of these conditions they are not caused by poor hygiene (I have great hygiene and it would still occur), as these fungi get their moisture by causing water leakage from sites of colonization, and cannot be eradicated with cleaning products, and even pharmacological treatments take weeks and months and also do not prevent reinfection.

No matter gender, most adults are chronically colonized by dermatophytes, and symptoms like redness, itchiness, rough or scaly skin, and dark veins of the inner thighs, scrotum, penis, vulva, labia, perineum, and even the anus are symptoms of chronic dermatophyte colonization, and these sites will also redden more noticeably than surrounding skin on sexual arousal or exposure to sunlight, and the skin of the entire pelvic region should not redden, even during sexual arousal, which is instead caused by these fungal pathogens and is a highly causal reason for many symptoms of metabolic disease. These dermatophytes prefer lower temperatures, and produce ammonia to disrupt the normal pH, lower circulation to the groin and reproductive organs, and inhibit the immune system, and the resultant hypoxic environment increases aromatization of testosterone in the testes. The upcoming chapter on skin health details how to eliminate these dermatophytic infections which will be required to do if presenting with these symptoms to recover full health of the reproductive organs.

As discussed in the chapters on pathogens and skin health, yeasts achieve colonization of the human body in part through production of oxidized lipid products such as *oxylipins* which are normally inhibited by vitamin E, and one mechanism of action of oxylipin is to impair chloride transport which then causes chloride deficiency, so colonization with dermatophytes is an obvious symptom both of vitamin E deficiency and deficiency of chloride, even if the diet is high in salt since absorption of salt is actually required to benefit from it. Even when the diet is high in vitamin E a deficiency can still can also still occur due to saponification of fats and fat soluble nutrients in the gut by other opportunistic pathogens as discussed in the chapter on calcium (which is a problem in turn of calcium dysregulation and low dietary oxalate), although this is fairly easy to also control using foods high in oxalate which binds calcium in the gut to prevent pathogenic access. Almonds for instance are high in both vitamin E and oxalate, and sprouted, roasted, salted almonds are extremely delicious but also actively promote chloride repletion since they have all the required factors to achieve this. Purslane is a widely used vegetable that happens to be extremely high in chloride, vitamin E, and oxalate, and when eaten regularly can also easily promote chloride homeostasis. Those with severe metabolic illness such as diabetes, cystic fibrosis, and cancer will find more rapid resolution when using a small dose of natural, supplemental vitamin E with salt mixed into juice or sugar water (after having also addressed saponification and ammonification of the gut). Such rapid restitution of sodium and chloride can sometimes contribute to problems like hypertension and restless leg syndrome (discussed in the chapter on sleep) if also deficient in potassium and boron, which should also be prevented and treated by consuming high potassium and boron foods like an abundance of fruit or a low dose supplement of each.

Early in my recovery I used topical vitamin E to the genitals to inhibit aromatization of testosterone to estrogen, as vitamin E is shown in studies to downregulate the enzyme aromatase, but it turns out its primary mechanism was from the inhibition of oxylipin produced by opportunistic dermatophytes that specifically target the urogenital tissues, and topical application is not the most effective route, but internally, accompanying salt or other chloride source which, over a rapid time, will naturally resolve the infections. Many people also have salt hunger, as discussed in the chapter on diabetes, which is another manifestation of salt malabsorption such as caused by microbial oxylipin and deficiency of vitamin E. There are also many claimed treatments for dermatophytosis, but mostly they are based on in vitro studies which are not at all replicable in vivo and do not actually work. One additionally strategy, however, is that caffeine is shown in studies to also disturb dermatophyte physiology and caffeine can penetrate into tissues to help more rapidly suppress dermatophytes, and use of caffeinated beverages is probably also a self-medication for resistance to pathogenic yeasts. But since it is chloride deficiency mediated by vitamin E deficiency which actually permits these conditions, other treatments are not ultimately helpful anyway and vitamin E and chloride homeostasis simply must be restored.

Generally when testicles are drawn up near the body this indicates lower testosterone production due to lower metabolic rate and cooler body temperature, and a relaxed scrotum indicates high metabolic temperature and thus high testosterone production. This behavior of the scrotum can be a great barometer for measuring male hormone production but older men's testicles droop all the time due to factors like dermatophytes and a high rate of aromatization which reduces total testosterone which the testicles attempt to resolve by increased testosterone production but which then simply sustains its aromatization to estrogen (which then just becomes a sustaining cycle) and thus also high estrogen circulation which further promotes parasites and other opportunistic microbes.

Unfortunately, most men don't realize the importance of maintaining erection health until we've lost it, but we can help other men by not being embarrassed about stupid things like erectile dysfunction and health problems. Show your confidence in the face of adversity, which is actually a real characteristic of manhood unlike the pretended and chauvinist attitudes of those who are insecure. Warn and speak up about sexual health, help those who are burdened by sexual compulsivity, and stop the encouragement of unhealthy habits like starvation, excessive exercise, alcoholic bingeing, sex-shame, misogynistic attitudes toward women, and the mutilation of children's reproductive organs with circumcision. Many women assume their premature loss of libido is just a natural state for women, which it absolutely is not, and sexuality should be enjoyed for many decades of adulthood, and a healthy endocrine system can promote pair bonding and increase feelings of attraction toward partners and help stabilize marriages and romantic unions. Fortunately you can, as I did, restore your boner powers pretty easily simply by addressing pathogenic colonization and dietary deficiencies as discussed in other relevant chapters of this book. GABA therapy discussed in the upcoming chapter on sleep is especially effective at regenerating the glans and other parts and functions of the reproductive organs.

For those with predatory sexual compulsions, the roots of this burden are born in unfortunate childhood traumas and excess nitric oxide which compels sexual arousal and can be resolved through continuous, daily supplementation of cinnamic acids to suppress inducible nitric oxide along with practice of inventory therapy as discussed in the chapter on spirituality to resolve resolve control behaviors within the subconscious which underlie such predatory behavior and thus relieve motivations to cause harm, as may also those who are victims of sexual abuse and trauma to find freedom from it which themes are explored more deeply in my book on psychology, *The Perfect Child*.

Hepatitis viruses can be transmitted through sexual activity (although some of them can be food-borne too), and they can cause permanent liver damage which itself can be life-threatening. I knew someone who died at the age of thirty-four from drinking too much because he had hepatitis, which impairs the liver's ability to detoxify things like alcohol. So it's very important to get vaccinated for hepatitis when young adults begin sexual activity.

Also, penis size is commonly a point of insecurity among men, even when they're not actually small, but this is not entirely a social construct as many people might characterize, as being an upright walking human shifted the genitals to be forward facing and thus a directly observable characteristic (as were the breasts). Insecurity is never solved by eliminating the thing which makes us insecure, for instance many lean and thin people are constantly insecure about their appearance, and even those with big penises are often insecure about the perception of their size. Such shallow insecurities are a result of trauma and fears of rejection as what underpin human evolutionary psychology as discussed in *The Perfect Child* and are *only* resolved through the resolution of unresolved trauma and our conceptions of self-worth, but the penis does in fact grow or shrink according to several specific health parameters, and when ill the penis can get smaller while those which are healthy but also possessed of very specific nutrient and health factors will experience an increase in penis size both of the flaccid and erect states which both function generally as an advertisement of physical health. This does not mean that those with large penises are inherently healthy, because health can always be lost, but for each person with a penis the size and quality will change relative to each person according to the fulfillment of those requisite states. Besides having adequate testosterone, the primary factor for overall penis size is the quality of the immune system as described in the chapter on immunity, where penis size is primarily an advertisement of robust immunity and thus ability to resist contraction of disease which can and does occur in sex. The flaccid size is a function of dietary anthocyanin, which increases endothelial nitric oxide production to relax cardiovascular tissue such as what composes nearly the entirety of the penis, which also likely serves an evolutionary purpose to reduce loss of penises to frostbite by pulling them closer to the body at times such as winter when fruit is not available in the environment, and may or may not affect people in varying degrees depending on genetic heritage.

Lastly, morning wood is different than sexual arousal, although its eventual disappearance as a reliable indicator of youth can catch men off guard when they suddenly wake up one morning without that rock hard erection digging into the mattress. Women also get morning wood, but a penis makes it more obvious, and morning wood is a reliable indicator of reproductive function and cardiovascular health that should be used as a diagnostic for health status. But morning wood is different than sexual arousal, and is the process of regeneration for the genitals which facilitates blood flow to cells to supply them with oxygen and other nutrients as needed for restoration. Engorgement of the reproductive organs with blood is facilitated by relaxation of contractile muscle that otherwise contract constantly (much like sphincter muscles) to keep blood out so that we aren't walking around 24/7 with an erection, and otherwise must be stimulated to relax during arousal. At night the rise in GABA and CO_2 production also stimulates relaxation of these contractile muscles to allow increased blood flow for regeneration of the organs, so morning wood thus begins to fail when excessive calcification of soft tissue from reduced respiration and CO_2 output as discussed in the chapter on calcium prevents relaxation of these muscles by keeping calcium-dependent contraction pathways chronically turned on. It is entirely possible to have full sexual arousal erections but not have morning wood, but it should be restored as it is a direct indicator of declining metabolic respiration and the required output of sufficient CO_2 to stay healthy. This CO_2 function in turn is primarily a function of the oleic-acid stabilization of the cytochrome oxidase respiratory enzyme as discussed in the chapter on calcium, and thus is also an indication either of too little oleic acid consumption, problems with digesting and absorbing fats such as saponification or selenium deficiency, or vitamin E deficiency caused by factors such as dermatophyte colonization since vitamin E is required to protect fatty acids like oleate from peroxidation, and addressing those problems can rapidly lead to restoration of morning wood.

There is no reason to persist with erection difficulties, and doing so is usually just a consequence of naivety and willful ignorance. Improving health through the restoration of a good diet with some simple nutritional and metabolic aids and restoration of the cardiovascular system as discussed in the chapter on vascular insufficiency is easy to do and can rapidly restore the ability to bone.

CHAPTER 20
CURING INSOMNIA

When I graduated High School in 1999 I found myself in limbo over the direction of my life. At a time when most young people are preparing for college, as a young Mormon boy I had been expected, without discussion, to instead serve a mission for their church. Even applying for college would have been a sign of unwillingness to serve, since my birthday was so soon after graduation, so I seemed to be waiting in place, paralyzed by a fear of disappointing my family and friends but not knowing what else I could do to progress since the religious counselor to which I had confessed being gay also denied me the opportunity to go, even though I had never even kissed another person, citing my habit of jerking off when other boys who had already engaged in full sexual intercourse with girls were already in the field. My nineteenth birthday came and went, and my friends suspected I was not actually going on a mission. Invitations to hang out rapidly dwindled and loneliness began to creep in from the cracks.

One rare night when our entire crew was together someone proposed we travel to a hot springs near a lake by our town. They had heard it was a good time so we piled into cars with our suits and towels and headed off. It was a thirty-minute drive, which for our small town was quite a ways. Eventually we found a turnoff onto a dirt road, no lights or signs to mark our arrival except for a handful of other darkened vehicles. We then trudged gleefully through the damp, barren lowlands, single file though a well-worn path among dry scrub and brush before suddenly coming upon a large clearing, a park of trampled, brown clay surrounding an embossed depression filled with murky water and four men conversing jovially.

The group of us were loud and rowdy and clearly a shock to the other swimmers who had been enjoying their solitude and looked bewildered as we jumped in. One of them appeared to be around our age, or just a little older. He was very muscular, with a beautiful smile plastered across a striking face accented with dark hair and bright eyes. One of the girls in our group immediately honed in on the gorgeous young man standing in waist-deep water where the top of his bare hips were just visible. I could hardly take my eyes off him, but dared not join my girlfriends for fear of betraying my quickly beating heart and sudden difficulty breathing. "Where are you from?" our friend asked shortly into their conversation. "Lehi," said the boy. It was a town nearer the springs with a reputation for being a little more redneck than our community, which only served to inflame my attraction by roughing his smooth edges. "This is our first time here," she continued, drawing close enough that she reached out to touch his arm in the way that girls do when they are enamoured. "I'm not wearing anything," he said quietly in warning. "WHAT?" screamed my friend as she jumped away. "You're *naked?*" The boy smiled even more as everyone turned to look his way, especially the girls who each took their turn glancing toward the line of water at his hips *as if they couldn't even*. My entire being succumbed to lust and I cursed the presence of my friends, suddenly recognizing them as the insufferable prudes they really were. What was wrong with being naked? I longed to step out of my life and join the strangers, who in their casual way seemed unbothered by the kind of misery inflicted by religion. Alas I could not gather the courage and I left later that night without ever learning his name.

For weeks afterward he haunted my dreams. Autumn was bearing down and though my adulthood loomed ominously on the horizon my situation had become no more certain. After fulfilling a challenge from my religious councilor to abstain from jerking it for thirty days with the promise of signing my mission papers he reneged on his part of the bargain. But his duplicity finally thrust the realization that this man was guided not by the Holy Spirit, but by bigotry, unconcerned with my actual wellbeing and had never intended to allow me to go. Unaware of my predicament my father dangled the carrot of paying for college if I attended their religious university, but which also required the approval of that same prick that prevented me from going on a mission, whom I later learned had harassed my sister and accused her of being lesbian because no boys ever asked her out but who in reality was so beautiful that every boy in our school was terrified to approach her. I had always assumed I would go to college on a swimming scholarship, and with excellent grades and a twenty-eight on the ACT there was no reason I shouldn't win easy acceptance to a wide choice of schools. Yet here I was, eighteen, graduated, and had applied to exactly zero and had no financial plan or resources to go either. This stalemate was caused all the more by the growing realization that soon I would not be welcome in the very society in which I was raised, and putting off any action for the course of my future was just an attempt to delay the horrifying reality which awaited. It would be a lie, though, to say I wasn't relieved at the realization that I *didn't* actually have to go on a mission. I finally did not believe at all in their church, though I had tried all my life to understand what they were all talking about, and my motivation for serving rested solely on the fear of angering my parents and other recriminations which would follow.

The reality of my situation became clear—I could persist in dishonesty, exhausting myself in the appeasing of people and institutions that never truly cared for my wellbeing, or I could come to terms with my quirky sexuality and see what life really had in store. Toward the end of that summer on my way home from my last meeting with the counselor I found out that I had yet again been forgotten by my friends who were all gathered at someone's house and had not bothered to extend an invitation. Arriving home I found only two of my younger siblings and my father in the house. The rest had gone to their friends', my brother with his new girlfriend with whom he now understandably spent more time than us. My parents had argued and my mother left in anger, so I made some food and asked my dad if he wanted to watch a movie with me. He had work to do, he said.

I was about to hole up in my room and feel sorry for myself when suddenly the image of the beautiful boy from the hot springs sprang to mind. The idea of being naked in nature with a boy as beautiful as him was overwhelming. For the first time I realized that people like me most likely existed, and that he had probably been gay. After all, he'd been more charming and sweet than other boys. Perhaps if I returned to the hot springs I could meet him, or someone else just like me. "I'm going to John's," I lied to my father, not really caring for permission anymore but for some cover to get away unquestioned. I resented my family for their instability, their indifference. I resented my church for not caring about me. I resented my community for their backhanded hypocrisy and callous disregard for those in need. I resented my friends for being two-faced and disloyal. There was in fact no good reason to preserve *anything* about my life as it was. Before me instead was sudden-ly a future in which I looked out for myself, went after what I wanted, and lived an autonomous and adult life.

Shaking with excitement I snuck my swimsuit and a towel to the car and drove off. My heart pounded in my ears the entire way there, my erection scraping the inside of my jeans (I also thought it was a good occasion to try going commando). Hardly able to breathe I found my way to the parking spot, left my suit in the car and made my way nervously through the murky path, grateful for the darkness to obfuscate my painfully apparent inexperience and vulnerability. The springs were completely vacant when I arrived, but I was grateful for some solitude in which to adjust to my nerves. I took off my clothes and neatly folded them into a nearby tree before stepping into the warm, sulfur-scented water which felt particularly soothing against my naked skin. The moon danced on the dark ripples as my feet sank into the thick mud beneath, the thrill of adventure stopping my breath for a moment. Meandering through the maze of languid rivulets I was amazed at the feeling of a freely floating cock, no cloth to conceal my manhood from prudish eyes, the sky overhead cut by overhanging skeletons of trees already bare of autumn leaves.

Before long two boys and their girlfriends showed up, uncouth and coarse it was clear these people were less warm and friendly than the ones we had met, so I kept my distance. Soon after a solitary man then arrived. He must have been ten years my senior, large and well built with a stomach that advertised a healthy appetite for beer. He too avoided the couples. "Hello," he said when he saw me back among the thicket. He had a deep voice, handsome, but his eyes were apathetic, uninterested in the soul of anyone who presented themselves to him. Still, one person to talk with was better than none and we talked for some time. Soon the pair of lovers abandoned us to the silence of the night, and the man moved closer to me. Though he was not as striking as the one I had fallen for last time my body trembled with anticipation. I had never been so near a naked, grown man, nor ever touched another person, and the promise of an encounter overpow-ered any sense of reason. "Are you gay?" I finally blurted out. The man smirked, "No." I averted my eyes, embarrassed that I had jumped for an opportunity and revealed myself, to have potentially put myself in danger. I almost turned away to leave. "But I'll jerk you off, if you want," he said.

Suddenly I felt reviled and lusting all at once. My dreams of a smoldering kiss beneath the moonlight on a warm autumn night with a boy who took my breath away were in a moment dashed by a crass, impersonal offer of a hand-job. But holding a thick cock in my hand was incredible. Here was a man who not only let me touch him, but wanted it. The feel of his large hand wrapped around mine was even more amazing than I'd ever imagined it could be. He didn't look into my eyes but down at the water where his hand slowly pulled at my erection. I wished even more it had been the other boy, and felt a sting of shame at giving in to my needs so haplessly. The spectacle was short-lived and I thanked him as any nice Mormon boy should and immediately exited the water. It was entirely the antithesis of romance and yet exactly as I had imagined. During the long drive home I was filled with an unexpected excitement. It had not gone at all as I had hoped—I felt gross and dirty and yet had taken the very first step freeing myself from the prison of my youth, full of post-orgasmic lust and excitement for what the future might hold. If an encounter like this had made me feel this way, imagine what the embrace of someone I cared for was going to feel like? I crawled into bed that night knowing my life with these people with whom I grew up was nearing an end and that a new, exciting world was opening before me which, for the first time, held a promise of happiness. I had officially left childhood.

I became more defiant at home, short-tempered toward dismissive remarks and their haste to harass me. My parents finally asked me to leave. But being on my own did not go the way I intended. My family helped me set up an apartment on the condition it be near home, not because they wanted me near but to prevent me going full-heathen, as I only saw them occasional on a weekend or two here and there though I wasn't in school and only working an entry level design job. Sadly, I found the same harassment from roommates in three different apartments in that town, because everyone was Mormon, and they belittled, rejected, and called me names for not attending church. Though I didn't know what it was at the time my insomnia had started at home, and now isolated from my family and friends whom even attended school down the street I found myself increasingly depressed and tossing and turning at night when I laid down to sleep. I befriend-ed a girl who had a crush on me, discovering for the first time how appearance can be used to secure companionship. But it was not a true friendship and I was unsettled in this community of hateful, isolated people. The one or two friends I found were not enough to stem my anxiety and loneliness since most of my living was done inside my head, alone, fearing to reveal myself to anyone. My insomnia began waking me in the middle of the night. *There must be more boys like me even in a place like this*, I thought. An add on *Yahoo!* personals led me to find a men-for-men section posted with brazen, unapologetic ads which described boys just like me who longed to meet, although much of it was much less romantic than I had expected. Two contacts I made on this site seemed to stand out—one, a guy my age who was lean and cute with a boy-next-door character about him, and another twenty-years older than me, manly, with a well sculpted, hairy chest and a deep, resonating voice (we chatted on the phone). The man had me hands down. I agreed to travel to his home for a date, but when I arrived a man answered the door who was not the one in the photographs, with severely greying hair and a sad, drooping body and eyes that avoided direct contact. He must have been forty years older than me and clearly deceitful in his representation of himself. But being raised Mormon I had absolutely no skills with which to protect myself and did not even realize until years later that I had been taken for a fool, that he had probably counted on my naivety to take advantage on purpose, so instead of confronting him or leaving as I rightly should have, so as not to hurt his feelings I let him give me a toothy, painful blowjob before finally making an excuse to escape, crying in the car all the way back to my lonely apartment.

Terrified by my inability to stand up for myself and ashamed at wasting my first two encounters on unemotional exploits I resolved next to meet the younger boy and attempt a proper date. He proposed we meet at a burger joint. I was prompt and waited expectantly at a booth in broad daylight, horrified when he walked in and sat across from me because if anyone I knew should happen upon us they would immediately know I was gay just by seeing his mannerisms and appearance. Still too "nice" to leave, I stayed put—He was cute, after all, and seemed kind and earnest, and soon I found myself relaxing in his presence. After inquiring if I was "out," he then asked the million-dollar question—"Are you hung?" I had never heard this term and if I had known it indicates a person to be shallow and emotionally unavailable I would have left immediately. Instead, my naivety continued to be a disservice. "What's that?" I replied. He explained that hung meant you had a big dick that hung from your body. Embarrassed, I replied that I wasn't sure. I couldn't believe there were people who wanted to ask about my penis only ten minutes after meeting. We kept talking and soon I told him about my previous two experiences, and also revealed that I had actually yet to kiss another person. Hearing this his eyes lit up. "I'll teach you," he said.

An hour later I was in his apartment. He drew me close and began to explain the intricacies of kissing. "Put your lips out a bit," he said, "but don't overdo it. The worst kissers try too hard, but don't be limp either." He brought his face close and pressed his lips lightly against mine. It was the warmest feeling I'd ever had—*my first kiss*. By lowering the stakes this academic pretense made it fun. "Biting is good, if it's light," he said before pressing my lower lip gently between his front teeth. But his instruction soon trailed off as he began to kiss me with feeling, occasionally looking into my eyes with sweet, yearning glances. It quickly stirred us to more. Our shirts came off, then furiously the rest of our clothes. He was beautiful naked and when our bodies pressed together I knew for the first time what it might be like to do this with someone I loved, or at least imagined what it could be, and to be loved in return, and for the first time in my life I knew what it meant to be happy.

Our wrestling grew more passionate. He reached to the nightstand for a tube of lotion. I had long used vaseline for a similar purpose, so I was not surprised as he lathered my erection in an off-green colored paste and did the same to his own. It was electric. Overwhelming. Then it began to sting. "Is it supposed to burn?" I said shyly. He grabbed the tube and turned it over. It was foot exfoliator.

Our date ended instead with a long, long shower waiting for the stinging to pass, laughing and talking. Though I never saw him again I was overjoyed to have actually connected with another boy just like me with whom I shared more than just being used, now with an arsenal of kissing skills to embolden my foray into the world of sex, and that night I slept more deeply than I had for years.

I finally decided to confide in a friend that I was gay. I chose her because I thought they were more open-minded than the rest of my friends and indeed she reacted with joy and surprise and told me of some of the other gay boys in our community (including sadly one who had tried to kill himself after being sent home from his mission for fooling around with another missionary), but she also betrayed me for the chance to be a center of gossip and during a rare visit with my friends at a party to see off another missionary I realized none of my friends would make eye contact with me. I pulled aside one of my best friends and asked if he knew about me. He replied that pornography had been a problem for him, and that I could get over my addiction too. My face grew red hot with embarrassment and when the moment allowed I slipped away from the party, never to see or hear from them again.

By the time my forced outing occurred I knew I was not interested in being friends with people like them anyway. Self-centered, disloyal, social cannibals I had never truly felt safe or comfortable around them. A few months later I finally made it out of that hellhole and moved to Salt Lake City, but soon my family surprised everyone and announced they were moving back to Hawaii. I found some conditional acceptance in the gay community in Salt Lake but soon realized my loneliness had only increased, and the stress of life was compounding daily. My insomnia became as regular as going to work. Tossing in bed was too aggravating to stay there, so I would get in my car and make a drive around the freeway loop to visit the *Kripsy Kreme Doughnuts* at the other end of the valley. I became such a late-night regular that to get rid of their expiring doughnuts the employees would load a dozen or two into my car completely free of charge. After a few doughnuts and the relaxing drive back I would get home and finally fall asleep (not under-standing how the doughnuts were treating the stress of dieting and low-carb eating). But my insomnia would gradually worsen night after night, from being a reasonable one a.m. on Tuesday, two a.m. on Wednesday, three a.m. on Thursday and so on until finally I could not sleep until the sun came up, would call in sick to work, fall asleep around noon, and the pattern would repeat in a seeming endless sisyphean curse, and I always expected it to get better, somehow, though it never did.

Over the years my sleep at times seemed to come more easily, such as after doing a heavy-metals cleanse or after exercising excessively, and always when there was another boy in my bed. But insomnia always came back and by the end of my twenties nothing at all seemed to work. I gave up coffee for months at a time, tried sleeping pills, anti-anxiety pills, melatonin, natural remedies and diets, jerking off, not jerking off, turning off my electronics, reading, walking, exhausting myself with exercise. Sometimes these seemed to work, most of the time they did not. Pills didn't cause sleep, they caused unconsciousness and it is not the same thing. I always slept best with someone in my bed, but then my ex shook the room with his snoring and at the slightest sniffle my eyes would shoot open wide awake in frustration. Alcohol put me to sleep, and I became a raging alcoholic, but then came the day when even alcohol could not make me sleep. By then I had developed thyroid cancer and my insomnia was permanent—I could never sleep until the sun came up, and in spite of my exhaustion only ever managed a few hours during the day at most. Insom-nia even began to *hurt*. I never ate junk food, hardly ever ate processed food, and avoided sugar religiously, and other than alcohol I considered myself a healthy eater, active, disciplined, and yet here I was suffering something that others ignorantly derided as a choice, influenceable by behavior and morals. The most infuriating part was going to visit someone who spent eight years in medical school only to be told to quit coffee or turn off the lights. *I already tried that, asshole.*

Sleep is such a natural part of our biology that there is no instruction on it in schools or scripture. It is regarded with inconsequence, because it seems so natural, so easy, until it leaves you like a jilted lover, no explanation, no way to resolution, and you lie in bed thinking he's about to come back until suddenly it's five in the morning and your alarm is going off at seven and it's going to be a painful day; at least there is coffee, thank God. I would spend most of my insomnia drawing, playing video games, reading, watching TV, whacking off, or writing, and the verse which begins this book was written in Los Angeles while newly sober but still sleepless, listening to Northern Mockingbirds chirp solemnly outside my apartment at two in the morning, alone, putting my life back together at the age of thirty-four when, as a young man, thought instead would be well into a marriage, raising children, moving into our second home.

Fundamentally sleep problems are also caused by problems with pathogens, in the gut and oral tissues, which produce harmful products like ammonia, histamine, lactic acid, and other metabolites which imbalance the nervous system, endocrine system, and other pathways which participate in circadian rhythms, so resolving chronic gut dysbiosis, parasitism, and oral disease can easily restore normal sleep. But though people think of sleep as simply not being awake sleep is actually a high-metabolic state requiring sufficient metabolic energy to induce just like any other activity such as running, sex, or digesting food. When cells in our body lack enough energy they also cannot properly manage *calcium*, as well-energized cells keep calcium largely to the exterior of the cell while limited amounts are allowed in to participate in production of cellular products and energy, after which it is then pushed back out in a perpetual-motion type, chemically powered process. It is here that sleep troubles begin and end because when cells begin to lose their high levels of metabolic energy they lose this ability to manage calcium which then begins to saturate cells more than it should which disrupts normal cellular function and thus impairs the ability to sleep. It just so happens that opportunistic microbes also exploit this unregulated calcium to colonize the human body, so problems with sleep are always accompanied by other illnesses like parasitism or gut dysbiosis which also serve to worsen sleep issues, and since calcium dysregulation is the stimulant for pain conditions like insomnia become literally painful as the body falls deeper into metabolic illness. Because calcium is required to suppress parathyroid and restore normal calcium function sleep can often be rescued by something high in calcium like ice cream or a warm milk tonic with cinnamon and sugar while restoring calcium metabolism through oxalate, vitamins K and D, and the ATPase channels which exchange calcium for sodium as discussed in the chapter on calcium.

When I was younger and not extremely ill I would often have a very large coffee at night, expecting insomnia anyway because why the hell not, only to find myself suddenly waking the next morning from a blissful night's rest. My experience, as has anyone who has used coffee to stay awake on a long road trip only to find themselves nodding off is that coffee does not actually interrupt sleep. When I gave up coffee in an attempt to fix insomnia it had absolutely no effect on my ability to sleep and only served to make my days more miserable. Caffeine promotes increased intracellular potassium and phosphate which helps the body to manage cellular calcium through increased sodium flux in opposition to the effects of pathogens and dieting, but coffee also contains a small amount of cinnamic acids (like caffeic acid) which helps scavenge the hydroxyl radical to restore ATPases, so it also helps us adapt to problems with calcium and metabolic energy production. But calcium dysregulation worsens as we age and negative effects of caffeine are in reality the loss of our ability to metabolize calcium properly due to factors like microbial hydroxyl radical production and loss of potassium and digestion, or insufficient intake of vitamin K as discussed in the chapter on calcium which most strongly impairs sleep and underlies the most disturbing sleep disorders, and the increased use of foods and beverages high in cinnamic acids can strongly help maintain ATPase function to promote the normal flux of calcium, sodium, potassium, copper, etc., through cells (which can also be supported by making sure to take enough sodium, including supplementation if required).

Because sleep is as much dependent on the production and availability of energy, *sugar* is extremely effective at lowering stress and promoting energy to help promote good sleep, so long as calcium metabolism is working properly, which is why we often feel sleepiest after a large meal since carbs and salt so strongly lower stress hormones. But states of diabetes can and does prevent normal sleep due to fructose malabsorption and loss of sucrase which impairs our ability to digest sucrose. After many years of irregular sleep I finally experienced a stretch of deep, slumberous sleep for a week straight consuming (admittedly low quality) chocolate covered almonds which caused this effect because of the high oxalate, tannin, cinnamic acid, and added high fructose corn syrup which was rapidly absorbed. As mentioned in the chapter on diabetes, fructose inhibits hyperglycemia caused by the release of glucose from glycogen storage by adrenaline, so fructose deficiency (from not eating enough fruit or sugar) or fructose malabsorption or impaired sucrose digestion results in strongly elevated heart rate and metabolic stress which not only can and does prevent sleep but also rapidly depletes glycogen storage which then deprives the body of glucose required to maintain a steady supply between long periods without eating such as occurs during sleep. A healthy liver can store up to five-hundred calories of glycogen, which can help us sleep for very long periods of time, but in those who are very young, very old, or metabolically ill it is far, far less and inadequate to sustain the body between long periods without food, so preceding sleep with a source of fructose and restoring fructose absorption and sucrose digestion can help suppress glycogen release to prevent excessive metabolic activation and prolong stores of glycogen to last all night.

Many grown adults who exercise and diet also wake naturally very early in the morning and are often quite proud of themselves for it because of our productivity obsessed brainwashing in service of capitalist masters who demand our productivity to line their pockets. But in fact waking very early in the morning is a symptom of very low blood sugar and steep rise in cortisol which follows depletion of adrenaline or glycogen to tear down lean tissue in order to release their sugars and amino acids, and the discomfort of this state then wake us from sleep so that we can go out and acquire more food, not money, which is why then eating breakfast can and does result in the overwhelming return of sleepiness since you actually did not sleep long enough and breakfast has now lowered stress hormones. As discussed in the chapter on depression, stress hormones like high adrenaline and cortisol serve the function of making us restless by design because it compels an organism to get up and go do stuff which, in the process, may result in the discovery of food or novel resources. This is the cause also of ADHD, OCD, and other restlessness which is not a defect of human function but a symptom of high stress hormones which act to motivate restlessness on purpose. As a young man I loved going to the movies but within five minutes of sitting in a theater I would be so restless all I could think of the entire time was the relief of it finally being over. This restlessness along with waking very early in the day resolved entirely after finally learning to keep my blood sugar sustained and restore my body's ability to form glycogen (which besides simply eating enough carbohydrates is primarily a function of low pathogenic burden which otherwise cause its continued release) and the healthy state is instead to feel languid and relaxed (not tired, but relaxed) at all times of the day, especially when waking in the morning.

Little kids and babies have very small livers and thus cannot store very much glycogen at all, and since a sharp rise in stress hormones adrenaline and cortisol results from glycogen depletion waking in the night is common in toddlers and other children who do not get dessert before bed (infants will always wake repeatedly during the night because their livers are basically incapable of storing enough glycogen no matter how much they eat). One of the reasons teenagers can sleep in so long is because their larger, healthier liver is finally capable of storing huge quantities of glycogen, but unfortunately this also helps to facilitate eating disorders like skipping meals if they think calorie deprivation will make them fit, which then over time causes the reverse due to the harms of starvation stress on the body and eventually become adults who cannot sleep even when they are exhausted. But if children are fed dinner in the early evening and don't eat again the rest of the night their liver has already started using up glycogen stores by the time they go to bed and it is inevitable they will wake during the night. Many frustrated parents will ignorantly refuse to give their children ice cream or other high-calorie, sweet food if their children wake during the night because they stupidly and cruelly think it would "reward" their child as if the child *chose* to wake up during the night which they did not you absolute fucking morons (who chooses to wake up????), where a child given a bowl of ice cream or other high-calorie, carbohydrate rich food will instead get tired again more quickly because of the stress-hormone lowering effect of sugar and calories and thence be able to stay asleep much longer and then you as well. Fructose is most efficient at restoring glycogen anyway so one of the best ways for parents to get a good nights rest is to never feed children yogurt because lactic acid blocks sugar uptake into the body and lowers the metabolic rate, nor common wheat which causes inflammation, nor foods with allergenic gums like carrageenan (*lots* of ice creams contain it), and to *always* feed kids something substantial, sweet, and of high quality before bed like fruit, smoothies (blended on low speed to avoid aeration), or well-made, high quality dessert.

There is also a difference between sleep and restful sleep, which those with insomnia aren't aware since the inability to even sleep at all makes any sleep achievement worth celebrating, and lacking deep, restful sleep is a problem of oxidative stress which literally causes damage to tissues and prevents the body from engaging the deeply restorative pathways. Often those with this type of poor sleep mediated by oxidative stress will also present with *bruxism*, which is a chronic clenching of the jaw and grinding of teeth which can also occur unconsciously during the day, which results in waking with a sore jaw that feels like tooth infection but is in fact the stress caused by chronic, unconscious clenching and grinding. Problems like bruxism occur because during metabolic stress the nervous system tries to stimulate fatigued cells through increased neurological stimulation similarly to how a heart defibrillator is used to restart a failing heart, and this overstimulation meant to resuscitate cells also overstimulates muscle contractions such as in the jaw to cause unconscious grinding and clenching. When I had bruxism my dreams often featured shattering teeth, which was quite disturbing, and waking with aching teeth and gums and feeling unrested or having dreams about teeth are obvious symptoms of bruxism.

Most people think this kind of sleeplessness is caused by emotions or mental thoughts but you will remember that emotions and thoughts are hormones and reflect the status of the endocrine and neurological state, not the state of mind, although mental stress can and does make the problem worse. Oxidative stress is most commonly initiated by opportunistic pathogens which disturb our antioxidant pathways such as depleting sulfur, selenium, manganese, copper, and zinc required in glutathione, glutathione peroxidase, and the superoxide dismutases required to consume superoxide and hydrogen peroxide. Oxidative stress might sound like a problem of excess oxygen, but in fact a deficiency of oxygen delivery to cells such as in states of anemia or low *boron* since boron acts as a chaperone for oxygen delivery to mitochondria (hypoxia) is a severe cause of oxidative stress and results in the formation of more superoxide and other reactive oxygen species. Mitochondrial silicon deficiency as discussed in the chapter on cancer is a common problem in metabolic disease which also impairs respiration, but restoration of mitochondrial silicon increases mitochondrial respiration which then in turn also more rapidly depletes oxygen and boron to ironically promote more hypoxia which can result in greater oxidative stress if boron deficiency persists. A common sleep issue caused by this deficiency of boron and state of hypoxia is restless leg syndrome in which legs will sometimes even twitch and kick spontaneously from an overwhelming urge to move, which can drive people mad since it makes resting impossible even when we are exhausted. I believe restless leg is ultimately caused by retroviruses (such as those which cause leukemia), and increasing chloride absorption through the use of vitamin E can actually make restless leg syndrome temporarily worse as the immune reaction causes an increase in reactive oxygen species and hypoxia at the site of their colonization. As discussed in the chapter on immunity, retroviruses are easily eliminated in the normally high-oxygen state (normoxia), so restless leg syndrome and severe insomnia represent a deficiency of boron which causes poor delivery of oxygen to mitochondria. Studies how that restless leg syndrome is related to low vitamin D, but boron deficiency also causes active catabolism of vitamin D through an increase of 24-hydroxylase, further indicating boron deficiency as the cause of this problem. So restless leg syndrome and severe insomnia problems are ultimately a problem of oxidative stress and poor immunity such as is reversed by repletion with boron, which can be done through the low-dose, consistent use of high boron foods, a boron supplement, or even small doses of widely available borax (such as 1/8 tsp in water or juice, making sure not to use a product that contains cleaning adjunct chemicals). If this symptom is a common occurrence, use of boron should be consistent even after the apparent resolution of symptoms in order to fully eradicate retroviruses and maintain normoxia as a prophylactic against hypoxia.

Excess neurological stimulation is also mediated through histamine stimulated by the presence of pathogens and exaggerated by the presence of microbial amine producers in the gut (which always includes histamine producers) is one major driver of this restlessness, and in the short term a nightly, low-dose of first-generation *antihistamine* about an hour before bed can help (many over-the-counter sleep aids are in fact antihistamines). But the enzyme *monamine oxidase* which consumes histamine is also copper dependent, and over the years a dose of cocoa powder often helped induce sleep which occurred because cocoa is high in copper and oxalate which helps to promote copper assimilation. Occasionally the use of iodine would also help because of its role in both thyroid function and immune suppression of opportunistic pathogens such as those which produce histamine, but this would not always work because of copper dysregulation caused by these opportunistic pathogens.

Sleep apnea is a common symptom that accompanies severe insomnia and is a direct consequence of poor CO_2 production as a result of poor mitochondrial respiration since CO_2 helps maintain normal oxygen tension, and in sleep apnea the CO_2 tension is so low that breathing actually slows or stops in order to retain as much CO_2 as possible, to prevent death, which then causes a person to wake from sleep, gasping for air. This problem is ultimately mediated by the dysregulation of our primary respiratory enzyme, cytochrome oxidase, which is also dependent on copper, where copper dysregulation is caused in turn by dysregulation also of calcium due to the effect of calcification on pH which mediates copper chaperones, because respiration results in the abundant production of CO_2 which helps sustain respiration and pH function in the Borh and Haldane effects that are required to maintain oxygen delivery to cells.

When sleep apnea occurs it reflects such extreme deficiency of boron, oxygen, copper, and thus CO_2 pressure that we are in danger of having severe and sudden health episodes such as stroke or heart attack due to poor oxygen status. Since vitamin A stimulates mitochondrial biogenesis dietary carotene can also strongly promote an increase in CO_2 production so long as delivery of oxygen and carbohydrate to cells is also adequate. But, as discussed in the chapter on calcium and respiration, the cytochrome oxidase enzyme is also stabilized by *oleic acid*, and the generous consumption of dietary oleic acid such as from olive oil, tiger nuts, hazelnuts, butter and dairy, or high-oleic sunflower oil (mayonnaise made of these oils is especially convenient) can especially strongly stimulate CO_2 output if there is adequate boron and copper. Oleic acid also comes from endogenous production from stearic and palmitic acid in addition to dietary sources, all of which also require normal digestion and packaging into cholesterol which can also be impaired by low selenium and sulfur due to sulfate and selenate reducing opportunistic microbes which cause those malodors of the breath and feces characteristic to metabolic decline (and such malodors always accompany apnea). Restoring the digestion and absorption of oleic acid as discussed in the chapters on calcium and immunity can result in so much CO_2 production from simultaneous ingestion of carbohydrate (if replete in silicon) that breath holding can actually result in temporary heart palpitations from retention of excess of CO_2. Naturally high CO_2 is actually protective of mitochondria, however, so palpitations from high CO_2 rather than low CO_2 are far less dangerous and is caused ironically because we are so used to breath holding it prevents proper ventilation of CO_2, which simply requires taking normal breaths to ventilate and will normalize within two or three weeks as oleic acid intake and digestion are sustained and cellular respiration is consistently supported by the principles in this and other chapters.

These same problems of CO_2 pressure and hypoxia also underly states of anxiety, which is why those with sleep problems often experience anxiety, and why panic attacks often stimulate hyperventilation as the body tries desperately to breathe in more oxygen, but since oxygen entry into cells from hemoglobin is mediated by CO_2 and boron, hyperventilation does not work but is why bag breathing can help rescue a panic attack since this causes recirculation of CO_2 and thus a temporary increase. Anxiety often results from behaviors like dieting or other dietary stress because deprivation of carbohydrate is the most effective way to impair mitochondrial respiration and lower endogenous CO_2 production. CO_2 also reacts with ammonia which helps detoxify it through urea so many people find relief from insomnia or other feelings of disease from drinking carbonated beverages, which effectively supplies more CO_2, and while this is a useful strategy many commercial carbonated beverages are also made with harmful ingredients and almost never contain tannin. This also does not reverse the underlying problem of deficient CO_2 production which absolutely must be reversed in order to make a permanent healing.

Since silicon repletion is also required for the synthesis of healthy connective tissue, and helps impair microbial ingress into tissues, repletion of silicon will also result in improved airway function, structure, and reversal of these problems, but requires proper digestion and acidification of silicon and will not work simply from a supplement, since acidification and bioavailability of silicon is the primary factor which determines repletion. As mentioned in previous chapter on immunity, repletion with silicon can also increase the rate of *sweating* due to increased respiration, heat, and production of ATP. Anyone experiencing metabolic disease regardless of age can and will also experience spontaneous and uncontrolled sweating in the evening or at night when trying to sleep, or during any physical exertion, including sex, or even sometimes when not doing anything at all, and misunderstand this as a function of the body overheating, especially since this problem is commonly associated with menopause and hot flashes (which is covered in the upcoming chapter on hormones). But when I found myself sweating in my early thirties for no reason every time I went to sleep I usually pushed away my boyfriend from embarrassment when he tried to hold me during the night, which he mistook for disinterest, being too insecure to explain to him what I was going through (though he had also proven himself unsympathetic to my wellbeing at that point). The problem with sweating and hot flashes is that it *feels* like we are heating up, and many people will drink cold beverages or even eat ice to cool down, when in reality a hot flash or other excessive sweating is the body suddenly *losing* heat through the skin, so the heat passing through the skin feels hot but because the core temperature is also falling, and adding cold beverages or ice to this problem only serves to further lower the metabolic temperature to then worsen metabolic health, since our body requires nearly 100° F (37.7°C) for optimal metabolic health.

A more physiologically appropriate coping behavior for hot flashes and spontaneous sweating is to take a nice, long, hot shower or bath, to relax and allow the body to heat back up to normal while the water can wash away sticky sweat until the problem can be resolved. Sweating itself is mediated by *calcium channels*, so excessive sweating is thus also a problem of calcium dysregulation and excessive calcification of soft tissue such as occurs during aging and metabolic illness. Doctors often treat sweating disorders by *parathyroidectomy* (removal of the parathyroid gland) which thus prevents the body from mobilizing calcium, but parathyroidectomy is incredibly debilitating to future wellness as the body is then unable to mobilize calcium for calcium dependent pathways (calcium citrate taken with dietary oxalate and dietary vitamin K can help those missing their parathyroid). Iodine occasionally relieved me of this sweating nightmare because of its role in immunity and thyroid, but was not consistent. But excessive sweating, regardless of the occasion, is also a problem of boron deficiency induced hypoxia, which is exacerbated by raising the metabolic rate since increased metabolism uses oxygen at a higher rate, and sweating instead lowers the body temperature in an attempt to also lower the metabolic rate and thus reduce consumption of oxygen. Since boron also participates in hormone homeostasis as discussed in the chapter on erections, hormone dysregulation and deficiency of vitamin D also always accompanies problems with excessive sweating since these problems also increase calcium influx into cells as a regulatory mechanism to lower the metabolic rate. Sometimes extra salt can help with sweating since sodium is required to efflux calcium from cells, but it is boron through the increased delivery of oxygen to mitochondria, which then results in greater production of ATP and inhibition of retroviruses, and restoration of vitamin D and hormone homeostasis which can ultimately reverse sweating problems.

Exercise can often cause healthy people to sleep fast because the increased production of CO_2 from metabolism of more carbohydrate and fats has this beneficial effect on cellular metabolism, but exercise has many of the same effects of insomnia or consuming lactic acid, especially in those who also diet, so in those experiencing any health problems no matter how seemingly trivial exercise will oppositely cause an increase in problems like insomnia due to the negative effect of adrenaline and other stress hormones on glycogen and cellular respiration. In severe insomniacs it is necessary to avoid all exercise until insomnia is entirely resolved because the excessive stress, production of lactic acid, and loss of electrolytes and depletion of glycogen will otherwise make it impossible to recover. The rule for exercise is that it should always be *fun*, and if it is not this is a symptom the body cannot handle it and will result in excessive metabolic stress and worse health problems. Because sodium also helps to restrain adrenaline by helping to increase the metabolic rate without stress hormones mild sleep problems can often be treated by simply dosing a small amount of salt in some juice or using salt heated in a high tannin beverage for better absorption. Being dependent on ATPase channels as discussed in the chapter on vascular sufficiency, however, this function can be interrupted by pathogenic production of the hydroxyl radical as discussed in the chapter on immunity, and because ammonia also inhibits sodium uptake this will only work when suppressing or resolving parasitism or other ammonia producers and is better to dose separately from meals rather than using more salt in food since salt remaining in the gut can and does instead promote amine producing microbes which make adrenaline analogs that worsen insomnia, but resolving those issues can restore the normal uptake and transport of sodium to promote more restful sleep.

Unlike exercise, stretching produces energy, which is why stretching *feels* so good. Just like exposure to sunlight, the manual elongation of cells stimulates the production of free energy in the form of ATP. I believe this effect of stretching is nature's way of harnessing the latent energy inherent in gravity and leverages it for our benefit much the same way electric vehicles regenerate energy from braking, converting kinetic, inertial energy into useable energy storage. The best stretches are thus those which utilize gravity, rather than strength, and stretching can produce huge amounts of energy to stabilize cellular respiration and promote relaxation and sleep. I often found that when sleep evaded me, even after using vitamins and other sleep aids it was stretching that made me suddenly zonk out. I cannot overemphasize how helpful stretching is for inducing sleep. ATP is also the "receptor" of magnesium within cells, so by generating more ATP stretching actually sucks magnesium into cells and thus helps reduce cellular excitation and promotes sleep. This obviously also requires magnesium which those with conditions like diabetes and autism will be deficient which requires heating magnesium in water with tannin to bypass the effects of pathogenic gut microbes and microbial ammonia as discussed in the chapter on parasitism. If replete in magnesium, a daily stretching regimen rather than simply waiting until insomnia starts (and instead of exercise) can also be a preventative measure and treatment for not only insomnia but also other issues of metabolic energy and wellness.

Melatonin is colloquially associated with sleep, with many melatonin products for sale as sleep aids, but melatonin is actually an adaptive hormone of stress which helps us handle the stress of darkness, and there is absolutely nothing natural about taking melatonin as a supplement which in fact can actually worsen sleep problems as well as contribute to infertility, hypogonadism, depression, and cancer since melatonin actively downregulates the metabolism and sex hormone production. Melatonin is a hormone of hibernation which rises in response to light deprivation, but we humans do not hibernate and instead of simply losing this hibernation response we evolved an *anti-hibernation* response in response to high melatonin which is achieved simply by a concomitant further rise in adrenaline which counteracts the state of torpor mediated by melatonin. This is why a long day at the beach in bright sunshine can and does result in profound desires to sleep but being indoors in the darkness for long periods of time is oppositely and ironically accompanied by restlessness and insomnia. Because the expression of melatonin is also cyclical with our circadian rhythms many insomniacs find the only time they can truly sleep is during the day when melatonin is actually very low. This change in the body which is regulated by light exposure is often termed '*dark adapted*' or '*light adapted*,' and when melatonin is excessively high and 'dark adapted' exposure to bright sunlight causes lots of blinking and trouble seeing in bright light, where the opposite 'light adapted' state does not cause blinking in bright light and can be used also to diagnose melatonin levels which are lower when light adapted.

Because sex hormones in adults are responsible also for our sense of wellbeing and self-sufficiency (testosterone does not only stimulate arousal but is the primary agent of motivation in general) people with extremely elevated levels of melatonin are also those who find themselves living in their parent's basement, jobless, lacking motivation, depressed, restless, and tired but unable to sleep. Like all other used hormones melatonin is also later secreted into bile for elimination from the body, and in excess also stimulates the activity of pathogenic microbes which promote not only insomnia but also dangerous conditions like appendicitis as discussed in the chapter on immunity which only develops during the night, darkness, and prolonged light deprivation stress and other immune dysfunction. This is in part why we can sometimes feel fine and restful until we actually try to go to sleep, which indicates an increase in harmful microbial production of metabolites like endotoxin, ammonia, and harmful forms of indoles which increase under the influence of excess melatonin during the night, whose activity can be strongly suppressed by consuming foods high in oxalate right before bed since many of these pathogens employ calcium to colonize the body and resist the immune system.

For these reasons insomnia usually originates in wintertime, which is a significant stimulant for melatonin excess, but which also happens to those who spend too much time indoors simply for the artificial replication of wintertime conditions and its harmful effect on our commensal microbiome which require vitamin D to supply Thaumarchaeota archaea and support local microbial B12 synthesis. This problem cannot be mediated even by having an office window, especially since most windows nowadays are tinted, as this requires unobstructed exposure to bright, direct sunlight on the skin and bright, indirect exposure to the eyes. Deficiency of the commensal microbiome (especially of the skin as discussed in the chapters on parasites and vitamin D) can become so severe that none of the strategies in this chapter will work if dysbiosis is extremely severe or extremely prolonged, and restoration of sleep is absolutely dependent on sun exposure, frequent dietary carotene to protect the skin microbiome, and interaction with the natural environment to collect commensal microorganisms. Histamine for instance is a potent and irritating inhibitor of sleep and produced in abundance by amine producing microbes in the gut during dysbiosis in the presence of high protein and unabsorbed salts which is degraded by monoamine oxidase. Loss of morning wood (which occurs in women too it's just a little more difficult without a penis to be obvious), is also a symptom of health problems that affect sleep since adequate blood volume is required for morning wood to occur and a function of electrolyte balance, the skin being the primary storage site of sodium and a significant producer of glucocorticoids which help maintain electrolyte status and water balance. If drinking plenty of water does not restore morning wood this is an excellent symptom of low blood volume stress, sweating during the night indicating skin microbial dysbiosis since sugar and ammonia in sweat is meant to cultivate commensal microbes.

Mitochondria do not only supply energy, they can and do also supply heat which is required by our body as a mammal to maintain normal metabolic function. One of the purposes of this heat is that it helps the body organize water in cells into structured alignment much like molecules in a crystal which then facilitates life and metabolism, and reduced body heat then makes it harder for the body to organize water molecules and maintain adequate metabolism. This is also why spending time in a sauna without causing heat stress results in feeling better as it supplements heat thus requiring less to be made by the body. But during the night and the state of blissful, restful sleep the production of heat is taken up instead by cellular organelles called *peroxisomes* which consume fatty acids (and other substrate) in *beta-oxidation* to produce an abundance of heat and CO_2 (but not energy) to provide heat for the body to maintain life during sleep. But metabolism of fat results in greater production of reactive oxygen species and during aging and metabolic disease the ability to metabolize fat without causing damage to the body becomes impaired so that peroxisomes can no longer safely provide this robust heat production which must instead be taken up by mitochondria and promotes greater fat retention to better insulate against heat loss.

Like mitochondria, peroxisome metabolism results in reactive oxygen species like superoxide which is highly damaging and must be controlled by superoxide dismutase. While in mitochondria this dismutase is primarily one based on manganese as described in the chapter on immunity the dismutase used by peroxisomes is primarily of copper and zinc, and because dysregulation of calcium, sulfur, molybdenum, and ATPases disturbs copper metabolism this then impairs the ability of peroxisomes to metabolize fatty acids for the production of heat to thus impair the normal, restful quality of sleep. As related in the chapter on immunity I often used cocoa powder or dark chocolate as a remedy for insomnia because (unknown to me at the time) cocoa is very high in both copper and oxalate which helps promote copper homeostasis by also restraining free calcium. Those with Wilson's disease present with excessive copper retention due to an inability to even discard it, which is a problem of copper ATPase and inhibition by the hydroxyl radical which much be suppressed by a diet high in cinnamic acids and molybdenum while taking care to suppress microbial hydrogen sulfide producers, as one of the symptoms of Wilson's disease is severe insomnia. Our primary respiratory enzyme which helps produce ATP, cytochrome oxidase, is also copper dependent, however, so the normal, generous production of ATP which would allow mitochondria to rest during sleep is also impaired by this copper dysregulation.

Peroxisomes are activated by the true arbiter of relaxation and restful sleep, GABA (*gamma-aminobutyric acid*), which causes cells to become hyper-polarized which then slows down cellular metabolism and gives mitochondria time to rest and repair. Because GABA is powerfully relaxing a whole host of mimetic drugs have been designed to promote or mimic its function, but are also why they are also highly addictive, not because they are addictive but because they replace the function of GABA in those who are deficient whom, unlike those whom aren't, find the only way to achieve relaxation is through drugs. Alcohol is also a GABA mimetic, which is a primary reason for its anxiolytic (anti-anxiety) properties, but GABA is in turn made from *glutamate* which is initially made alternately from glucose or glutamine and another reason low-carb dieting is so harmful, where glutamate is the metabolic opposite of GABA and stimulates wakefulness and alertness. Melatonin is a backup and adjunct for GABA, especially during times of stress, to downregulate the metabolism to prevent cells from over-consuming nutrients which would in fact actually cause us to die during sleep if we ran out of nutrients and did not have these regulating functions. Melatonin and GABA have a generally inverse relationship, with high light exposure such as during the summer upregulating GABA and lowering melatonin while low light exposure upregulates melatonin and lowers GABA, which is why the greatest sleepiness often occurs in the afternoon or after a long day at the beach. Melatonin is also thought to be an antioxidant and is promoted as such by purveyors, researchers, and nutritionists because studies show melatonin to greatly reduce oxidative damage, but melatonin is not a true antioxidant and accomplishes reduction in oxidative stress simply by inhibiting oxidative respiration in the first place, preventing oxidation pathways and the robust metabolic processes by which our higher metabolic functions for energy production are facilitated but which also result in oxidative stress, and so lowers oxidative damage by stopping the processes which create it but which are also required for healthy and restorative sleep otherwise accomplished by GABA.

Because GABA shifts consumption of energy to heat production to help promote cellular regeneration it is dangerous to use GABA mimetics since the body requires ATP to live, and using them in excess such as occurs during abuse causes potential for serious illness and even death because of their inhibitory nature. GABA function is never, ever, ever, ever achieved through the use of drugs or supplements but instead the restoration of normal metabolic health, alleviation of ammonia and pathogenic colonization, and restoration of glutathione and adequate exposure to sunlight. Potassium most strongly promotes GABA function and one of the primary reasons for GABA deficiency is potassium deficiency caused either by low potassium intake or factors like ammonia which disturb normal sodium and potassium homeostasis. When GABA is even mildly functional potassium repletion or use of a low dose of *potassium citrate* is one of the strongest promoters of sleep. But as discussed in the chapter on vitamin D and cardiovascular disease, potassium uptake to cells is a function of ATPase channels which are inhibited by the hydroxyl radical produced by opportunistic pathogens, and this channel also requires ATP, so problems producing ATP such as what accompany diabetes, aging, metabolic disease, and chronic colonization by pathogens impairs potassium uptake to cells, so even high potassium intake can fail to reverse potassium deficiency and promote proper GABA function. What's worse is that too high of potassium intake without effective cellular uptake increases the risk of heart attack and other problems as high extracellular potassium disturbs the normal electrochemical potential of cells, and using a supplement of potassium should always also be accompanied by carbohydrate and sources of cinnamic acids (cinnamon, nutmeg, peaches, apples, turmeric, ginger, etc.) to promote ATPase function. This is why potassium citrate is so useful, because citric acid itself directly promotes ATP production, where potassium chloride is shown in studies to actually cause potassium loss (likely because of the direct delivery of chloride to cells). Potassium is also required to store glycogen, so a high potassium diet and use of potassium citrate taken with these steps before bed can address most sleep problems.

Lysine has been shown in studies to assist in promoting better sleep as lysine also has anxiolytic properties and potentiates GABA function, and while it has not been demonstrated in studies I personally believe lysine functions as a GABA reuptake inhibitor and that repletion with lysine promotes relaxation and better sleep by raising GABA expression. Lysine is also the necessary precursor to synthesis of another amino acid called carnitine required in the beta-oxidation of fatty acids both in peroxisomes and mitochondria, but the problem is that, like many nutrient problems, lysine deficiency is not really caused by dietary deficiency but instead by pathogens such as *Candida* which actively degrade lysine because lysine increases sensitivity of *Candida* to the immune system (and antibiotics). Lysine is also synthesized by healthy gut microbes, and competition with microbial producers of ammonia and hydrogen sulfide is likely the primary cause of lysine deficiency which contributes to insomnia. Instead this is also a problem of immunocompetency and our body's ability to inhibit opportunistic pathogens like *Candida* or *C. difficile* which disturb our body's natural functions. As discussed in the chapter on immunity the most important factor for immunity is *copper* which sensitizes pathogens to oxidation by the immune system, but copper is also required in the zinc, copper superoxide dismutase required by peroxisomes to prevent peroxidation stress from the metabolism of fatty acids for the production of heat during sleep. But copper is also a cofactor for diamine oxidase which degrades histamine, and histamine is one of the strongest stimulators of wakefulness which is also produced by opportunistic gut microbes, so interference of copper metabolism by pathogens also results directly in oxidative stress and stimulated wakefulness which causes restlessness and irritation when trying to sleep, and production of histamine by gut pathogens under the influence of melatonin when we are deficient in copper is the specific reason for not feeling sleepy once you go lay down to sleep.

After resolution of these impairments to GABA I have found *valerian root* to be useful for increasing GABA even further during sleep which can profoundly stimulate cellular regeneration, as valerian contains the eponymous *valeric acid* which, along with acetic acid, is shown in studies to activate genetic transcription (oppositely inhibited by methylation). During GABA release cells take up high quantities of chloride to cause hyper-polarization, so this also requires repletion with chloride such as by resolving ammonia excess and supplementing some salted water boiled with tannin, but this also means that profound GABA function is actually inhibited by metabolic stimulants like caffeine and nicotine, so in addition to the previous steps in this chapter the use of valerian root will not work if exposed to any stimulants like tea, coffee, and even chocolate within days of using valerian (three days abstinence seems like a sufficient amount), or the continuation of high adrenaline or other factors which reverse GABA-activated chloride channels. While giving up stimulants can be foreboding, the effect of valerian activated GABA is as powerful as an illicit drug and can produce an overpowering sense of relaxation and desire to sleep equivalent to GABA mimetics like *benzodiazepine*. Specifically it should result in an obvious rise in body temperature and feeling of euphoria, and if this does not occur it means valerian is not working and should not be used until the previous steps can be accomplished (if valerian fails to induce sleep its effects can be reversed with a dose of niacinamide and aspirin to restore mitochondrial energy production). Especially in those who are older the use of valerian can instead produce "cold brain syndrome" which occurs during aging anyway and can be mistaken for senility but is in fact just excessive metabolic inhibition of the brain by deficient production of heat and energy. For this reason valerian should not be used in older persons or anyone who does not have an adequate metabolic rate until after these problems are addressed. Because it can induce sleepiness it should only be used before bed, and valerian also lasts in the body for several days so do not use it more than once or twice a week, and higher doses will absolutely not work better but will just more strongly inhibit mitochondria, so never exceed 1 gram per dose. Because tea is a primary strategy for achieving tannins in the diet, the use of nuts with their skins or herbal tea high in tannin such as from Indian bay leaf (*not* bay laurel) are great alternatives.

This is also a good time to mention that when restoring a healthy metabolism it is common and expected to feel sleepy and languid both in the morning and mid afternoon which most people mistake for being tired and view as negative because of our merciless preoccupation with productivity and materialism. An adequately fed and stress free body produces more GABA generally and being sleepy in the mornings and afternoon around nap time is actually a positive sign that stress hormones are low and GABA function high and should be expected as health improves. Taking a nap in the afternoon can be nice but is not necessary, and wakefulness is promoted by light exposure, so getting sun in the morning or afternoon can help promote alterness required for being active, and you can also use coffee and food to keep from having afternoon lethargy if necessary.

Finally, our modern technology can also interfere with sleep, but not in the ways which are often ignorantly cited such as looking at a screen. When I relocated to Palm Springs at the age of thirty-one I had not yet hit the height of my insomnia, but still was never able to sleep before one or two in the morning, every single night. Palm Springs seemed a reprieve from the stress of life and I thought it might finally help me get my health under control. My first night there I fell asleep at nine p.m. and didn't wake up until nine a.m., and it was the first time in ten years I had slept so well and I was excited for many more nights of blissful slumber. I spent the day setting up the house—the furniture, the electronics, etc., and though exhausted was very disappointed the next night to find myself again tossing and turning. For the next three years my insomnia was constant, and I would try to sleep and be woken by agitation and fits of coughing (which I would later discover to be cystic fibrosis), or my snoring partner, and spend hours on the couch watching TV or reading a book only to grow sleepy, retire to the bedroom, and wake immediately every single time. Sometimes I fell asleep on the couch and I could not understand why there was a difference between there and my bed and began to think it was my partner's snoring that made me agitated and restless.

But one day almost three years after living in Palm Springs we purchased a new wifi router which was more powerful and had a broader range and would reach all the way to the pool deck. That night after turning it on my insomnia became unbearable. It actually HURT, physically, like nothing I had ever felt, and I could not feel relaxed even on the couch. I suddenly realized the wifi station near our bedroom had been a primary cause of my insomnia the whole time, and my first night in Palm Springs it had not yet been connected. I got online and did some reading and sure enough found many studies showing the deleterious effects of wifi radiation on human physiology. I turned it off immediately and for the first time in years slept well again. But my boyfriend hated having the wireless off even when we were sleeping during the night, so it was difficult to keep away from wifi, and I started sleeping in the living room simply because it was further from the wifi and I could actually get a few hours of sleep if I became sufficiently exhausted. But I began turning off the device when he fell asleep, and when he left on a business trip I turned off every signal-emitting device in the house and for three nights alone slept soundly, not even waking to use the bathroom, even though I was still very sick with cancer and cystic fibrosis.

Wifi makes sleep troubles *worse*. The radiation reacts with copper and iron in our cells just as it does the copper in a receiver's antenna and stimulates cellular activity which prevents them from shifting into sleep mode, and probably reflects deterioration of the myelin sheaths which normally line and insulate nerve cells which then permits radiation from sources like wifi and cellular to reach them (though cellular is far weaker). Wifi is microwave radiation, the same power that heats your food in ninety-seconds or is used in induction stovetops, and is also energizing your tissues and causing interruption to cellular processes which all function on principles of energy management through the direction and flow of electrons. Much later after having made this discovery I still desired it to not be true and after a year of sleeping well in an apartment far away from any wifi sources moved to one surrounded by more than twenty wifi signals. I spent that entire year with nearly the same kind of insomnia, except now that I was healthy it no longer hurt so badly. When we were still together I even observed my boyfriend snoring more loudly when his cellphone was parked near the bed, which makes sense because snoring is a problem of metabolic fatigue of the nasopharynx tissue and energy stress from microwave signals would simply further fatigue those tissues. If you are having sleep problems you absolutely *must* get away from wifi signals at night, but reversing peroxisome dysfunction and copper dysregulation can help a great deal and at this edition of this book am able to sleep more deeply than in all my entire adult life while surrounded by many, many other wifi stations in this apartment complex but still must turn off my own since it is in such close proximity to my bed. Wifi has a very strong falloff rate so it isn't totally necessary avoid *all* exposure, but if there is one in your home turn it off when you're not using it and put it as far away from your bedrooms as possible, especially those of children, and go back to using ethernet cables, which are faster anyway.

Insomnia is only difficult to relieve because of the way we live our modern lives, away from sunshine, over-stressed and under-fed, suffering from malnutrition, and exposed to all kinds of ungodly radiation, pathogens, and toxic contaminants from industry and materialism. Just like the tobacco industry suffered major political and economic consequences after the harms of cigarettes were finally acknowledged by the public, communications companies will suffer a similar fate for ignoring the physics of electromagnetic radiation on the human body. There are too many studies which have conclusively established a negative effect of such radiation on human physiology as the technology currently exists and the absolutely insane number of human beings currently suffering insomnia is caused by this widely adapted technology. Future technology such as LiFi will probably be better, and is faster anyway, if it doesn't affect eyesight in humans or animals and might be a promising reprieve from this problem.

Sleep can once again be satisfying and easy to come by, requiring only some compassion for the body, feeding it well, and avoiding those modern impediments to human biology. Of course, none of this guarantees these conditions will not recur, which can happen if the body is placed under the same kinds of stresses which cause them in the first place, which includes dietary stressors, pathogenic infection, and insufficient exposure to sunlight. But since you're already reading this book you are perhaps unlikely to repeat many of those behaviors.

CHAPTER 21

PERMANENT WEIGHT LOSS, POSTURE, CHRONIC FATIGUE

"What are you doing?" came the voice of one of my sisters at the other end of the basement. All four of them had piled downstairs unnoticed and now stared at me disapprovingly. It was less a question and more an accusation, as if I had been doing something wrong, and I didn't help my situation by quickly yanking down my shirt. "Nothing," I lied, feeling the hot flush of shame rising in my cheeks. I walked past them as if I wasn't completely mortified at having been caught admiring myself in the only large mirror in our house. In the dim light of the basement of the eighteenth house in which we had lived I had seen for the first time the striated lines of my muscles running from my ribs down through my belly button and tapering into a line before disappearing into my jeans. Flexing them, I had realized I could make my muscles appear more pronounced. *This is how men have muscles,* I realized, suddenly excited at the very first signs of becoming a man, pulling my shirt up I saw this definition was on my chest too. I flexed them, imaging how big they might get as I grew and the attention it might win.

Of course, it is not their fault that my family was also brought up in such an oppressive, shame-based community which denigrated the experience of being human and humiliated us for having a body, but it was nothing but a downhill slope from there, a mine-field of religious and cultural reasons to mistrust and deplore my body. Yet as a human male I am *severely* perceived or admired based on my body, and the quality of my health can even (unfairly) improve or destroy my social and economic situation. Boys new to manhood post photos of their lovely bodies online and find instant success, happy to indulge in the delusion that they, and not nature, are responsible for their devastating appearance and demigod muscles, nor succeed in understanding the shallow and impermanent interest from others equally ignorant to our basic animal instincts. Women too have similar struggles and triumphs, though I cannot write from their perspective, and we all find the various stages of life either supported or sabotaged by the body because the body is who I am and how I experience life, and everything the body does has a purpose.

When I finally fell in love the second time it was with a boy I had seduced for a hookup. The sex was so good we kept meeting, and suddenly Valentine's day arrived and we were still spending time together so I asked if he'd be my Valentine. I bought new clothes, set the table with wine and candles, and cooked duck and duck fat fried rice which did not turn out because we got drunk before the meal was ready. He kindly pretended to like it but I ordered Brazilian delivery instead and then we fucked the rest of the night. It was an unexpected relationship, one that came out of nowhere and fit perfectly into my life. I have never had so much fun with someone as I did that boy. We spent almost every day together, and rarely argued.

But it was the first time my weight began to be an actual problem instead of just an annoyance, and I also held back more than I should have on account of a deep fear of intimacy. By Christmas he was giving me quick pecks on the cheek, coming over less often, and his eyes wandered when we were alone. We broke up but then tried to get back together. Things continued to get worse, and as I left to go home for Christmas it was clear he was not interested in continuing our relationship, and suspected him of being unfaithful.

I was grateful when driving into Park City during a heavy snowfall to get away from the bustle of Los Angeles and burrow away into the snowy blankets of the Rocky Mountains. My struggle to stay lean and the failure of yet another relationship weighed heavily on me, made worse by the religious firewall which stood firm between me and my family to whom I was still not allowed to discuss nor involve my romantic life. But just a few hours into the visit as my parents were discussing the specifics of orchestrating that night's dinner my father pulled me aside. "I wanted you to know you're welcome to bring anyone home for the holidays now," he said. "Oh," I replied, not expecting to be welcomed as a full member of the family without a heated discussion, tears, and heartache. How strange it was to finally be accepted, more or less, when my relationship was now looking down the barrel of a shotgun. Knowing that I was in love with someone had probably softened his opinion. *Thanks but your timing is lousy,* I wanted to say. *My boyfriend doesn't like me anymore and we're breaking up.* "Thanks," I said instead.

Depressed, I decided to get on a dating site. I was tired of feeling lonely and constantly rejected by people to whom I was loyal and affectionate. I was not on there for ten minutes when a message came from a devastatingly handsome boy also my height, sporting a well defined six-pack, pecks, and a smile that would knock you out cold. His eyes sparkled with the newness of romantic conquest, not yet deadened by heartbreak, an air of confidence infecting everything about him. Half worried I was cheating and half that he would turn away immediately at seeing me I found myself accepting his invitation. But I also lacked a car and was staying with my parents with a few of my newly married siblings. How we could meet exactly was not an easy thing to figure out.

"Want to go to a movie tonight?" said my mom while I was in clandestine conversation with this boy. God apparently wanted me to get laid. "Actually, an old friend of mine wants to meet up." I lied, "He was going to dive up here, is that okay?" "Sure," she said.

They finally left and I paced the house, palms clammy, sweating profusely as I waited for him to arrive. Even though my online pictures had been taken only hours before I was sure he would turn away immediately when he saw me, and then I could enjoy a quiet night in my sweats drinking spiked cocoa alone by the fire and not worry about silly things like romance.

Finally the doorbell rang. It is rare in my life to look right across at someone, let alone to also instantly fall in love. Of course, it wasn't really love, as my heart still belonged to the boy who no longer wanted me, but his smile nearly split his face in two, it was also genuine and kind, and I was smitten. "Hi," he said kindly, and before I could invite him inside added, "You're cute." "Thanks," I smiled, desperately relieved as I shut the door behind him and took his coat. My nervousness quickly gave way to excitement as he asked, "What do you want to do?"

"I thought we could hot-tub."

"I brought my suit in the car," he said. I gave him a wry smile, since I did not live here and this was not a real date threw all caution out the door. "I don't think we need them."

He stepped over and gave me a kiss, then we took off our clothes and ran with towels out to the hot tub. As he climbed into the water his well-defined butt muscles tensed, the smooth, defined haunches of an athlete. After months of despair and frustration I couldn't believe this was happening. We slid into the steaming water amidst the descent of silent, heavy snowflakes, the dim light from the house casting a warm glow across the deep snow all around us. He beamed as if being with me was the thing he'd been waiting for all his life. After talking a little bit his hands drifted through the water to find my leg. My fears of being rejected were not being realized, at all, even with my spare tire and saggy appearance. It was more than cathartic. It was affirming.

His hand slid inbetween my legs, then we kissed for a while as the snowfall grew heavier. After another conversion he rose up out of the water and took a seat on my lap, smiling down at me as the snow touched his beautiful face, his massive erection sticking straight up in front of me. We kissed some more. "Want to go inside?" I asked. He nodded.

Ten minutes later we collapsed on top of each other. At this point my health had already begun to decline and erectile dysfunction was sadly now the norm whenever I got nervous. He finished right away, and I quietly waited for him to excuse himself and depart, to put put me out of my anxious misery. "Want to go get ice cream?" he asked instead.

We got dressed and headed to Park City's Main Street and slipped and skidded our way into a coffee shop and ice cream parlor where he told me more about his life and ambitions to relocate to Los Angeles. He asked about my life, my dreams, and life in L.A. I told him about my failed relationship. His attention drifted at times and I was readying myself at any moment for this dream to end, but two hours went by before he finally suggested that the storm might prevent him from making the hour drive back down the canyon.

The drive home was muffled by waves and waves of snow, that otherworldly quiet which the dead of winter brings. Every once in a while he stole a glance my way. "I wish I could spend more time with you," he said. "Me too," I replied.

"Actually, I am going to be in L.A. for New Years."

"Really?"

"Yeah, I wasn't going to say anything, but I'd love to see you again. Can we spend New Years together?"

My boyfriend and I had made plans, before things had gone under. Unsure whether we still would and being a person who kept commitments even when I shouldn't, I hesitated. "I don't know if I'm going to be single or not," I said. "I want it to work out."

"Okay," he replied with a disappointment that made me feel desired. "But if things don't we can," I said.

Nearing my parents house he slowed down on a stretch of abandoned road and pulled to the side. "I need to kiss you more," he said, before throwing himself at me once again. The snow quickly covered the entire car, wrapping us in a warm, dark igloo of hot romance. Our clothes came off and a short while later we both finished all over my chest. I had never seen so much come in my life. Laughing, and kissing we tried to clean up but the only option was my shirt, carefully hidden beneath my coat after he finally dropped me off as I made my way with excuses to my bedroom, in no hurry to get rid of it.

Returning to L.A. I had two resolves—one, to get back in shape and two, to make things as great with my boyfriend as it had been with this boy from Utah. But it quickly became apparent that a one-sided effort did not have much fire as when shared. He even declined to come home with me on New Years so the next day we parted ways with the revelation that he had indeed cheated on me.

I began running every morning, spurred by the use of the exciting new supplement, resveratrol. I quickly lost weight, and over the next few months the boy from Utah would fly down every weekend to be with me and look for jobs. We talked about taking trips together while lying in bed covered with sweat and boy juice, fucking two or three times a day. I woke up one morning to him watching me sleep. It was a little creepy, but deep down I loved it. No one had ever been as interested in me as this athletic specimen of man, and I was still flabby and out of shape. He talked to me constantly, even when he was not in my city, and being with him was easier than anyone I had ever dated. I began to relax and enjoy my long extended weekends with him.

Soon I was back in my thirty-six-waist jeans. My old confidence returned and this new supplement gave me more energy than I'd had in some time. Sure, I felt jittery and restless (due to it's unknown side effect of strongly increasing cortisol) but things were going so well there was little reason to worry. After a few weeks I couldn't believe it when I needed to buy thirty-four-waist jeans, which I hadn't worn since I was eighteen, as it seemed not only had I lost all my body fat but my pelvis had actually thinned as well. For the fist time I also had a partner who liked me for who I was, since he had fallen in love with me when I was fat and at a low point. Life was finally going to be the way I wanted it.

But of course, life is not like that, and the day before I was to fly to Utah for Valentines and surprise him with a beautiful hotel room to spend the weekend the tone in my new love's voice changed. He had been so excited about being in love he came out to his family, but they rejected him entirely and demanded he attend conversion therapy. I fell to pieces. He agreed to see me for dinner but my heart broke a second time in six months as I sat across from him, robbed of his warmth and affection which had been so freely given now sterile and indifferent as a stranger. His last trip to Los Angeles he told me he was falling in love with me, and worried that I had scared him by not returning the same I assured him I too was falling in love. I told him about the hotel room I got us, and he agreed to spend the night but insisted he was straight and refused to touch me. I was sure my presence would draw him out of this nonsense but he refused to kiss me, to even look at me, and slept beside me all night on the other side of his bed in his magic Mormon underwear.

Still rent from my failure in my last relationship I collapsed in a pile of misery and self-loathing. I turned to heavy marijuana use to subdue the exceptional squall within that would not be silenced, tossing and turning every night due to the effects of dieting, excess exercise, and use of resveratrol unless I was totally obliterated, tormented by the dream of his luminous eyes and bright smile and warmth of his large, muscular body. He didn't even give me the pleasure of closure, refusing my calls and texts as soon as I boarded the plane back to Los Angeles. The emotions in me were the most violent and unsettled I had ever experienced, and I wrongly harassed him until he finally gave in and talked to me one final time, saying plainly he was no longer interested.

Though heartbroken and mad with frustration I was determined not to let this deter my first resolve, to become active and fit again, so I did not abandon my routine though the emotions nearly drowned me. I returned to swimming and grew more fit than I had perhaps in all my life. Yet I appeared to be losing the bulk of my muscle, finding it more difficult to retain mass than was usual. It was also during this time I tried other supplements to stifle the disquiet in my soul which grew at each passing day. *St. John's Wort* and *5-HTP* promised great improvements in mood and happiness, but the frightening episode of arrhythmias one day at practice made me think perhaps all these things I was taking were contributing to it, so I abandoned them all (including resveratrol). Suddenly my emotions improved and my muscles began to grow again, without adding any unwanted body fat.

Years later the first man I was ever able to bring home for the holidays asked me to marry him on Christmas day in front of my entire religious family. This was our third Christmas together, the second with my family since his would not even acknowledge my existence, and as we had ascended into Park City through freshly fallen snow the radio (which we never usually listened to) announced that the law prohibiting same-sex marriage in Utah had been ruled unconstitutional. I should have known it was coming too because every single one of my five, already-married siblings had their phones out and pointed at me as I slowly emptied my stocking after a long Christmas morning unwrapping presents with all our boisterous nieces and nephews. The ring was at the bottom of the snowman stocking my mother made for me years earlier when I hadn't come home for Christmas, beneath a mess of tinfoil chocolates and tiny, wrapped trinkets. It was shiny, silver, a *Tiffany* engagement knot. It was a tight fit, though, and proved a struggle to slip on. He had craftily taken my ring measurement six months earlier while getting a neck-lace repaired. I was twenty-pounds lighter then, and fifty since we first met, again struggling with my weight, even more severely than ever. On the drive to Utah he had remarked how fluffy my new vest was, which I embarrassingly corrected him was not the vest, but my gut. While on his knee my soon to be fiancé accidentally asked me to be his wife. I said yes without a moment's hesitation but my joy was tainted by thoughts about how much better it would have been if I was lean and fit in all those videos of our proposal. I would only have one and now an important event was forever marred by evidence that I could not control my body. It was okay. When we got back to Palm Springs I would start an even more ambitious diet. So what if I didn't look my best during my only marriage proposal? Love isn't really known for its good sense of timing. At least I will have a husband. I made up my mind to go to boot-camp three times a week to burn it off. I could make up for it by being fit at my wedding.

I turned the ring around and around for the rest of our trip and the entire drive home, beaming with the joy of certainty in love. I got back to exercising and a calorie-restrictive diet, but my weight problems were persistent, and increasing my efforts not only failed to slim me down they began to exhaust me strangely, as if my body was running out of gas, and I even continued to put on weight. One day in the gym, jogging on a treadmill I grew obsessively frustrated with the calorie counter on the bike. It ticked *SO SLOWLY* in spite of the high speed at which I pedaled. I became fascinated with the power of one calorie. According to the machines I could run with so much effort for a long while and only expend a few measly calories of energy. At most a few hundred could be burned but that required an hour or two, energy which I definitely did not have, and I must have needed to burn *thousands*. How was this possible?

Instead of romantic bliss my fiancé began regarding me with open contempt, commenting negatively on my appearance and even making fun of me at times. I grew terrified he would leave and so I redoubled my efforts, but every workout, every diet seemed to take a little more life from me. Eventually my health would decline to the point of being unable to sleep at night, at all, ever, and the physical pain became so severe I medicated myself with copious amounts of alcohol, pain killers, and spent many hours each night either in a warm bath applying epsom salts or breathing into a paper bag on the couch trying desperately to get air into my lungs. At a pound shy of *three-hundred* and my fiancé transformed into an outright adversary, and entirely dropped any pretense of being my ally.

I topped at three-hundred-one when he finally left. But within six months of learning how to properly care for my health I rapidly lost sixty pounds, faster than I had ever put on weight, not only without exercising but also while eating three to four pounds of sugar a week and a diet regularly exceeding four-thousand calories (since I am so huge), finding also improvements in the long and trouble-some illnesses I suffered. In addition to a huge calorie intake I consumed butter and ice cream regularly, foods many people regard with utter contempt even while enjoying them. Especially for someone who suffered severe alcoholism, cancer, thyroid disease, premature erectile dysfunction and aging to look the way I did from consuming so many calories and so much sugar and fat was nothing short of remarkable. A few years before I wasn't even sure if I was going to live, let alone fit into thirty-six-inch waist jeans again or regrow my lost hair, and all without any dieting. Unbeknownst to me at the time this benefit occurred in large part due to the inhibition of hyperglycemia by fructose, which then helps the body retain glycogen stores for longer and thus resolves any need for substantial fat storage, which was restored by a diet high in tannins, sugar, fruit, plenty of sun exposure, and eradication of opportunistic microbes which impaired digestion.

While I very much enjoy the legion of young, muscular athletes and models which populate social media their ignorance to metabolic challenges and the promotion of stress-based methods of weight loss are entirely antithetical to the true function of human physiology. Young, healthy men and women can envious-ly withstand considerable stress for a great period of time as the body possesses many resilient, adaptive survival mechanisms which spare us even from the stress we cause ourselves, but anyone who does not find success in such stress-based approaches to health and fitness are illustrations of the true function of human physiology which is one that resists stress but is still susceptible to it. Instead of wondering why success comes so easily to the young and athletic and not others, even when those others expend far more effort against debilitating conditions with which healthy persons do not contend, most people who use stress methods simply exclaim that everyone else isn't trying hard enough, which is an entirely asinine precept considering that those with metabolic challenges expend far more effort under more trying circumstances.

The healthy person who has never had health problems and finds exercise to be fun and invigorating is a clod for telling others with metabolic burdens that success only takes dedication and self will, and in truth their actions are motivated by the same fear held by all of us which is of those real limitations of life which cannot be ignored or willed into submission. Others witness the progress of these physical idols and regurgitate the same stupid inconsistencies even when it does not work for them, not because there is real truth in them but because it supports their personal worldview, trauma, and desire to ignore the limitations of mortality. My own attempts to improve or even maintain my physique using the stress methods sent me speeding toward total metabolic collapse and the development of serious thyroid disease and cancer by my early thirties because, having cystic fibrosis, my body was even less able to resist the consequences of merciless abuse, starvation, and overwork.

The stress methods of weight loss and athletic activity destroy the very metabolic pathways which support wellness, lean muscle, and athletic ability because they do not create energy, they only spend it. The facilitation of youth and wellness which includes effortless leanness and health requires an abundance of energy, and if we only spend energy and do not make energy we end up in an energy deficit. Calories are energy which keep us alive, so the idea that a calorie deficit produces weight loss is technically true, but it is because your body is dying from a deficit of energy. Death is the ultimate expression of energy deficit, and we drive ourselves toward it by purposefully depriving our bodies of the fuel required for cells, tissues, and organs live. This does not mean exercise and physical activity is bad, only that to facilitate such endeavors without incurring a metabolic debt requires sufficient energy production, processes which can be inhibited by dieting but also by pathogenic colonization and interruption of nutrient pathways, and rather than regarding such activities as a means to support health they should be regarded as recreation, facilitated by good health but never a source of it. Exercise should *always* be fun. If it's not fun it's because the body has not sufficient energy to sustain it, and so releases excessive stress hormones which foul the mood and promote restless irritation.

About a year before the tumors were discovered on my thyroid, during an unproductive doctor's visit where the doctor once again said there was nothing wrong with me except elevated white blood cells (oh, is that all?) a nurse mentioned when the doctor was out of the room that my blood results suggested pre-diabetes. Considering I was forty pounds overweight and suffering tremendously this didn't come at all as a surprise, but it also motivated me to engage in more exercise and dieting and eventually trying resveratrol again which this time not only did not result in weight loss it further worsened my symptoms and suffering and promoted even more weight gain. That I also had cystic fibrosis not diagnosed by the medical profession even after an emergency room visit for a severe, relentless cough which had been especially bad for several days and entirely prevented me from sleeping at all further emphasizes how narcissism, body shame, and destructive ideas about health and wellness cause us massive harm and the polar opposite results we want for ourselves or, more psychotically, for others to be fit and healthy in satisfaction of our own fears and narcissism. As a lifelong athlete familiar with training and hard work (unlike my partner whom instead spent his young life in the theater), I was absolutely mystified when after turning thirty no matter how hard I pushed my body I continued to put on weight and lose vitality until suddenly I was nearing obesity and dying of cancer and alcoholism.

Resveratrol caused its effects because it severely increases cortisol, which is how it caused me to slim down excessively when I was younger, even causing my bones to shrink, but when I was older and already sick it broke my body and actually made me *gain* more weight because cortisol forces catabolism of lean muscle into free sugars and amino acids in preference of fat which is actually the last storage site of calories on the body to be consumed by stress, since it participates in thermoregulation, and later promoted *more* fat deposition. The stress method of weight loss also deteriorated my skin and youthful complexion, caused stretch marks, and caused my hair to fall out and robbed me of my sex drive entirely in opposition to every proponent of exercise and diet as a means to health and fitness.

The way most people describe the calorie model of weight gain or weight loss makes it sound like we are a series of pipes through which flow calories. Everything in the pipe goes into us and stays there unless we are morally strong enough to do something about it. Thankfully, we are not a set of pipes, and our bodies are instead a complex spongey mass of biochemical pathways which respond according to chemistry and the environment, not discipline or willful resolve. To store calories chemical reactions must take place, as they also must to rid it. The major inconsistency in the calorie-deprivation, calorie-burning stress method of weight loss and fitness is that there really is not much difference between resting energy expenditure and active energy expenditure. Going on that run or spending an hour at the gym doesn't actually burn *any* more calories than your body already burns just being alive and sitting around all day. The brain burns the most calories of any organ in the body and a body at rest burns calories constantly—my body at rest burns at least three to four thousand calories a day which know because that is how much food I eat *every day* and I do not exercise and, unlike when I was younger and athletic, do not gain excess fat. After my recovery I mostly sat all day at work in front of a computer and still lost weight. The most activity I got was walking to get coffee or having sex (which honestly could have been a lot more often). When I got home from work I sat to read, watch TV, or play video games. Two or three times a week I practiced muscle control as discussed in the chapter on free muscle, which is standing in place and practicing muscle isolation and contraction and also just lied about how often I did it (I *wanted* to do it two or three times a week). There was a period during later research when self-infected with pathogenic bacteria I again gained weight, which was then again lost after their resolution, without dieting or exercise, directly demonstrating the role of fat in protecting us from the destructive effects of pathogens.

My problem in relationships was not that people kept leaving me because I struggled with my weight. Instead, my experiences of abuse and trauma from childhood conditioned me with a paucity of self-esteem and to feel comfortable in the presence of manipulative, shallow, and unreliable people because I could in turn control them if I submitted to their control behaviors, and would unconsciously seek out partners who were charismatic, controlling, and heartless and get myself into situations which were always doomed from the beginning. I also defensively used to think that weight loss and people who fixated on fatness as a marker of health were shallow but in truth most people don't actually know what it means to be healthy and the desire or fixation on looking fit and losing weight is just an ignorant shortcut for describing what they think is health. If you bought this book so you can be skinny you're also an asshole who has a lot to learn about life, and you probably treat other people just as shitty as you treat yourself and suffer from unresolved trauma surrounding your body image and self-worth which drives self-destructive behaviors that will ultimately lead to your death if you do not resolve that trauma as discussed in the chapter on spirituality and my book on psychology (The Perfect Child) because no matter how much we know about disease or the human condition we can never, ever, EVER extract ourselves from the immutable laws of mortality or cause and consequence. Being lean and fit does *not* equate to being healthy and most people utilize stress methods for managing weight which are, in the long term, very bad for us and will always lead to other problems like hair loss, heart failure, and even cancer because excessive exercise, low-carb and fad diets, and calorie cutting and starvation destroy our commensal microbiome, immunity, and endocrine system. Even young people whom are resistant to the severe effects of stress who can lose weight from stress methods will always, always experience emotional turmoil since stress hormones and deficient production of energy causes discomfort, which are the beginnings of aging and metabolic illness, and will always, always lead to serious consequences as we grow older.

There is one very simple biological pathway underlying weight gain, which is that all fat deposition is actually triggered by *water* influx into adipose tissue. You probably read that and think maybe you can stop drinking water and lose weight but again we are talking about biochemistry and not behavior and it is impossible to will the body to stop losing water from the bloodstream to fat. Specifically, ammonia such as is produced by parasites, yeasts, *H. pylori*, and *Streptomyces* chemically competes with water for entry into cells, and excess ammonia caused by pathogenic colonization is thus the primary promoter of fat retention. Inflammation in the body is water influx into cells, and since water dilutes electrolytes and dampens electric conductivity of cells excess water is toxic to vital organs, so one of the primary functions of fat besides thermoregulation is as a storage site to get water away from internal organs, to sequester water into fat (much like the proverbial camel hump which is in fact not proverbial as fat is in fact a water storage mechanism). This protective mechanism occurs more dramatically as the cardiovascular system becomes depleted of water as discussed in the chapter on vascular insufficiency because the bloodstream is normally our water reservoir which must be replaced when disease impairs the normal function of albumin and electrolyte metabolism, and because ammonia is also similar to water but is not water it is highly toxic, especially to the nervous system, the body must first eliminate excess ammonia to maintain nitrogen balance before it can also resolve water excess. Failing to drink water out of a misguided idea to deprive fat of water will instead only result in a heart attack or stroke as the bloodstream dries out, and this problem is instead entirely that of pathogenic colonization which must be addressed as discussed in other chapters.

Most people do not understand that most hormones are also made from fats, and one of the primary catalysts for extra fat storage on the body is the loss of dietary fat absorption due to colonization by opportunistic microbes for which the body then compensates by increasing the endogenous synthesis of fats from dietary carbohydrate while lowering the metabolic rate to prevent overconsumption of fats that are required for our metabolic survival entirely separate from the caloric function of fat. This is the reason why those with metabolic disease present with an increase in circulating triglycerides, fatty acids, and dysregulated cholesterol as discussed in the upcoming chapter on hormones since the body, still requiring fats for its survival, must resort to different strategies to obtain it. High triglycerides are a recognized marker of disease, because they are the body's backup to disturbed fat metabolism, but mainstream treatments for high triglycerides typically destroy the part of the liver which produce them which further deprives the body of requisite fats and results in worse, not better, overall outcomes in mortality and quality of life. As discussed in the chapter on gut health fat is also antimicrobial and during bile dysfunction (which serves to emulsify fat) the microbiome is altered which then promotes those which are resistant to fat exposure to further cause disease and promote lower metabolic rate and greater fat retention. While this can be mediated by avoiding dietary fat, which is a common dieting practice, avoiding fat still impairs synthesis of hormones, so only resorting gut health and normal cholesterol function (in the chapter on hormones) is the only way to normalize hormones and fat metabolism. Advocates of paleo or primal diets want to think of our species as mythical, violent warrior hunters who stalked and ate giant mammoths and other wild animals—Mostly we just killed and ate their babies, which is why they went extinct, but we also were *already* human when we became hunters, and we instead became human while subsisting entirely on fruit, blossoms, leaves, nuts, roots, insects, and mollusks with only the occasional fish or small animal, and our physiology is far more strongly regulated by plant biocompounds, specifically watermelon, and the role of fire and cooking than from animal products. Without plant foods we are ineffective at absorbing fats and fat soluble nutrients, cannot resist parasitism and colonization by hydrogen sulfide producing pathogens, and our metabolic rate falls because of nutritional profiles which resemble winter or famine, and since fat is necessary for steroidogenesis, thermogenesis, and heat insulation the body instead actively retains fat when nutritionally stressed rather than dump the very thing which keeps us alive.

Fat is also not lost during exercise because it is 'burned' into energy as is commonly assumed. Energy can never be created or destroyed and when the body engages in 'burning' fat as an energy source that fat is actually converted into *CO2* and *water*, which releases energy, so fat lost from its active metabolism is actually lost through breathing and peeing it out. CO2 promotes mitochondrial fission (they split into new mitochondria), and since mitochondria are the energy centers of cells this means an increase in energy too when metabolizing fat. But, mitochondria produce far larger quantities of CO2 from carbohydrate oxidation because carbohydrate is rapidly metabolized where fat metabolism takes longer (and also risks more reactive oxygen species), but dieting, excessive exercise, low-carb diets, and anything else that promotes "fat burning" forces mitochondrial fusion instead (they combine to reduce mitochondrial density) because the absence of carbohydrate and nutrients required for its oxidation signal to the body the reduced seasonal availability of nutritional resources, and reduced mitochondria means a lower metabolic rate and thus preservation of nutrients and calories. It is through this mitochondrial regulatory mechanism that excessive exercise and undereating (and other metabolic stressors) actually *promote* weight gain as the body ages or succumbs to metabolic stress and why ignoramus athletes and self-righteous blowhards usually have absolutely no fucking idea what they are talking about when discussing fat, fitness, and calories, and especially *never* conditions like diabetes, obesity, and heart disease their rhetoric actually serves to promote, not resolve.

Exercise itself also induces fatty acid oxidation pretty rapidly after starting, and the more metabolically ill someone is the more fatty acids they release during physical exertion. But those who are most ill release fatty acids even when they aren't moving at all. Animals like canines or cetaceans whose ancestors had to constantly be on the move for survival are far better at metabolizing fat as an energy source, and canines (which are true distance hunters) can run for hours and hours and even days without tiring because their body does not suffer metabolic consequences from high fat metabolism, so in humans exercise itself can actually induce mitochondrial dysfunction and sustain and even promote metabolic illnesses rather than relieve them if mitochondria are not properly supported, and those who do find relief from metabolic illness through exercise benefit simply from the increase in CO2 produced during exercise which helps to maintain the body's pH and respiratory capacity which can and are instead better supported by diet and absence of pathogenic colonization. Exercise routines are also typically begun in tandem with a healthier diet or behaviors like going outside which are far stronger promoters of CO2 production and mitochondrial health than exercise, especially because sun exposure so strongly upregulates mitochondrial respiration by removing nitric oxide from cytochrome, where those who are naive to human biology assume it is the exercise rather than just being in the sun or eating more fruit or sources of oxalate which is responsible for their experience.

What makes this even more amazing is that someone who is fit, young, and healthy produces so much CO2 and ATP from so much working mitochondria that exercise for them is actually easy and enjoyable because they are able to produce enough energy to support the physical demand of exercise, while someone who is overweight or sick with metabolic disease produces so little CO2 and ATP their efforts are truly herculean compared to those who are already fit and healthy, and why misguided ideas about biology and physical wellness are so harmful and unproductive and causes those who are already ill to become even more ill as they push their bodies further into deterioration due to incorrect and harmful propaganda perpetuated by people who have absolutely no fucking qualifications to talk about biology the way they do.

Another primary function of fat stores is to capture sugar (glucose) during hyperglycemia (high blood sugar) when we are unable to store that sugar as glycogen. As discussed in the chapter on sleep, a healthy liver is able to store between 400-500 calories of glycogen, but during fructose deficiency such as occurs either from dieting, low-carb diets, sugar avoidance, or impaired sugar digestion as described in the chapter on diabetes the absence of fructose causes such extreme release of glycogen stores from even small amounts of adrenaline that it can even wake us from a dead sleep due to the resulting increase in metabolic rate, racing heart rate, sweating, etc., (this is usually from amine producing microbes in the gut, however). The body does not want to lose those valuable calories, however, and since it cannot store them as glycogen due to the chronic absence of fructose it instead deposits them as fat (fat cells also store glycogen, however). All throughout my young adulthood I prided myself on not consuming sugar but, like every normal person, also enjoyed caffeine, and in addition to the many emotional adrenaline triggers in my life (due to unresolved trauma and volatile interpersonal relationships) the use of caffeine without any fructose was causing near constant total glycogen depletion which not only made it difficult to feel rested and satiated but which also promoted an increase in fat deposition which I then treated by even more dieting, causing even worse hyperglycemia and glycogen depletion in a self-defeating cycle of stress and dieting where instead the chronic consumption of fructose, especially from healthful sources like well-ripened fruit, use of invert sugar (especially before caffeine use), and restoration of normal sugar digestion and absorption helps prevent hyperglycemia, excitability, weight gain, and glycogen depletion (large amounts are not required, but instead benefits from consistency).

As was the theme of Ray Peat's work, energy production is what facilitates the proper organization of cells and gives them the ability to be strong, flexible, and resistant and the reason that many of the therapies in this book help to improve health is through the facilitation of energy production which then empowers cells and tissues to properly construct and arrange themselves, not by force but by a rational understanding of biological pathways, and the gentle coaxing back to health through good nutrition, behaviors, and elimination of pathogenic organisms and stress, and the same factors which promote weight gain also cause chronic fatigue due to consequences like the impaired mitochondrial silicon (discussed in the chapter on cancer), poor immunity (chapter on immunity), and insufficient thyroid function (thyroid chapter) which directly regulates the production of energy. Reversing gut dysbiosis and restoring mitochondrial silicon, immune function, and thyroid function will also address problems like chronic fatigue.

Posture problems are also a consequence of cellular energy production since energy is needed for muscles and connective tissue to retain their support of the body, and posture is never, ever a function of the conscious mind but instead a reflection of cellular integrity, and rapidly in my progress back to good health found myself more easily and unconsciously sitting and standing more upright simply through the increased production of more energy from a generous diet and purposeful promotion of cellular respiration. Nearly equal to loss of silicon in problems with energy production is the function of *copper* in the respiratory enzyme *cytochrome oxidase* in the mitochondrial electron transport chain to produce ATP. Restoring copper before silicon or otherwise promoting mitochondrial respiration without restoring silicon can result in an increase in electron leakage from mitochondria, but after reversing mitochondrial silicon deficiency the restoration also of other factors required in the electron transport chain like copper, vitamin C, oleic acid, sugar, and sunlight can result in massive energy production as mitochondria suddenly become once again stable and efficient. Formation of *thiomolybdate* from interaction of microbial hydrogen sulfide and dietary molybdenum is a toxin that reacts with copper dependent enzymes like ceruloplasmin as discussed in the chapter on immunity, and because copper is required in the immune reaction this copper dysregulation promotes pathogens like oral infectious microbes which access the bloodstream and consume sulfate and connective tissue, reducing vitality, promoting fat gain, and deteriorating posture. Copper itself is also involved in the synthesis of elastin and collagen which hold together tissues, skin, bones, muscles, and organs through the function of the enzyme lysyl oxidase.

Swayback disease is a condition of posture deterioration and was once only thought only to concern livestock, but human swayback is extremely common and is marked by a forward pitching head and chin, exaggerated spine curving, and tilting pelvis which is a particular consequence of colonization by hydrogen sulfide producing through deficiency of copper by the formation of thiomolybdate (which also causes deficiency of molybdenum used in oxidase enzymes). Because cystic fibrosis impairs copper transport as discussed in the chapter on immunity I presented as pigeon-toed and knock-kneed most of my life which was adorable and added to my uniqueness as a person, but restoration of copper homeostasis through restoration of calcium metabolism and endogenous malate production with supplementation of copper (taken with dietary tannin and malate such from mixing with some sumac) at the age of forty-two allowed for the first time in my life to obtain a more normal gait and proper alignment of the pelvis, legs, knees, neck, and feet, especially when walking which subsequently then required learning how to walk and train muscles which were underdeveloped due to the shifts in posture caused by cystic fibrosis (specifically my quadriceps and abdominals handled most of the walking and standing upright that should be a primary job of gluteus muscles), and also eliminated tension on the *vastus lateralis* and *iliotibial band* which since my late twenties had frequently resulted in significant lateral knee pain. In my late twenties my ankles started popping and cracking with every step because of both misalignment and stiffening joints, but now in my mid forties and even heavier they don't make a sound.

A very easy way to thus diagnose copper dysfunction is also poor posture, especially in conditions like swayback, scoliosis, aging, or other metabolic disease. It should *never* be required to consciously move the head over the spine nor to right the pelvis nor to walk with a normal gait, and when the body has sufficient energy the pelvis should orient naturally upright when standing, to cradle the intestinal organs which in human swayback instead spill forward against the gut wall and produce a protruding gut which is often stupidly mistaken for fat, although this does also then stimulate fat deposition around the abdominal wall to support the constant stress of the intestines spilling forward. With swayback, bending over is also more difficult since the strain of doing so requires the activation of muscles which are atrophied and misaligned, and even moderate physical exertion can be fatiguing. Swayback and thus copper dysregulation is something that should be checked regularly at doctor's visits by simply observing the patient standing when taking their height, and a chin that protrudes forward any more than normal is a primary and easily identified symptom of copper dysregulation (and since halitosis and malodorous feces are a symptom of toxic hydrogen sulfide producers which interrupt copper metabolism this is very easy to diagnose). But since doctors are almost never interested in diet and nutrition it wouldn't do much good until the medical profession fully embraces diet and nutrition origins of disease (and without bias). Those with scoliosis are shown to present with higher levels of copper in hair which means the body is not using copper properly which is most strongly disturbed by soft tissue calcification which impairs copper binding and function in copper associated proteins like ceruloplasmin, metallothionein, and cytochrome oxidase at the root of these issues.

Because of the complexities of copper metabolism most people have no idea that simply taking a copper supplement can actually be toxic and even result in liver failure as free copper is highly reactive. As oral pathogens also consume connective tissue which further impairs posture and structural integrity, restoration of immunity and normal function of copper, calcium, vitamin C, molybdenum, sulfur, and halides as discussed in the chapter on viruses and immunity is the key to resolving these problems. Improvements can be quite rapid if done correctly, however, since we don't require an enormous quantity of copper, and the body is quite adept at capturing and retaining dietary copper if there are no intervening factors, and copper repletion should result in natural improvements to energy and posture, and if this does not occur it indicates continued factors which impair copper metabolism that are not a function of copper itself. Once recovery starts it may require some conscious effort to train and strengthen muscles in new positions which can be most effective through the practice of muscle control discussed in the next chapter on muscle, and practice walking with the pelvis rotated back to its upright rather than forward tilting, but this should feel easy and not require force if energy production has been restored.

Proper posture diagnostic is also often incorrect and leads to misdiagnosis. Tilting the pelvis to its upright position when standing and walking will naturally, without effort, also cause the legs to rotate outward and reverse knock-kneed or pigeon-toed orientation, with the tail bone rotating downward, which will and can even result in being 'duck-footed,' with the feet splayed outward rather than pointing forward. The feet are designed to push outward, not down, using the ball of the foot and big toe as means of motive force at an angle to the ground where going over top of them instead results in less force and ambulatory efficiency. There may also be some gender differences in foot position, with males having more outwardly splayed foot position that is in fact natural and should not be corrected, and females having a more forward position of the foot, but none being in fact exclusively forward or inward pointing which instead reflects waning energy production and fatigue of supportive muscles and connective tissue that has nothing to do with the mind or effort but biological production of ATP by mitochondrial respiration. Practice of muscle control will strengthen muscles rapidly and help promote stronger posture, but only if normal copper metabolism has been restored.

Another important function of fat which I have not really discussed is its structural role—When tissues age, become weakened, overly stressed, and misaligned such as what occurs during chronic fatigue, metabolic disease, and distended guts the body will actually pad these areas with extra fat in order to help support the structural integrity of that area, since mitochondria can no longer support sufficient energy production, which is why fat also accompanies these changes of posture which accompany aging and metabolic disease. A classic demonstration of this can be seen in older people who develop a hump across the back of their neck alongside swayback condition, which is almost entirely made of fat. Oftentimes extra fat around the waist, arms, neck, pectorals, etc., is there simply for structural reasons because metabolic decline and factors like hydrogen sulfide which interfere with mitochondrial respiration impairs our ability to generate energy for making protein and building lean tissues, which is why raising the metabolic rate and resolving pathogenic infection can reverse fat deposition as muscles and connective tissue strengthen and regenerate.

Vitamin D is the primary regulator of fat retention, and when we are replete with vitamin D the body automatically sheds fat pounds because vitamin D is a signal to the body that there is enough warmth and nutrition in the environment to risk dumping the insulating thermal layer of fat which otherwise keeps us warm, and this is likely a function of calcium scavenging properties. In support of this concept, studies show that vitamin D actively shrinks fat cells and acts as a mineral-sparing diuretic, promoting increased removal of water (fat being also a storage site for water) without losing electrolytes.

This is of course *not* achieved by supplementing vitamin D but by the complex biochemical pathways that create and manage vitamin D as discussed in that chapter. Vitamin D is so effective in promoting effortless weight loss that inability to lose weight can also be used as a diagnostic for vitamin D status, and when replete with boron, sun exposure, sugar, and carotenoids extra fat should simply come off the body at a slow, noticeable, daily pace. As discussed in the chapter on vitamin D, sugar also spontaneously causes fat detoxification through the liver and removed in feces but this pathway contributes to fatty liver if there is insufficient sulfur (either due to poor intake or hydrogen sulfide producing pathogens) because sulfation is required to keep fats water soluble and constrained to the feces after detoxification which are otherwise reabsorbed continuously back into the body due to opportunistic microbes during vitamin D deficiency. If this does not occur, more knowledge and implementation of those pathways must be addressed.

One of our only true "fat-burning" functions which can contribute to the loss of excess fat in a healthy way is the oxidation of fats which occurs at night, during sleep, under the expression of GABA which promotes a shift from cellular respiration to fatty acid oxidation by *peroxisomes* rather than mitochondria to generate heat from fat to keep the body warm while mitochondria are given an opportunity to rest and regenerate, and addressing GABA dysfunction and sleep problems can and does also result in noticeable loss of body fat every night simply from sleeping. Anthocyanin is also shown in studies to increase heat production from fatty acid metabolism, and an increase in skin heat can be directly felt when consuming regular sources of anthocyanin (this is not the same as a hot-flash, however, which instead feels uncomfortable and stimulates sweating) which can help support this function. In this sense, true, restful sleep really is one of the best and healthy ways maintain a normal, consistent, and healthy weight because it helps the body regenerate and restore itself, which cannot be achieved by pharmaceuticals which force sleep since this pathway is required to achieve restful sleep in the first place.

Weight loss is not about discipline, and certainly isn't about "burning" anything. It is about facilitating a body free of stress through healthy practices, good whole foods which are appropriate for human physiology (especially fruit, vegetables, and sources of anthocyanin), resolving gut and oral microbiome dysbiosis, promoting mitochondrial energy production through factors like sunlight exposure, vitamin C, and healthy digestion. If you are someone who derives self-esteem (or lack of it) from your body, this is a result of negative experiences and trauma as a child which deprived you of understanding your individual worth as a person, and unresolved experiences of abuse and trauma tend to cause focus on our body as a point of orientation to which we can anchor our sense of self (which is especially pronounced in those who suffer from narcissism). But the body ages, and is unreliable, as are those with whom we associate which fit into our control and coping mechanisms that result from trauma and reinforce negative ideas of self worth. You may be able to get sexier and solicit more validation, but you will never resolve the insecurity and self-doubt which underlies this poor valuation of self-worth without also resolving experiences of childhood trauma as discussed in the upcoming chapter on spirituality and my other book, *The Perfect Child*, to establish a conception of the self which is not reliant on such fleeting realities of existence as the human body.

CHAPTER 22
FREE MUSCLE

As I recovered from cancer I found putting on muscle to come so much more easily than it had any other time throughout my entire life, even during the many years of training as a young athlete. Ironically, a sedentary lifestyle proved to make muscle gain easy and effortless. This occurred because the primary problem with building muscle is not actually building muscle, but keeping it. Hormones and pathways of *anabolism* build muscle, but *catabolic* hormones and pathways tear muscle down to convert muscle into useable sugars and amino acids, so people with high metabolic stress also have high catabolic activity which makes building muscle much harder, and a sedentary lifestyle with a great diet and healthy environment instead lowers catabolic stress to promote retention of muscle growth.

For this same reason bodybuilders everywhere have also recognized the association between muscle mass and low cardiovascular training, or the inverse when cardiovascular training is high, regardless of strength training since the effects of stress and stress hormones on the body are immutable. This is also why runners have such little muscle mass in direct correlation to their degree of training and exertion, since chronic physical exertion more rapidly depletes liver glycogen and then requires muscle catabolism to access muscle glycogen to prevent the heart and brain from dying. Athletes have thus devised elaborate and detailed strategies to harness and control this correlation through patterns of 'bulking' and 'shredding,' but because the majority of nutrition and fitness concepts are still based on a misguided pain-equals-gain, stress-based approach to 'fitness' with complete ignorance to the problem of pathogens on metabolic health the true nature of muscle building is completely misunderstood and effort is far more excessive and extremely less efficient than what is necessary to achieve and maintain great musculature. Usually interfering with it, in fact.

We are monkeys. Well, great apes to be exact. And no other species of great ape hits the gym. Gorillas, the most muscular of all primates, sit on their butts *all day long*. They don't lift heavy things or move much in the search for food, and yet they possess *huge* amounts of muscle. So where'd it all come from?

The formula for building muscle is this: *protein + unopposed testosterone = muscle*. The key to this formula is *unopposed* testosterone, meaning that elevated testosterone is not always effective as is the case when enough stress hormones exist to counteract the effect of testosterone, promote its aromatization into estrogen, or such as when nitric oxide is so excessive it inhibits mitochondrial respiration and thus the process of anabolism. In humans, males grow bigger muscles than women because of our naturally higher levels of testosterone, though testosterone is still required for women and deficiency can be just as detrimental. If women supplement more testosterone they suddenly grow large, masculine muscles (as well as other masculine traits). Transgender men experience this change if they choose to transition because hormones have the same effects in all human bodies regardless of gender, and the reverse occurs for transgender women, and all aging humans experience decline in gender characteristics as they age and very often engage in gender reaffirming medical treatment like hormone replacement therapy. Most people believe ignorantly that the human body is static and constant, but you can see how hormones dynamically and constantly affect body composition in a continual process at all times that is subject to change, disruption, or enhancement, not only through pharmaceutical processes but also by our diet, environment, behaviors, pathogens, and metabolic health. When hormones change, even from moment to moment, they also change the character of the body, because that is what hormones do. A beautiful, young, muscular man would in the course of just a few weeks lose the *entirety* of his muscle should the flow of muscle-forming hormones suddenly cease and high quantity of stress hormones surge. The idea that the character of our bodies and identity are permanent simply because we have stopped growing is nothing more than an illusion performed by consistently working and present biological processes much like the air in a hot air balloon which, if allowed to cool, would immediately fall from the sky.

Because plants never cease growing their primary hormones are *estrogens* because estrogen is a hormone of growth, not a hormone of femininity, and in fact no hormone has gender qualities at all and gender is instead a function of the ratio, quantity, and balance of certain hormones to others. Estrogen functions to promote cellular division, proliferation, and water influx (which also stimulates fat deposition) by stimulating the process of *mitosis* which causes cells to swell with water which triggers duplication of chromosomes and division of the nucleus and then the cell to thus achieve cellular proliferation and multiplication. This is why the cycle and pregnancy are associated with high levels of estrogen, to support growth of the uterine lining or a fetus, but also why estrogen is also associated with cancer, and many transgender women and aging cisgender women who use hormone replacement therapy suffer health problems, especially as they age, from using only estrogen which is mistaken to be the primary hormone of womanhood when in fact it is the higher ratio of progesterone to testosterone and estrogen that accomplishes femaleness. Many transgender women seeking to inhibit testosterone take pharmaceutical diuretics which inhibit testosterone, but this is achieved by the inhibition of *all* sex hormone production and so they often fail to grow breasts, a feature easily accomplished by aging cisgender men due to the increased aromatization of testosterone to estrogen, even while taking large amounts of estrogen because of the absence of progesterone, not understanding that estrogen is in fact made in the body from androgens and that taking aromatase *promoters* while also supplementing progesterone would in fact eliminate the need to even take estrogen in both cisgender and transgender women and would result in greater femininity than what either are able to achieve in current strategies of hormone replacement therapy.

Progesterone achieves its function in the body because it helps to both regulate and prevent the growth effects of estrogen where it is inappropriate, in men as well as women, and part of the aging effects of testosterone aromatization in males is because of naturally lower levels of progesterone which decline even further during aging which thus fail to protect the body from the growth-stimulating properties of estrogen. Testosterone and other androgens are anabolic, which describes growth not in the sense of cell division and quantity but where cells actually increase in bulk, glycogen, fibers, mitochondria, etc., which is not achieved by inflammation and swelling as occurs from estrogen, but too much testosterone such as occurs in the use of anabolic steroids for bodybuilding results in massive aromatization of testosterone to estrogen especially since exercise and dieting behaviors strongly lower the metabolic rate, and because men naturally lack high progesterone the use of steroids in amounts typical of bodybuilding then results in overgrowth and enlargement of the head, navel, nipples, mammary glands, and ironically loss of hair since growth pathways turn off mitochondria (as discussed in the chapter on hair loss). Most ironically the use of anabolic steroids also causes the shrinkage of testicles and penis as the body tries to rescue itself from high aromatization by lowering the endogenous production of testosterone, achieved through involution of the testes which is why all those enormous, roided bodybuilders never fill out their tiny, tiny posing briefs. Where instead the normal production of high testosterone in males such as is achieved by low-stress, a good diet, and other factors which promote testosterone as discussed in the chapter on erections achieves its effects more through the process of *differentiation* where cells and tissues develop the secondary sex characteristics of adulthood, which for males includes large muscles. For instance if a child were exposed to the type of differentiation promoting hormones which support adult physiology they would also evolve directly into fully differentiated adults but at the size they currently stood, and the reason we do not mature for many years is to allow time for the body to grow a substantial foundational of size and resources before it then transitions into the differentiated specializations of adulthood secondary sex characteristics, changing from *quantitative* growth to *qualitative*.

Melatonin is the primary inhibitor of sex hormones and as such it is generally more elevated in children, and when it rises in adults due to sunlight deficiency or supplementation it similarly inhibits sex hormones and thus inhibits muscle growth, and one of the primary difficulties men and women experience in fitness and muscle growth besides starvation which increases catabolization of muscle is an excess of melatonin which inhibits its growth in the first place due to excessive sequestration indoors and attitudes such as that ten to fifteen minutes of sun exposure a day is enough (lol). Muscle only grows if the actions of testosterone are *unopposed* by oppositional hormones like melatonin because muscle is expensive (though not as expensive as fat) so the body attempts to reduce muscle when under stresses that indicate low availability of nutritional resources, in order to prolong survival, such as from low carbohydrate or winter (or artificial winter from being indoors all the time).

Certain foods like polyunsaturated fats in corn, soy, canola, and fish oil can also trigger declines in testosterone and negatively affect muscle growth. Fish oil is actually algal oil from algae, which is highly unsaturated because of the very cold temperatures of the environment in which plankton grow, and in the very hot environment of the human body these polyunsaturated fats easily undergo peroxidation damage and since hormones are also fats they are in turn directly affected by peroxidation due to diets high in polyunsaturated fats. Because it produces such strong inflammation common wheat gluten is also an effective inhibitor of muscle growth, especially in those who are also aging or suffering metabolic stress. Deficiency of anthocyanin impairs steroidogenesis since, as earlier discussed, anthocyanin is a nutritional regulator of blood flow and inducible nitric oxide which otherwise inhibits mitochondrial respiration required for high hormone production, and the reason why young specimens of men who inflate almost effortlessly with muscle even when doing very little exercise is due to a totally unopposed androgenic system because of a good diet low in stress with daily sun exposure which occurs not from genetics but family dietary and behavioral traditions which promote such healthy behaviors (and exposure to healthy microbes).

Because the entire function of *cortisol* is to actually catabolize muscle into into useable sugars and amino acids it is the most consequential inhibitor of testosterone function and muscle growth. Cortisol results most strongly by periods of hunger, especially prolonged, low blood sugar during insufficient consumption of carbohydrate, after adrenaline has exhausted liver glycogen and because the longest period going without food is typically during sleep the practice of avoiding breakfast such as I did frequently throughout my youth is the fastest way to cause enormous cortisol spikes which not only results in massive catabolism of lean muscle but also severe psychological stress as the brain is then deprived of sugar required to produce energy for it to run well and be healthy. Cutting out only carbs in attempts to slim down which works in healthy people by causing an *increase* in cortisol still reduces muscle mass even though other foods are still being eaten because cortisol is most strongly released in response to blood sugar levels and *always* breaks down muscle first to release its glycogen. Infection with *Clostridioides difficile*, the microbe which induces chronic glycogen release, can also keep cortisol chronically elevated, especially if the diet is very restricted, which is a primary reason for conditions like bipolar disorder and schizophrenia, because cortisol release always follows adrenaline release once circulating blood sugar begins to fall. As cortisol also dissolves other organs such as the thymus, thyroid, liver, etc., this does not only affect muscle, and the effect of cortisol is also cumulative, successive elevation causing more and more damage as it peels away layers of internal organs and lean tissue. The supplement resveratrol works in part by strongly blocking sugar uptake which then causes massive cortisol production, so I experienced an extreme loss of both body fat, muscle, and even bone but also extreme restlessness, agitation, and insomnia as cortisol is also the hormone of anxiety. When I used it again in my thirties there was no fat loss at all, only muscle loss, because by then too much cortisol had entirely destroyed my thyroid and adrenal glands and impaired my ability to even metabolize carbohydrate at all which in turn promoted an increase in fat retention and loss of even more muscle mass.

In contrast, my recovery included a sedentary lifestyle, too ill to engage in physical activity, yet even so I lost more than sixty pounds of fat and six pant sizes while also experiencing an increase in the musculature of my arms, legs, and chest from consuming up to four pounds of sugar a week in fruit smoothies in addition to all the other food and calories of regular meals and snacking (the amount would be more like two pounds of sugar for a regular sized person). Just because exercise *can* make a person lean and build muscle *does not mean it is the only way to do it*, nor even the best way to do it. Muscle also isn't only for looking good—being able to move through life, avoid or reduce injury, engage in sex, care for children, endure a workday, and let's not forget important muscles like the heart are all reasons to be concerned about muscle health that are not aesthetic, which as well rely on healthy methods of muscle gain to avoid the devastating crises which occurs from stress methods and their deleterious effect on anabolic pathways. As I experimented further with infectious pathogens they caused a significant decline in my physical strength which prevented me from even being able to bend over or get on the floor to clean my apartment, and as I discovered the cures to those illnesses my physical strength came back significantly and I was once again able to care for myself more effectively which never had anything to do with exercise or training since muscle is a natural feature of the human body, not something that must be earned.

As a young man I put on twenty-five pounds of muscle in just a few months once I began swimming competitively because it also stimulated an increase in hunger which I satiated through copious amounts of pasta in addition to my normal meals. I would come home from a workout after school and with nothing else to eat would just boil a package of pasta and dump on a large amount of marinara sauce which would cool down the pasta, heat up the sauce enough to eat, and inhale it before going to take a nap and having dinner later with my family. Though made from common wheat which caused other health problems it was a good source of both protein and carbohydrate as most grains are also very high in protein, but this progress was also reversed the following two years as my neurotic coach doubled our workouts and caused excessive metabolic stress and thus the catabolism of muscle as our bodies struggled to keep up with the carbohydrate and caloric requirements for such extreme physical activity. Similarly, the stress methods of muscle building—exhausting muscles, the "tearing" of fibers (which isn't a thing), and working to failure achieves muscle growth by stimulating an influx of water into muscle cells, through inflammation due to stress, and the appearance of anabolism but not true anabolism. This is most easily seen in those body builders who are puffy and stiff, as if stung by a bee and in a perpetual allergic reaction, i.e. musclebound which is a term that does not mean muscular but instead bound or inhibited by muscles so stiff they restrict range of movement. This occurs because the extreme amounts of inflammation promoted by the stress methods also causes stiffening of connective tissue and an increase in fat deposition as water excess is redirected away from internal organs (as much as is possible), and this type of growth happens because the stress of exhaustive, repetitious movement stimulates the release of stress hormones like estrogen, serotonin, and growth hormone whose purpose it is to make cells take up water to repair the damage caused by such stress. But this excess water also slows down metabolic respiration and electrical conductivity of cells which reduces their overall metabolic rate and thus requires even more effort to achieve the same results from the same behavior, and muscles wrought by stress methods thus means they are formed by an increase of water within a cell, not by anabolic growth, and because the body is also not interested in maintaining inflammation or stress hormones it constantly tries to heal this inflammation, so "muscle" wrought during the stress-methods of bodybuilding deflates *very* rapidly as the body actively sheds this inflammation to reestablish homeostasis, which means rapid loss of muscle gains which then requires constant maintenance through even more stress to sustain the inflammation and prevent the decrease in water influx. In short, the reason most people find it difficult to put on muscle is because their body is constantly trying to "repair" the muscle and reverse the inflammation which makes their muscles appear larger which are in fact not real muscle gains at all but simply water retention inside muscle tissue.

Steroids also accelerate this problem since estrogen is the primary mediator of water influx into cells during inflammation as part of the repair and growth phases of cellular function, which is exaggerated and enhanced by constant inflammatory stress caused by relented exercise and dieting behaviors. The artificial increase in estrogen then also causes thickening of tissues and risks development of cancer, tumors, and necrosis of vital organs (such as is a common side effect of steroid abuse) because the chronic water uptake by cells stimulated by excess estrogen also suffocates them, and this stress has not just an effect on muscle retention, however, as the systemic inflammation caused by such activity spreads to the rest of the body, diluting electrolytes and slowing down the metabolic rate of the skin, hair, eyes, brain, liver, kidney, heart, and every other internal organ, which is why those who use steroids often develop internal organ failure and why those who really abuse steroids turn shades of purple as their body literally loses the ability to transport oxygen to keep tissues sufficiently oxygenated. Over time the stress method of body building then also leads to dull skin, hair loss, eventual fat deposition, and other more serious illnesses like cancer and heart failure. A couple I once knew who went on a short course of steroid use both had catastrophic liver and splenic failure and were hospitalized for a period of months.

Real androgen anabolism stimulates muscle growth that is neither transient nor based on water influx and inflammation. The testosterone influence on cells stimulates sustained intracellular increases in cytosol, glycogen, mitochondria, and other organelles and nutrients which compose the cell as well as supportive connective tissue to also support increases in strength, and the actual factor which stimulates the growth of muscle cells is the electrical stimulus which triggers contraction, not weight, exhaustion, or tearing of anything, which means that muscle growth can and does also occur simply from contraction of muscle and doesn't even require weights. Anabolism, rather than inflammation, is one of constructive metabolism where cells create structures which are persistent and lasting and best of all do not even require chronic elevation of stress hormones to maintain (in fact it requires a reduction in stress). Often when I was younger I found increases in muscle mass when casually going to the gym or working out, then motivated by my success resolved to be more dedicated but find my results slowed or even reversed, because casual exercise reduces stress, where excessive causes it. Many young men still teenagers suddenly without intention find themselves the object of much desire when they develop athletic bodies simply from eating and playing, then finding validation in that attention seek more by purposefully dieting and exercising but end up finding it difficult and often antithesis to being fit and healthy when ironically they weren't even doing any of that when they became hot in the first place, because muscle and sexual attraction is a feature of health, and dieting and stress destroys health, and thus also sexual attraction and muscle. Methods for building muscle then which do not solicit the release of stress hormones through exhaustion and fatigue cause muscle to grow much, much faster and more easily but also result in longer lasting, larger, and more easily maintained and better looking muscles with more definition and firmness than the puffy, marshmallow muscles of overworked bodybuilders simply because of the compositional effects of hormones and reduced catabolic stress which also preserves the integrity of the skin, hair, eyes, brain, and other important body parts and prevents the aesthetic collapse of the entire body, which also has implications for metabolic disease like cancer and aging resistance (so long as the body is free of pathogenic infection) caused instead by metabolic torpor and stress.

The retention of electrolytes promoted by reductions in stress and inflammation caused by dieting, excess exercise, and colonization by pathogens also increases the contractile power, strength, volume, hardness, and responsiveness of muscle cells, making them feel firmer and contract faster, harder, and longer. This occurs because the contractile stimulus of cells is electrical in nature, facilitated by electrolytes but which in turn is inhibited by inflammation, which is water that dilutes electrolytes in solution. Many body builders have large muscles but are not comparably strong to actual athletes, because of the influx of water caused by estrogen which results from steroid use that inflates muscles but simultaneously dilutes their electrolytes and thus conductivity. Connective tissue like the extracellular matrix, ligaments, and tendons are also dependent on chloride and bromine as cofactors in their synthesis, but because physiological stress also promotes the increased loss of these electrolytes the body then also has a difficult time even synthesizing healthy connective tissue required to support muscle growth. Since chloride and bromine are also used in the immune reaction, parasitism and other chronic colonization by opportunist microbes also directly impairs the conductivity of cells and synthesis and growth of tissues. Reductions in stress combined with supplemental lithium, sodium, chloride, and potassium with sources of sugar such as fruit juice, lemonade, or even sugar water to promote the channels which uptake and transport electrolytes is very noticeable as muscles almost immediately begin to feel harder and contract more strongly and responsively with very little neurological stimulation, and contraction can be maintained for a much longer duration before fatiguing (taking these before a workout is always better than after). The intimate relationship of tyrosine, adrenaline, and sodium as discussed in the chapters on depression, immunity, and hormones is particularly important for muscle strength, as excess stress which stimulates and depletes adrenaline and cortisol directly promotes loss of both tyrosine (from which adrenaline is made) and sodium, through its increased use and then loss through urine and sweat, and since sodium is the primary regulator of cellular metabolism and conductivity the loss of sodium through stress and stress behaviors which lead to the depletion of stress hormones is the greatest impairment of muscle strength and growth.

Incorporating an understanding of muscle growth into an active life can get even greater gains in physical health which last and are easier to maintain than using the stress methods, and if real muscle was a function of effort, strain, or "tearing," of the fibers women who workout just as hard as men would grow muscles as large as men. But they can't because muscle growth has nothing to do with exercise but everything to do with hormones, stress, and nutrition, and muscle will grow even without training, even while just sitting on your ass, by preventing catabolism which is the entire battle for muscle in the first place. Women do have more androgens than estrogens, the opposite idea a common misconception, and if the endocrine system of women is health they build muscle too but it stays lower in volume and density but will still be strong and fit. Some exercise does increase testosterone further, as long as it is not excessive, women having a natural limit on its production. Primarily, a good diet and sun exposure increases testosterone. But more important than increasing testosterone, a good diet also lowers those elements which *oppose* testosterone, thus increasing the amount of it that is unopposed, making the testosterone more effective and thus the formula protein + *unopposed* testosterone = muscles.

When I was recovering from cancer I kept a sugary, fruit-filled protein shake with me at all times of day and this kept my blood sugar up constantly which in turn strongly inhibited the release of stress hormones, which fluctuate greatly in relation to dietary carbohydrate, so I never lost any muscle and even the tiniest bit of muscle growth resulted in a net increase in muscle bulk even while sitting at my desk job and being nearly inactive. But emotional stress also increases adrenaline, even more potently than sugar deprivation, because the brain is one of the primary regulators of the endocrine system and responds to our life experiences by prepping the physical body for stressful situations we encounter. This can even be potentiated by unresolved childhood trauma in which our perception of life is more negative, paranoid, and fearful and thus results in exceptional levels of adrenaline and cortisol regardless of whether we have volatile emotional experiences and so resolving experiences of trauma can and do also promote muscle growth simply by resolving psychological stimulation of stress. Drugs and factors like acetaminophen and ibuprofen can and do also inhibit muscle growth by overly suppressing inflammation since inflammation is the process by which muscle growth is stimulated but also because hormones like testosterone must be sulfated for transport throughout the body and xenobiotics like pharmaceuticals rapidly deplete sulfate (especially if colonized by hydrogen sulfide producing microbes). Fructose such as I consumed daily from sugar and fruit also fuels the sex organs and is required by the Leydig cells of the testis, while saturated and monounsaturated fats such as from butter, ice cream, cocoa butter, hazelnuts, chufa, olive oil, etc., stabilize mitochondria and facilitate testosterone production because they are stable in the high heat, high oxygen, environment of increased metabolic rate and promote mitochondrial respiration and cellular integrity.

Many stresses to the androgenic system come from environmental contaminants such as endocrine disrupting dioxins in pesticides, chemicals in soaps, and industrial food additives like soy, gums, some preservatives and even certain food colorants which all lower testosterone or raise oppositional hormones and prevent natural muscle growth. Unfortunately while marijuana can be beneficial for some heath conditions it can and does also prevent muscle growth because marijuana's promotion of relaxation is achieved by blocking the function of adrenaline which oppositely lowers blood sugar, which is why it stimulates hunger, and oppositely raises cortisol (this corticosteroid effect is why it can help manage pain, though, but this can also cause muscle wasting). Pot can be fun to use and can even help spare tyrosine required for the immune system and reversing depression, and small doses on occasion would not seriously impair muscle, but used chronically in high doses and not supported by generous carbohydrate consumption always raises cortisol which then catabolizes hard-won muscle bulk for its glycogen content, especially in those who are already prone to metabolic stress and dieting, which is why it can and does sometimes result in paranoia (which is the feeling of excess cortisol).

As discussed in the chapters on immunity and erections, parasites like *Trichomonas* are specifically interested in our sex hormones, especially estrogen, for their own reproductive purposes. They thus also shift our hormone profile to greater estrogen, especially when colonizing the prostate, testicles, and breast tissue. Most men do not know we all have completely intact mammary glands and breast ducts, and colonization of male breast tissue by parasites due to a poor diet and insufficient sun exposure is the cause of gynecomastia (breast tissue enlargement). The greatest cohort of gender confirmation care are cisgender young men and surgical treatment of gynecomastia, but topical and supplemental application of low-dose lithium followed by sun exposure and a diet high in lithium such as from leafy greens, legumes, fruit, etc., can rapidly eradicate the parasites and thus restore normal physiology of the breast. Full-body light exposure after low-dose lithium to help restore the function of the genitals and other mucosal organs will further support long term recovery of normal musculature and testosterone production.

While testosterone is highly anabolic it is the active form of testosterone, *dihydrotestosterone*, which is responsible for the strong secondary sex characteristics in males like leaner muscles, larger vasculature, bigger forearms, and the most masculine body hair patterns, so while many males can achieve an increase in muscle mass from working out they do not have sinewy, cut muscles and mistake this as a problem of calories rather than hormones. As discussed in the chapters on immunity, thyroid, and hormones, free copper which occurs in chronic colonization by pathogens also inhibits the enzyme 5-alpha reductase which produces dihydrotestosterone, so restoring hormone production, resolving pathogenic colonization, and restoring vitamin C (thyroid chapter) which scavenges free copper can increase the masculinization of the male body and muscles.

The inhibitory effect of estrogen on muscle growth itself is achieved through the increase of inducible *nitric oxide* inhibition of mitochondria, and while dietary citrulline is required to grow muscle through the synthesis of arginine and glutamine, stress and factors which impair healthy nitric oxide function result in excessive inducible nitric oxide and deficiency of endothelial which oppositely increases blood flow. Sunlight, thiols (sulfur), sugar, and anthocyanin support muscle growth in part by removing inducible nitric oxide from mitochondria, but using pre-workout products, especially when failing to promote mitochondrial respiration, accelerates the production of inducible nitric oxide to inhibit mitochondria and thus promote muscle atrophy rather than promote muscle growth. Erectile medications also very strongly promote excess nitric oxide and accelerate muscle wasting and aging. I can grow and retain significant muscle mass without working out *at all* simply by manipulating and blocking excess nitric oxide and promoting an anabolic hormonal state even though my lifestyle is entirely the most sedentary it has ever been because the stress hormones which catabolize muscle are simply not present, and even fractional gains in muscle are more effective in the long run simply because they are never lost, just as what occurs in our animal relatives who also do not need to go to a gym to get big and strong.

It is also easy to unknowingly neglect and misunderstand the other part of the muscle formula, *protein*. In fact, most people who hesitate to eat do not get enough protein to build muscles, especially if chronic dieting or fasting is part of the regular diet, but protein also requires carbohydrates to properly metabolize and assimilate, and eating enough carbs and fat will make a person feel satiated where only consuming high protein will not satiate for long as the body induces cravings for carbohydrate which is required in the first place to metabolize that protein. Thankfully, many foods have protein and deficits mostly occur only due to dieting, fasting, fruitarianism, etc., and other stressful behaviors which are easily remedied simply by eating a good diet. Many plant foods like nuts and grains contain plenty of protein and it is not even necessary to use animal products to get enough. In fact the consumption of high protein without protective factors like tannins and carotene can instead result in the pathogenic production of ammonia which directly inhibits muscle growth, as while ammonia can be sequestered into the amino acid glutamine which is used as an an energy source, an excess of ammonia and deficiency of sugar strongly impairs absorption of sodium required to lower adrenaline and sustain the metabolic rate to then increase torpor and catabolism of muscle. The first time I ever tried whey protein powder at the age of thirty was also the first time I ever experienced brain fog, unknowingly colonized by *Streptomyces* microbes which impair biotin and thus the breakdown of the branched chain amino acids required to package ammonia, and symptoms of high ammonia like changes in vision, brain fog, and constipation also indicate high ammonia and poor assimilation of protein required for muscle growth. Many studies show an increased requirement for protein in aging and ill individuals, but this is caused by high catabolism of protein by opportunistic pathogens, using our dietary protein to produce ammonia, hydrogen sulfide, toxic amines, etc., which reduces the amount available for our bodies. Taking higher quantity is then not sound advice which instead further promotes pathogens and problems like ammonia. The bodybuilder pot-belly, now a regular sight in gyms and social media which was never something that used to occur in lifters, is a consequence of the introduction and popularization of protein powders lacking any protective nutrients like dietary tannin, giving free and abundant access to opportunistic parasites and other microbes. Adding in high estrogen from the use of anabolic steroids and dieting which further promotes microbial overgrowth many body builders soon find the only positive thing about their health is the quantity of muscle (not even quality).

Most people also do not know that the healthy gut microbiome produces a constant supply of healthy amino acids like lysine, tryptophan, alanine, etc., which is also probably required for good health and good muscle growth since no dietary source of protein is made of ideal compositions of amino acids. Lysine is one of the strongest promoters of muscle health, so foods like dairy or peas which are high in lysine can be very productive, but the gut microbiome is proven in studies to also produce lysine, and likely do so from plant foods that feed healthy microbes, when pathogens which suppress these microbes are resolved. This function is also not vague or nebulous, as cravings can be used as a diagnostic for the state of the gut microbiome, where craving plants and feeling satiated by healthy food means an ability to break down plants, and cravings for meat indicates an inability to effectively break down plants and an inability to benefit from them. A plant based diet does contain less protein, but this simply requires consuming more calories of fruits and vegetables so more protein and other muscle building nutrients can be synthesized by commensal microbes, and a plant diet is never achieved through willfulness but restoration of physiological factors which naturally increase preference for plant foods.

While many people may think they do not have significant sources of stress hormones which promote muscle loss, a major cause happens every single day. At night. While we're asleep. The lack of food (protein and sugar) during sleep causes a sharp and sustained increase in adrenaline and then cortisol nightly, especially if dinner is eaten early which can cause a period of up to 12 hours without food. Unless measures are taken to specifically prevent the rise in stress hormones while sleeping it *always* occurs, even in those who are healthy, because the body simply cannot go that long without eating. Most healthy people can store between 1,500 and 3,000 calories of glycogen in their liver, but in those with high stress hormones, low natural muscle mass or without effortless muscle retention it is likely that the liver is not storing nearly enough glycogen which then results in greater muscle catabolism during sleep. By eating some good protein and carbohydrates immediately before bed such as casein protein, a good mozzarella (you can make your own from good milk), nuts, ice cream, fruit (apples are excellent because their high pectin prolongs digestion and production of short chain fatty acids that contribute to steroidogenesis), or pea protein the muscle which would be lost in sleep will remain and thus contribute greatly to gains. In fact, sleep is the primary cause of muscle loss, simply due to the stress of poor diets and dietary behaviors, especially in those who utilize stress to build muscle since sleep so strongly resolves inflammation and promotes healing. Even if only a tiny bit of muscle is saved it very quickly adds up to a lot when behaviors are maintained to prevent drops in blood sugar, including during sleep.

Protein is also not only for tissue building. The amino acids from which protein is built are also used to create hormones, enzymes, neurotransmitters, other metabolic products, and to remove toxins from the body through sulfate via methionine and cysteine. Tissue catabolism can produce the stress hormones, but very little of the healthy androgens. Having good protein in ample amounts (supported by generous carbohydrate intake) will not only help build muscle but support overall health as well. Plant protein also always has a better balance of amino acids but plants are harder to break down and require an intact and health microbiome, and if my ravenous pasta consumption as a teenage athlete had instead been from safe sources of grain such as spelt, einkorn, or kamut as discussed in the upcoming chapter on bread I would have avoided the health effects caused by common wheat and thus greater gains in muscle bulk, strength, and overall energy and wellness. Protein structures like collagen the body makes to support strong muscles are also destroyed by the activity of pathogenic oral microbes as discussed in the chapters on immunity and oral health, and their enzymes weaken connective tissue which in turn prevents taught, springy, strong muscles and can be a major factor in poor posture, protruding gut, hernia which is mistaken as an injury from physical activity, and muscle weakness which is a greater liability the older we get and is the very reason for weak muscles associated with aging. Resolving the influence of these bacteria can quickly help muscles and connective tissue to strengthen, thus promoting strong posture and easier, higher-quality physical development.

It is important to stay ahead of your hunger. Every time you are hungry it is too late, and the body has already released adrenaline and cortisol to catabolize muscle and lower the metabolic rate. If the gut is free of pain, bloating, and constipation and you are fed, testosterone is rising and those which oppose it are dropping, especially if there has been sufficient sunshine exposure. Testicles should also hang low as discussed in the chapter on erectile dysfunction, which will generally indicate testosterone production, and testicles which are usually high and tight indicate high stress and lower testosterone production because aromatization results from lower metabolic rate which lowers temperature thus bringing testicles closer to the body.

Exercise techniques for building muscle are beyond the scope of this book but I very much recommend the discipline *Muscle Control*, developed by Maxick (Max Sick) which is an old-school, bronze era method of muscle building which is more effective than any other I've tried. It is also highly meditative and relaxing and helps rebalance and strengthen alignment of the body and is so effective at building muscle one session can produce as much as three or four times at a gym, because the pathway which grows muscle is not weight but electrically stimulated contraction of muscle cells. Muscles in fact have no idea how heavy weight is when lifting and training, it is purely the strength of contraction which grows muscle, which can be done more effectively through targeted practices like muscle control. Some people have tried to capitalize on this technique and sell Maxick's book with what they call *isometrics* which is just not the same as muscle control, which I enthusiastically endorse and not isometrics.

Also, in the chapter on sleep I recommend stretching as a method to help induce sleep, because stretching utilizes the force of gravity to generate free ATP in cells, which accounts for the flood of relaxation which occurs post stretching, where the act of exercise consumes ATP, and the smaller benefit which does come from movement is in fact the stretching of muscle and connective tissue, which instead produces energy, which can be used to rehabilitate muscles and produce energy and wellness. Especially in those who are metabolically ill, but also in those who are well, a daily stretching practice which uses gravity rather than contractile poses can more effectively maintain and promote muscle health, strength, and mobility than an actual exercise routine.

Muscle growth is not hard, and in fact requires that we treat our bodies with compassion, reduce stress, and be well fed. Not only will this give us a tremendous amount of progress and muscle gain, it will also improve our overall health and wellbeing, both physically, emotionally, and materially. As all tissues including muscle produce energy from the function of cellular mitochondria, improving the function of mitochondria can make muscles stronger and more resilient in addition to increasing energy for better physical performance, endurance, and stamina.

CHAPTER 23
GOOD BREAD

One quiet Sunday after church when I was ten-years old my dad drove us to our restaurant which he had finally opened. It was build as a massive English-style manor home set back from the road in a country town between patchwork farms, now sadly replaced by a parking lot for a Popeye's Chicken, but when we were children and corporate America had yet to bulldoze one of the only treasures that crappy town ever had we played on the restaurant grounds with the freely roaming geese and chickens or tended the pheasant coop or visited the quickly growing pig in his pen. As part of their religion my parents chose not to do business on Sundays, so it seemed out of place when arriving at his work, especially without the bustling energy of the large staff to enliven the enormous kitchen now strangely dark and quiet. We were immediately ecstatic though realizing we were not there for his work but for *our dinner*. It didn't matter that I was only ten, and the youngest only two, my father made each of us a full half-pound, medium-rare, cooked to perfection angus beef hamburger with made-from-scratch garlic buns and fresh, thick-cut English-style chips and gourmet salad served on pewter plates and root beer in pewter goblets. Though we gorged ourselves there were a lot of leftovers to take home and we spent the rest of the afternoon playing hide-and-seek in the enormous, empty restaurant. That day, our family eating together in a giant, industrial English kitchen all to ourselves was one of my fondest memories. Our food culture growing up was often like that, no small feat for a lower-middle class family of eight. Of course there were lots of *Lucky Charms* and macaroni with hot dog slices, but my favorite food was my father's fresh-baked bread which rarely lasted long enough to cool down, eaten with huge slabs of butter (after margarine finally died the death it deserved) usually accompanied by admonishments of *"that's too much."*

I often caution against the consumption of grains, not as an edict since life without pizza and chips can be admittedly boring, but as a generality. As humans

we have not really evolved to be efficient consumers of grain. There are long histories of dietary plagues cause by grain-based diets like the Pellagra epidemics in the
early Southern United States, where white settlers ignorantly consumed incorrectly
processed corn as the cornerstone of their niacin-poor diet. Indigenous Americans
had long understood the need to process corn with lime to make it edible (not the
fruit lime, this is referring to limestone and its high calcium content), the irony
their assistance would have been to those who murdered and displaced them
clearly karmic. But in fact nearly every grain traditionally consumed by the entirety
of our ancestral predecessors involved some kind of processing. Our grandparents
didn't make white bread because they were slothful and ignorant, they made white
bread because the phytic acid contained in the hulls of whole grain tastes bad
because it causes malnutrition. Of course they didn't know the science of it, only
that they faired better when things were done a certain way and used the tongue
as a guide and tool for survival. In fact, the much lauded saying *"the whiter your
bread the quicker you're dead"* does not in fact refer to refined flour but originates
from Victorian England when white flour was considered a status symbol and
thus frequently cut with toxic bulking agents like chalk or alum by unscrupulous
vendors, greatly harming people's health and giving rise to the phrase. In fact,
most of humanity which has existed before us contained a richness in food smarts
we in the Western world have complete ignorance of, an ignorance which has cost
a great many lives and compromised the standard of living for countless more.
While many modern agricultural practices have enabled the feeding of so many
people, key lessons learned by those who have come before us are having to be
relearned, sometimes painfully.

"Well, what about bread?" Is often a response I get after cautioning against the
consumption of wheat. This is a legitimate question. I often wondered the same
thing. Why did bread, which my ancestors have eaten for a thousand generations,
give me such horrible stomachaches and illness? After I found out serendipitously
the constant sinus infections I suffered in my twenties were caused by gluten and
iron fortification in common wheat it didn't take much effort to give it up and the
relief was rapid, total, and undeniable. And yet I missed bread. Once in a while,
after going months or years without eating wheat I would indulge in some pizza or
hamburgers only to be reminded exactly why I had stopped in the first place.

While iron fortification certainly wasn't in my ancestor's bread, gluten
certainly was. Did they all have those horrible reactions? Unlikely, else it would
not have become the dietary staple it did. And gluten is a protein, so why isn't it
digested into amino acids? What changed? For one thing, the hybridization to
promote the growth of wheat as a cash crop. Hybridization has been used often in
our agricultural history. Corn, for instance, used to look more like a stalk of wheat,
dainty and grass-like. Over time it was bred by Americans (and further bred by
white colonial Europeans) to produce bigger and better fruit (seeds) and thus more
food. There is actually a huge variety of corn types which are being lost because of
the industrial unification of one solitary monoculture. Purple, blue, fat, skinny, and
more tasty varieties. In fact, many crops have been lost to widespread monoculture
and the consolidation of agribusiness away from family farming. Farming used to
be a literal cornucopia of a wide range of heirloom plants and animals raised and
sold locally by residents to their neighbors, but now vast tracts of land are planted
with only one, highly homogenous and sometimes even genetically modified
isolate of any one food type, often diluted of its nutritional density in favor of size
and resistance to handling, leading to severe limitation of dietary and nutritional
diversity. When common wheat was hybridized to better resist the growth pressure

of artificial fertilizer it also resulted in tougher gluten more resistant to environmental stress but thus also human digestion, preventing the gluten proteins from breaking down in the gut, especially in people with compromised digestion, and in turn now wreaks havoc in the body. The addition of iron which I have discussed previously merely added insult to injury, inflaming the inflammation and cementing the great gluten avoidance craze that has now gripped Western civilization.

So you will be surprised to hear that I have been eating bread again. Yay! But how? It's really obvious if you think about it. My bread is made from grains which did not go through excessive hybridization. If bread is made from safer varieties of wheat like spelt, einkorn, kamut, or emmer varieties it means it contains gluten which is more delicate which we are actually equipped to digest. This eliminates any gluten reaction, unless you are extremely celiac, because the gluten is actually digested and reduced to its component amino acids. These flours are also not usually fortified with harmful iron and other inappropriate additives. Also, unlike plain grain flour products, bread is special because it is processed by the inclusion of the yeast, which helps to break down and predigest grain even further, making the starches, proteins, and fats in the grain even easier to digest, and it is *yeast* which is the very reason why bread has held such status in the annals of history.

I have mentioned before in chapters like *Niacin Therapy* about the importance of endogenous *niacin* production. Ultimately the purpose of all variants of niacin is for the purpose of synthesizing nicotinamide adenine dinucleotide which is extremely important for our biological health as it facilitates the transfer of elections between biological processes. Where niacin and most variants require a handful of enzymatic steps to make NAD, a form of niacin called *nicotinamide riboside* merely requires one, and guess where the *only* natural source of this valuable niacin variant originates? YEAST. It turns out that the importance of bread and its place it our human evolution hasn't much to do with wheat at all, but the production of nicotinamide riboside, apparent also to the wide array of yeast-cultured foodstuffs which permeate the cultures of man. Bread has the special advantage also of being low in lactic acid because yeasts do not produce lactic acid (sourdough bread has bacteria but contains mostly acetic acid, similarly to traditional kombucha or apple cider vinegar), and niacin is also highly heat resistant so it is not destroyed by baking. This also explains why other wheat products which are not fermented can cause digestive distress and don't impart as many health benefits as do yeast-risen baked goods. Not only does my homemade bread not give me deleterious health effects, it helps improve my overall health. I have increased energy, brighter skin, and feel fuller and more satiated because of the type and abundance of vitamins imparted to the bread by the yeast and the mineral, carbohydrate, and protein richness of the grain which is made more bioavailable because of the yeast but also because yeast actually synthesizes other B vitamins. Humans became the intelligent and wide spread creatures we are as much for our symbiotic relationship with this simple organism as fire or tool use because it provides us with such a surplus of NAD precursors, and may itself be the real reason we have such large brains as animals.

For similar reasons, the fermentation of other foods can be helpful or make them digestible. For instance, soaking and fermenting wholegrain rice in water or cooking liquid for twelve to twenty-four hours will activate its natural phytase enzyme to break down phytate, and the natural yeast and bacteria on the rice to break down the anti-nutrients and improve its nutritional profile. This not only also makes rice taste great but helps with its digestion and prevents some of the problems associated with rice consumption (do not drain after fermentation as this will pour out the B vitamins and enzymes synthesized by the microbes). Other fermented products are not always helpful, however, such as yogurt or sauerkraut which contain excessive amounts of lactic acid or bacterial species that can interrupt the gut microbiome and are not always safe to consume, where our more friendly fermentation products come from yeasts and acetogens. Oftentimes sources like the internet will claim a ferment is lactic acid, such as sourdough bread, when in fact the predominant acids in sourdough are short chain fatty acids like acetate, where ferments with yeast and dominated by short chain fatty acids rather than lactic acid are highly useful. Lactic acid fermentation generally requires calcium, so low calcium ferments like bread or kombucha are instead primarily short chain fatty acids, not lactate. Bread is also medicinal in the sense that it contains lots of glucans from yeast, if it is fermented properly for long periods of time, where glucans can inhibit the translocation and activity of pathogens in the gastrointestinal tract, further explaining the traditional role of bread but not necessarily grains in support of our general health as a human animal.

Sprouting or soaking is also a helpful and important strategy not only to make grains more digestible but to also actively improve their nutritional benefit. Studies have shown, for instance, that sprouting grains and seeds increases their vitamin E content *more than 500%*. Since vitamin E is important for many metabolic systems, especially cardiovascular health, reproductive health and virility, skin health, to slow the aging process, and even for restful sleep, sprouting grains, seeds, and nuts is one of the best ways to do this. Throughout our history as a species vitamin E came largely from the consumption of seeds and nuts, but as grains became more common and thus foods such as bread and pasta, nuts became more of an afterthought, snack, or treat, especially because they tended to be more expensive. Now, almost the entirety of vitamin E supply comes from wheat or other grains, and when I cut out wheat due to gluten allergy my vitamin E intake incidentally plummeted which contributed to the rapid decline of my wellbeing. Refining wheat only removes about 40-50% of vitamin E, not all of it, unless it's bleached in which case that ruins pretty much all of flour's nutritional value (safe grains and organic varieties are in practice never bleached). Because vitamin E is an important chain-breaking antioxidant (meaning it stops the cascade of oxidization caused by reactive oxygen species such as are created by the immune reaction), this in turn leads to a rapid increase in metabolic disease when vitamin E stores are finally depleted. Vitamin E is one of the most powerful antioxidants in existence, but as a such a supplement of vitamin E should have near miracle-healing effects, but it doesn't have this function because vitamin E must also be continually recycled in the body for real benefit which in turn requires other nutrition and dietary habits and whole food sources, and once steps are taken to address these deficiencies as discussed throughout this book dietary vitamin E is more than sufficient to supply the needs even of someone as large and metabolically ill as I was. So using sprouted spelt, einkorn, kamut, rice, oats, or pumpkin seeds, sunflower seeds, almonds, hazelnuts, etc., has the most powerful vitamin E activity achievable, even from just a few slices of bread per day if you're already healthy, even more than supplemental vitamin E.

The primary reason grains are not best for us is their generally high arginine content which is a primary substrate for ammonia producing microbes. Any amino acid can be metabolized to ammonia, and arginine is very important for our health and growth, but arginine also has more nitrogen than all other amino acids and thus is a primary target for opportunistic microbes which use ammonia to alter their environmental pH (including that of our body). Very often when people embark on dieting behaviors they commit to cutting out carbs and sugar and so in turn cut out a great deal of grain and thus dramatically reduce the consumption of arginine which then greatly reduces ammonia burden and allows the body to more effectively resolve hyperammonemia, but then mistake the reduction in carbohydrates as mechanism of action when in reality it was reducing dietary arginine and thus microbial ammonia production. In fact, avoiding carbohydrate while reducing arginine intake is a missed opportunity to more effectively resolve metabolic health, because CO_2 produced from carbohydrate metabolism also helps acidify and dispose of ammonia, and there is no faster way to get better than dramatically reduce arginine exposure by limiting the intake of grains, meat, and nuts, and instead consuming more root vegetables, fruit, and leafy greens while also making sure to eat plenty of cucurbits (for their citrulline which in turn helps metabolize ammonia into endogenous arginine production). This is effective in restoring health by restoring absorption of sodium and chloride and all the pathways which are in turn dependent on sodium and chloride, but because of problems like the internal circulation of excess arginase by cellular exocytosis caused by pathogens as discussed in the chapter on pathogens and metabolic disease it is not possible when suffering metabolic disease to resolve hyperammonemia without also addressing arginine exposure in the first place.

Otherwise, safe, sprouted grains can be a healthy dietary staple for generous quantities of dietary vitamin E so long as they are not eaten in excess and problems like ammonia excess is addressed. Sprouting makes foods perish more quickly so most products are not already sprouted, but there are some available (sprouted oats are somewhat common). If you are not able to find these, you must practice sprouting yourself, and whole-grain foods that are not sprouted or fermented like whole grain pasta should never be eaten and instead only use their refined flour products. If soaking and sprouting seems arduous to do so, understand that actively sprouting and soaking grains, seeds, and nuts to increase their vitamin E content is one of the most medicinally beneficial strategies for improving metabolic health. Soaking is literally also so easy and only requires filling a jar or bowl with whole grains or nuts, pour water over them, and then wait twelve to twenty-four hours. It takes no more than a few seconds of effort each day, and the only reason it seems labor intensive is because we are not accustomed to it as a practice. Because of the synergistic nature of nutrients, such as vitamin E and magnesium (which is high in spelt) the direct improvement of nutritional quality of such properly prepared foods cannot be replicated by supplements, but since we also must eat it makes the supplement of nutrients through such practices more convenient and cheaper than using lots of commercial supplement products.

They who bake bread will never bake alone. But to have bread which improves health instead of destroying it there must be these requirements: made of safe varieties of wheat (einkorn, kamut, spelt, emmer, etc.) refined is great but soaked and sprouted whole grain is more useful for health (and no, neither organic common wheat nor common wheat sourdough is safe—organic just means it's grown without pesticides and glyphosate and has nothing to do with the species). It should also be properly fermented, where most commercial brands of bread raise their dough with chemicals which then does nothing to predigest the grain nor provide for nicotinamide riboside and other B vitamins, and even commercial yeast bread is sometimes risen too fast to really affect the grain very much or aid in digestion. I do make my own bread, and if you can't find such bread anywhere near you, you have to learn to make it yourself and it would be well worth the investment (there is a great recipe on my website, and whole sprouted berries of spelt, einkorn, and others can also be consumed as breakfast cereal or in savory dishes for their vitamin E).

Because grain is always high in silicon, making bread with Swiss cheese culture or even just adding B12 to bread can actively help address many metabolic problems because of how B12 promotes the microbiome as discussed in the chapters on gut health and cancer and can do a lot of great things like promote healthy growth, restore vitamin D synthesis (due to microbial short chain fatty acids), and support reproductive and cardiovascular health as well as recovery from cancer. Because most dietary B12 sources are of animal origin, B12 bread is also a more humane way to acquire B12, but is also more potent since it also comes with the very substrate, indigestible carbohydrate, required to benefit from B12 and the production of short chain fatty acids and other B vitamins by the microbiome. B12 bread can also be a convenient source of B12 during times of vitamin D deficiency such as winter or what occurs in aging. I also use these flours to make yeast-risen pancakes, cake, or cupcakes, which are easier than bread, although bread is a lot easier to make than you might think. Foods like pasta or pie dough are tastier with refined flour, and it's just fine to not use whole grain sprouted flour when making these, and do not buy the whole grain products of such unless it specifically states that it is sprouted, else you will consume enough phytic acid to block the nutritive benefits of eating it in the first place.

Bread does have an important part to play in human health. Just as wolves eat meat and birds eat seed, yeast is essential to human wellness and prosperity. Bread just happens to be the best way to supply it, and properly made bread can also lower your food bill because it provides better nutrition than a lot of other food products, by supplying the unique form of niacin and extra B vitamins it makes us and our children more satiated more often and thus less requiring of other foods. But to reap those benefits it has to be made right, or you will be doomed to repeat mistakes we have no reason to repeat, since we cannot digest grains without properly preparing them. Nicotinamide riboside is available as a supplement, but there are far more nutrients in properly made bread than you could ever hope to supplement, and to reduce food to its mere flagship vitamins is to continue suffering ill health. Whole food, prepared correctly, is key to restoring or maintaining normal, robust health, and as this chapter illustrates there is no reason to starve and deny yourself to achieve good health. Oppositely, the hedonistic consumption of a broad array of nutrients from safe and appropriate foods is medicinally supportive of a healthy body, mind, and spirit. So enjoy some well-made bread.

CHAPTER 24

HORMONES

In 2014 while living in Palm Springs with my ex my health issues went from bad to worse. But I woke up one morning to find not myself but my partner of four years and supposedly soon to be husband if we could set a date writhing in agony. This wasn't the first time it had happened, so I was not as alarmed as I should have been, and he refused when I suggested we go to the emergency room. After some insistence I got him to agree to visit an urgent care. This had happened three other times over the last four years, and he was either suffering kidney stones again or another case of *gastroenteritis* as had been (wrongly) diagnosed by the emergency room six months prior. But something really wasn't right and as I waited in the empty reception of the urgent care watching the door through which he had disappeared a deep dread gripped me. Sure enough he returned much too soon to have had any real examination and before even seeing the fear on his face I knew it was serious.

We rushed for the car, him holding his side as if his guts might literally spill out, his anguish finally released in a burst of tears. While I had seen him cry histrionically and manipulatively many times over the years I had never seen him cry for real, and it scared me so much that I was also surprised by how scared I was. I drove as fast as I could without being reckless, ran a red light, and flung his door open as we reached the emergency room of what would turn out to be one the worst hospitals in California. Mistakenly I thought our terror was about to end but after parking and running inside found a nurse telling my pain-stricken fiancé he had to fill out paperwork before even being admitted even though he could barely stand up and had no control over his arms. I nearly yelled at her but there was a security guard with a gun nearby so instead I held my crying fiancé with one hand and furiously wrote for him with the other. After another fifteen painfully long minutes we were finally admitted, and almost an hour after first arriving at the hospital he was finally drugged up and smiling and tentatively diagnosed with appendicitis, waiting for a free doctor to operate.

I went out to call my mom. The sobs were a shock. I thought I'd been holding it together. Really, I was terrified. She helped me calm down, and after calling my fiancé's brother returned to find my Love finally high and making jokes with a nurse (drugs are glorious, aren't they?) while his body steadily fell apart on the inside waiting for those incompetent doctors to attend him. *Three hours later* he finally went into surgery. Then the operation went twice as long as expected and the doctor finally emerged to inform me that his appendix had burst on the table (of course it did you waited three fucking hours to get him into surgery). They let me into the recovery area and I was so relieved to finally see his dopey face in the dark of the recovery room but the hospital was literally under active construction in the rooms next door (I wasn't being hyperbolic when I said they were the worst) and the banging and construction equipment made the entire experience feel like a post-apocalyptic video game and not reality. He fell back asleep and I went out for flowers and soda to there when he emerged from the fog of anesthesia.

While I was in the store my phone rang. The number was unrecognized but the area code was from my partner's hometown, so I answered. The woman on the other side of the call was my fiancé's evangelical mother whom for the last three years had refused to even acknowledge my existence but now suddenly knew my name and talked to me as if calling me was the most normal thing in the world. She asked about him and I told her the nice version of what had happened. Then she informed me they were flying in and had already bought tickets, and my precious relief suddenly turned again to dread, this time of the socially diseased. Maybe it would be good? Maybe they would see how much I cared for him and it would soften their hearts?

I spent all the next day laying in my partner's hospital bed with him, watching *Bob's Burgers* and *Archer* on our iPad and slowly walking him around the floor as directed by our nurses. His feet once stuck to a sticky pad for catching construction dust and would have fallen over if I had not been there, but the jolt injured the fresh incision and he fought hard to hold back more tears as we continued to literally trudge on through this nightmare.

A few days later his parents walked through the door and their icy, detached stare at the sight of me laying in the bed with him sucked every bit of joy and hope from that hospital room. Looking back I can see how it was the beginning of the end for us, but of course my ex loved his parents and having them come to his side was good for his morale, though not his healing nor our relationship. Over the next few days his parents managed to make insulting remarks about our dogs, our house, my cooking, but lifted not a finger to wash dishes or assist with food prep, treating me like wait-staff, and at nearly every turn tried to swing the conversation to politics. They refused to stay under our roof even though we had a really nice guest bedroom, and I was regarded with no more admiration than a caterer and spoken to like a civil acquaintance, except when his mother strangely flirted with me to ingratiate herself and manipulate me which was especially strange considering that not only was I uninterested in women, I was her son's lover.

Having delivered their otherwise stoney repudiation of us and eaten from our table finally left us in what would have been peace but my ex's long incision of a traditional rather than laparoscopic operation because the doctor *"didn't perform those,"* meaning he had never trained for it, was bulging and red so we went back to the hospital and on seeing the unsettling development our doctor had as much fear in his face as my partner when we first arrived a week ago and shuffled us once more into the emergency room, this time through a back door which we found out later was to avoid his poor surgical work being reregistered as a return emergency room visit which would otherwise cause the hospital regulatory scrutiny, and I watched as he and four other doctors immediately put my partner out right there in the emergency room and opened him up (so they could do emergency surgery right away after all?). When they finally finished they called me over. Confused, because why would I be required to participate in surgery, I had to be beckoned again. They showed me his open three-inch incision through which I could see the layers of skin and the bloody, striated tissues of my Love's inner abdominal wall. I felt faint but tried to keep it together. Because it had been infected, they told me, the wound now had to remain open, to heal from the inside, and a nurse wouldn't be dressing it twice a day. I would.

We finally returned to a quiet home. Only, it wasn't so quiet. My fiancé's ordeal and the visit from his parents triggered something in him and he indulged even more violent outbursts and emotional fits than normal. That someone could survive several years of undiagnosed appendicitis and shout and flail so furiously after major abdominal surgery was a testament to his vitality, but something in me finally broke. My health had been declining for the last three years but one day about a month after his surgery I realized I could no longer feel like I was actually going to live much longer. Sure, I'd had debilitating insomnia, my hair was falling out, I had a cough that hadn't gone away for a whole year, I couldn't get warm if I stepped into fire and my extremities swelled just from walking around the block with my dogs, but before my ex's appendectomy I'd always believed and felt like I was about to get better any time now. Something changed. It wasn't emotional, it was physical. Breathing was almost impossible. I couldn't get air into my lungs. I was gasping for air nearly every moment of the day. Being cold was now a chill. My own skin felt icy and numb except for the infuriating itch all over that never went away and somehow traveled into my spine when I laid down to sleep. My extremities were pale white. The pain was excruciating. Meanwhile my ex grew stronger every day. The color came back to his face, and so did his lust for life. Mine did not. I was not going to make it.

After learning about the potential benefits of the hormone *progesterone* from the work of Dr. Peat I ordered some and tried it right away. It immediately made me feel good and had seemed to rescue some of the worst symptoms. But afraid it might "lower my testosterone," I stopped because progesterone is known as a female hormone. It had also made me put on more weight, but finally realizing my relationship was doomed anyway I no longer cared what my partner thought about my appearance, I just didn't want to die so I started it again and this time in much higher doses. Immediately my low temperatures rose from an alarming 95.1° F to a safer 96.5° F, and it improved my pulse as well (yes, my temperatures were so low I thought the thermometer was broken). I finally stopped shivering in the Palm Springs heat. It also had the welcome effect of making me *feel* good too as if reducing my tension and anxiety, something I hadn't felt in at least three or four years. It lessened that insufferable itch and gave my extremities the feeling of having blood in them once more because progesterone also helps the body retain blood volume. At that same time I finally got to a good doctor and was finally diagnosed with multiple growths on my thyroid including several large nodes, one a full centimeter long growing on the isthmus, which is itself only 4 to 5 millimeters, and effectively one-hundred percent chance of cancer. But progesterone had finally started to bring me away from the brink, one day my constant cough finally slowed, then the eczema on my cheeks disappeared, and I started having massive erections like I'd not had in years.

But my weight didn't change, and my fiancé couldn't see the improvements though they filled me with hope. He said he had only asked me to marry him so I would change, then one day he left and never came back. I heard later he told people he had stopped loving me two years earlier. That was before I'd gotten fat. Before he'd asked me to marry him. He was sober most of our relationship but somehow in all the chaos I had missed his relapse back into cocaine addiction sometime toward the end. Alone and with nothing I moved back to L.A. and started over, with no insurance or healthcare, sleeping on couches and getting around on public transit while trying to heal from debilitating thyroid cancer and reassembling something of a life. I stopped drinking with the help of a twelve step program, and now sober and with progesterone and other health tools many of my health issues really began to rapidly improve. I began to lose weight and went from 301 pounds to 280 in just two months. During that time I had my first full nights sleep in three years because progesterone helps promote functions like thyroid to produce sufficient energy which then helps cells relax. It was amazing, and actually restful. Along with other strategies and nutrition one-by-one each of my cancer related symptoms began to subside, along with my depression and other health problems. For the first time in many years I saw real hope.

But then I encountered more erectile dysfunction, because progesterone can in high doses inhibit testosterone, although I didn't know at the time this is actually not a harmful thing and progesterone will continue to improve overall health even if specifically male functions are suspended temporarily, but it can be demoralizing if you are male and ignorant to why it is happening. Since I was desperate not to die it didn't matter how well my sex drive worked, and the relief progesterone otherwise brought far outweighed the negative aspects, but I also felt like my weight loss stalled so I kept my other strategies and dropped progesterone. I lost more weight during that summer and health improved steadily, now supported by even more tools and strategies, including the regrowth of hair in some of the places I had lost it and resumption of much of my normal hormone production due to the effects of an actually healthy diet, consistent eating habits, and resolution of opportunistic microbial colonization. As mentioned in the chapter on libido young men who are healthy produce as much progesterone as young women not on a cycle, as progesterone is in reality more a hormone of youth and wellness and is the healthy version of cortisol which helps to coordinate and mobilize minerals and active metabolic function, strongly promotes thyroid health, blood volume, muscle, hair, reproductive health, and other related functions.

Women also experience conditions like *endometriosis*, which is a growth of uterine tissue outside the uterus, or *polycystic ovary syndrome (PCOS)*, which are poorly understood by clinicians, but endometriosis is exactly the kind of problem caused by infection with *Trichomonas* which results in low progesterone because progesterone protects our bodies against unrestrained growth effects of estrogen, which is why estrogen is involved in tumor growth and why progesterone can be therapeutic to cancer. The body does not randomly grow cysts, which are instead symptoms of parasitism, and polycystic ovary syndrome and endometriosis are, I believe, the result of parasitic colonization which results in chronic immune activation and excessive stress hormones (adrenocorticotropin) which also upregulate androgens (via dehydroepiandrosterone), which thus inhibits progesterone but not the aromatization of androgens, and when androgens aromatize spontaneously they tend also to convert into less helpful forms of estrogen such as estrone. Many parasites are shown to alter the composition of sex hormones (another point of evidence for cystic fibrosis being parasitic in nature), and diseases like PCOS and endometriosis are direct consequences of eating disorders, poor diets, exposure to endocrine disrupting dioxins and pesticides, or sexual abuse which can and does also transmit opportunistic pathogens to children. Progesterone itself is in fact antiparasitic, because it directly opposes the function of estrogen in the reproductive cycle of parasites which colonize our bodies for our sex hormones, and part of its therapeutic mechanism of action is likely through the direct suppression of opportunistic parasites as demonstrated by conclusive studies. This means, however, that conditions like PCOS and endometriosis are in fact conditions of parasitism and that conditions of parasitism like diabetes, autism, and even cancer are also symptoms of progesterone deficiency, and one of the primary therapeutic mechanisms of progesterone is likely the inhibition of parasites which otherwise impair the immune system and promote secondary colonization by other opportunistic pathogens like viruses, bacteria, and yeasts. Because it does inhibit testosterone in high doses, progesterone can also be very useful for aging cisgender women and transgender women seeking gender affirming care, and to treat PCOS, endometriosis, diabetes, and cancer (as recommended in that chapter).

Fertility is also primarily maintained by progesterone regardless of gender, and specifically prevents the uterine wall from contracting during pregnancy which would otherwise dislodge the uterine lining as occurs during the cycle. Problems conceiving or carrying to term are easily treated by daily supplementation of natural progesterone if dietary changes as recommended in this book support its use. Progesterone is also, however, the hormone of *empathy* and is the reason for greater emotional sensitivity in women, especially during a cycle or pregnancy, so taking progesterone or restoring natural, endogenous production also results in the *increase* of emotional tenderness and sensitivity, and since many of us also do not like our emotions mistake this as a negative side effect. Understandably many women end up preferring the less emotional, numbing state that accompanies low progesterone, even if it does come with worse physical health, and I often have to repeatedly remind those taking progesterone or restoring health than an increase in emotional sensitivity is an expected effect of progress and that dislike of emotions and preference for numbness is a symptom instead of unresolved trauma which teaches us to dislike being alive and prevents us from effectively handling the chaos of life, which can be unlearned through inventory therapy as discussed in the upcoming chapter on spirituality or my book on psychology which can instead teach us to derive uncommon joy and spiritual experiences from emotions and the human condition. Because progesterone is the hormone of empathy it is also very useful for treating apathy, anhedonia, sociopathy, and psychopathy as it mediates the connection between actions and feelings that is missing in such conditions, which are at their root conditions of poor progesterone production catalyzed by stress, trauma, and parasitism and pathogenesis. This is not to excuse sufferers of those conditions from their behavior, as many people with these conditions do not engage in harmful behavior to others, which is instead simply used as an excuse for it. But resolving the underlying factors like diet, environment, trauma, and pathogenesis and using supplemental progesterone can help restore a normal endocrine system and thus emotional state.

Progesterone is required and useful for health (supplemental or produced by the body) not only because of its direct effects on human physiology but also because progesterone is the precursor to corticosteroids like *aldosterone* and *cortisol* which mediate resistance to stress and regulate electrolyte status. Studies also on *premenstrual syndrome* (PMS), which is a state of severe discomfort preceding and accompanying a cycle, show highest associations with insufficient production of cortisol which, since cortisol is made from progesterone, indicates progesterone deficiency which then increases the effect of estrogen on cells to cause cramping and discomfort since a primary function of cortisol is to provide sugar, electrolytes, and amino acids from catabolized muscle to fuel the internal organs. Most often problems with the menstrual cycle are direct consequences of dieting and dieting behaviors due to the traumatization of women (and men) under systems of patriarchy which teach us to see value only in the state of our physical body for the benefit of others rather than that value inherent to our innate existence which is for our benefit alone. All hormones are made from dietary fats, sugar, and protein (and require other nutrients like the elements, carotene, etc.), so any problem with the body can never be restored during dieting behaviors.

Alternatively, the hormone *pregnenolone* can be used for very similar benefits of progesterone and without some of the unwanted effects as pregnenolone is the master hormone of the body from which most hormones are made including progesterone, estrogen, dehydroepiandrosterone, testosterone, cortisol, etc., and taking pregnenolone also results in its ample conversion to progesterone if butyrate status is sufficient. It does not have overt effects itself in the way other hormones do which also makes it more useful to take as the body can then make any in which might be deficient without risking the specific side effects of those hormones, for instance such as taking testosterone which in slow metabolisms can and will aromatize into estrogen and ironically shrink testicles and promote weight gain and hair loss. Pregnenolone is extremely useful in treating many symptoms of metabolic disease and very specific symptoms of pregnenolone deficiency are fatigue at the end of the day and social anxiety because pregnenolone deficiency results in less resistance to stress, even mild ones like being awake, and especially social stress, because of impaired ability of cells to respond to and meet that stress. Even being awake requires constant hormone production so even a simple desk job without any physical exertion can still cause significant fatigue if there is not enough pregnenolone to regulate normal endocrine function, and by the end of a day leaves us feeling run down or exhausted. Because other humans are some of the biggest triggers of the flight or fight response, social occasions result in an increase either of dopamine or adrenaline which mobilize sugars from glycogen storage and sodium flux, but aldosterone and cortisol help to prevent sodium loss from the body and provide sugars when glycogen storage is depleted (which is chronically true in anyone with metabolic stress), so deficiency of pregnenolone and thus aldosterone and cortisol cause increased anxiety from social interaction, even the prospect of social interaction, and those who are deficient in pregnenolone (most commonly due to dieting behavior but also factors like parasites) will experience anxiety even at the thought of going to a party.

Pregnenolone supplementation is so effective in treating symptoms of daily fatigue or social anxiety it is obvious from even the first few doses, and about 25-50 mg taken every morning can help prevent daily fatigue, while a large dose of about 200-300 mg can also be taken several hours before any expected social event to reliably alleviate social anxiety. Because pregnenolone converts to cortisol, however, it absolutely *must* be supported by consistent maintenance of blood sugar and adequate intake of calories, protein, and fats otherwise taking pregnenolone will oppositely cause an increase in cortisol which can then cause feelings of unrest, anxiety, and discomfort since cortisol is highly catabolic. This problem is not common and usually occurs only in those whom are extremely lean because this reflects an existing excess of catabolic stress from excessive cortisol, and reversing dietary stress, dieting behaviors, and eating constantly before beginning the use of pregnenolone can prevent this side effect.

A woman once asked about some serious side effects she was experiencing from the use of pregnenolone, and after some further investigation it was eventually mentioned she was also on *beta-blockers* due to a misguided idea that blocking adrenaline would be helpful since she had heard that adrenaline was a stress hormone and excess adrenaline contributes to poor health. But adrenaline functions to release glucose from glycogen storage and the purposeful inhibition of adrenaline prevents glycogen release which then motivates massive escalation of cortisol, and since cortisol (like many other hormones) is also made from pregnenolone its supplementation directly resulted in massive cortisol spikes. This illustrates another way in which we become so desperate for health we do more harm by not exercising reason and common sense as beta blockers are in no way ever part of normal human physiological function and their use is a consequence of distrusting and condemning the body (and worship of the pharmaceutical industry) rather than having compassion and empathy for our biology and human condition. Any kind of health problems which affect the endocrine system and disturb normal hormone production can directly benefit from supplementation of pregnenolone if endogenous production is not sufficient, and the symptoms I experienced in my thirties are the same as women experience during menopause because in reality anyone of any gender can go through menopause at any stage in life if factors disturb the normal production of hormones. In men the condition of menopause is usually called andropause even though it's the exact same condition and there is no reason for genderization because they have the exact same conditions, causes, and symptoms. Many women are also recommended estrogens or phytoestrogens like isoflavones for the treatment of menopause but because pregnenolone is the master hormone of the body from which all the other can be made supplemental pregnenolone is the more effective route to address symptoms associated with menopause, supported by all the dietary, behavioral, and environmental strategies that affect metabolic health as discussed in this book (especially the chapter on libido) as well as the resolution of chronic pathogenic colonization.

Natural, endogenous production of pregnenolone and progesterone are also easy to restore, as most hormones are made from *cholesterol* which is in turn made primarily from dietary fats. Fat malabsorption due to gastroinestinal colonization by opportunistic microbes is the primary inhibitor of normal pregnenolone production, so chapters on parasitism and gut health while restoring a healthful diet usually results in an increase in wellness, energy, and endocrine function specifically due to increases in endogenous pregnenolone synthesis. The mechanism of inhibition is specifically from ammonification of the gut which disturbs stomach acid and healthy populations of microbes which produce the short chain fatty acids required to in turn acidify dietary silicon as discussed in the chapter on cancer. Before fats and fat soluble nutrients are packaged into cholesterol for distribution in the body they are captured by structures called *micelles* and *liposomes* dependent on bile and, while widely studied by science, micelles and liposomes are not fully elucidated and their formation and structure remain somewhat nebulous. Because of my research into mitochondrial silicon and cancer and the role of silicon in the lipid mitochondrial bilayer I realized silicon probably also plays a role in the formation of micelles due to its dual nature as a semiconductor when activated by acetic acid and likely helps to make the dipolar bridges that help solubilize fatty nutrients into these structures in the watery environment of our gut and bodies. Studies on topics other than human biology do show that silicon lends itself to micelle formation, so this confirmed role would definitely occur in the environment of the gut from digested food substrate when silicon and acids are present. This also means that foods high in silicon are required in the diet in major part because they promote the normal digestion of fats in the presence of acids (including bile) for healthy cholesterol and hormone homeostasis through formation of micelles and liposomes, so long as other principles of digestion and the microbiome are also addressed such as production of stomach acid and inhibition of microbial ammonia producers. What's more, studies have found that silicon can restore normal cholesterol homeostasis, increasing the "good" cholesterol HDL while lowering amounts of "bad" LDL cholesterol and triglycerides, which are simply backup strategies for failing HDL, and it is very likely then that silicon also plays a role in HDL cholesterol formation and may also be a significant transport mechanism for dietary silicon. So restoring silicon digestion as discussed in the chapter on cancer while also consuming good sources of fat like butter, coconut oil, olive oil, and nuts with dietary sources of silicon like green beans, sprouted oatmeal, spinach, dates, raisins, plantains, cucumber, pineapple, mango, sprouted whole grains like rice and spelt, corn, etc., can and will result in an increase in progesterone production and other hormones through production of endogenous pregnenolone.

Progesterone synthesis is also shown to be upregulated by butyric acid, produced specifically in the gut by butyrate producing commensal microbes such as *Clostridium* species dependent in turn on dietary *boron* such as occurs in foods like grapes and raisins and the *Prunus* family such as apricots, peaches, nectarines, etc., but also many other plant foods. It has also been mentioned previously that coconut oil is high in *lauric acid* which strongly upregulates endogenous pregnenolone, and stimulus of pregnenolone by coconut oil is so strong in fact it can rapidly deplete vitamin A if there is not sufficient dietary carotene (this led me to experience a drop in libido and to mistake coconut oil as harmful when instead an increase in dietary carotene with coconut oil instead promoted robust libido), and consuming healthy fats with sources of silicon will not only result in the greater uptake of healthy fats and thus promotion of hormones like pregnenolone, progesterone, testosterone, DHEA, etc., but also fat soluble nutrients these foods contain such as vitamins K and E and carotene. Conversely, this heretofore unrecognized requisite for silicon in the packaging and absorption of fat and fat soluble nutrients is the reason why eating 'healthy' can sometimes seem unproductive since dietary sources of silicon are not necessarily consistent even in healthy foods—for instance brassicas, nuts, sweet potatoes, potatoes, peppers, and fruit juices are usually low in silicon, which is also further inhibited by ammonification of the gut. Adding a little plant-sourced silicon to tea for drinking alongside foods low in silicon (never add silicon to dry foods as solid silicon is extremely hard and will chip and score tooth enamel) can help resolve this deficiency and promote normal fat digestion and hormone homeostasis and should be practiced by anyone with metabolic disease—do not use excess, however, since silicon spontaneously polymerizes would only be useful in a low to moderate dose (like 25-50 mg). When experimenting with this strategy I felt the same increase in feelings of empathy as I experienced from supplementation of progesterone, so its efficacy was undeniable. Because the skin is a site of hormone synthesis coconut oil and other fats do not always need to be eaten but can also be applied to skin, which can also help especially with injury, metabolic illness, or skin disorders as the skin readily absorbs fatty nutrients, but making sure to consume dietary silicon with dietary fats and sources of fat soluble nutrients while addressing pathogens and ammonification will reverse hyposteroidogenesis and replenish normal levels of pregnenolone and progesterone and other hormones thus resolving any requisite for their supplementation. Coconut oil is very low in oleic acid, however, so it should not be the only source of dietary fat, but using coconut oil can be an especially helpful method for restoring pregnenolone if also replete with carotene and zinc. As many other functions discussed in previous chapters such as cardiovascular health and even parasitism benefit from progesterone, this strategy of consuming some silicon with dietary fat can be even more productive than taking medications and supplemental hormones, helping to resolve parasitism and promoting expansion of the blood volume and retention of chloride and other halides required for the immune system.

Because progesterone is also antiparasitic this decline in cholesterol function is a primary catalyst which allows parasitism by parasites like Trichomonas which require sex hormones for their reproductive cycle. Sterols such as cholesterol are fundamental elements in biological life, and part of the unique niche we inhabit in nature is the very particular hormone profile of human biology which while promoting human biology also actively impairs microbial pathogens that are permeable to fatty molecules like sterols, and part of the aging process which occurs to all animals is the eventual impairment of normal cholesterol function due to stresses in the diet or environment which then allows ingress by opportunistic pathogens as discussed earlier in this book, so consistent, daily effort promoting good cholesterol function through dietary silicon, good fats, and inhibiting ammonia and restoring stomach acid and bile acids should also result in eradication of symptoms associated with parasitism such as problems with reproductive health, cystic fibrosis, weight, hair loss, and even cancer.

Of course, vitamin C is also antiparasitic and is required as a cofactor for cholesterol synthesis, and promoting silicon uptake as discussed in the chapter on immunity synergizes to restore many biological functions through vitamin C repletion including the increase in cholesterol, bile, digestion, tissue regeneration, metabolism, thyroid, etc. But vitamin C also promotes hormone production by protecting cholesterol from oxidation by free copper, and studies show that both the oxidized and reduced forms of vitamin C chelates free copper (which likely also helps our body properly metabolize copper into protein chaperones), even liberating cholesterol from copper that has already reacted to it which likely helps reverse atherosclerosis (heart disease). After restoring vitamin C repletion through the strategic combination with silicon I also began seeing an increase in masculine features I had lost over decades of being ill, because free copper inhibits the enzyme *5-alpha reductase* which converts regular testosterone into its active form, *dihydrotestosterone* (DHT) responsible for the most male characteristics like lean musculature, large forearms, increased vasculature, and a centralized body hair pattern (which is why gender affirming therapy for males cannot only consist of regular testosterone but must also include DHT). This chapter could also just as easily be titled *vitamin E therapy*, since vitamin E is so crucial for inhibiting the lipid peroxidation of fats which prevent cholesterol and steroid synthesis. As discussed in the chapter on viruses and the immune system vitamin E is crucial for a properly function immune reaction and prevents oxidation chain reactions otherwise caused by the immune reaction to infection, allergens, and includes pathways like sulfate synthesis and xanthine catabolism. This nature of vitamin E also protects cells from the stress of cellular excitation, calcification, general metabolic fatigue, and also protects hormones directly from oxidation and is extremely useful in promoting metabolic wellness and arresting conditions of aging and metabolic disease, but vitamin C also protects vitamin E in circulation from oxidation by copper and helps promote vitamin E renewal, so restoring vitamin C as discussed in earlier chapters also helps restore vitamin E status. Intracellular vitamin E is regenerated by glutathione which means that vitamin E deficiency is also caused by hydrogen sulfide producing microbes since excessive hydrogen sulfide directly impairs glutathione status (so vitamin C also helps promote vitamin E by promoting catabolism of hydrogen sulfide), and while a supplement of natural vitamin E can certainly be helpful it is only helpful inasmuch as the normal recycling of vitamin E can be restored, after which dietary sources like nuts and leafy greens are more than sufficient, especially if consumed with dietary sources of silicon like green beans or plant-derived silicon added to some tea before boiling to promote the increased formation of micelles and liposomes (sprouting nuts and grains can also increase their vitamin E content up by up to 600%) which can also help potentiate the use of pregnenolone, progesterone, or dietary fats restore normal hormone production. Many natural progesterone products are already formulated with vitamin E for this purpose, but since fat soluble nutrients are primarily distributed by cholesterol its dietary form accompanying dietary silicon is most effective.

Weight gain is often a supposed side effect of supplemental progesterone, such as I experienced in my recovery, though this is not really an effect of progesterone but consequence of pathogenic colonization and resultant excess of ammonia which disturbs the normal transport and metabolism of water as discussed in the chapters on gut health and parasitism, as by participating in mineralocorticoid management of electrolytes progesterone better helps the body sequester water away from the internal organs, which helps them run better as excess water lowers electrical conductivity of cells, but which increases water deposition in fat until such time as the body can resolve ammonia excess and properly eliminate water excess. Weight gain with use of pregnenolone or progesterone is always a sign of pathogenic colonization and excess ammonia which must be addressed if health problems are to be resolved. One condition which could likely benefit significantly from supplemental progesterone is *cerebral palsy*, which occurs from ischemic injury most commonly from premature birth and is shown definitively in studies to be associated with immature hormone changes as a result of underdevelopment. Studies have explored the use of supplemental estrogen and progesterone together for treatment of cerebral palsy but progesterone alone would be the more appropriate hormone for use of non-gestational persons since progesterone can also be converted into estrogen as required by growing tissues. Progesterone restores the plasticity of nervous tissues, which are dysfunctional in cerebral palsy, and could likely help regenerate those tissues and thus regulation of neurological function, as well as the topical application of coconut oil (not in excess—once a week would be sufficient) and a nutritive diet including carotene, zinc, silicon, vitamin E, etc.

Progesterone should always be limited to natural products, however, as synthetic progestins *do not* work the same as the natural form no matter what your doctor may say, and studies which show negative effects of progesterone are done using the synthetic type. I also learned that some prescriptions of synthetic progesterone are even injected which is insane considering that progesterone rapidly transfuses across all tissues of the body and injection is entirely unnecessary. Mucosal tissues of the mouth, digestive tract, and vaginal walls are especially receptive to hormones, but it can also be added to the skin when mixed with a little olive oil or coconut oil since the skin also readily absorbs fatty nutrients (which is why exposure to endocrine disruptors in clothing, bedding, and other textiles is oppositely so harmful). Many progesterone products (including those which are natural) sometimes contain harmful ingredients like parabens, poly-acrylamide, soy, or exotic oils from seeds and plants and herbs which might sound great except that such "essential" oils and herbs are the very kinds which exacerbate symptoms and promote estrogen by causing depolarization of cells as discussed in the chapter on oral health, and should contain as little ingredients as possible. I strongly advise finding a product made entirely without soy, and if a product does not indicate from what it originates it is likely soy (the vitamin E) and another should be used instead (if that's difficult it's fine to use a soy product while restoring endogenous production which shouldn't take more than a few months). While supplemental hormones can be very useful, restoration of endog-enous, natural production should be the primary goal no matter your gender as supplements never resolve the underlying causes of illness which will continue causing health problems if they are not addressed.

Many reproductive issues such as menstrual pain and discomfort or prostate inflammation are also treated with NSAIDs like acetaminophen and ibuprofen, but while these are effective painkillers they are also highly toxic to the human body and risk significant liver damage, rapid depletion of sulfate, and impair healing since healing pathways are mediated by inflammation. Because it is common for women to receive ibuprofen after labor this can and does significantly delay recov-ery and can even induce postpartum depression and psychosis. It's okay to use a little of these pain meds if they are really needed but should only ever be used if absolutely necessary, quit as soon as is possible, and instead use aspirin, sugar, and topical magnesium chloride and coconut oil for menstrual pains, recovery from labor (which will double). Because menstruation is a condition of heightened estrogen and progesterone production, severe menstrual pain is a symptom of low progesterone and pregnenolone production likely due to dieting or impaired fat absorption due to a diet low in silicon, fat, and fat soluble nutrients. During menstruation organs like the corpus luteum and the uterine lining are regen-erating and menstrual pains can be thought of as growing pains for the female reproductive system, which are uncomfortable in direct proportion to deficiency of progesterone, and so require an abundance of nutrition and hormones. Remember when using supplements to always avoid additives like silica, gums, carrageenan, and other problematic fillers which can contribute to metabolic problems instead of reversing them. It is in the consumer's best interest to practice due diligence in reading product labels and identifying good-quality manufacturing, since most supplements are made cheaply and risk of buying an inferior product is high, and long term health is never a function of supplement use but of dietary habits and strategies to restore normal biological functions with supplements merely supporting those efforts.

Using progesterone in high doses which are useful for therapy can also shift the menstruation cycle since this tricks the body into thinking it is pregnant. For this reason progesterone can act as a contraceptive but is not entirely reliable, especially since progesterone also strongly promotes fertility. In women with a cycle who want to become pregnant progesterone is best used only in the second two weeks of the cycle to avoid shifting it, but shifting and inhibiting it isn't a problem any more than it is when pregnant and can be taken all the time if desired and not attempting pregnancy. One of my sisters who was taking progesterone at my advice to address severe metabolic sickness became pregnant after being unable for some time, because progesterone promotes fertility by promoting wellness, and though they had not been trying to get pregnant they also weren't trying to prevent it, thinking wrongly because it wasn't occurring that it wasn't going to. Fearing out of ignorance that progesterone might affect her pregnancy but not asking me for further advice (due to sex shame and other traumas of being raised in our family and religion) she stopped supplementing it and then miscarried because her body was still too ill to maintain its own progesterone production (this was before I understood how to restore it through diet and the microbiome). Normally the placenta takes over production of progesterone but this does not occur until about week twelve or thirteen of pregnancy, and after finally notifying me of her miscarriage I explained what had happened and how to avoid it in the future by not stopping progesterone until the second trimester. She used progesterone again, got pregnant, and carried my very healthy baby niece to full term. Progesterone falls during lactation after delivery, though, to allow for the estrogenic, prolactin mobilization of calcium required for milk production, so it should not be used during breastfeeding, and can actually stop lactation, which is another reason why it is so important to be healthy naturally through strategies outlined in this book which will eliminate the need to use such supplements in the first place and enable the body to do these things on its own if it is treated well and absent of stress and disease.

Being alive is the greatest effect I got from progesterone. I don't think I would have made it otherwise. But it goes further than that, and has many profound and easily attainable benefits that no other known medication has, except maybe aspirin, and can be used in many ways to help rescue severe health issues, especially cancer and other metabolic diseases. Progesterone's most attractive feature is the low cost and wide availability of natural products which makes it easy to access, and again it should be the natural form of progesterone. Some studies are even using it to cure brain trauma and restore paralysis and when accompanied by a good diet, sun exposure, and resolution of pathogenic colonization and use of high dose progesterone along with other healthy dietary behaviors discussed in this book (including restoration of vitamin D) could help some people with neurological damage or limited paralysis regain some function (when used as a supplement, not natural production, as artificial intervention would be required to raise progesterone to levels which would achieve this). But it won't make up for poor health choices, so make sure to take an overall approach to health and progesterone can help bridge the gap.

The Leaf

A little green leaf lit down in June. "What's this?" cried the leaf. "It's too soon to be hewn!"

"I'm sorry!" said tree, "I have too many leaves, and your presence was sucking the life out of me!"

The leaf, without legs, found nothing to do but lie on the ground, he started to stew. "I don't deserve this!" he thought over and over. "To be cast off like garbage, on my own, with no tether."

It seemed like a time long and listless advanced, but was only an hour since given this chance, when a breeze came along and blew the leaf off, "Now where will I go, unwanted?" he scoffed.

The leaf blew along without any companions, felt sad for himself, that he had been abandoned. But shortly the wind brought him near others who tumbled and blew and seemed fine without tethers.

"Who are you?" asked the leaf. "Aren't you lost and afraid?"

"No," said the leaves, "can't you see? We've got it made! A leaf is not meant to stay with its tree. In fact you must fall to become what you'll be. Now we're on this long, joyous journey together and the end will be sweeter for lack of a tether."

The leaf was now happy, though his plight was the same, 'cause it's all in the journey, and opinion of pain. If falling is hard, and loneliness double, ask what you can do to think different of trouble. One thing is for certain—life is harder than not. So be like this leaf, no matter the plot.

CHAPTER 25

CURING ALCOHOLISM AND DRUG ADDICTION

One Saturday when I was fifteen our family was driving home from my dad's office buildings where we earned extra money doing janitorial work instead of having normal summer jobs, and I was staring out the window like a proper brooding teenager, dreaming of all the ways life could be better than it was while my five siblings, tired from the day's janitorial effort, were silent and nodding off in the back. Actually, I clearly remember fantasizing about a fire-breathing dragon flying along our car, I was just insecure about sharing that. "Nathan," my dad's suddenly authoritarian tone broke the hypotonic drum of the Suburban's rolling tires, "we know what you're doing when you take long showers."

WHAT? I thought, completely in disbelief this was happening, in front of my whole family no less. "You're no longer allowed to be in the bathroom more than five minutes."

My face turned red. I didn't reply and just glared out the window. What could I say to something like that? Who would even say something like that, to their own children, in front of others. "No long showers," agreed my mom, who then looked at dad in a way which revealed this to be a premeditated attack. Why they thought a good time to address my masturbation habits was in the car with my entire family present seems insanity to me, except they most likely did mean to embarrass me, to inflict the greatest level of shame possible.

This was just another example of the kind of constant emotional abuse in which I grew up, not half of it from just my parents, full of religious threats and debasing shame for simply being alive. Exploitation of experiences common to all humans such as sex, weight, desire, loss, and fear is a common feature of religions and abuse not for any real concern for our wellbeing but because, being common to all humans, become the most convenient point of vulnerability for purposes of control. The irony was that I hated whacking off in the shower. Water is a terrible lubricant, as any boy knows. I did all my masturbation under the covers or while streaking around naked the forest near our house under cover of darkness. No, I loved taking long hot showers because it was the only place in the house where I could get away from *them*. Unlike the rest of my life a shower was peaceful, quiet, a sanctuary. I found out later that children and adults with thyroid problems instinctively shower hotter and longer to self-medicate a reduced body temperature so it was literally also medicinal to my medical problems. But wellness wasn't something that concerned my parents nor the community at large, and as is the experience of many teenagers, my life seemed nothing more than one emotionally assaulting experience to the next. Real relief finally came when I was nineteen, on a date with a handsome, kind boy at his apartment when he asked if I'd like a glass of "red or white."

"Red or white, what?" I replied, was how little I knew of alcohol, how efficient my insulated upbringing. He chose for me and brought a glass full of red wine. I remember how acidic and fruity it tasted. I did not get a buzz but there was something about it which felt instantly freeing, as if for the first time I knew what life was like without pain and inhibition, for a moment free and mature, happy, unencumbered by the neuroses and insecurities under which I suffocated, and all in a beautiful glass of pretty red liquid. From that day out alcohol freed me every time, from ever-present stress. It made my life enjoyable, brought fun and companionship, the kind of life other people get to live without it—the kind of life I always wanted.

But even when alcohol proved detrimental to my life I was never able to connect the dots. Actually I was, but deeply in the back of my mind, inaccessible, a very real fear that alcohol was ruining my health, as though the person who knew this was trapped inside the body of a person who drank liberally. In Los Angeles I would meet models, actors, and athletes who refrained from drinking even on a rambunctious night out. I saw their example and longed to join their ranks—but the tequila was just too good. Actually, I longed for them to join me and prove that alcohol was compatible with such beauty. They never did. Not even crashing my car into a concrete wall going fifty miles an hour on the freeway while drunk and high on marijuana was I able to understand that I was an alcoholic. But when my life finally fell apart at the age of thirty-four I was standing alone in a three-bedroom house in Palm Springs shared with my fiancé of four years which we would soon have to vacate, wondering why my life was such a shambles. Of all the things a white male my age and privilege should have—a job, a car, a place to live, money, a lover, friends, I had not a one. A few days prior after a party during which I drank copious amounts of tequila I had said to one of our guests, "I'm so hungover." "Really?" he replied, "We didn't have that many drinks." I was surprised by his response, as it was the closest anyone in my entire life had come to even suggest I had a drinking problem. I recalled the events of the previous night and how I repeatedly returned to the kitchen to pour clandestine refills of tequila gimlets during moments when our guests were outside, or in the bathroom, or watching the TV intently, and after everyone had gone to bed. Because I am so tall I always assumed that everyone was always watching me, but I was so good at sneaking my alcoholism that not even my partner with alcohol and addiction problems of his own knew the quantity of alcohol I was putting away.

Desperate for a way to hold on to my life as it was I asked for help from someone I had never met but knew was sober, who was a friend of my fiancé. My motivation was that he might help preserve my relationship, as my partner had also relapsed into cocaine addiction from which he had been sober several years, but the conversation did not go as I had anticipated. He did not join in my commiseration, and though he allowed me to vent he then explained that there was nothing I could do except to help myself. This was something I had never thought of, but it was not his words which made an impression on me. Rather, he spoke with a calmness I had never heard before, as if he was familiar with pain and heartache and knew the secret of life and accepted its changeableness and instability. I would later come to know this as serenity. But right there on the phone as he suggested I try a program for codependents of alcoholics (Al-anon) I finally realized that *I* was the one with a drinking problem. Suddenly the plagues of my life all made sense. "*I am a drunk!*" I thought with glee as we began to wrap up our phone call. My pain and desperation suddenly lessened. I hung up the phone and contemplated my situation. My problems became quite clear. It was not that I couldn't manage a relationship, hold a job, be financially responsible, or avoid bad partners. I had a disease which made the accomplishment of these things impossible, because it always got in the way and assumed priority over everything else. Initially I thought that identifying as a drunk would save my relationship. On Valentine's Day I prepared a warm welcome for my partner who had returned to get some clothes. I apologized for my self-centered behavior and acknowledged my alcoholism, and promised that I would no longer drink. "That's great," he said in a chummy tone not used between lovers. "Are you going to meetings?"

Meetings? I thought. *Oh, he means Alcoholics Anonymous.*

"I don't need them," I said defensively. As the words left my lips I knew I was lying. I was not good at life. I had failed utterly. How was I going to get my life back in order when I did not even know where to begin? Sure, things could be yet worse but that was no standard to live by. I had no idea how to be an adult, how to run my affairs, how to find success in relationships and business or to deal with the suffocating uncertainties which are the garb of mortality. I would not survive if I did not learn how.

I didn't say as much, though. Suddenly I did not want him there anymore. I felt it was a real chance for me to get out of old patterns of behavior entirely if I only reached out and grabbed it. My misery turned to excitement, and as soon as he left I ran to the computer and looked up the very next meeting I could find.

A few hours later I walked into a small building with no signage in a half-empty commercial development. Blinding florescent lights made the few old men gathered appear decades older than they were. None of them looked at me or even acknowledged my presence. After I sat down, a crazy lady sitting to the side asked me why I was there. I told her my fiancé had left. She said it was not a good reason to be there. It was obvious that she was no person from whom to take advice, so I ignored her. Then a man twenty years my senior walked in. He saw me and paused, then stepped forward with an outstretched hand and introduced himself, and asked if I was new. I nodded and introduced myself, my emotions an equal mix of overwhelming joy and sadness made it difficult to speak without my voice catching. He offered his help and phone number. The meeting started. The attendees went around the room declaring their names and length of sobriety. They did not care that I cried when I said I was an alcoholic. They encouraged me to return but did not indulge my self-pity, giving advice on good meetings and encouraging me to pursue the program. I stuck with it, even as I moved back to Los Angeles and struggled to put my life back together, and within a few months found myself on the way to an entirely better future.

One day while working on my cancer situation and sober for half a dozen months I was reading a paper written by Ray Peat on the nervous system discussing the neurochemical *acetylcholine,* and Dr. Peat's description of what acetylcholine does for the human body suddenly made me realize that a lot of the things I had been using to treat my cancer had also been treating my alcoholism because of their influence over acetylcholine. I had been having an amazing time in recovery, having incredible and life-changing experiences with no trouble staying sober, and happy though others who entered the program at the same time were depressed, despondent, and relapsing. I had thought I was just good at being sober, but having made this realization I researched more about acetylcholine in terms of my hypothesis on its possible role in alcoholism and addiction and experimented with therapies informed by that research. I quickly confirmed my hypothesis through my own experiences and finally understood what causes this condition and thus how to cure it.

Attempting to share this cure with other alcoholics and addicts was sadly unproductive and demoralizing, assuming that like me others would be eager for a resolution to our shared torment. But I learned that many people do not actually want to get better, feeling more comfortable with the pain they know and the control that makes them comfortable rather than the unknown. But I also realized that some unconsciously understand the concept of a cure to mean not relief from the condition altogether but no longer being able to use drugs or alcohol for their therapeutic effects. To be clear, this accomplishes total relief from the underlying conditions of pain, suffering, and illness which are the cause for abuse, and alcohol and drugs are not actually the problem in addiction and alcoholism and are nothing more than the available medicines to treat the underlying condition. I also find it poorly effective to prescribe this chapter directly to those who are very ill as their cognition, fear, and insecurity usually prevent them from understanding this complex biology and nutrition, let alone incorporating it into their recovery, and will be most useful for medical professionals, policy makers, or friends and family members of those who are doing very poorly. As the underlying mechanisms also relate to other metabolic pathologies it is valuable to anyone with an interest for their own health to understand this information whether or not they also have the disease, since all of our biology operates in the same way and thus all of us, especially children, are vulnerable to developing it.

To understand why we use drugs and alcohol we must first understand the most basic nature of these substances. Because alcohol is a type of sugar it helps cells make huge amounts of energy, and this why we so often use it, especially if we are stressed or want to feel better, since alcohol helps to easily and powerfully run fatigued cells. Because of ridiculous ideas on health and wellness I met a lot of stupid alcoholics and addicts barely sober who thought they should also give up sugar. Guess how well that worked out for them? Even if you believe sugar is addicting (it isn't), if it means you're going to have an easier time staying sober shouldn't you probably choose the one which doesn't impair your cognitive function? People who don't want to believe alcohol is bad for our health, even if they're already sick, often hail the witless tripe of some things working differently for different persons, as if some of us are different species or something. One dolt commented on an article I wrote on alcoholism that Europe had a strong tradition of drinking and was an example of a peaceful, functional society, conveniently forgetting both World Wars, the Holocaust, the Albanian genocide, Brexit, etc., and the reason alcohol can harm our health has nothing to do with morals, religion, or spirituality, and many of us who should probably stop drinking do not want to because those who told us not to drink because it was immoral would then be right, not only about the drink but about our character, while also depriving us of a very useful and widely available therapeutic treatment of the pain and discomfort we suffer. Unfortunately, alcohol is still incompatible with health, but only because of biochemistry and not because our abusive parents or religious leaders say so. In fact, because of their biases and prejudices those people have stood in the way of a cure, and are explicitly responsible for the untold numbers of addicts and alcoholics which have lived and died and the damage caused by this condition over the past many centuries as religion antagonized scientific progress. As a former alcoholic no one wanted alcohol to be healthy more than I did, as it helped me cope with the frustration of being unable to control my drinking, but if I've learned anything it is precisely how much life absolutely does not care what I want to be true. Sure, maybe you won't get cancer from alcohol. Maybe, like me, you can manage your drinking for many years, but that doesn't mean you are a superman with your own laws of biology and chemistry. It's okay. Alcohol helped me think I was exempt from life a time too, and the good news is that alcoholism and addiction are real physical diseases which have nothing to do with self-control or willpower, and the callous disregard by those who condemn us for our condition will have to answer for their own behavior and the harm they cause to others.

In the mid nineteen-hundreds a man by the name of Curt Richter was studying rats and their response to stress. He noticed that when rats were subjected to a painful stimulus (torture) while being fully restrained the rats would quickly surrender and cease to struggle. Rats given even one chance to escape during the torture continued to attempt escape every time. The rats with no chance to escape suddenly stopped trying to escape, and would not even attempt to escape when given a later opportunity to do so. They had acquired an inability to perceive hope, and when put in a swim test where a healthy rat can and does swim and stay afloat for two or three days without drowning, as well as the rats allowed to escape, the rats who developed hopelessness had heart attacks within an hour and drowned. This acquired response to stress, marked by an inability to perceive hope and which resulted in the permanent inability for rats to survive challenges to their physical safety was termed *learned hopelessness.*

When I was twenty I could not bring myself to attend college even though I really wanted to go, and had applied and been accepted for a second time. I was not yet drinking regularly but I would look forward to occasions when one of my friends threw a good house party so I could have a drink. I wanted to be sociable, affable and charismatic, and able to hit on guys and be good at my job (and be able to stay at one) and face life and people without fear, without feeling paralyzed. I wanted to have hope for the future. But as hard as I tried I could not. I could only be any of these things when I'd had a drink (or had one not too long ago). I was not conscious of the connection between drinking and my desires until my drinking reached epic levels. Drinking had been an unconscious reaction for much needed self medication just like my long showers as a kid. When I did finally become aware of it I was without explanation, or recourse. How do I acquire the ability to function the way I wanted when it had proved so beyond my physiology to do so? Of course I sought help. I tried therapy, both psychological and psychiatric, I got into yoga and mediation, tried antidepressants and nutritional approaches. Read books. Asserting my willpower. None of these approaches came close to the freedom afforded by alcohol, nor did they relieve me the need of it. Even a small drink seemed to free me from the bondage of my condition, yet it was also limiting since I couldn't drink at work, or in the morning (not yet anyway), or for too long without some kind of side effect. I was trapped between a rock and a hard place.

Eventually I developed cancer, and lost important parts of my life.

The condition of learned hopelessness exhibited by those rats happens when our natural learning process becomes a negative feedback loop. Normally, the parasympathetic nervous system and a chemical called *acetylcholine* are responsible for the imprinting of learned behavior. When functioning rightly, acetylcholine is integral to our learning and development. A pianist becomes good at controlling ten separate fingers simultaneously because of acetylcholine. Repeated exposure to a piano, music, and instruction trains the pianist's mind and body to respond while being exposed to the stimulus of the keys, sounds, sights, instruction, etc. Because of acetylcholine, when the fully practiced concert pianist lifts their hands over a keyboard their body instinctively knows how to respond. In the same way, a basketball player learns to instinctively control a bouncing ball without even looking at it. Chefs learn to distinguish between foods and more deftly form works of art. A teacher also learns how to better control or inspire their students. But acetylcholine functions in even more subtle ways. It teaches us what body posture to adopt when among friends and which to adopt among enemies, things which we aren't always conscious of learning, like how fast to move when crossing the street or which kind of dogs make us relax and which make us nervous, or what to say or do around our parents to avoid getting beaten. In the condition of learned hopelessness the parasympathetic system (or in other words, *us*) has learned that escape or hope of escape during broad stimulus like life and people is nonexistent. I must always hide who I am or be rejected by my friends and family. My parents do not love me. I was abandoned as a child and no family will take me in. Men will take advantage of me and I must always be on guard. Physical violence is everywhere. Paying this bill will make me even more afraid of my bank account. But since stressful stimuli also increase the expression of acetylcholine, and acetylcholine also increases stress and the expression of stress hormones, hormones which induce torpor, malaise, fatigue, and pain, which further amplifies the suffering and physically destructive conditions of the disease, and the elevation of stress hormones in turn increase acetylcholine sensitivity so a person with the condition becomes stuck in a negative cognitive feed back loop that is in effect, a paralysis of our vitality. Stress increases acetylcholine. Acetylcholine increases stress. When negative perceptions of life are the lesson learned from this disease the reaction to life is quite simply emotional and social paralysis. Because this condition involves the nervous system and its excessive activation by stimuli and the overexpression of neurochemicals, learned hopelessness is thus a neurological disorder.

Invariably, every mainstream idea about addiction and alcoholism, especially those coming from the medical community, see addiction as a problem of willpower and indulgence, but a fundamental problem that all alcoholics and addicts have is a universal *inability* to actually enjoy themselves. Just like the rats in Curt Richter's experiments, those who are not alcoholic or addicted grow and develop in an environment which contains at least some enrichment, fun, and enjoyment, with other humans demonstrating compassion for them (usually parents or other older humans) as well as skills of self care, recreation, interests, hobbies, pursuits, and other skills for seeking out and practicing behaviors which bring fulfillment. I once saw an article on a reputable news outlet from an establishment psychologist urging people to abstain periodically from fulfilling activities like sex or eating great food so they could retrain their brain to be less dependent on dopamine. This person had absolutely no understanding of the function of dopamine in a human animal because its role as a hormone is not to indulge human excesses and provide temptation but to teach a human animal what behaviors facilitate a successful human life—you know, things like eating, or having intimate and fulfilling relationships. All alcoholics and addicts I have ever known or worked with fundamentally do not know how to enjoy themselves, and activities for normal people which feel indulgent like eating a bowl of ice cream or having really great sex is, for those with with this disease, always accompanied by guilt, shame, or embarrassment and do not produce dopamine the way they do in those without addiction because of the effect of stress on draining dopamine, and so drugs or alcohol are required for them to enjoy even the simplest of normally rewarding activities.

Since acetylcholine is a chemical it can also be influenced by environmental and nutritional factors and an excess may not even be related to social and interpersonal dynamics. Nightshades which include potatoes, tomatoes, eggplant, and peppers contain powerful poisons called *glycoalkaloids* which are meant to deter pests like nematodes, by inactivating the enzyme *acetylcholinesterase* which is supposed to regulate and balance acetylcholine, and these poisons kill those pests by overstimulating their nervous system with acetylcholine. Since we are much larger than nematodes these poisons do not usually kill us, and in fact are hardly noticeable except that they still effect this enzyme which is supposed to inactivate excess acetylcholine and so artificially elevates it and thus promotes agitation, restlessness, and activation of learned hopelessness. Some agricultural pesticides also block this enzyme to kill insects through the same pathway, and then we consume these pesticide saturated foods. Since stress also increases the expression of acetylcholine a child in an abusive home will be more effected by acetylcholine than a child in a peaceful home, and a child in an abusive home will be more effected by the abuse if *also* fed a diet which increases the effect of acetylcholine. But a child in an abusive home with a great diet can grow up without the disease, and a child in a peaceful, loving home with an incorrect diet can still succumb to it. This is why alcoholics and addicts have heretofore appeared to share no common demographic denominator, and come from all walks of life, backgrounds, gender, and ages. Either way, a child developing the condition of learned hopelessness becomes more and more sensitive to stress, and every stress reaction, environmental or nutritional, increases acetylcholine until the point that acetylcholine is chronically elevated, chronically learning that stress is everywhere and everywhere creates stress, even from the most seeming mundane of stimuli, and a child spends their childhood simply trying to survive it rather than learning what makes them unique and life fulfilling. A child who grows up with threats of rejection from their family because they are attracted to the same gender is a child who is constantly exposed to stress and elevated acetylcholine, even when the abusive parents aren't present. When the child becomes an adult, just like when the concert pianist encounters the conditions of sitting at a piano and acetylcholine stimulates their mind and fingers to do their thing the alcoholic and addict (or learned hopelessness adult) experiences their conditioning, which is not to impress adoring crowds with soaring music but that there is no hope of escape.

At this point you may have guessed what alcohol does to acetylcholine. That's right, it turns it off. In fact alcohol inactivates acetylcholine so well that in excess it completely erases acetylcholine, and since acetylcholine is what creates learning, which is in essence memory and consciousness, its absence causes a total blackout. With enough alcohol memories cease forming at all, both mental and physical, and a person wakes up to find themselves lying on an unfamiliar lawn in an unfamiliar neighborhood with no recollection of where they are or how they got there or driving into a concrete wall on the freeway without any recollection of starting the car. And this is also why alcoholics constantly return to the bottle in spite of negative experiences, because the very presence of it entirely reduces the effect of acetylcholine, which is required for learning, and thus very little imprint or learning from lived experiences. Alcohol is thus its own cloaking device. Little or nothing is learned or retained while it is present. It is why I could not remember the last few years of my relationship between Christmas vacations, when whole years seemed to disappear in a matter of days, or why even crashing my car into a concrete wall was not enough to help me see my own alcoholism, because so much time was spent drunk or recovering from drinking that my ability to remember life itself was destroyed, even when traumatic. But since the majority of acetylcholine is eliminated with alcohol so is the state of learned hopelessness and memories of trauma and thus provides relief to the alcoholic. Since acetylcholine can also be effected by diets, cultures which traditionally have a high rate of nightshade consumption like the Midwest (potatoes), Russia (potatoes), and Mexico (tomatoes and peppers) have correspondingly higher rates of alcoholism because their diets are higher in chemicals which elevate acetylcholine. Eggplant is highest in solanine (draining eggplant with salt probably discards much of it) and there are some traditions in places in Europe and the Middle East with justified notions that eggplant can cause insanity because solanine can raise acetylcholine so much it can actually destroy neurological function. Alcohol just happens to be the most powerful medication for treating excess acetylcholine, cheap and widely available. Alcohol is the medicine alcoholics use to relieve themselves of the symptoms of learned hopelessness. As such, alcoholism and addiction are in truth a neurological disorder. Because of course it fucking is.

Though drug users may or may not also use alcohol they do suffer from the very same neurological condition of learned hopelessness, and where alcohol works by directly antagonizing acetylcholine the way in which drugs like marijuana, Xanax, methamphetamine, or heroin ease the suffering of this disease is instead either by blocking acetylcholine release in the first place or increasing other hormones or chemicals which antagonize the *effects* of acetylcholine rather than acetylcholine directly. Acetylcholine, for instance, lowers dopamine but methamphetamine and many other drugs directly raise dopamine, reversing the debt caused by excess acetylcholine expression. By increasing the neuroinhibitor GABA, heroin and opioids help cells resist the negative effects of acetylcholine and that associated suffering of learned hopelessness. Marijuana interferes with acetylcholine production and lowers adrenaline production (but since adrenaline is what releases glucose from glycogen storage blood sugar falls which then causes the munchies). All forms of substance addiction center around the activity of this neurological chemical to relieve sufferers of its negative effects, regardless of the substance used. The reason that some drug addicts don't abuse alcohol, besides using drugs which accomplish similar effects, is because their gut microbiome still produces acetic acid, so there are no cravings for acetic acid substrate, but the excess of acetylcholine is still a problem, hence addiction. Alcohol and drugs also antagonize pathogenic organisms like *C. difficile* and *Candida*, but many drugs like cocaine, nicotine, and opioids are are also alkaloids which inhibit parasites, and part of therapeutic nature of drugs and alcohol is to treat infectious pathogenic organisms which destroy metabolic health, and why restoring a healthy microbiome and addressing chronic infections is so important for the entirety of our wellbeing. Cocaine is a widely abused drug which very specifically inhibits helminthic parasites, as it is derived from leaves of coca plants and like many plant chemicals is an evolutionary defense against microbes and other threats to plant wellbeing. In fact, cocaine is often adulterated specifically with an antihelminthic drug called Levamisole, which can be fatal to humans when used like cocaine, but mimics some of the medicinal benefits that cocaine has in treating parasitic infection. I never dared use cocaine as a young man but was perplexed why so many of my friends and acquaintances who did seemed to more easily stay fit and youthful even as I aged and struggled with my weight, but it was precisely because of drugs like cocaine are purine alkaloids just like caffeine and nicotine and thus also treat pathogenic infection and thus metabolic disease. Unfortunately, because it also disrupts our endocrine system and neurological pathways, especially suppressing hormones of shame and guilt, cocaine abuse eventually leads to severely destructive behavioral problems and long term metabolic deterioration in spite of its limited medicinal uses, so in fact much drug abuse is actually also self medication of widespread parasitism as discussed in chapter on pathogens and metabolic disease.

Drugs and alcohol also only work while they are in the body, which is why sufferers of these conditions continually turn to them for relief, because they don't effect permanent cures, and eventually cause social and physical consequences from dependency. For years I believed I was no longer suicidal, but when my life fell apart I saw I had been committing suicide long and slow through alcohol abuse, the only two choices available to either drink or to die, because to live with things as they were was not possible, literally, for the disease which I suffered would not allow any other option. The biological systems which construct a life and personality had for me formed an ugly view of the world, and no matter how much I tried and wanted my perspective to be different, no matter how many pleasant things went on around me or much I wrested, fought, and pleaded with God, the world, or my own self control there was no way I could ever have treated such a disease on my own with the tools which were available to me. That boy who gave me my first glass of wine was murdered in his adulthood. Also a victim of this disease, he was in a situation no sweet, loving person such as him would ever willingly place themselves in if we weren't suffering such a debilitating illness. No person, even homeless and destitute from addictions would chose to be there if they weren't victims of this disease. That this even has to be explained is incredible to me.

I once read an article decrying Alcoholics Anonymous for being the only primary treatment of alcoholism, given that there are some adjunct medical therapies available as well. The subtext from the author was really a beef with the concept of God and one could strip everything about A.A. from the article and not have lost the message they were putting forth. I get it. God was an integral part of the torment which I was subjected to as a helpless child. Though not actually a God, of course, but adult men and women who hurt me in the name of their idea and concept of God. A more patient person might frame them as well-meaning, but I know adult behavior and people who use God to control their children are hateful, lazy, and traumatized adults who resort to fear and intimidation because they are powerful tools, with little regard to the eventual outcome of their actions and are more concerned with their own benefit than that of their young charges. No, that author is not wrong to despise the concept of God when authority is tied together with the very nature of learned hopelessness and our abuse as children. It is from these very people who were Gods to us that the excruciating condition from which we suffer came.

And yet twelve-step programs can work to relieve alcoholics and drug addicts from their enslavement, if actually done (doing six steps of a twelve-step program is not doing a twelve-step program). So if alcoholism and drug abuse are a neurological disease, how can recovery programs work? Because learned hopelessness is a process created by neurological learning pathways it can also be *unlearned.* Learning is a neurological process. But that is also the key word—unlearned—a process of facilitating new experiences which can replace the old ones to in turn empower an addict or alcoholic to take care of themselves, and since all addicts and alcoholics basically lack self empowerment, the process of learning new skills to replace the absence of any can bring the new kinds of experiences which will give an addict the confidence, pride, and self-esteem they lack. Because of an insufficient childhood we were not taught how to do these things for ourselves, how to care for our own wellbeing or seek out fulfilling life experiences, how to enjoy our time on this earth not in spite of life's mundaneness but because of it, and as a result feel helpless to affect life in ways which would be productive and empowering and bring fulfillment, which does not come from being disciplined or balanced but from enjoying ourselves and other people. Learning skills that bring empowerment such as conflict resolution, self-care, fun and leisure, goal accomplishment, making real friendships and maintaining them, cooking, forgiveness, restitution, professional skills, etc., can supplant those feelings of helplessness and, if supported by the nutritional guidelines of recovery, will be more productive and permanent. Most with whom I work don't even cook themselves regular, delicious meals, which is a great place to start.

This relearning is cemented by abstinence, however, because concomitant drug and alcohol use still antagonizes acetylcholine which is needed to form new replacement experiences and positive associations, to facilitate new life experiences and the practice of self-care and self-fulfillment. Of course, there is a lot of dogma in recovery programs. My own experience was a mostly positive one which exposed me to new life skills such as how to amend broken relationships and care for my own wellbeing, but to provide more neutral therapy which more directly addresses the psychological origins of this condition I have appropriated these therapies and altered them for more effective resolution of past trauma, outlined in the chapter *God and Spirituality.* My other book, *The Perfect Child,* is also more specifically focused on experiences of childhood abuse, how to resolve it, and how to prevent it as a parent. Such therapy is absolutely required for alcoholics or addicts to overcome past negative experiences and to learn how to care for ourselves, or to prevent the disease in our children, and these versions more effectively resolve the psychological aspects of this disease without dogma or reliance on recovery programs, especially since recovery institutions do not focus at all on the biological and psychological factors which participate in the etiology of the condition (mostly because nobody has heretofore understood them), and every alcoholic or addict who wishes to escape their hell must engage in this kind of self-relearning, self-care, and self-empowerment to find the confidence we lack, else the feelings of fear and insecurity will continue to be too great to ever get real enjoyment out of life, which is entirely possible and more wonderful than you can ever imagine.

Because acetylcholine is a physiological substance it can also be altered the way it is with alcohol but with healthier, more effective, and more permanent therapies which make it much easier to abstain as is required for effective psychological healing. One of the best and most available to treat excess acetylcholine are first-generation *antihistamines.* I find this hilarious, as will anyone familiar with the program, because the program which was made decades ago regards alcohol as an allergen (which is not). Antihistamines work to combat alcoholism by blocking the destructive effects of excess acetylcholine and have been used unknowingly for this purpose for years in rehab clinics and emergency rooms to protect against the effects of severe withdrawal because the rebound of acetylcholine during severe alcoholism can be so intense it can actually kill a person. But antihistamines only block the destructive *effects* of acetylcholine rather than eliminating it like alcohol, and as such help facilitate the relearning process of unlearning learned hopelessness while still providing relief, and unlike alcohol the worst side effect is drowsiness. This is why recovery was so relatively easy for me because all the while of practicing inventory and being supported by the program I was using antihistamines to address my cancer, since excess parasympathetic nervous activity also contributes to cancer, but was also blocking the negative effects of elevated acetylcholine and making me feel great without requiring the use of alcohol, which made abstinence comparably easy.

Incidentally, first generation antihistamines also function as sleep aids and can be very useful since many alcoholics also suffer insomnia. At the outset of my recovery from alcohol I was taking *doxylamine succinate* to help combat my cancer and aid sleep. Not all over-the-counter antihistamines are actually antihistamines, though. Some are steroids or other compounds and will not at all provide this benefit. *Diphenhydramine* is another type, and there are yet more which are available, also some through prescription. Excessive use can overload the liver and isn't necessary, so they should not be used long term but are fine until a person is healthy and feeling better. Small doses also do huge work and I would break a tablet in half or even one-quarter and take once before bedtime for several months. An antihistamine will relieve an alcoholic of the activation of their learned hopelessness while assisting recovery from it. On taking one you may notice a slight reduction in the severity of the emotions which can lead to relapse. After several weeks the real benefit will start to kick in, which is sort of a sense of the pattern of negative emotional cues starting to vanish altogether, and moments are taken as they come rather than in anticipation.

Acetic acid is actually the end metabolite of alcohol metabolism, and since acetic acid is also the substrate for many important biological pathways including cholesterol and steroid synthesis alcohol produces the effect of making a drinker feel calmer and more confident during and after drinking, when we wonder why were even drinking so much in the first place and feel like we can quit, only to find ourselves just a day or two later suffering cravings. One study I found showed that drinking increases brain acetate by two-fold, and since acetic acid is so important for fundamental metabolic pathways like the citric acid cycle it easily supplies this necessary substrate. Because of this, one of the strongest etiological causes of alcoholism and addiction is the loss of acetogenic bacteria in the gut as discussed in the chapter on gut health, as acetic acid is supposed to be synthesized by our gut microbes, as well as avoiding carbohydrate required for gut microbes to metabolize into acetic acid as described in the chapter on gut health. Because of dieting and stress, alcoholics and addicts often have disturbed gut function and thus less short-chain fatty acid production. Not only that, but alcohol is also usually antibiotic to many types of opportunistic bacteria which colonize the gut due to dietary stress, so alcohol also becomes therapeutic to conditions of chronic infection which then makes it difficult to give up as it literally disinfects, temporarily, the body from those opportunistic agents. Because alcohol is antibacterial this also destroys healthy gut microbes, and it is required to resolve gut health and chronic microbial infection as discussed in earlier chapters to promote commensal gut microbes and restore local production of acetic acid from dietary substrate like pectin from fruit and other indigestible and digestible carbohydrate.

Specifically, supplementation of *sodium acetate* as described in the chapter on gut health and even the supplementation of acetic acid substrates like powdered pectin added to beverages *can and does severely relieve the impulse of cravings.* I actually discovered this by having many of my readers relate to me their reduced desire to drink, especially to excess, after regularly using sodium acetate I had recommended to assist in gut health. When I did start drinking again after three years of total sobriety I was amazed to find that instead of desiring an entire bottle of tequila or two or three bottles of wine I would actually feel like stopping after just one or two beers, and that hard liquor was now so powerful I didn't really like drinking it, and when I did drank like a normal person sipping on a very small amount for a long period of time, and now go months inbetween drinks because my mind doesn't even think about alcohol and I get to enjoy it when I do. None of this is because of willpower, but from healing my physical, emotional, and psychological health as described in this book. Sodium acetate effectively relieves cravings when used with consistency (especially when mixed into sugary drinks like juice or lemonade with added sugar to better promote sodium absorption), and can prevent drinking in excess if taken an hour or two before drinking but can also making sobriety bearable and productive. One alcoholic I tried to help would actually purposefully avoid sodium acetate when they wanted to drink because they knew it was so effective in serving the purpose of drinking in the first place (some willpower is required but for most people their behavior is not that ridiculous).

Deficiency of B12 due to poor *Thaumarchaeota* is the primary reason for deficiency of acetic acid, and including B12 once daily in a meal such as breakfast (mixed into, not taken alongside) can help reducing cravings. Alcohol is highly antibiotic and many who abuse alcohol are also self-medicating chronic pathogenic colonization which promotes extreme discomfort by causing high ammonia and hydrogen sulfide which disrupt neurological function and impair steroidogenesis and the immune system, so resolution of pathogenicity and restoration of a healthy gut microbiome is key to long term, normal gut microbiome production of acetic acid. Vinegar can also be used culinarily such as in salad dressings and sauces or supplemented in fruit juices to get yet more acetic acid, but acetate is consumed as an energy source in the absence of carbohydrate consumption so this therapy works far better when ceasing dieting behaviors and blood sugar is consistently sustained such as by not going more than two or three hours without eating, and actively choosing carbohydrates regularly, especially fruit which is an ideal substrate for acetate production by gut microbes. Interestingly, many alcoholics take a liking to kombucha which is traditionally made with acetic acid producing bacteria (it does contain a small quantity of alcohol, which is fine). Some brands add lactic acid bacteria to their brew now to control excess alcohol so commercial kombucha isn't a best source, and sodium acetate is far more effective. This function of acidification by microbes producing the short chain fatty acids and supplementation of vinegar or sodium acetate is also strongly complimented by the dietary use of foods high in silicon with dietary fats as discussed in the previous chapter to promote normal steroidogenesis, as acetate is a primary factor also in the synthesis of cholesterol from which hormones are synthesized, and loss of hormones due to factors like ammonification which disturbs digestion of silicon, or a diet low in silicon, raises dependence on alcohol and drugs to endure the stress caused by low steroidogenesis. For instance, progesterone is like the healthy version of cortisol, and as steroidogenesis declines due to factors like low dietary silicon or ammonification by pathogens (or dieting) the body produces more cortisol to make up for progesterone deficiency which causes wasting and increased loss of electrolytes, blood volume, immune function, etc. Ironically beer is often very high in silicon due to the use of hops, but its not very bioavailable due to its alkaline pH, which actually increases loss of silicon due to polymerization in the gut. Instead, having good dietary fats like butter or coconut oil with high silicon foods like green beans, dates, pineapple, mango, raisins, sprouted oatmeal or other sprouted whole grains, etc., will help increase steroid production which can help promote faster recovery of both the mind and body (or increased resistance to developing dependence in the first place).

The overuse of alcohol is especially problematic because before alcohol is metabolized to acetic acid it is first metabolized to highly toxic *aldehydes* which are most responsible for the toxic effects of alcohol. Aldehydes are in turn detoxified to acetic acid by *molybdenum* dependent *aldehyde oxidase*, and so molybdenum depletion due to excessive alcohol intake also impairs other oxidase enzymes such as sulfite oxidase required to metabolize sulfur for pathways like detoxification, hormones, and glutathione and taurine which protect cells from stress, or xanthine oxidase which helps protect us from parasitism. A diet high in molybdenum rich foods like the cucurbits (cucumbers, melons, squash) and peas can be very useful to prevent this problem, but molybdenum deficiency is primarily a problem of microbial hydrogen sulfide as described in the chapters on immunity and thyroid which results not only in the depletion of molybdenum but also formation of toxic thiomolybdates which in turn poison copper dependent enzymes and thus worsen health. In the chapter on thyroid I also discuss how dietary cyanide is transported in thyroid hormone along with iodinated thyroid in order to help regulate metabolism in the body and defend against pathogenic colonization, and many studies show that hypothyroid disease strongly correlates with states of alcoholism and addiction which occurs because disruption of cyanogenic thyroid hormone is required to prevent overactivation of cellular metabolism and promote normal feelings of relaxation. Iodinated thyroid raises cellular metabolism by increasing chloride channels and alcohol directly inhibits chloride channels (which are also stimulated by acetylcholine), and intoxication by alcohol is a direct function of chloride status which is why post-drinking often includes strong cravings for food since most food is heavily salted and a great source of chloride which counteracts the effect of alcohol. Metabolism of cyanide which otherwise helps normalize the metabolic rate and prevents overactivation, agitation, and irritation requires its conversion first to thiocyanate which is disturbed during colonization by hydrogen sulfide producing pathogens. Since dietary cyanide reacts with toxic thiomolybdate which converts it back to molybdenum required for oxidase enzymes and forms thiocyanate required for thyroid and immunity, alcoholism is also more prevalent in those with diets low in carotene, molybdenum, and cyanogenic foods like brassicas, almonds, yuca, etc. Even corn and carrots contain some cyanide so when we are free of hydrogen sulfide producers there is plenty of dietary cyanide in a good diet to support this function, but after colonization by hydrogen sulfide producers, which is evident by malodors of the breath and oral cavity and feces and flatulence (masking with oral care products does not make this problem go away), it is required to actively suppress and resolve hydrogen sulfide producers as discussed in the chapter on immunity and support cyanogenic thyroid as discussed in the chapter on thyroid, and it can be especially helpful to consume dietary sources of molybdenum and cyanide together which will result in greater uptake and availability both of molybdenum and thiocyanate.

Vitamin C is especially helpful for recovery and always depleted in those with severe progression of addiction and alcoholism because vitamin C is a cofactor for the synthesis of dopamine and adrenaline that help us to feel well and function properly (although restoration of vitamin C as discussed in the chapter on immunity can result in temporary excess of adrenaline and thus intense feelings of anger since adrenaline takes priority over dopamine). Long term abuse of drugs and alcohol eventually also deplete vitamin C since it's a cofactor in synthesis of dopamine and adrenaline, which then causes encephalopathy of the liver and hyperammonemia. Vitamin C deficiency is actually a major contributor to heroin and opiate abuse and is a primary driver behind the current opioid epidemic in the United States. I once suggested vitamin C to someone recovering from heroin addiction who, like many people, had decided to become sober because his addiction was finally taking a serious toll on his physical health. But in taking vitamin C he recovered very quickly and promptly returned to heroin abuse since he did not do any work addressing his trauma. But for this reason, vitamin C restoration as discussed in the chapter on immunity can be a powerful tool in addressing addiction and alcoholism (temporary anger can results from restoration of vitamin C though too, so be cautious of that and have patience with your feelings until adrenaline repletion also results in dopamine repletion). The reaction of vitamin C with bacterial and dietary nitrite also results in the production of small quantities of nitrous oxide (laughing gas), which is a natural potent opiate and which shows how healthy people are literally low-key high *all the time*, and hypocritical in their judgement of addicts as nitrous oxide helps induce things like normal sleep, GABA expression, calmness, a healthy libido, and other benefits they self-righteously mistake to be characteristics of superior moral fortitude. Using vitamin C is crucial in recovery to calm the nervous system, promote sleep, and regenerate damaged tissue.

As mentioned earlier, *niacinamide* can also be very useful for helping to promote the abstinence required to cure addiction because it directly promotes NAD and thus helps to increase energy which in turn promotes relaxation. Many men and women with substance abuse problems suffer also from eating disorders as discussed in previous chapters which you will remember are caused by high torporific hormones, and alcohol in these states is often used as an alternative source of calories instead of eating real food because alcohol is a sugar, in which the use of niacinamide can help to treat eating disorders and thus make recovery more possible since adequate caloric and carbohydrate intake is absolutely required for recovery. Because niacinamide helps to lower the torporific hormones produced by the raphe nucleus, using niacinamide daily for anyone in recovery can greatly relieve some of the emotional and metabolic stress associated with addiction and alcoholism.

Also as discussed in the chapter on depression, anxiety, and PTSD, the area of the brain called the *dorsal raphe nucleus* is damaged and directly involved in the development of learned hopelessness, which is why depression and other psychological trauma always accompany addiction and alcoholism. The raphe nucleus is the center of neurological serotonergic function and during events of inescapable stress such as what result in alcoholism and addiction, PTSD, depression, etc., the function of the raphe nucleus becomes deranged and begins to chronically elevate levels of serotonin which in turn cause chronically elevated levels of acetylcholine and a decline in metabolic health and wellness. Studies on learned hopelessness have also shown that it can be reversed by exposure to *bright light*, which is how I designed the light therapy as discussed in the chapter on depression, and its efficacy confirms involvement of the raphe nucleus in the condition which underlies alcoholism and addiction. The therapy to permanently remove learned hopelessness is so surprisingly simple I was even more giddy when figuring it out because

I had removed my own condition and thus experiencing life in a way I had never even thought possible. Using the same light therapy described for treating the dorsal raphe nucleus in the chapter on depression, directing a bright light such as from a 300 watt warm-spectrum bulb (*not* heat, but color temperature) onto the back or sides of the head for a minimum of two or three hours a day for at least two weeks can stimulate the dorsal raphe nucleus to increase its metabolic rate and thus reduce the output of serotonin and restore normal metabolic function. As long as the light source is fairly powerful light will travel through the skull and stimulate the dorsal raphe nucleus (and also the pineal gland) and thus reverse the excessive serotonergic condition of learned hopelessness. This also requires vitamin C to start and raise the metabolic rate and to promote normal dopamine synthesis, and other tools which increase the metabolic rate like fructose, fruit, B vitamins like niacinamide, and sun exposure should precede light therapy to benefit from the effect of increased metabolism on lowering of torporific hormones.

Light therapy does not remove the preconceptions about life which have been created over a lifetime due to this condition, such as a fear of people, finances, remorse, guilt, shame, etc. as is addressed by trauma therapy in the chapter on God and spirituality—What is does is remove the chemical depressors which facilitate the overwhelming negative emotions which impair healing and motivate substance abuse in the first place. If done correctly, results will be noticeable within just several sessions of light therapy as the body begins to feel more relaxed and less urgency felt around life, and should be continued as directed in the chapter on depression until the condition is permanently resolved. If all other factors are addressed this light therapy will guarantee a complete and total recovery and is not optional for full recovery. Although total abstinence may not be required for this recovery process it is absolutely required during light therapy, and because most alcoholics and addicts also delude ourselves about the amounts and frequency of substance use it is better to practice total abstinence during the entire recovery phase for at least 6 months to a year, using the tools in this chapter to make abstinence both bearable and successful.

Many drugs which are now illicit like LSD and MDMA, drugs which currently plague many people suffering from substance abuse were originally developed specifically to treat many of the symptoms and conditions similar to or involved in learned hopelessness, and mainly work by increasing factors which combat the effects of elevated acetylcholine rather than targeting the chemical directly. Unfortunately they too ended up having too many side effects to be considered by doctors as viable for standard treatment, because our fundamental physiology and appropriate environment and nutrition must be addressed to solve these problems, not through further pharmacological intervention, which will never succeed in doing what is required by nature. There is often research into these drugs for psychological therapy and often present amazing results when used in a clinical setting. But chemical intervention in psychological wellness is never successful long term because it does nothing to address our experiences of trauma which underlie stressful conceptions of self-worth and life in general, so although many people do experience initially positive benefits of psychological drug therapy due to their chemical interference in these pathways it is no different than abusing drugs, dependent on chemical intervention, and will fade with time as our perception of life remains constant and informed by past experiences of trauma. For this reason it is absolutely required to practice introspective trauma therapy such as is accomplished by inventory trauma therapy discussed in the chapter on God and spirituality or *The Perfect Child* for permanent resolution of the symptoms of learned hopelessness. Other conditions which appear like addictions such as gambling or excessive video game consumption are not addictions at all but are instead coping mechanisms which are borne out of a near total lack of fulfillment in personal relationships mediated by defensiveness and distrust in drawing close to others which, while supported by healthy endocrinological function is entirely a function of such trauma and can only be alleviated by personal introspection such as what inventory therapy accomplishes. As mentioned also in the chapter on erections there is no such thing as sex addiction, which is instead a biological reflex to metabolic stress which must be separately addressed as discussed in that chapter.

There is always the possibility of regressing back to conditions of addiction during times of nutrient stress or insufficient light exposure such as during the winter or with excessive sequestration indoors, but all that is required then is to merely repeat this process and take care of your body, and recurrence can be entirely prevented by guaranteeing a good diet, high metabolic rate, and addressing factors which impair the immune system as discussed in that chapter to prevent colonization by opportunistic microbes which disturb the endocrine system and our nutritional status. After the body has fully healed drinking may even be resumed safely, and amazingly a former alcoholic or addict will find themselves able to drink like a normal person so long as they actually complete this therapy properly, which will first require a long period of abstinence which, if not easy to do, means that restoration of the endocrine and nervous system as required for recovery has not yet been accomplished. Glycoalkaloids like solanine in potatoes are water soluble so while boiling peeled potatoes and discarding the water can cause some loss of potassium and other nutrients it is also safer for those with alcoholism and addiction if nightshade vegetables like potatoes are pre-boiled and drained (after recovery has been achieved, not during, and I still avoid having potato or tomato sauces which concentrate tomato and thus glycoalkaloids more than two or three times a week).

The condition of learned hopelessness was later renamed by an enterprising psychologist to the less appropriate term *learned helplessness*, and indeed most of the current literature available refers to it by that name. I take issue with this for a number of reasons—that the condition has nothing to do with helplessness. A sufferer of this disease is no less aware of the options and ability to overcome stress or to rise to the challenges which come easy to healthy individuals. The condition truly is one of *hopelessness*, where the very point to go on is lacking rather than the means of doing so. In addition the term helplessness implies a sense of personal responsibility for the condition, which could not be further from the truth as it is a disease and largely beyond the control of those who suffer it, and in fact the major contributors to the work on this condition continue to regard the solution as one of personal choice, which completely fails to comprehend the nature of our biological function and the root source as a neurological condition as well as the nature of reality itself, which is often beyond our control. The terms also do not fully describe the nature of the disease nor its distribution and distract from the causes and cure. In addition, the researchers who renamed it experimented by torturing dogs, and while all animal abuse and experimentation unsettles me I find it impossible to believe that a person capable of electrocuting dogs could possibly comprehend the condition. I propose that the collection of symptoms of learned hopelessness be reclassified and renamed to something which appropriately and succinctly describes the full scope of the disease, defined as the excessive and chronic elevation of acetylcholine and causing impairment of social and personal care and wellness as arises from an overactive parasympathetic nervous system. Levels of acetylcholine and acetylcholinesterase can be measured objectively in a doctor's office to establish morbidity, supported by outward manifestations of behavior and suffering and history of abuse, trauma, neglect, and dietary factors which contribute to the condition. Such a term could encompasses the true nature and effect of the disease, remove stigma, and provide a singular and specific path for achieving cure and treatment of all symptoms. While alcoholism and drug abuse are considerable manifestations of this disease they are only some outward symptoms, so this term would also include those who suffer the disease but have not passed into self medication, with treatment being as simple as the use of antihistamines, sodium acetate, improved diet, and appropriate trauma therapy to help the person relearn positive associations with the conditions of life.

Fixing the disease which underlies drug and alcohol abuse is really a lot easier than it has seemed, and only seemed difficult because the pathways involved were very elusive and current research heavily infected by bias and prejudice. Cravings can start to return if stress becomes excessive or certain dietary, environmental, or gut conditions are not fully remedied, or from excessive nightshade consumption (potatoes), but these therapies effectively eliminate the causes and can simply be used again should symptoms recur. By fully understanding the factors which contribute to its development a person with alcoholism and addiction may now be empowered to help themselves since a true healing can finally be made through easy, accessible, and actionable steps and finally get to live the kind of life that those without this condition take for granted.

CHAPTER 26
CURING HAIR LOSS

One Sunday morning as a teenager I was awoken by my mother. She was angry. Groggily, I began to piece together the night before. I had been at my best friend Will's house late, after hanging out with other neighborhood friends, eating cereal in his room playing Zelda and other old Nintendo games. For some reason that night I realized that I was seventeen and had never had a haircut of my choosing. "I hate my hair," I had said to him. "I've never had a haircut I wanted." Without even thinking and with the enthusiasm which was one of the reasons I loved him so much my friend proposed we buzz it off. I hesitated. To be free of the same hair I'd had all my life promised more than a new style—I'd always had the haircut my parents wanted, wore the clothes they chose, took the classes they picked, listened to the music they listened to. How was it that I had only one year of High School left and never even discovered what kind of music I liked? Taking off my hair would be a rebuke of my parent's authority, a rejection of all they had done for me.

So I agreed.

"I hope you're happy," said my mom in a surprisingly less disapproving tone than I had expected, though still seething with resentment. When she left my room I smiled from ear to ear, not entirely because of my rebellion but also since I had finally done something for myself, truly made a decision that reflected my desires and not of others. Soon my hair grew out to a clean, tight cut and with it came a small increase in confidence (and attention).

I never thought I would mourn aging, nor hair loss, being a rationally minded person I knew I would grow old one day. But when that day came twenty-years earlier than I expected it was more traumatic than any of the accidents and injuries I had ever gone through. When my hair began to recede it catapulted my apparent age far into the future, as if stealing the years of my yet unfulfilled youth right from under my feet. I had my first grey hair at the age of twenty-one, because cystic fibrosis causes people to grey prematurely, but now was threatening to take the rest of it. Worse, this outward loss of youthful vitality came with debilitating illnesses which in practice made me feel even older than I looked, and the hair loss and early greying was just a constant reminder.

If anyone in life deserves love more than others it's those who are sick. Not many would really disagree with this, but when did you last ask an obese person out for a date? How about someone balding? Elderly? Physically disabled? One day while at a recovery meeting I noticed two strangers sitting next to each other. The first was an old man who looked very sick. He had little hair and his skin was inflated like an old, soggy sponge and red in places it shouldn't be. His eyes bulged out of his head like someone had their hands around his throat, and his posture was agitated, without any trace of confidence. The other man was young and striking in appearance, his smooth skin framed with dark hair and a thick, deeply colored beard. He had wildly passionate eyes, well-formed muscles, a thin waist and strong, hairy forearms. He sat in such a way as to project an excess of self-worth. I was drawn to admire the young man, spinning fantasies of a date and of late nights with him in my arms. The bliss of falling in love. Such thoughts about him came easily, almost by reflex. I looked again at the old man and wondered why I did not have similar feelings for him, whom of all in that room was probably the most in need of love who in all likeliness will never again have a chance at finding it. On the face of it the reason seems obvious—one is attractive, the other not. But there is more going on than these superficial sentiments. As a Libra I fall in love with almost everyone, but there are limits even to that. Why do our instincts steer us toward youth and health even when we ourselves aren't up to par?

When I was still in my early twenties I was approached by a man who very much wanted to be in a relationship with me. He was short and fat but seemed kind and charismatic. At first I was not inclined to go along with it, but it struck me that someone with an unenviable appearance might be kinder to me and easier to date, so I relented and decided to give it a chance. One day shortly into what turned out to be a tumultuous relationship he reprimanded me for gaining some weight, even though I was still entirely a twink and incredibly skinny. *You've been* fat *the whole time we've been together,* I thought angrily. In hindsight I recognize his behavior as abuse and narcissism, although at the time I felt it was just criticism. But this illustrates how many of our insecurities about health and wellness can be destructive and hypocritical, and lacking empathy for ourselves we then do not show it to others, and since mortality is the only constant in life everyone will eventually reach a point where they are forced to come to terms. If this does not occur until your deathbed you have indeed missed out on life.

Of course, it is possible to love those who are no longer young and healthy, or even those who are not good people. But the all-too-typical human response is the rejection of those who appear unhealthy as if they deserve it or do not measure up to our unrealistic standards even when we ourselves do not even meet our own expectations. Most people come to my book and work (indeed any health regimen) simply from a desire to be loved. But those who love us because of our physical appearance do not know love. It is instead desire, something entirely different than love and which in turn exposes us to jeopardy should anything come to mar it.

As we age or decline in health our appeal to other human beings generally begins to wane. The physical manifestation of metabolic or infectious illness interrupts attraction in others because most illnesses are caused by pathogenic microbial ingress into the human body, and for those enslaved to baser instincts the impulse to avoid contact with disease is stronger than their ability to empathize. It is the great paradox of human love—that those who need it most are the least likely to find it. While devastated by Andre Aciman's exquisitely written book, *Call Me By Your Name* the cynic in me kept thinking that had the story not been centered around a beautiful young man it would not have be published, nor even written, though the same story would be no less beautiful (don't mistake me for being altruistic, I *loved* the book). Lovingly, at one point in the story the sagely father points out that with age comes a time when no body wants to look at your body, let alone come near it. When I was dying of cancer—fat, sick, losing my once thick and lustrous hair I was abandoned by the love of my life (clearly he wasn't, right?) and by friends and family also, even doctors, thrust into the dark alleys of social ostracism. My experience of illness was one of complete rejection, as it has been for many who have lived on this earth such as the thousands and thousands of lovely young gay men who died lonely deaths during the AIDS crisis, abandoned by everyone but the lesbians and occasional allies who cared for them, often even their own mothers, because of this very tendency we have to expel those who succumb to the realities of mortality.

I later had a few encounters with good-hearted boys which were enough to keep my hopes alive, and a month after my life fell apart while still overweight and sick a chance and unexpected encounter in a steam room with a handsome face, washboard stomach, and taut butt who afterward said I was beautiful began a process of untangling my internal self worth from my aesthetic state. I contemplated the meaning of suffering, and why it is that most of us so callously withhold our affection from those who truly deserve it, which I was also guilty of doing. I found that up that point in my life I had been using my romances, both short and long-term, and other relationships to support a narrative about myself which played in my head on a loop, to combat the fears instilled in me as a child, which went along the lines of *I am of value and there isn't anything wrong with me*. This narrative was a way to cope with a lifetime of abuse, neglect, and rejection both by loved ones and strangers alike. But this narrative was false. There was and still is *a lot* wrong with me. I had depression. I was dying of cancer. I was often afraid. I made mistakes and was deeply ashamed of them. I have difficulty keeping friends. Some behaviors controlled my life more than I wanted. Then I was alone and abandoned, failed at life, not much value to *anyone* even myself, let alone a romantic companion.

Adults should technically not have to take care of each other. That is the definition of adulthood—the ability to provide generally for one's own physical, mental, and emotional wellbeing. Adults do, and should, care for each other during times of need, but most adults carry the scars of childhood with us in spite of our best efforts, unable to heal the damage of pain, heartache, and loss, and life becomes immeasurably more difficult and the idea of taking care of another adult who needs so much themselves in addition to everything else is just too much. To spare ourselves of that burden we reject those who carry wounds openly, the same ones we harbor deep within, because the prospect of enduing someone else's pain on top of our own is simply too great.

The truth is there is no problem with having wounds. It is okay to be incomplete, and is in fact confirmation of our humanity, though most of us don't think about our weaknesses like that. Whenever I feel myself stooping from shyness I reproach myself and wish I were like other men standing tall and strong and alluring. Going to great lengths, often unconsciously, we project images of completeness as much as we think we can for fear of becoming a victim to the very same self-preservation tactics employed by others which we in turn employ ourselves. Life is perceived in a way which is convenient for our psychological coping, to marginalize or excuse our shortcomings, to ignore things over which we feel powerless precisely because we feel incapable of addressing them, confusing sexual attraction for love we then fear the loss of youth, never realizing what love really is until by our own behavior we chase it away.

This coping behavior involves the rejection of anyone who impinges upon our personal narrative. The most extreme example of this kind of rejection is that which exists between differing faiths, where those on either side of a religious divide reject the other, or those without any, even though it advantages them nothing and makes no tangible difference on their quality of life, nor whether their belief is truly valid, or not, or beneficial, or not. Like many I was raised in a community from which I learnt to consider imperfection a defect, the repetitious correlation of sin with imperfection enabled no victory over defects but it did foster overwhelming shame and dissociation from friends and family. No matter the affiliation nearly all the religious people I know live at constant arms length from one another, even among themselves, because letting others in would disrupt a carefully balanced card trick, living entire lives having never known the sweet, stinging joy which comes from the baring of one's soul to another. I adopted their view of imperfection for my own thinking and went about life trying to be whole by appearance, since I could not in practice. It is a silly idea to value an absence of imperfection, in any aspect of life, and a betrayal of higher ideals. Imperfection is virtuous, meek, and rational. It is acceptance of reality, and of our station in the universe. Without excusing wrongs, which itself is an act of trying to be perfect, it is our very imperfectness which defines us each, the very thing which makes life worth living in the first place, without which there would be no journey, no savor, no progress.

Nonetheless I condemned others and rejected them, to my own detriment, if who they were or what they did threatened my personal narrative, which included their physical appearance as well as the quirks of personality like silliness or weirdness that threatened to expose my own fears of inadequacy or the frightened, embarrassed, and inept person I am. To support our personal narratives we do horrible things to other humans—persecuting, harassing, even killing each other to maintain these ironies, even when such actions do nothing to alter our own reality, and even when it inconveniences us or carries consequences we don't actually want like the loss of friends and family or incarceration. But the pain of realizing we have caused pain to another person is so great it is easier to pretend we are not the source of it, which is why people double down when faced with the consequences of our actions, because it risks destroying our personal narrative that we are not defective, not the bad guy, the foundation of our entire identity and worldview.

Many men and women leave our partners when mortality becomes too real for our liking. This of course does not alter our own mortality but serves only to entertain delusional ironies a little longer. I employed these tactics of rejection in many ways, exploiting the mistakes of my partners and their feelings of obligation to me in order to support my own narrative, that I am special and worth loving (of course they did the same to me too, but from the same motivation). I used to believe I was a nice person which was a part of my personal narrative because I was raised to be a nice person, and so it was impossible for me not to be nice and nothing I ever did was never not nice because I was and am a nice person. But of course I was often not nice at all, entirely unkind and cold when called upon to demonstrate compassion for others, and it was only when I was thirty-four when the consequences of lacking useful life skills piled too high to ignore did I realize how not nice I really was.

A surprising truth about these misguided self-perceptions is that only the threat of impending pain is unbearable. When my personal narrative was finally destroyed it was incredibly freeing and wonderful, no longer enslaved by the frantic need to prop it up. In the end my effort to protect this self-perception cost me what I wanted most, and learned, as many others have, that life has its own parameters and cares not for our sentiments, beliefs, or morals. We can accept this and find peace and harmony not only with ourselves but also our fellows, or continue to fight everything and everyone and reap that unending frustration which comes with it. The insistence that fate follow *our* rules not only fails to improve anything about us or the circumstances of our life, it actively puts us at odds to the fulfillment of our own desires. A girl I used to know rejects men, public figures, actors, friends, and boyfriends who show the slightest deviation from total stereotypic maleness. Will she ever know what it's like when a man truly bares his soul? Probably not. The only men who fit in her life are those who are at all times guarded. Likewise, a man who shames or rejects others for being fat must live in a world where romantic options are limited to the perfect, one in which he himself can never gain weight and where no happiness lasts since deterioration of the physical form is inevitable, and which limits his experience to a temporary, transient, and shallow aspect of human physiology and sexual attraction which also makes romantic conquests self-limiting for the constant fear and sentry of imperfection. Likewise, the rejection of those who are gay creates a reality in which no one can show a departure from gender stereotype, and must at all times censure themselves for fear of being a victim of the very prejudice they help create. The shaming of addicts is a life in which that person can show no dependence of any kind, but since we are all dependent are cut off from the joy and relief of being vulnerable to and needing others.

The worlds we create for our self-centered views do not actually exist, so we exhaust extraordinary energy convincing ourselves that they do. When I was younger I often had men approach me with exuberant declarations that I was the embodiment of their dreams. I always fell for this, because it played into my own delusional narrative of being especially unique and thus worth loving, and in spite of an increasing list of failures from such prospects I continued to ignore the nagging feeling I shouldn't engage with such people, who only wanted to insert a pre-formed fantasy into my physical shell, with no real love or concern for the person I really was. It devastated me, and I took from it not the lesson to refrain from falling captive to those men but that something was severely wrong with who I was, to bury myself even further while continuing to date these types of partners—who stop trying to figure you out very soon into the courtship, no longer asking probing questions nor sharing much about themselves because to do so would disrupt the fantasy, and to preserve their delusion they clam up and start complaining before you even move in together that he just wants to sit in silence and use his cell phone even though he doesn't even know what your favorite book is or about that time in High School when you forgot to tie your speedo because it was five in the morning and it disappeared in front of the entire team when you dove in the water.

Now that I have finally regained most of my health I once again find myself the occasional target of a yearning glance or effervescent conversation. Surprisingly this comes even when I carry extra pounds or my grey hair screams out my age. After getting well I found there is only one characteristic of the physical body which really draws people in which has nothing to do with how much you weigh or even whether you have acne. When we become ill and our metabolic rate falls the muscles and ligaments which hold the eyes in place begin to weaken and the eyes slip back into the head which in turn causes the eyelids to fall since the eye is not propping them up correctly, and this gives the eyes a smaller, duller appearance which advertises metabolic stress and illness. This is the only physical trait by which *all* humans are unconsciously aware when it comes to physical attraction. Reversing metabolic disease oppositely strengthens the connective tissues of the eye socket, holding the eye properly and promoting bright and expressive eyes which in turn reflect the vitality behind them (hyperthyroidism problems can hold them too tight which causes the opposite condition of bulging). Even being out of shape or aged beyond what we might consider desirable does not really matter to most other humans, but it is instead the eyes, the windows to the soul by which others are drawn to experience you.

Having been on both sides of physical appearance I no longer enjoy the naivety of first contact. There is a burden of waiting for someone who does not already have a definition into which I should fit, no role for me to serve. Although the waiting is fun (and I certainly take advantage of opportunities) I also realized that I am able to wait and pass on certain options because I am finally free from fulfilling those expectations which come from supporting that delusional personal narrative, to which I came not by self-will, altering my attitude or mindset, but by practicing inventory therapy discussed in the upcoming chapter on spirituality to resolve my past experiences of trauma and loss. Now I no longer define life, and every joyous moment, every setback comes and goes as simple life events which I can take in stride.

It may seem like I have been rambling about a lot that has nothing to do with balding. In truth I have been describing the foundation for the first requirement of hair restoration—*reality*. Though there is one primary cause for hair loss there will *never* be a pill or simple treatment to reverse it, unless it reverses all metabolic disease, because hair represents the basic function of our biology. It is a reflection of the inner metabolism and overall wellness, which is why it is so intrinsically connected to our sexual identities, why it is one of the first characteristics to suffer when facing metabolic decline. In order for hair to grow and be of high quality the entirety of the body must be in good working condition. This is why attention to reality is so important, as the state of the metabolism is easily upended by any of a number of behavioral, nutritional, and environmental stresses. Unless we adhere to the realities of biochemistry hair will *absolutely not* return. If that sounds a little ominous, take heart. It's actually not too difficult and, unlike current pharmaceutical options, it also helps to invigorate the entirety of health, and reduce physical and emotional stress and improve overall quality of life. Other than abstaining from a handful of harmful behaviors the process of hair restoration is actually a bit hedonist. Before attempting to restore hair it is important to restore at least a decent metabolic rate as measured by the temperature and pulse diagnostic. Without a good metabolic rate the body will not be able to execute the metabolic pathways which I will be discussing that relate to hair. Hair growth also requires full repletion of all B vitamins, especially biotin, and because our B vitamins are largely supplied by native gut bacteria gut dysbiosis such as is described in the chapters on gut health and diabetes can prevent hair growth simply for a lack of these essential nutrients and the presence of those which interfere with metabolic health. Especially important for hair is biotin which is well known to benefit hair, skin, and nails but which is inhibited by avidins in eggs and produced by microbes like *Streptomyces* for which simply taking biotin is not an effective long term solution. Inhibiting avidins through the strategic use of acetic acid (vinegar and sodium acetate) such as with eggs which are a potent dietary source of biotin as discussed in those chapters does help restore biotin, however, and can thus directly support normal hair growth. Once the metabolism is running again and the gut is in better working condition only then can one expect this therapy to work.

The prominent but now defunct theory of male pattern hair loss was that elevated levels of the active form of testosterone, *dihydrotestosterone* (DHT) caused hair loss. This theory was not based on real evidence nor properly formulated clinical trials but formed simply from the correlative observation that DHT is elevated in the scalp of all men. Products were then formulated to reduce DHT, which failed to restore hair and should have indicated that this theory of hair loss was not correct. If our active form of testosterone is the culprit it would mean reducing our active testosterone-ness, and indeed the side effects from such drugs produce effects like depression, muscle loss, erectile dysfunction, and development of accidental feminine physiological characteristics. One male I knew who adhered to his hair-loss medication presents with enlarged nipples, difficulty building muscle, compromised erectile ability, and serious depression because even women have testosterone which promotes motivation and vitality, and though he does have hair still (he's only in his mid-thirties) it is thin, dry, and wispy because DHT is what makes men look like men and helps support vitality and drive, and without it we lose those characteristics the hormone imparts to our physiology. Destroying DHT is akin to cutting off the testicles. Yet they insist on taking it, taking evidence of retaining some hair even if it becomes thin and lifeless that the medicine is working, in spite of the glut of horrible side effects, and even while still actively losing hair not in spite of being on such medication, but because of it.

The identification of testosterone as the cause of hair loss without real evidence is yet another symptom of the religionist influence over our healthcare, the body deficient and subject to animal instincts and the deterioration of mortality. Surely the hormone of lust must also be the culprit for debilitating hair loss, right? There are lots of other metabolic identifiers elevated in the balding scalp which have not come under scrutiny but which are even more obvious interrupters of metabolism. Some of the metabolic products which are elevated in the scalp, including the one which I have discovered to be the cause of hair loss, could be addressed with powerful and financially profitable medical products, but the bias which infects research prevents such insight. The real purpose of dihydrotestosterone in the scalp (and elsewhere in skin) is to thicken the structure of men's hair. It stimulates hair to be thicker and stiffer, to grow upward a bit on the scalp and producing a sort of crown of hair above the skull as a sign of male virility, which is why we continue to sculpt hair upward across centuries of fashion, while female hair tends to fall more naturally down around their features. This characteristic of human males is the equivalent of a dark mane in lions or the widened face of male orangutans, and it goes hand in hand with the increase in forearm size and hairiness that often accompanies manhood, the dimorphic differentiation from female characteristics. All humans respond very strongly to a grown man with a bit of height in his hair because it triggers deep, psychological desires for protection from a virile male (even in straight men). So it is true that DHT is involved in the pattern of hair loss, because DHT demands more growth activity from those hair follicles than others, but removing DHT as a means to "cure" hair loss means you are removing the very thing responsible for the robust and healthy growth of that hair and so removing it does nothing to restore it. Doing so is like adding water to gasoline in an attempt to make your car get better gas mileage. It is illogical and contradictory to the growth function of hair.

Since hair loss has heretofore seemed so mysterious a condition, research has been stymied also by the expectation of an equally elusive and mysterious solution which then leads to ever more ludicrous, ineffective treatment strategies. But the cause of hair loss is actually much more simple and thus less difficult to remedy. Another elevated yet ignored metabolic product present during hair loss is the amino acid *tryptophan*, which appears in increasing quantities among the hairs and scalp of thinning, greying, and absent hair, with a direct and consistent correlation in age and gender from children to seniors. In healthy, working metabolisms tryptophan is not stored in tissues but is converted either to serotonin and melatonin or to the beneficial vitamin *niacin* (vitamin B3) and thus NAD through the *kynurenine pathway, where serotonin* and *melatonin* are hormones of torpor which slow the metabolic rate and niacin oppositely drives the metabolic rate acting as an electron transfer intermediate and cofactor in many enzymatic functions. Most of our daily supply of necessary niacin comes from internal synthesis—or should in healthy and well-fed individuals. In the hair follicle it is the disruption of the kynurenine pathway which is the true cause of hair loss, which then leads to the excess deposition of tryptophan which is then converted to serotonin which actively slows hair follicle metabolism and eventually prevents the growth of hair. Since NAD is the mechanism by which cells shuttle electrons around and enable metabolic function it makes sense that an interruption to this would limit or restrict the function of such robust metabolic processes such as occurs in hair growth. As the principle of the kynurenine pathway is discussed in the chapter, *Niacin Therapy*, that chapter is essential for understanding how and why hair loss occurs and requisites for the kynurenine pathway must also be satisfied for hair growth to occur.

While a pharmaceutical could possibly treat kynurenine pathway deficiency in the scalp it is largely dependent on the overall state of health and thus dependent on the diet and metabolic wellness, and this is also so easy to accomplish that spending money on a pharmaceutical would be unnecessary as well as less effective. Firstly, the greatest disruption to the NAD pathway in hair follicles besides starvation and dieting comes from polyunsaturated fats, especially the omega-3 fatty acids EPA, DHA, and ALA which have been shown in studies to bring the kynurenine pathway to a screeching halt. The mere presence of these fats altogether not only stops our endogenous production of NAD, they do so at a phase of the kynurenine pathway which results in the formation of the neurostimulant *quinolinic acid* which in excess is toxic to cells and the nervous system which overdrives cells and causes the overconsumption of spare nutrients as the body attempts to forcefully resuscitate failing cellular metabolism. As discussed in the chapter on niacin therapy, quinolinic acid is intended to increase cognitive function for creative problem solving by an organism under stress, but over an extended period of time induces neurodegeneration, mania, and hair loss by exhausting cells of their nutritional resources.

But while avoiding concentrated sources of dietary polyunsaturated fats is most important for reversing hair loss, polyunsaturated fats which interfere with NAD synthesis are also synthesized internally from other dietary fats as discussed in the chapter on niacin therapy, which is largely regulated by local temperature because saturated fats easily solidify in cooler temperatures like butter in a refrigerator which then makes it impossible for cells to transport them, and in the presence of reduced temperature fats are desaturated by *desaturase* enzymes into more unsaturated forms. To give you an idea of how important heat is for our metabolism I once ordered some pure steric acid, one of the most stable and abundant fatty acids in our body, and at room temperature it is a solid wax and required heating on the stove to melt it. The skin is always several degrees colder than the core of the body so fats in the skin are normally desaturated by *delta 9-desaturase*. During zinc deficiency and low metabolic rate failure of desaturase enzymes cause skin conditions like styes and chalazion as discussed in niacin therapy which require repletion with zinc and raising of the metabolic rate (and a warm compress) to resolve. In the skin delta 9-desaturase normally makes *sapienic acid,* a fatty acid entirely unique to humans, from palmitic acid in the sebaceous gland of a hair follicle which promotes healthy hair follicles and is antibiotic against pathogens. But if the polyunsaturated omega-6 fat *linoleic acid* is present, which comes mostly from sources like vegetable oils, fish oils, etc., and tempera-ture is low, instead of sapienic acid delta 9-desaturase produces the omega-3 fats which most strongly stop the NAD pathway at the point of quinolinic acid synthe-sis, not only causing NAD deficiency but also excessive cellular excitation of cells by synthesis of quinolate which actively causes hair loss by exhausting cells of the nutrients required to make hair. So the combination of low (local) temperature and a diet high in polyunsaturated fats directly leads to hair loss, and this is the primary cause of hair loss. As discussed in earlier chapters, interference by sulfate reducing microbes with detoxification also causes reabsorption and recirculation of detoxified fats which also potentiates this problem to cause long term, systemic kynurenine dysfunction, even if the diet is low in polyunsaturated fats to begin with since the body also produces polyunsaturated fats as a means to more easily detoxify them out of the body since they are more water soluble than saturated fats. So the problem of hair loss is systemic and complex and not easily reversed by simple interventions but instead by holistically treating the entire body.

The reason men present with increased rates of hair loss compared to women is also not because of DHT but because women have higher amounts of *progester-one* which increases thyroid activity, protects cells against the growth stimulating effects of estrogens, expands blood volume, and promotes increased fat deposi-tion which helps insulate the body from heat loss. As oft discussed in this book, estrogen is a hormone of growth, not femininity (gender traits are determined by hormone quantity, ratios, and patterns, not because hormones are gendered), and aging or metabolically ill men have much higher rates of aromatization of testos-terone to estrogen since estrogen is required to regrow stressed and injured tissue. One the effects of estrogen is to increase *inducible nitric oxide* during a deficiency of iodine and thiocyanate due to problems with thyroid and immunity which helps protect cells against pathogenic colonization and oxidative stress, so progesterone helps maintain mitochondrial respiration even in the presence of estrogen and lacking high levels of progesterone makes men more susceptible to the estrogen-ic activation of inducible nitric oxide which then also impairs NAD production, function, and mitochondrial respiration. This regulatory effect of estrogen is the reason why those who use steroids often present with hair loss. As discussed in the chapter on hormones, progesterone is also antiparasitic as well as antagonis-tic to estrogen, so those with low progesterone such as aging males or a higher ratio of estrogen due to the massive increase in aromatized estrogen from excess supplementation (injection) of androgens then also present with hair loss. Those who use steroids often have behaviors like dieting and excessive physical exer-cise which which increase aromatization, since stress lowers the metabolic rate to further increase aromatization and inevitable hair loss in those who vainly pursue aesthetic goals through harmful and artificial means like starvation and steroids. The misunderstanding of DHT, testosterone, and estrogen prevents aging men and transgender men from using DHT for fear of losing their hair when in fact DHT has less tendency to aromatize to estrogen than regular testosterone and is responsible for the more male-associated characteristics like coarser body hair, lower voices, larger forearms, and less body fat. Because progesterone promotes expansion of blood volume it also helps to deliver more heat to the scalp (as well as oxygen and other nutrients), but progesterone also directly promotes thyroid function, so women and young men have an easier time maintaining scalp temperature, metabolic respiration, and immunity which prevents the enzymatic synthesis of the omega-3 fats that disrupt the kynurenine pathway and prevents parasitism of the skin. Healthy young men have in fact as much progesterone as young women not on their cycle, which is why youthful males also maintain more fat retention (especially in the skin) than aged males, which also helps to retain body heat to maintain a higher metabolism, and older men with thinner skin which better reveals underlying muscle is not a feature of a high metabolic rate but of lower metabolic rate and severe metabolic stress as the skin is catabolized as a reservoir of fat, amino acids, salt, glycogen, and hormones to replace that which is missing from the diet (or caused by pathogenic colonization).

As would logically imply, women then have less tryptophan residue in their hair and scalp than male counterparts at every age because their increased heat transfer to the scalp helps maintain conversion of tryptophan to niacin and NAD. But women can and do lose their hair, and hair loss in women represents major nutritional deficiencies or pathogenic colonization since they do not so easily loose it. Eating disorders are some of the fastest ways to cause hair loss, but I have also worked with women suffering chronic hair deficiency who did not realize they were parasitized and since parasites and secondary opportunistic pathogens so strong-ly interfere with nutrition, hormones, and energy production hair loss in women without eating disorders is a good indication of parasitism. Eating disorders result from early childhood abuse and trauma being raised in patriarchal societies which exploit and objectify women and girls and can be very difficult to treat, but coun-seling, use of low dose niacinamide, and trauma therapy such as discussed in the chapter on spirituality to find self-worth and learn self-care behaviors will help resolve this problem. Undereating and dieting behaviors in all humans promotes hair loss simply because it reduces body temperature and elevates stress hormones which constrict peripheral blood flow to better maintain core temperature, and hair restoration can never occur in anyone who regularly fails to maintain their blood sugar and pulse and temperature rate, regardless of why.

As discussed in the chapter on niacin, omega-3 fats are purported to increase mental acuity in children but it does so through the increase production of *quinoli-nic acid* and thus overexcites and overstimulates the brain and nervous system, and there has long been a recognized correlation between intellectual occupations and hair loss because quinolinic acid, although stimulating mental acuity, also inter-rupts hair growth because it is a product of incomplete kynurenine pathway meant to increase cognition and thus better problem solving abilities such as finding food sources as an evolutionary human which would then resolve the deficiency. But in our contemporary societies with unnatural environments, diets, and absence of support the rise in quinolinic acid can become so extreme and chronic as to entirely destroy a person's mental health and wellbeing, à la the film *A Beautiful Mind,* and quinolinic acid is why hair loss is also associated with an increased risk of mental illness. This is also the reason why intelligent people are often observed to be less happy than their counterparts, which has nothing to do with intelligence but is instead caused by the underlying excess of quinolinic acid and deficiency of NAD which both stimulates stress and the increase in cognition. Quinolinic acid also promotes a significant increase in intracellular nitric oxide (nearly 200% in one study) which suffocates mitochondria and lowers the metabolic rate (in order to preserve spare nutrients). In societies such as ours which pride achievement over wellbeing this stress passes as increased mental function, even when signs of distress are obvious. Low quinolinic acid is also why manual labor occupations, especially those which are out of doors, are oppositely correlated with hair retention as sunlight helps promote completion of the NAD pathway and removal of nitric oxide from cytochrome oxidase.

The autonomic nervous system also plays a large role in promoting hair loss because quinolinic acid which results from low NAD production strongly stimulates the nervous system and increases acetylcholine expression as the body attempts to stimulate failing cells (much like a defibrillator) but which in turn exhausts their already deficient nutritional resources and thus promotes failure of features like the hair follicle. The nerves of the scalp extend along the direction in which hair tends to recede in so-called male pattern baldness, and looking at the map of neurological architecture of the scalp it is easy to observe a correlation of typical balding patterns along the direction of nervous system structure as they travel from the central nervous system. Short-term antihistamine therapy such as what is required to reverse addiction and alcoholism can also block the neurological stress that causes overstimulation and exhaustion of hair follicles, but this is also a function of thyroid hormone as discussed in the chapter on thyroid in which iodine and cyanide function to both stimulate and inhibit metabolic respiration, respectively. Loss of thyroid function is a major mechanism of aging not only because loss of thyroid increases stress pathways (like adrenaline) but also because thyroid is a primary transport mechanism for iodine and thiocyanate used in the immune reaction which then makes us vulnerable to colonization by pathogens. Hair-eating mites like demodex colonize the scalp and eat hair in the same way sea urchins eat kelp, which I believe to be the likely cause of alopecia and most male-pattern hair loss, because iodine is otherwise deposited at the root of hair which is a defensive mechanism that keeps microscopic organisms from consuming or living in hair follicles and skin pores. In previous editions of this book I used and recommended the mixing of potassium iodide in some stable fat like shea butter to apply to the scalp, after seeing anecdotal reports of topical iodine promoting hair regrowth and recognizing the effect of fats which inhibit the kynurenine pathway on iodine status. This worked because restoration of iodine helps not only to kill pathogens which inhibit hair growth but also to reverses the production of inducible nitric oxide which, while produced to kill microbes, also inhibits mitochondrial respiration, and when trying this method I saw the return of many tiny vellus hairs and regrowth of lost scalp hair. While this was useful and can be used to jump-start hair regrowth, this is not the natural way by which fats and iodine reach the scalp and thus does not cure hair loss in the long term without restoration of normal thyroid and immune function as discussed in those chapters (and is also very inconvenient). Discovering how to fully restore thyroid function, especially the heating of iodine in water with tea or other tannin source, not forgetting the role of cyanogenic thyroid, finally eliminated any need to apply topical iodine or fats and was also more effective long term in reversing hair loss, including the effects of dietary phytoestrogens and inducible nitric oxide and also eliminating the need to avoid legumes which, when prepared properly, are in fact very healthy and useful in the diet. The yet unrecognized role of dietary cyanide in thyroid health and its distribution to sites like sweat glands is important to suppress opportunistic microbes like mites and fungi which colonize the skin, which is why hair loss accompanies thyroid disorders, aging, and metabolic illness, and alopecia and hair loss are almost always accompanied by poor dietary behaviors, but deficiency of iodine and cyanide can and does easily occur due to industrialized food system and pathogenesis.

Hair loss is also not only a problem for the top of the head and aesthetic reasons but also relevant to our sense of *hearing*. Hairs in the interior of the ear receive and transmit sound-waves, and hearing loss is caused by the same factors which which promote scalp hair loss, including pathogens like mites. This is also why significant temperature drops can cause painful earaches, because temperature drops in the ear are so dangerous for our hearing due to the formation of polyunsaturated fats by desaturase enzymes in the presence of low temperature. When I was thirty-five I one day rolled over in bed in the morning and suddenly started hearing a bird chirping I had not heard in my other ear, and realized I had suffered significant hearing loss of the higher registers in one ear. I'm not sure when this problem resolved but at the age of forty-four now have no hearing loss in either ear, and sometime in the interim of then to now the same therapies used to restore my hair loss also resolved my hearing loss, probably especially through the restoration of thyroid which then helps support immunity throughout the body. While this was admittedly a small hearing problem it also occurred at a ridiculously young age due to such significant health stress and is probably a direct consequence of copper dysregulation as discussed in the chapter on immunity which then impairs the immune response to pathogens such as those which colonize the skin and impair hair growth. Copper is also required for normal hair pigmentation, so conditions of aging which also present with both hair loss and greying hair likely result from the inhibitory effects of calcification on copper status, and after reversing calcification the restoration of copper homeostasis such as through the complimentary combination with tannins (such as in tea) could more rapidly reverse problems with hair loss related to pathogens such as what also affect hearing. I suspect ear tissue of being a primary site of parasitism by some yet unrecognized parasite which accounts for enlargement of ear tissues as seen in the aging process which also contributes to hearing impairment.

Because polyunsaturated fats also impair vitamin D binding protein which is required to transport vitamin D throughout the body for local extraction of citric to prevent calcification of the endoplasmic reticulum of cells this means that the practice of swishing and swallowing a source of saturated fat such as coconut oil or butter as directed in the chapter on niacin therapy also functions to promote hair regrowth by promoting vitamin D mediated extraction of citric acid from the citric acid cycle which prevents calcification of the endoplasmic reticulum which is a major site of synthesis for proteins, peptides, enzymes, etc., so it makes sense that calcification of hair follicles directly promoted by the presence of polyunsaturated fats is reversed by niacin therapy. One study in fact showed that inhibition of endoplasmic reticulum stress prevented both hair loss and hearing loss in mice, validating this principle, where this is not achieved by pharmaceutical intervention but by maintaining a diet, gut, and behaviors which satisfy these metabolic pathways, and preventing calcification as described in the chapter on calcium.

While it may theoretically help to keep ambient temperatures raised or wear protective clothing like hats during cold weather to prevent desaturase enzymes from creating polyunsaturated fats this does not provide nutritional substrate for the kynurenine pathway, promote internal metabolic production of heat, support blood volume, resolve inducible nitric oxide, nor address chronic pathogenic colonization, which is why strategies designed to simply increase blood flow to the scalp do not on their own restore hair growth. One of the only hair restoration medicines which sometimes works to regrow hair does so by increasing blood flow to the scalp, but it also forces this reaction, not by coaxing or facilitating biological pathways, and so is just as likely to promote hair loss when cells are forcefully exhausted of requisite nutrients, and the only way to regrow hair will only ever be the proper support of our nutritional needs and resolution of stress and pathogenic colonization because the underlying pathways are simply too complex for any quick fix drug or treatment to achieve.

Because it is an indication of environmental nutritional abundance, *anthocyanins* (which are the purple, blue, and dark red pigments of foods like berries and red cabbage) as discussed in the chapter on erections oppositely shifts nitric oxide from inducible to endothelial and helps liberate mitochondria to respirate while also helping to increase blood flow to peripheral tissues such as the skin, and daily consumption of even a small amount of anthocyanin (equal to like a handful of berries or one or two purple plums) can strongly reverse mitochondrial inhibition and promote blood flow to the scalp so long as all the other factors here are also addressed. Anthocyanins are so effective in shifting nitric oxide imbalance they can effectively stop hair loss entirely if metabolic illness is not too severe. When I was first developing niacin therapy and accidentally experienced a regrowth of my hair from use of progesterone, niacinamide, and daily sun exposure I was also consuming regular packages of frozen mixed berries in my smoothies, and being such a commonplace food item I did not at all suspect berries to be something which could be required to regrow hair. During some later financial stress and accidentally breaking my blender I stopped having smoothies and neglected my anthocyanin intake and began again to experience hair loss which fully underscored the importance of anthocyanins in hair regrowth. This role of anthocyanins makes a lot of sense in evolutionary terms as berries and other fruits high in anthocyanin are the most common and widely available fruit in nature, and anthocyanin appears in many, many foods but not those common to industrial food systems and certainly not from diets high in grains and animal products (black rice being the one exception), and we would only have access to such foods during warmer seasons when it is safe to also risk increased blood flow to the skin, and this function of anthocyanin is a signal to nutritional abundance in the environment which regulates nitric oxide function to in turn control heat loss or retention which directly affects things like skin health and hair growth. Anthocyanin also increases heat production from fatty acids (this is also mediated by nitric oxide), a pathway which would be logically downregulated during times of food scarcity and cold such as wintertime to prevent caloric loss, but this also means more heat can be generated in the body for distribution to the scalp, which is also increased by the vasodilating effects of anthocyanin. Without regular consumption of anthocyanins, those who are losing their hair are unlikely to find regrowth very rapid. As I was consuming about half a bag of mixed berries two or three times a week it definitely does not require generous amounts, only regular consumption, and they can be fresh, frozen, dried, canned, or juiced.

As discussed in the chapters on diabetes, vitamin D, and erectile dysfunction sun exposure to the skin directly increases local endothelial nitric oxide synthesis and moves inducible nitric oxide from mitochondria to the bloodstream where it promotes vasodilation rather than mitochondrial inhibition, so sun exposure directly to the scalp is therapeutic for hair loss. This benefit of light on endothelial nitric oxide is secondary to anthocyanin and nutrient dependencies, however (and also dependent on citrulline). Similarly, melatonin which is increased by deficiency of sun exposure is mostly a stress hormone and accomplishes its function by doing the exact opposite of NAD and promoting inducible nitric oxide synthesis, and since melatonin is made from serotonin which, like niacin, is also made from dietary tryptophan the increased production of melatonin triggered by deficiency of sunlight reduces production of NAD. Hair loss in most people is primarily a problem of light deficiency because of inducible nitric oxide and excess of serotonin and melatonin and can never be resolved without generous, daily light exposure (without getting sunburned). While supplemental niacin or niacinamide can help promote hair regrowth they also cause downregulation of tryptophan catabolism and thus increased deposition of tryptophan in tissues when used in excess without addressing kynurenine pathway dysfunction, and long term resolution of hair loss cannot only be addressed by a supplement. Even though it is vital for health, tryptophan normally has a very low rate of deposition in the body because its very presence is more likely to promote excess serotonin and melatonin production, which is why its increased presence in the scalp and skin is so curious and suspect, and why it promotes aging, so the effectiveness of niacin therapy is more about the catabolism of tryptophan through facilitating the NAD pathway in the skin and scalp and reducing deposition of tryptophan and the production of serotonin and melatonin.

Fructose is shown in studies to reduce formation of the hair-inhibiting products of desaturase enzymes. This occurs because fructose fuels cells, upregulates respiration, and is involved in a lot of enzymes and metabolic processes but especially in male-associated biological pathways like spermatogenesis and Leydig cells where testosterone is made. As discussed in earlier chapters a healthy body can actually synthesize some fructose from glucose as needed for enzymatic processes, but in health compromised people, especially those experiencing hair loss, weight gain, and erectile dysfunction the body is no longer able to synthesize fructose, inhibited in a similar manner by polyunsaturated fats in order to inhibit the metabolism and spare nutrients from overconsumption, and so dietary fructose becomes a necessity for restoring hair growth. But, as discussed in chapter on pathogens and metabolic disease, fructose malabsorption due to the presence of ammonia in the gut prevents absorption of fructose and sodium which further depletes the body of fructose stores and sodium vital to metabolic processes like the kynurenine pathway and blood volume (while also promoting gastrointestinal bacterial overgrowth from unabsorbed sugar and salt). Sugary foods are associated with warmer seasons and an increase in nutrient availability which in combination with light exposure signals to the body that it no longer needs to downregulate the metabolism, which in turn helps promote factors which encourage hair growth.

Other behaviors that activate the autonomic system are starvation, fasting, excessively strenuous exercise, and social stress like fearfulness, avoidance, isolation, narcissism, etc. If you for instance are someone who stole my book or have done other harmful things to other people you have unresolved trauma and control behaviors which cause mental and emotional stress which contributes to health problems and poor decision making, and it will be impossible to regrow hair until you learn to take responsibility for your behavior such as is achieved by inventory therapy discussed in the chapter on spirituality (and my book on child abuse). Fear, anger, resentment, anxiety, contempt, arrogance, sociopathy, psychopathy, and self-pity are all mediated by stress hormones like adrenaline, cortisol, and serotonin which constrict peripheral blood flow and lower the metabolic rate. Learning to make amends and developing healthy life skills and the ability to take responsibility is empowering and oppositely lowers stress, even when facing the consequences of our actions. It is otherwise extremely difficult to regrow hair or fix other health problems when burdened by harmful behaviors, not only because of the biochemical consequences of psychological tumult but also behavioral coping mechanisms like dissociation, denial, and poor impulse control which prevent acceptance of reality and changes to behavior required to reform and rehabilitate the endocrine system. For instance, a person obsessed with success and money may not get sufficient daily sunlight exposure, or combative spouses who revile their partners and families and blame their problems on everyone else are unable to cultivate healthy relationships which would otherwise lower stress and raise the metabolic rate. Those afraid of death and disease will be constantly disappointed by the mortal limitations of life.

Perhaps you don't have any fears related to mortality, and if this is the case it can be easier to regrow hair, but the autonomic nervous system is still overactive from all stresses whether they are nutritional or psychological and it will be difficult regrow it if fears and insecurities continue to dominate our existence. Other signs of an overactive autonomic nervous system are insomnia, irritability, restlessness, depression, apathy, anger, anxiety, and reduced social vitality. Practicing light therapy, rehabilitating the nervous system (as discussed in the chapter on alcoholism), and empowering the mind through inventory therapy will help reverse neurological stress that contributes to hair loss. Work less hours, date nicer people, eat plenty of good food, become less self-centered, and take yourself less seriously and take responsibility for your choices and behavior. Stressing out about hair loss should stop—It is a mere trait of mortality, and we all age and die so that we may experience the full breadth of mortality and the true meaning of life. The fear of being undesirable due to physical deterioration mistakes attraction for love, and the practice of inventory can help enlighten your mind to deeper realities of existence than such superficiality. Love and attraction are not the same, and everyone can be loved in spite of their physical appearance, but only if we offer it also to ourselves as well as others. Real love supplants fear of rejection, and thus worry over silly things like hair loss.

CHAPTER 27

THE ENDOCRINOLOGICAL ORIGIN OF INSTITUTION AND SOCIAL DISCORD

I'm not sure if the prevailing sociopolitical climate portends a sea-change toward the integration of humanity as one or a world in which subversive forces have a larger reach across the world. Perhaps some of both. One thing is for certain, that the underlying causes of things which separate or unite us as a species are becoming more clear and important, and access to social inclusion through instant engagement platforms is without a doubt having a more positive impact on the world that I ever could have imagined. For the first time in human history young people have access to other people and cultures the world over, and support from many more friends and strangers which help to fulfill our developmental and social needs, most importantly when our families cannot provide for those, and access to limitless information and educational opportunities.

While many of us think about other humans in terms of culture, social dynamics, or psychological personality everything that makes us who we are is in truth determined purely by biology. Goodness, empathy, violence, bipedal, diurnal, social, moral. Even institutions which constantly materialize to support or plague the society of man all originate from our biological makeup, since even our psychological characteristics are themselves based on physical and biochemical biology. Dictatorial leaders rise to power because people with deranged endocrine systems (to which the thyroid belongs) instinctively seek to subdue their heightened sensitivity to emotional stress and fear by amassing control over their surroundings, which includes people and society. Conditions in such a life have persisted in a way as to mangle their normal, healthy, and constructive endocrine balance to produce one of extreme agitation and restlessness. A kind and loving person will never seek out the power of a dictator because a kind and loving person has a healthy, balanced endocrine system resistant to the stressors of life and thus unmotivated to seek any salve which otherwise motivates such behavior, not because they deserve to be healthy and happy but were lucky enough to grow in an environment which facilitated it. This evolution of the endocrinological state is not vague nor furtive. It can be evidenced from physical appearance as well as the outward behavior of individuals. It is no coincidence that corrupt, power-hungry, ruthless people always present with a deterioration of the physical form—fat, saggy, hair loss, wild-eyed, an appearance of an old leather purse stuffed with a neurotic amount of diversely shaped trinkets, easily angered and short on warmth and friendliness, combative, secretive, bound tight as a rattlesnake are all conditions of the reduced vitality which creates such personality types.

Hormones are not signaling molecules as they are so commonly described. Hormones *are* the very quality which they impart to a personality, just as granite is hard and water wet. As I mentioned previously, if hormones could be personified they would be the very essence of the qualities to which they are attributed. Testosterone would be confident, aggressive, and anabolic. Progesterone would be kind, empathetic, and stabilizing. Cortisol would be agitated and manic. Serotonin would be lethargic, morose, and ashamed. Hormones lend their chemical nature to that of the cell which they saturate, influencing it to bend toward that of the hormone itself. It is not a mundane, mechanical signal but the very qualities of life itself.

Moralistic demagogues, obsessed with sexual themes, spending precious energy to condemn others suffer from deranged reproductive functions themselves, hence the orientation to such themes, with exaggerated fixation on sexual natures because the particular blend of endocrinological imbalance such as excess nitric oxide and low GABA compels over-activation of their sex drive, as well as low satisfaction from sexual activity, made worse by depressive lows of insufficient dopamine. This tumult causes them much personal consternation, especially if past experiences taught them to feel shame for sexuality and their God-given bodies, and the outward vomit of shouting and anger is really their way of trying to come to terms with emotions and situations they find understandably difficult to bear. Liars have exaggerated responses to the flight or fight response of adrenaline which occurs during confrontation, because to survive as children in the homes of opportunistically abusive parents they had to employ strategy to avoid undue pain and suffering and now as adults do everything in their power to continue avoiding those situations which do still elicit the same endocrinological response their body learned in youth. Lazy and lethargic people are simply deficient in sex hormones, which are the motivating element of a personality. Unfaithful romantic partners are discontent in the bonds of a relationship because heightened nitric oxide from a poor diet and elevated stress hormones results in the manic stimulus of sexual activity, which at the same time blocks a normal, loving imprint which should normally result from intimacy. Of course, a moral resolve can prevent petty behaviors which accompany emotional discord. Or can it? Perhaps a person able to act well in spite of internal conflict is merely less afflicted than those who act in harmony with destructive tendencies? After all, none of us is more powerful than biology, which is why we eventually pass from this life.

People with healthy endocrine systems are content. They live happy lives with whatever resources they have, aren't threatened by life, and focus on their own improvement instead of others' not because being healthy is a moral consideration but that they were luckier not to encounter the conditions which caused deterioration in their fellows. Abuse and trauma victims often become abusers and perpetrators themselves because the toll of the event or accumulated events wreaks havoc on the endocrine system. But because factors like parasitism and chronic colonization by other opportunistic microbes actively derange the immune system, endocrine system, and cause nutrient deficiencies on which our healthy endocrine system and neurological function are dependent, much social discord and geopolitical turmoil is also mediated by microbes and their effect on our health and wellbeing. Because deficiencies of vitamins K and D strongly disturb calcium metabolism, for instance, increased rates of parasitism in populations that consume high quantities of dairy but low fruit and vegetables more strongly alkalinizes the body to impair immune hypohalous acids and promote parasitism which then purposefully disturb the endocrine system to promote their reproduction using our sex hormones. The deficiencies in carbohydrate and salt absorption caused by these microbes drives up stress hormones to strongly agitate infected persons and literally drive them insane. It is in our nature as humans to gather and work cooperatively, so there will always be social dynamics which construct our communities, and being together to accomplish life is built into our very biology. Without such bonds we suffer emotionally and physically, and in fact feelings of social insecurity are rooted in a deficiency of pregnenolone. Whenever I have anxiety about attending a social event I supplement some extra pregnenolone and my anxiety disappears in minutes, and resolving chronic pathogenic colonization strongly resolves emotional turbulence and promotes clearheadedness and peace, then learning empowerment through inventory therapy helps teach new life skills that alter fear and insecurity to instill greater confidence and personal effectiveness, not just those which are tangible like how to talk to others or maintain friendships or employment but those of the mind and soul in recognizing the true meaning behind the events through which we live.

Many moralistic people recognize the personal benefit in service and helping our fellow man, but most regard this as a past-time or religiously associated with sacrifice and discipline. This view is absolutely incorrect when it comes to our biological nature. Full human satisfaction and happiness *depends* on the constant engagement in service to one another. Our biology is not oriented toward selfishness, with a mere capacity for selflessness as most religions proclaim, but is instead naturally oriented and required to engage in regular assistance to our fellows in order to be whole. We would never have thrived as we have as a species if not for cooperation. Serving others is merely the biological impulse for cooperation, and in so doing fulfills deep, primal instincts which are unable to be satisfied through other means though we try with impressive dedication. Failure to serve others results in restlessness and dissatisfaction, no matter what or how much we have, which is why so many rich people run about the world causing mayhem. It is no wonder that self-centered lives descend into discontent and tangential distraction. Without the connectedness and achievement that comes from selfless orientation toward one another the human condition remains unfulfilled. Service does not have to mean venturing to skid-row to feed the homeless, although more of that would be helpful, but it can mean helping our family members with their lives, assisting friends on a less superficial level, listening to others without intent to respond, being employed as a teacher, counselor, or using that law degree to help those who are oppressed, mentoring younger associates without ulterior motives or regardless of your attraction to them, or supporting coworkers in life and not just business such as a colleague of mine who once drove me to get my car after it had broken down even though I could have gotten a ride-sharing service.

My religion growing up preached service to others as if it were a morally superior thing to practice, and so service activities were always shallow demonstrations of condescension to elevate one's own sense of repugnant self-righteousness and validation of ideological beliefs rather than any real interest in making the world a better place or truly helping other humans. But the biological impulse for connectedness through selflessness is the real foundation for religious association, as any casual observer can see, where most people don't really believe their chosen religious affiliation but rather yearn for the companionship and togetherness which forms through a group of like-minded others gathered in non-competition. It is why religious proselytizing finds success among the poor and downtrodden—the promise of fulfillment of this biological deficit is overpowering. It is also why gay, lesbian, intersex, and transgender and other different-gendered children suffer so horribly when ostracized, because they are robbed of opportunities to fulfill this biological necessity of belonging and the ability to contribute. Fortunately we often find support among chosen family and other ways to be a part of society, but such setbacks often lead to a selfish refocusing to mere survival which in turn impairs the opportunity for selflessness and service to our fellows and thus real intimacy with other humans, which is a source of contentment and emotional prosperity. For any human to achieve the peace and happiness which completes a healthy endocrine system it is not only necessary to support the physical health through diet but to fulfill our biological impulses to associate and serve each other.

Human beings are actually not that smart. We think we are smart because we are, in comparison to the other creatures who live on this planet who cannot design cars or rocket ships or build cities. But that does not mean we are smart. Even the smartest among us is actually quite stupid and severely limited in our ability to make good choices, see the bigger picture, or comprehend reality. We are but a lower form of intelligent life, an infant species in the very dawn of its existence in the universe, barely progressed beyond our ancient ancestors who are incorrectly portrayed by art and science as several leagues beneath our supposedly modern day mental and cultural prowess meant only to bloat our own unintelligent ego, apparently intelligent for the mere cumulation of knowledge across vast stretches of time and countless individuals, without which we are no more advanced than the parents who lived at the dawn of fire, easily swayed by personal biases and biological programming divide ourselves from each other according to personal beliefs which are actually exactly the same as everyone else's, trapped by mythological excuses to justify our own existence and the horrible things we do to each other, our coarse dialogue and competitiveness the result of an inability to comprehend real truth, truths which could have freed us long ago from the chains by which we still are bound. Maybe in another hundred-thousand years we will be somewhat smart. But right now we are not, and because of that we must make extraordinary effort to recognize how we come up short, that we may better provide not for humanity as a whole, but for our own sakes.

Many studies demonstrate how an imbalance of the endocrine system contributes to crime, including domestic violence. The brains of criminals and abusers suffer from deranged endocrine systems which results in clouded mental functioning, aggravating the dominance of various stress hormones. Thieves are deficient in hormones which impart vitality and relaxation, and so resort to the action of taking and risk of consequence to stimulate a rise in thrilling hormones which temporarily improve their endocrinological and metabolic state. This does not only mean the stereotypical impoverished thief but also those who are wealthy and exploit labor, steal wages, and swindle people of their money in the name of profit, to wreck businesses, saddle them with debt, collecting fees as they destroy lives, productivity, and stability of the economy, or lie and mislead to market unnecessary and even harmful medical or health products on unsuspecting, trusting consumers. One former employer of mine was quite open about personal resentments and demonstrated manic and unstable behaviors. This person also went to great lengths to deceive employees and clients alike, promising positions or promotion or services we could not perform only to fire people once his mistakes wrought consequences. The deranged state of their hormone balance, excitability, quickness for vengeance, and rash mentality caused them to operate in ways which were exploitive and ethically unsound, challenging personal and professional relationships for the transient relief brought by this excitement in scheming and conflict but which resulted in many destroyed relationships, broken trust, and lost productivity as well as economic hardship not only for their victims but their own business as well. Many businesspeople pride themselves on being aggressive, scheming, and "dominant" or "A-type" personality when in fact they are just psychologically ill and believe their ability to cheat, exploit, steal, or deceive employees, customers, and government is good business strategy rather than the depraved and immoral behavior it actually is. Such behavior is always motivated by an unstable endocrine system which cannot afford to relax, which disconnects from other people, because the agitation of those hormones make it impossible to be content or to form real bonds. A true pinnacle of personhood is one who is cool and collected, even in the face of adversity, able to see the larger benefit for all which in turn benefits them rather than the limited scope of self-interest which in the end always undermines even that by sabotaging the inexorable interdependence on which every life and institution depends. But even this is not motivated purely out of altruism, it is because they are possessed of a healthy and balanced endocrine system and thus undistracted by the tumult of one out of step and can see how the whole is affected by the parts.

The antidote to crime, especially in the United States, is often thought of as law enforcement institutions like the police and prisons. But even as the United States maintains the highest rate of imprisonment in the world and the highest funding of law enforcement it doesn't change the rates of crime because law enforcement does not actually prevent crime, it only persecutes crime. The function of police is to prosecute offenders. The idea that law enforcement stops crime assumes the threat of arrest, jail, or legal consequences is what reduces crime, but only honest, law abiding citizens care about laws and law enforcement, and people who engage in lawbreaking are motivated by self-preservation, need, want, greed, or other self-centered factors which result from trauma which don't account for personal responsibility nor the community, and law enforcement does nothing to address those factors and can in fact promote them by disenfranchising at-risk people. The rate of crime in the United States plummeted during the 1990s and early 2000s in direct correlation with the advent of the internet and video games because connectedness with others is a primary factor which neutralizes stress and thus crime and stabilizes communities. Engaging in crime is a risk that humans do not naturally want to take, and it is only after significant trauma or absence of effective life skills that individuals will risk so much for so relatively little. Lithium deficiency in municipal water supplies has also been shown to correlate with violent crime, because lithium paralyzes parasites and helps the body defend against parasitic colonization which would otherwise result in severe mental health conditions and high stress hormones and fear which drive criminal behaviors. But I also believe that ammonification of the gut and body by diets high in commercial beverages and refined foods low in tannin and other polyphenols which accounts for the development of metabolic conditions like diabetes, autism, and cancer also account for emotional instability and discontent since ammonia producing pathogens also disturb the normal metabolism of dietary silicon required for the normal digestion and absorption of fats and fat soluble nutrients required for a properly functioning endocrine system. This is not to say those who commit crime aren't responsible for their actions—all crime is motivated by animus, anger, hatred, greed, etc., and we are behoved to act with personal responsibility in spite of our emotions and desires without harming others. But in those who lack the skills to manage their own feelings and affairs the risk of criminal behavior is increased by metabolic disease such as is also caused by poor diets of nutritional or economic origin. No parent would stand by and watch their children starve just to be law abiding, and it is absurd to expect institutions like the police to resolve problems that are economic, nutritional, and environmental which instead must be solved through community action and empowerment, such as with the knowledge contained within my work.

Police are often also infiltrated by criminal elements because of the power the institution gives to its members. In the United States many racist nationalists, sexual predators, and authoritarian adherents join police because they desire empowerment as an agent of these institutions to empower their control behaviors. This desire for control is one of the major reasons police are so ineffective and oftentimes actually violent themselves because most police are, in the first place, also fearful of violence and crime and use their empowerment in such an institution mandated with violence to in turn control that fear. It's why police fail to intervene in school shootings and have abysmally low rates of crime prevention because fear is the primary driving motivation for membership, and fear is a very poor motivator for doing what is right. I once posted on social media that police should be disarmed, to protect them as much as their frequent victims because police are often attacked because criminals know they are armed. A cop I once dated was shot just for driving through a neighborhood, and a cousin who is a police officer responded angrily to my post that without armed police there would be disorder and society would fall apart. This is laughable because we have not had police for most of human history, and many countries do not have armed police but have far less violence than the United States. Because guns inspire fear American police are themselves more likely to be shot at, a fact they are aware of which further increases their fear and so in turn themselves more likely to shoot as well. The sheer ratio of citizens to police also completely invalidates such arguments— the Los Angeles region has *twelve million* residents, and the number of police in the city of Los Angeles is only 0.002% of the population and yet has a lower rate of crime than most smaller towns and cities in the United States. Human civilization is not orderly and stable because of authoritarian institutions like police but because people are naturally cooperative, kind, honest, love family, and desirous of peace and prosperity. Oppositely, those like my cousin who join police, especially when it is heavily armed and empowered, do so because of their personal fears and desire to control that fear, because the endocrinological hormones adrenaline and cortisol which rise in response to fear are so uncomfortable to endure. It just so happens my cousin is obese and suffering from diabetes, and my old love interest was mercilessly abused by his father during his childhood. Feeling in control can and does bring stress hormones down but since they are originally mediated by dietary and environmental stresses and childhood trauma and so are not resolved by wielding power, which can often also exacerbate fear and cause irreparable harm.

Society does need forms of law and law enforcement, but the most important function of such institutions is the formal documentation and exposing of crime for people to bear witness and receive justice, in place of feudal systems in which facts are obfuscated and violence arbitrary. Because calmness and cool-headed wisdom which results from a well-functioning endocrine system also imparts a quieter, content, and contemplative personality, candidates for leadership, law enforcement, and other institutional positions which would actually be most effective are usually ignored because the flailing mania of charismatic, vociferous, and agitating personalities of the unstable and traumatized attract more attention. This has repercussions in politics, business, and social organizations, leading to ineffective leadership by people who are only there because they were louder, but which also results from poor health which then ultimately compounds their ineffectiveness. A single politician or business leader infected with *C. difficile* can be unstable, drug or alcohol addicted, and foment anti-social behavior in their supporters also burdened with endocrinological imbalance and pathogenic colonization. Oppositely, diets high in good fats like butter, sources of silicon like green beans, sprouted oats, raisins, etc., sources of tannin like nuts, teas, fruit, and other requisites for good hormone homeostasis like daily sun exposure, vitamin c, and dietary iodine and cyanide can help people feel contented and happy in their lives and better resist parasites and other pathogens which underly metabolic and cognitive decline, and empowering people with knowledge and resources to effectively care for their own wellbeing can change behavior and resolve political instability and heal the mental illnesses which have driven volatile human political patterns throughout history.

There is nothing wrong with being unintelligent, and those who think it a problem are unintelligent indeed. In truth it is what we do with what we have which is most important, and the only true marker of intelligence is curiosity. But metabolic disease and its causal traumas can cloud the mind and prevent curiosity which would otherwise lead us from our problems. While becoming a better person does require a resolution to internal moral conflicts, it is more easily facilitated by the restoration of endocrinological integrity through proper diet and nutritional therapy, to calm the hormones, oxidation, and chronic immune activation which results from a destroyed endocrine and immune system. Emotions once unstable and turbulent become easy and constant, removing the emotional distraction which so often prevents a calm and objective understanding of one's predicament and possible resolutions. Being good comes easy when a person is healthy, especially if they are empowered with effective tools by which to live their lives.

My own hubris led to thoughts of my work being used to extend the lifespan of unsavory individuals without whom the world might be better off, but in reality if those people were to heal their body, and thus their endocrine system, the mind would improve and their susceptibility to love and compassion and guilt for wrongs committed would actually increase, for it is impossible to be at once healthy and unwhole. It is one of the reasons why teenagers and young people are so often openminded and generally more tolerant of others, as they are still healthy their endocrine system does not easily motivate unsocial behavior. The same is true for adults if they can heal and restore the integrity of their own endocrine systems. Because geopolitical turmoil results from metabolic illness, poor cognition, heightened stress hormones, and insufficient access to resources, taking care of everyone's health by empowering individuals with knowledge of human biology as well as addressing experiences of trauma and abuse as discussed in *The*

Perfect Child will help prevent conflicts which might otherwise arise from future overpopulation and neuter the power of corrupt and dishonest actors.

The *otherism* in which many politicians and religious leaders engage is a primary source of the kind of childhood trauma which underlies social instability and risk of criminal behavior, but even individual parents and caregivers can infect their children with fear of others as what occurred in my conservative, religious childhood where we were taught to think ourselves better than others and fear those who were different. Most people do not realize that engaging in otherism primarily imperils our own wellbeing, not that of others, as our own behavior limits what we can do, where we can go, and with whom we can build relationships. When I was forty-one-years old, during my last attempt to repair my relationship with my parents, I one day told my mother about a romantic affair I once had in my twenties with the handsome son of an old Hollywood heartthrob, and she cut me off and told me she didn't want to hear about it. It was deeply troubling considering I had been partnered with someone for nearly five years during which she had got to know him and invited him into our family, but she had only done so because she did not want *him* to think she was the homophobe she truly was and had been emboldened by his departure from my life and indulging so much conservative political media to treat me that way. I realized I was never going to be allowed a real relationship with her and finally stopped trying. On a global scale otherism deeply affects places like the Balkan peninsula where residents are confined to tiny, tiny states and limited economic prosperity and opportunities because of unresolved trauma and prejudice from generations of war and bloodshed. Going into the world saddled with debilitating fear of others was a handicap that took several decades for me to overcome, and trauma therapy as discussed in the upcoming chapter supported by an endocrine healing diet can remove fear and insecurity and help each of us become more empowered to care not only for our best interests but in turn others as well.

Institutions which have more relevance for the health and wellbeing of human societies like governments and religious organizations suffer from the same dynamics, but because they have more real impact on the lives of both the subjects and administrators of those institutions they are subject to more unstable malcontents seeking to satisfy the tumult within themselves, who fail to understand that the disquiet and raging in their soul is not a deficit of power, money, or fulfillment, but one of balance between dopamine and adrenaline, cortisol and progesterone. While the achievement of gain, whether in power or resources brings superficial relief of these struggles, the effect is transient, and so like an addict searching for stronger drugs their ambition increases until their destructive potential finally destroys them or the institution which has enabled them, not least of all because the peaceable, satisfied, and healthy people have taken their own prosperity for granted and looked the other way as yet one more maniac ascended unchecked.

As long as we continue to respond preferentially to the ostentatious characters of imbalanced personalities we will always be plagued by the negative aspects of institutions we need to support robust societies. Once we become cognizant of the true qualities of humanitarian giants, and have compassion on those with deranged endocrine states instead of electing them to office, will we be served by the better nature of humanity and find lasting success in institution.

CHAPTER 28
GOD AND SPIRITUALITY

On a warm day toward the waning end of 1988 I was baptized into my family's church. The uniform for the occasion was a white jumpsuit which zipped all the way from my little eight-year-old crotch to my neck, wrapping my body in a warm cocoon of clean cotton which my mother claims I wanted to wear all the way there, and I believe her, though she probably felt it was for the solemnness of the occasion and not because it was a finely-tailored, white jumpsuit.

Inside, the church changing room was dim and small, and grown men—the fathers of other kids being baptized—disrobed alongside us as they changed into their own white uniforms and prepared to baptize their own children. Their large, muscular forms were the first I'd seen without clothes. It would be many years before I understood my attraction to them.

My turn came to enter the baptismal room where my father waited already half submerged in water as an audience of family and strangers looked on from rows and rows of velvet-upholstered chairs. The chill of the baptismal font took my breath away. Aside from the plop-plop of water dripping back into the font, the room was eerily silent when I reemerged. I don't know if I expected applause, as Mormons do not clap or exclaim during services, but the quiet seemed to punctuate the absence of celebration.

We changed into Sunday clothes and the ceremony concluded with a particular blessing Mormons think is unique to them but is actually quite common among all the religions which also sprang up during the so-called *Second Great Awakening* (how are they great if they happen so regularly?) that occurred in the United States during the early eighteen-hundreds. Later that evening a party was thrown in my honor and attended by aunts, uncles and cousins during which I received presents and made cardboard wings and enjoined my uncle to fly me around in circles. We played board games and ate until we couldn't eat any more.

A few days later my mother sat me down at our dining-room table and placed an empty page from my journal to which she had taped a photo of me and my father taken right before my baptism, I in the white jump suit and he in his trim Sunday best. "Write about your baptism," she said. Pen in hand I set out to faithfully accomplish her request. *'This is a picture of me when I was baptized,'* I wrote. It was concise, truthful, sufficient. "I'm done," I announced. She took my page but the approval I anticipated was not forthcoming. «You need to write more," she said with a scowl. "Write about how you felt, about how special your baptism was. And you can't get down until you've filled the whole page."

What more could I write? Grown-ups had made me enact a ritual which meant nothing to me, had no real meaning or consequence except what was inherent to the observers. My mother would not like to see that on paper. Actually, it seemed I understood baptism exactly for what it was, but being eight I assumed there was something I didn't get, some secret of the universe which eluded my young mind. When my family came together to celebrate, the rare moment my distracted father was proud of me—*that* was the part about which I would write, if I could. Unable to be honest about my skepticism yet unable to lie I decided to play up my gratefulness to my father, *and* cleverly increase the font size to quickly reach the bottom of the page. It was an obvious cop-out but who would accuse an eight-year-old of writing too big? The look on my mother's face when I handed it in a second time was muted consternation. I had technically fulfilled my obligation but she was clearly frustrated in convincing me of the importance she thought I should weigh that day in my life. She didn't realize I perfectly understood it. I just didn't agree.

As my parents and leaders indoctrinated us I suffocated under the burden of my sexual orientation and the heteronormal ruse I felt obligated to perform. Religions reduce sexuality to obscene physical acts, mundane descriptions of our God-given bodies, invalidating the innocence of a person's ability to love another and robing participants from experiencing what it really means to love, even those who think they are doing what is right. The obvious reduction of women to mere physical roles is a serious consequence, but even straight men find themselves criticized for wanting to love someone, their God-given sexuality reduced to banal and disrespectful anecdotes. Robbed of an opportunity for real intimacy yet lacking courage to fight for themselves they then project their emotional isolation onto others in inappropriate ways. As a thirteen-year-old I once had to listen in silence to one of my child-abusing uncles describe a desire to kill a man who had hit on him while traveling, and watched in horror as my parents left such talk unchallenged though all of them had long suspected me to be gay.

Mormonism promised many things, but even before I left home I had discovered the emptiness of those promises and been hurt by every person important to me. Finally at eighteen I waded alone and inexperienced into the terrible world of humanity, to discover the harsh realities of life and no tools with which to survive or support group to catch me when I fell. The world beat me immediately. To what other conclusion could a boy like me come than that God didn't exist, or that he did and hated me? Either option meant no God, and so it was, as it is for too many.

Suicide was the solution reached by a tender-hearted boy who believed in everything. Surviving it, I found a determination to live in spite of my wounds and find a way to be happy. One thing became clear—I could not live life using the rules from my childhood. They had failed me completely. I had to find new rules which would actually help me live. I would spend the next fifteen years striving to discover what those could be. I would move to Los Angeles. I would make friends, lovers, and business associates. I would often act selfishly. Occasionally I fell prey to predatory individuals. I learned from meditation that peace comes when we are still.

Drugs and alcohol brought joy and relief. From love I learned where I belonged, and from heartache even more so. The more I lived the more apparent the fallacy of my religious upbringing, further reinforced by the struggle of siblings, parents, friends, cousins, aunts and uncles who continued to fight life and loved ones, grasping desperately for some pittance of consistency and relief only to find their happiness implode.

One day my own struggle finally culminated in the collapse of everything I had tried to build. Alone, abandoned without resources and friends (or so I thought), physically sick and headed toward death, few of my new rules held up. Like so many gay boys I had tried to be strong in the face of my adversity by excelling at whatever I attempted—school, athleticism, relationships, to show I was stronger than my adversaries but which brought further inexplicable demoralization. I had become alcoholic. One requirement of the program that helped me recover is to learn the true parameters of life, the exact bounds by which we are encompassed and not the ones which most of us wish to exist. The point was to accept whole-heartedly the conditions of my reality, desirably fallible and legitimately powerless. I did so, and no longer at the mercy of people, places, and things, for the first time in my life I could actually operate with success and without fear and sadness, logically within the limits of existence and stop stepping on the toes of everyone around me, no longer needing to force life to bend to my will, no longer a victim of my own expectations.

It was a daunting and uncharted direction, and worst of all the apparent validation I might give to the very people and institutions which had done me wrong, whom had all laid a claim to God. I made the decision anyway. Suddenly my life got easier. Before that time I had been responsible for nothing less than raising the very sun every single day. That's a lot to have on one's shoulders, especially when I can hardly remember to brush my teeth every morning, let alone excel at an impossible career, bend the favor of every man and woman I meet, or convince an unavailable parter I was worth loving. Previous to realizing the true nature of life I saw adversity as evidence of either no God or a God that disapproved of people. The reality I found is that God is simply the concept that we do not control the Universe, which is instead governed by forces we can only study but never control. God never forces any person to do anything, which is why terrible things are allowed to happen, and why the consequences of my own behavior piled upon my life whether I was trying or not. The wonderful truth is that I was *never* alone, even when I was trying my best to destroy my life I was always given opportunities for escape, to heal, to get better, even when I didn't ask for them and usually did not see them simply for the unresolved trauma of my past and the resulting control and coping mechanisms, and instead of the illusions put upon me from childhood I finally saw reality for what it was and found the ability to leave things as they are and focus only on what I am truly capable.

The most evil people I have ever met are those who say God is only available to you through them or their ideology. It is a lie which exploits our need to connect to something greater for the personal gain of others whom seek comfort in control and delusion. Believing them will rob you of a life full of joy and peace, which is even present in adversity. Like so many others I had confused religious institution for God, when they are in fact as separate as a bagel is from cream cheese. They can go together but are not actually joined (yes, God is the cream cheese in this metaphor). I am a gay ex-Mormon and I have more God in my life than any person I have ever known, and I never go to church or read archaic texts.

Because of my indoctrination into my parents' religion I always wondered how, if certain religions were supposed to be more legitimate than others, could adherents of other religions be more fervent or dedicated in their belief that the members of ours, and thus did that make theirs more or less valid as a result? In all likelihood my family, had they been born on the other side of the world, would feel as equally committed to another religion and its ideals though it differ entirely. Were the beliefs of our ancestors, in their druids and witches or devotion to polytheist pantheons lead by figures such as Zeus or Ra, any less zealous or valid than that of my own parents' simply because it was another religion, place, or time? Were they truly just more primitive and thus ignorant and heathen, or is man simply the same across the generations, given to similar patterns of behavior inherited with biology? How many hundreds or thousands of years earlier might we have discovered answers to diseases which have wiped countless people from the face of the earth; the untold suffering which results from superstitious substitution for facts of science and reality which are so easily discoverable? How much longer will the smartest creatures to have ever walked the face of the earth be vexed by their willing grasp of illusion, deceit, and subterfuge? If it is majesty you seek go out at night and watch the countless stars pass through the heavens—life is far more majestic than myth.

All this taken into account means either only one sect is right, which shows incredible hubris in the face of the collective history of mankind, and an inability to empathize with other human beings, or that all human beings are equally driven to fervent devotion to beliefs. The overwhelming likelihood that a person also adopts the same religious ideals held by parents rather than migrating in statistically significant numbers to any one particular belief (absent coercion or enticement) hints at deep psychological workings which rather promote and proliferate an offspring's adoption of parental guidance rather than any inherent truth to ideals and why people have complicated emotional responses when attempting to disconnect or sever themselves from those backgrounds, much as baby lions might feel about hunting and survival guidance passed down from their parents, with strong resistance to deviation as a biological mechanism which helps promote the survival of a species, even at the expense of the individual, but which in humans with our complicated social and intellectual capacity can take the form of esoteric, non tangible concepts, ultimately divisive and abjectly unproductive to the family of man.

When confronted with the fact that those with darker skin are the progeny of populations which lived closer to the equator and thus increased exposure to potentially harmful ultraviolet light, people who believe racist traditions of mythological origins of skin color clam up and avoid discussion on the topic in order to avoid the uncomfortable flaws and contradictions in their worldview. Modern religions like Christianity, Buddhism, and Islam all originated at the same time due to changing attitudes about polytheism, which had been the dominant foundation of religious traditions, because of cataclysmic plagues of ebola and other diseases which spread like wildfire through denser populations of humanity never before seen in human history and claimed the lives of enormous numbers of people. Fear drives people to believe in the divine, and I used to believe that the defects seen in religions were caused by those creeds and ideals to which their adherents subscribe, but after so many years watching from the outside I now know that people are the same wherever they are, and the behaviors which seem unique to religion are in fact just characteristics of humanity which are merely enabled or excused by religion. The child abuse rampant in Mormonism and Catholicism stems not from religious toxins but because there are adults who abuse children,

Personal Inventory

Resentment	Cause	Part(s) Hurt	My Part	Character Weaknesses
a person, idea, institution, event, obligation, problem, limitation, trauma, etc.	a brief description of every and all possible causes	(self-esteem, pride, emotional security, financial security, personal relations, sex relations, or ambitions)	our role in contributing or continuing to contribute	various character weaknesses revealed by the resentment

Samples

Resentment	Cause	Part(s) Hurt	My Part	Character Weaknesses
dad	never came to any but 1/2 of my swimming meets	self-esteem pride emotional security personal relations ambitions	continuing to resent him for it	inescure ungrateful resentful selfish arogant critical entitled
my boss	criticised my work. This triggers past expereinces of being criticized by my parents and teachers. could get fired.	self-esteem pride financial-security ambitions	didn't do as good a job as I could have. reacted defensively. chose to work here in the first place, continue showing up for work	inescure ungrateful arogant critical entitled lazy combative argumentative
boyfriend	said I need to diet and implied I'm fat. I can't control biology, my body is getting older, rejection sucks and I can't make people love me	self-esteem pride sexual relations ambitions	I starved myself for years and abused my body. Chose to date this asshole and argued with him about my weight which I didn't need to do	insecure overly serious defensive unrealistic timid fearful ungrateful argumentative

though the religion environment enables their behavior. Baptists and Evangelicals hate differently gendered people and those without religion not because their religion teaches them so but because humans are often afraid of those we do not understand. Islam promotes the subjugation of women (wait, they all do that) not because of religion but because all humans are inclined to dominate and control when they have been traumatized and one gender has literally greater physical strength to enforce their will. All religions harbor and promote racist sentiments because *all* humans have the capacity for racist prejudice, which is in reality a fear of competition, and need no help or encouragement from religion though they receive it bountifully. Even atheists believe they are different than the screaming pastors and angry housewives though they engage in the same demeaning, bombastic conjecture and antagonism. There is no substantive difference between atheists and those whom profess faith. Both are loud, pugnacious, wanting in warmth and peaceable discourse who seek to indoctrinate others to their respective versions of a higher-power, atheists' higher power being the absence of one.

Religion is not made for seeking God. It is made to entertain men who find a dearth of satisfaction from the perceived mundaneness of life, mundane only to those who cannot bond with people in their lives and find fulfillment in the every day. I knew many religious men who revel in books and discussion on myth and legend, experiencing the thrill of adventure in ideas of divinity taking part in the affairs of men, not because it betters their humility nor service but because it is an entertainment, a potent distraction from their daily lives and absence of purpose, no different than reading *The Lord of the Rings* or watching *Star Wars*. It was very confusing, as a child to see so many men exhaust themselves for religion yet emulating their behavior brought only emptiness and isolation. God was supposed to be in scripture and self-deprivation, but I could not find God in religion because God is not scheming and weaving intrigue in the backrooms of church administration buildings. Religious doctrine is a shelter for the failings of humanity, to excuse personal culpability, to comfort the selfish and self-centered who wish to hide from the failings of their past, present, and anxiety in the future. The religionist goes to extremes to convince himself he bears no responsibility for mistakes, even to the murder of those whose presence reminds him of such. Mormons joined the long tradition of relishing tales of genocide, a practice that never sat well with me as a child and seemed to compete with the nature of the God I unknowingly sensed.

Unlike every other aspect of life, connecting with the divine is a wholly and entirely personal and inward process. The outward affects of worship, religion, and institution are processes for control of peoples, and impair rather than facilitate spiritual development. It is one of the reasons why most successful spiritual practices involve solitary effort rather than that of the group, and why some religious creeds have decried the outward embellishment and promotion of conviction. Religions are social institutions which have supplanted our tribal structures, fulfilling instincts for safety, order, and togetherness normally provided by the hierarchy and bonds of family groups in which we were designed to flourish. Spirituality is what flows within us, the very energy of life that makes us alive. It is wholly separate and unrelated.

Religion also covers for lesser sins against our fellows. Lying, gossip, intrigue and conspiracy, hypocrisy, disloyalty, impatience and judgment, harshness and conflict are all qualities assumed by religious beliefs, for the convenience of the adherent, relieving them of responsibility for their actions. Of course humanity needs no excuse to entertain such defects of character, and it is truly hard to think we have perhaps caused grave injury to other people and have been the bad guy,

Fear Inventory

Fear	Cause	Effect	Better Way?
a person, idea, institution, event, obligation, limitation, or problem of which we are afraid	a brief description of what caused this fear	what is the effect of having this fear on our life?	how might we differently consider that which we are afraid?

Samples

rejection	rejection sucks and I need people who love and support me in my life. Been taught that rejection is bad and means I'm a bad person.	can't handle rejection. constantly trying to prevent it. don't relax and enjoy my relationships. resent people in my past who rejected me.	it's okay to be rejected, make mistakes, and even fail. others are affected by their own trauma the same as I am. there are awlays new opportunities, even maybe for someone better.
making mistakes (not being perfect)	other people can or might use my mistakes as an excuse to hurt or control me. I'm not perfect and mistakes are inevitable. was abused when I made mistakes growing up	I avoid things I'm afraid of not doing right, including dating or work opportunities. When I do fail, which is inevitable, I'm especially hard on myself and embarassed.	it's not possible to avoid making mistakes and that's okay! I usually try my best and am actually doing a great job. Life is hard and doing my best is enough.
conflict	arguments and fights are stressful and sometimes even scary. was taught to fear them and avoid them, to not let others control me, not empowered with effective conflict resolution skills	I avoid conflict all the time, even by lying or misleading people and can't handle when it does happen. I also don't share myself with others which creates a wall between us.	conflict is actually good! It helps people meet needs and needn't be so serious. conflict also doesn't mean there needs to be a loser— both sides can win and most conflict is just poor communication

especially to those we love. To assuage that horror by intervention of the divine is an intoxicating proposition. But of course there are consequences, as there is in all things. The religionist who increases in meanness and senility as their life-line wanes, who clings tighter to conservative tropes, media, and politics is feeling the weight of their accumulated wrongs, heavy indeed, less easy to push to the recesses of the mind, and the spirit bends under the weight, fatigued from a life spent running a closed rat-maze of justification and inconsistent morals. Having never rightly accepted mistakes and fallibility nor amended the fissures of a well-lived life is an incredible hardship, one that our mortal condition cannot well bear and which brings the dreadful consequences of a derelict mind which has painted itself into a corner. Angst lashes out in anger, hatred, resentment, and regret as death approaches because the disparity which exists between the belief of sins forgiven yet never having actually amended any wrongs scratches at the back of their mind like a rat in a sinking box. It is the conscience, prodding one to take care of things which need addressing. A fear of death is not a fear of dying. It is a fear of dying with yet unamended wrongs. To expire while still burdened with guilt. To never again have a chance to make things right. Before I practiced the twelve-step recovery program I had accumulated a list of many wrongs which, although none too extreme nonetheless weighed on me greatly and woke me often in the dead of night, gripped by a fear of dying. Upon my last amends I woke the next morning without even realizing I no longer feared it I had slept so well. The realization came to me one day much later when the absence of it was so persistent as to be obvious and the realization that my heart was light and free.

There is a much easier path in life. To contritely prostrate oneself to the indefatigable changeableness of the human condition is much easier than the mental hopscotch of pawning one's sins to the divine. To mend the chasms between friends and family, to pay respect to our shortcomings and the suffering of our victims, to take oneself less seriously, to restore confidence with peers and colleagues, to consent to the impermanence of life is a true salve for living, dependent only on one's own volition, without the need for God but whom looks on in hearty approval.

Because the failings and inconsistencies of religion are more plainly visible these days, young people more than ever are realizing how it fails to live up even to its own standards. Religion has a "youth retention problem," because many of us grew up with promises of humanity, love, and kindness watch in horror as our leaders used the sacred to defame innocent children, demonize kind and loving people, stoke racist tensions, and ignore mass murder. Is it any wonder the new generations eye these institutions with scorn, especially when God can be had without them?

The AIDS crisis of the eighties and nineties was not for gay men. Like all such calamities it was for our neighbors, our mothers and fathers, the association of man to measure their moral aptitude and capacity for compassion, to lay bare hatred and fear before the whole world and show whether they would protect the meek or turn on their fellows in prejudice. They failed miserably, revealed to be the selfish, pitiable mass of squirming terror they are and so set in motion the downfall of the very institutions which laid the groundwork for such callous disregard for those in need. Such calamities occur karmically for the exposing of those who work in secret, in the dark, against the family of man. The child abuse scandals of the Catholic Church, or the exposure of police brutality toward those with dark skin, a final, public revelation that abuse and racism are still bred in this country and fed by the religious houses of vanity and self-serving intent. All of this is meant to pound to dust the walls which have been separating us from each other. Closer to home we see parents banish our beloved brothers and sisters, cheat, bicker, complain, and revere money. Adults heave lawsuits at each other, destroy families and reputations, and then sit in church and praise God. Bigots, racists, and fear mongers are welcomed with open arms but the meek and humiliated are shunned. The incongruity is obscene. It can be papered over no longer, and the world entwined by social media has seen this.

That to be content and without fear requires an explanation for life is contrary to belief in a higher power. Men and women who exclaim for a deity do not actually believe their own desperate protestations—exaggerated tirades are tantrums of a tormented soul, unable to find rest, seeking courage in shouting from the battlements, throwing cover for emotions which make them feel inadequate and afraid because they do not believe in God else they would be content with the answers he gives. Instead they seek magic to change their unhappy circumstance, and God does not do that so they persist in fomenting struggle. It is no coincidence most adults I've ever known who make obvious capitulations to religion are also the very ones guilty of child abuse, spousal neglect, secret lives, and overwhelming self-pity, because they have rejected reality they cannot form natural relationships with those around them and so disconnect from life, finding no pleasure nor satisfaction in the company of love, nor the mundaneness of the everyday, and so must seek excitement and purpose in fantasy and mythology, in conflict and extreme emotions, but which leaves them ever wanting for its superficial irrelevance, and the circle of recrimination chases itself without end.

The secret is we are all afraid, but it is through each other that we find courage. God does not test us. The trials of life are not retribution, vengeance, or punishment, but simply experiences to taste the meaning of life, without which we would not know the full breadth of mortality. Some experiences are for growth, to teach us that our behavior goes against the grain of love and kindness, to reveal to us those actions which are in opposition to life. Others are opportunities to learn valuable compassion, such as when we are abused, to understand how pain can derail even the best intentions. Terrible things happen because without them our life experience as a mortal would be insufficient. God allows our actions to have consequence, not because we deserve them but only because it is the natural order of logic and reason from which we may better learn how to survive, if we are paying attention.

A prayer *never* goes unanswered, but it is often not the answer we want and, like my family and myself who prayed for me not to be gay, pretend God has not answered us even though he has very much done so because *no* is an answer. Prayers which ask for ourselves show little belief in God because if God exists they know already what we need and want. If you pray to God *only* ask to know God's will and have the strength to carry it out. Whenever I hear religious people pray they barrel through an oration, never ceasing the performance until they close and then immediately get on with whatever they were doing. Instead of talking *at* God during the entirety of supplication stop and listen to what God has to say to you. There is always a message, but you won't hear it you don't fucking shut up for a moment. For the legion of young gay men and women, and those who are trans and others who pray fervently to be relieved of being different God has already answered those prayers, by *insisting* you be different. It is not the answer many want but it is still his answer. He will not change our circumstance because everything is as it should be, even in the face of extraordinary persecution. For some reason unknown to us we are meant to experience the burden of harsh animosity, but from which we are blessed with the ability to show great love in return, the great lesson Christians and other religious adherents have forgot.

Real answers to where, and what is God are easily found not in religion but in *inventory therapy*. This practice makes complete sense and is really easy to accomplish, yet hardly anyone has ever done it, least of all our religious or political leaders because this practice is derived from twelve-step programs and my experience achieving sobriety. It diagrams life on a simple worksheet, making past trauma easy to understand by separating out the events which influence our path from the ways in which we influence it, highlighting the cause of our hurts, identifying who caused them, paying respect to the effect they had on us, showing what part we played (even if it only means holding onto pain) and finally revealing specific character weaknesses we wish to be rid of which cause us to do things like always dating the wrong person, worrying too much about things beyond our control, or always overdrawing our bank account. It gives both legitimacy to the things we have suffered while helping us separate ourselves from those events that may have been traumatic and saddled us with burdens we'd rather not have. It is hands down the most effective therapy I've ever encountered. Including our fears in the inventory practice remedies preoccupation with things like death, social anxiety, and self destructive behaviors. That ceaseless train of conversation that prevents our mind from getting rest finally becomes quiet when these inventories are made. It is enlightenment to *exactly* what parts of life we can control and what parts we leave to fate. This suddenly relieves us of bearing the burdens of institutions, shame, and rejection, and opens the space for peace, compassion, and love that we all so desperately need. While this practice has benefits for all, gay men and women and others rejected for being different may find it especially helpful for finding peace with themes of rejection, abandonment, violence, death, body image, sex shame, isolation, unrequited love, broken hearts, unmet expectations, and financial insecurity. Waiting for those who finish such a practice is nothing less than the promise of understanding the secrets of the universe and the purpose of life itself. By smelting out the clutter of conflict and resentment it opens the mind and frees the soul to see things as they truly are. *"God,"* goes the Serenity Prayer, *"give me the serenity to accept the things I cannot change, the courage to change the things I can, and the wisdom to know the difference."* It really is not a prayer, it is a mantra for life. It designates that there are things which we should not worry about, but instead take them and the lessons they bring into our experience, and that there are things which we can change but doing so is difficult. It acknowledges the struggle of living, the travails and hurdles over which we pass, acknowledging that we often confuse the two. This practice is the serenity prayer in action.

Most people buy this book because they are afraid of death and disease, but even if this or any book could forever solve all your health problems and keep you alive indefinitely (it can't do either), being healthy and living forever would still not cure the fear of death because a fear of death has nothing to do with death, but is a pathological desire for control, death being the ultimate subversion of that desire, and if you desired this book should give control over health and disease, well, you're an asshole.

But when we are confronted by hesitation or resistance at the task of resolving fears and becoming a better person it is not because we don't desire it. Even the worst among us is trying his best. Though perhaps it's not good at all it is probably the only way he knows. No, such resistance comes because we do not know what lies on the other side of our character. What will replace our control mechanisms when they are gone? Anger gives people the sense of power. What happens without that power? Sexual attraction and sexual predation give people a sense of domination. What happens if we are not dominant? Victims derive self-importance in reliving trauma. What happens when that trauma is gone? Belittling lends a sense of security by diminishing others' importance. How can we be loved or wanted if we acknowledge our own faults and mediocrity? The hesitation to clean ourselves up comes because we cannot see the other side of the clearing, a fear of the unknown, what it looks like to be without these various tools we have amassed to deal with life, to give up that control.

The key to beginning, I learned, is accepting what we already know to be true—that we really are in control of very, very little in life, and that it is also okay that we control so little. It is the way things are meant to be—can you imagine if we actually were responsible for making people love us, becoming rich and successful, raising children to be good and respectable, or even to stay healthy and never die? Just the thought of it stresses me out, as it does you, let alone trying to do it as so many, many people do every single day while life passes us by. Accepting that we have adopted behaviors to convince ourselves of the illusion of control, which exists solely for our own selfish emotional comfort, suddenly frees us to change because we no longer need to have control. Complete acceptance does not happen right away though (trying to control feelings *is also control!*). Practicing the inventory shows us on paper what to control and what not to control, in the form of an easy-to-read chart. It also shows us that our experiences are valid and where we need to make changes and amends—That awful thing we went through truly *was* awful, even though we felt the need to convince ourselves and everyone else that the pain was real. It shows where we had no power, over a person, event, or even ourselves, and the resulting damage was not our fault. It then shows us which things we do have responsibility for, and which, by the way, turn out to be more simple than the things we took on instead.

This practice also has implications for all aspects of our lives, even that which is physical. The absolute strongest stimulant for adrenaline release is not exercise, stimulants, or metabolic disease but emotional conflict. If a person is at odds with others in their life—a fat-shaming husband, a controlling wife, tumultuous relationships with siblings, coworkers, etc., self-hatred and body shame, regret and remorse for the past, or fear of the future each impassioned interaction or even just the anticipation of conflict releases large amounts of adrenaline which in turn cause dopamine deficiency, loss of electrolytes, vitamin C, and even catalyze destructive eating disorders. The trauma of our past can also produce a mind which is restless and sensitive to even the slightest threat, or one which ruminates constantly on the wrongs which we have suffered and adrenaline becomes chronic and debilitating for the overall health even if life is relatively calm and stable in appearance. If psychological stress is a regular occurrence in our lives it inhibits healing and recovery, both mentally *and* physically, because the body is never able to get out from the influence of stress hormones regulated by the mind in response to stress.

But while external stresses stimulate adrenaline expression a great deal of our stress is actually caused also by our *perception* of it. Most of us concerned with our health sorely fear death, believing if we can just figure out how to be healthy we can somehow cheat death, but since we can't actually do that we then spend a great deal of our life trying to avoid even thinking about it, but which in turn distracts us from actually living and causes great anxiety when it does enter our mind. Cheating death is not only impossible, it is not in our responsibility. In fact, our ONLY responsibility in life is to show up for opportunity and do our best.

Because inventory therapy is an actual, structured, actionable practice and not just some inspirational saying or catchy phrase all it requires is doing our best, and that in turn will relieve us of fears, insecurities, and control behaviors by empowering our mind with answers and solutions. These new skills of empowerment then not only alleviate stress and thus the expression of adrenaline but replaces them with confidence and hormones of reward such as oxytocin and dopamine, having acquired new life skills which empower us to handle the unknown, the unexpected, and the uncomfortable, so this practice can have as much relevance for physical health as it does spiritual by helping us accept reality rather than fight it, which is something we cannot do anyway and why that behavior reaps nothing but frustration and loss. But this is also because there is no separation between the spiritual and physical, they are one in the same, the energy which makes us alive is also what mediates spirituality, and they cannot be separated any more than time from space.

There are two parts to the practice of personal inventory—the personal inventory and the fear inventory. I have altered the format a little from the way it's presented in twelve-step programs to also provide therapy for those who do not suffer from substance abuse and to remove unhelpful dogma which impairs those programs. Though this practice originates from the founders of Alcoholics Anonymous it is really a therapy for simply being alive and has little to do with substance abuse. Because I do this practice regularly (whenever anything unpleasant occurs, within or outside myself) I write in a notebook, and the therapy absolutely must be written, by hand, because it functions by communicating with the subconscious, which does not occur without the act of writing. But the mere act of doing *is* the therapy, and does not require other steps than what is presented in this chapter.

To begin a personal inventory, copy out this five-column chart on a piece of paper. In the first column under the heading *resentment*, write the name of a person, institution, or idea which causes you any kind of consternation. Resentments are poison to life. They make us hate people, fear others, lose sleep, and become hurtful in return. But rather than stewing about them or tucking them deep into the back of our mind where they fester and undermine our spiritual integrity, we are here setting them on paper to be expunged. Sometimes we think we have no resentments because we spend our time ignoring or repressing feelings we don't like, or we might want to think of ourselves as lacking guile and malice from a desire to be a good person. Resentments are not bad and do not make you a bad person, they are a natural response to loss and misfortune, and if you errantly believe you have no resentments identify instead the areas of conflict which occur in your life and, if you are honest with yourself, you will find resentments within. *Anything* that causes you to ruminate, stew, obsess, cry, feel frustrated, remorse, or regret for the purposes of this therapy is a resentment.

Next, under *cause* write a brief phrase referring to the event or reason for the resentment. It is helpful to split up repeat offenders into each separate cause, rather than lumping many causes into one resentment. If a repeat offender should offend after doing inventory on our experiences with them, do new inventory to heal the fresh frustration. This is a *practice*, meant to be done repeatedly and often, a tool with which to improve life and our experience.

Under *part hurt* identify the parts of a self which were damaged by the event— these parts are the elements which make up our identity as a person which, when damaged, cause us pain and suffering. As human beings we all require certain things to feel whole and safe, things like food, shelter, love both platonic and erotic, community, or opportunities for accomplishment, and each of these needs correlates with a part of our self. Whenever we are denied these basic requirements for life a correlating part of the self is damaged. This then creates within us scars, painful memories, and defense mechanisms in order that we can be more vigilant and prepared for similar threats to our person in the future. These parts of self are not arbitrary but instead chosen from a list of options which are: *self-esteem, pride, emotional security, financial security, personal relations, sex relations, and ambitions.* A cause can affect one, many, or all of these parts of self, so choose whichever feels relevant for your personal experience. Sometimes we are unaware of which parts are hurt. For instance, many people try to compensate for past events which made them insecure about themselves or their value as a person by adopting confidence as a way to cope with the pain, and so will not choose pride or self esteem because they now view themselves as impervious to such disappointment, but this very act of adopting confidence as a defensive mechanism shows deep wounds to our pride and self esteem, and of course we are wounded in such ways. Clues to the parts of self which are hurt come directly from the preceding column, cause.

Under *my part*, list your actions which contributed to the event or *continue* to contribute to it. Not every event included our actions, especially those which happened to us as children. In that case our part is continuing to contribute to the event somehow, through obsession, resentment, or simply holding on. This column is for actions only, not emotions, feelings, and certainly not other people. For instance, emotions are not under our control, so the statement *I let their behavior make me angry* is absolutely not something you would write here. That would go under cause. Rather, *I shouted* would be something written under my part. Being especially self-honest during your part in resentments which we might like to believe we had no role will help free you of the burden of carrying it with you. This is not a judgement of our actions or value as a person. It is merely a sober analysis enlightening us to the ways in which we can and do effect our environment and life experience. Occasionally our part will consist of positive actions, such as standing up for another person. Generally, the things written in *your part* are actions and choices. Adjectives which are only one word or so go in the next column.

Lastly, in *character weakness* list character traits which we possess which motivate the action listed under our part. This again is not a judgment of our character or value as a person but a way to identify exactly how the events of our past caused damage to us as a person. For instance, if your parents were especially vindictive you might have naturally adopted lying and dishonesty as a way to avoid this abuse, or if you have ever been assaulted you might have developed fear as a character weakness, which is a natural result of such a traumatic event. Identifying exactly how these events have damaged our person allows our mind to resolve them and will replace them with the corresponding and opposite strength, simply through this writing process, so long as you are willing to let go of them. Examples of character weaknesses are things like selfishness, contemptuous, dishonest, unrealistic expectations, egoistic, and self-pity, which typically get in the way of our own wellbeing rather than promote it.

The first three columns of this chart are meant to show legitimacy to our life experience and the parts which we cannot control. Because of the ways in which we were hurt as children most of us spend a great deal of time trying to justify our feelings to ourselves and to others, expending a great deal of precious emotional energy simply trying to validate what we know to be our own experience, and this practice serves to relieve us of that burden by showing us that yes, we were hurt and those experiences really did damage to us as a person. The last two columns are meant to show how we affect our own experience and contribute to any given situation, and is the part which we actually can control. Knowing how exactly the events of our lives have shaped us helps us to finally find resolution and wholeness.

An example of a personal inventory entry might be a resentment against your father, because he didn't accept you when you first came out. Identifying that this hurt my pride, my self-esteem, and my personal relationships helps me to identify exactly how I was hurt by the event. My part was holding him to an expectation of perfection, having unrealistic expectations, not forgiving him for many years, holding onto the pain, making the choice not to tell him earlier, but also making the choice to come out. My character defects in relation to this resentment were frustration, unrealistic expectations, self-centeredness, and a lack of empathy.

The second part of this practice is the *fear inventory*. Fears are ideas about life that prevent us from living fully. They cause us to avoid situations, opportunities, and challenges. Often they motivate animus, and every character defect originates from a fear of something. For instance, people who fear financial insecurity may lie, cheat, steal, or coerce, agitate, or belittle their significant others, children, and friends in dealing with that fear. The fear of not having money comes from being afraid that no one is watching out for us, or not believing in some kind of higher power or purpose, that life is left only up to us. Other fears are more visceral, like fear of the dark, of violence, of men, of our mother, of natural disasters, impending doom or wild animals. These too can all be relieved by inventorying them. Laying them out on paper brings resolution to those fears, because all fears are simply caused by lack of answers and this practice answers why we have such fears. The fear inventory also gives legitimacy to whatever experience caused the fear in the first place. It then shows us how that fear limits our experience or initiates behavior we'd rather not have, before helping us to consider that perhaps there is another way to consider the thing we fear that is more reasonable, which will be more profitable to us in the long term. Chiefest is the realization of why bad things happen. We would never willing submit ourselves to experiences which crush our hearts and tear out our souls, so they must happen to us that we may understand what it is to have truly lived. There cannot be joy without sorrow, no health without disease, no life without death. It is the way things have always been, otherwise our earth would not exist, yet the contamination of God's reality by religion has made us afraid of death, of change, of heartache, making excuses for sin, fomenting self-pity, ironically causing life to be the more unbearable. Rather than removing the thing of which we are afraid, which is impossible, the knowledge of *why* we fear is the key to removing that fear.

To take a fear inventory is to accomplish this understanding. We begin by copying this form to paper. Under the first column titled *fear* write the name of any fear which causes any sort of suffering. Under *cause* we write from where this fear originates. Under *effect* write how having this fear has failed us as it pertains to a corresponding part of self reliance (self-esteem, pride, emotional security, financial security, personal relations, sex relations, and ambitions). Under *a better way* write an opposite approach to this particular fear especially as it pertains to trusting life to carry us through, or your personal concept of a higher power. For example, a fear of death may be caused by the simple fact that we do die and that some day it will happen to you and there is nothing you can do about it. You also may have been taught that death was a punishment or associated with shame, or that not knowing what happens after death is scary. The effect could be that it has prevented us from enjoying life and relationships by relying on our own pride to soldier through the fear, or that it caused us to often wake in the middle of the night, and a better way than a fear of death could be realizing that all people die, or that it's okay not to know what happens afterward, and because it's going to happen no matter what, trusting life or our higher power to carry us through to the next stage just as it saw fit to bring us into this one. Another example might be a fear of losing a job or the process of moving. The cause would simply be that people lose their jobs, that a fear of layoffs may be in circulation, or you are having to move and moving can be stressful, requiring energy, exertion, and stepping into the unknown. The effect of these is to cause daily anxiety, even when nothing is actually happening, merely in anticipation of it, making you tense, unhappy, maybe robbing you of sleep and peace of mind, or causing distance between you and those you love, because in your mind you feel that you are alone, relying on your own power as a single mortal human. A better way would be to realize that you are probably being given a great and exciting opportunity to realize your goals or better your life, even if it doesn't appear so, that God or the Universe is watching out for you and helping you along your life path, that you are in fact not alone, and also that you will most likely meet this challenge the way you have similar ones throughout the course of your life, and that after it is done you will perhaps be very grateful for it. The point in resolving our fears through this practice is not to pretend that things are okay when they aren't. In fact, it is the opposite, to speak the name of the problems and the unpleasantness—having to move, having to die, having to lose friends and loved ones. Paying respect to our struggle is part of the therapeutic nature of the fear and personal inventory. By facing the reality of life rather than ignoring it through pretense we find the anxieties and conflicts within us replaced with wisdom, gratitude, and peace.

Your inventory should take up *many* pages. Mine took five hours to share with another person. Someone took eleven hours to share theirs with me. The clutter of a well-lived life is long, and all that toil shoved to the back of the mind takes up a lot of space. It is no wonder this therapy is so healing. As the first things are gotten rid of, older memories will pop into your head as you're vacuuming or driving to work. Write them down and get them out. If the items in 'my part' involves any untoward or hurtful actions against others, you must make amends for that behavior or it will not be expunged from your mind. For instance if you hurt someone, no matter the reason, you will still be burdened by the guilt of your choice even if you do the writing practice, and so you must approach them and make an honest amends without any concern for your own ego, which means addressing only your behavior and not theirs, without excuse or marginalizing your behavior, so long as doing this will not cause further hurt. Do not use this practice to entertain self pity—but rather to enlighten your mind of the ways in which you can or cannot affect your own life experience. Sharing this information with a confidant is also therapeutic, as is meditating on the results and the new knowledge that there is a better option than quivering and obsessing now gives us the chance to change our lot, not by controlling life but by expanding our enlightenment and ability to cope with it. In fact, the last and final step of this practice is to communicate to the Universe your intention to let go of those fears and character weaknesses you have written down. Hesitation or refusal to do this will only cause you to cling to them as a drowning person does a safety raft. The water is only chest deep, and you must let go in order to be free, which thus requires the humility of prayer and supplication. Pray to your conception of God or a higher power about what you have written down both in the personal inventory and the fear inventory, inform them of your willingness to let go of these character weaknesses, ask for direction in so doing and to know their will and be blessed with the power to carry it out, always remembering that the purpose of prayer is not to ask for things or divine intervention but only for enlightenment and to spend time in communion with the spiritual. If there is much resistance felt when trying to do this practice I have found it helpful to recommend inventorying the resentment towards the practice! This will provide clarity about this resistance and thus help remove the barrier.

Today I understand what is required of me, and what is not. Life is immeasurably easier, but also richer and wonderful. The great acrobatics to discover reasons for God or for Not God are over, no one who hurt me is right and I get a great comfort in living without a desire to know the future or the past, even when things go badly, and especially when they are good. In the years of my struggle I believed the lie that God only exists in religion. Man is the author of religion, and man is pretty much all that religion offers. God is found elsewhere. I have a connection to the ebb and flow of the great universe I thought was reserved for leathery old white men, whom I now realize do not actually have it, and so my once resentment of them has given way to compassion, because where I live is more wonderful than I ever believed was possible, and they will likely go to their grave still trying to believe they are better than others. My upbringing said I had to be worthy of spirituality, but spirituality runs through everything. It is the undercurrent of all life, the power that brought us into consciousness is what we experience to be God. It is at our fingertips, and had easily through moments of quiet reflection and internal dialogue.

Our ancestors felt their spirituality no less powerfully than our contemporaries, not because any religious ideals are ever inherently right, but because whatever the divine is it clearly has no ego. It cares not for anyone's conception of it. Better for those of us who have been cast out by the seething masses it cares not what *their* conception is either. Sadly, evil men have always used lies and deceit to sway influence, and so it still is. It does not mean they know God, as anyone who pays a little attention can plainly see.

The future of spirituality seems quite exciting. For the first time mankind can counsel each other instead of relying on institution, because of the advent of social media and the connectedness it provides from the source of each own's personal relationship with the spiritual forces of life. Homosexuals and others of us who are different-gendered persons, brothers of Nisus and Euryalus to whom this book is dedicated, are a gift from God to families and societies who need us and our unique gifts and talents, a light in dark times and a support built literally into the biology of the human race. Indeed the only light in the harsh and tumultuous environment of my childhood were the songs and plays written largely by gay men like Howard Ashman and Steven Sondheim, and the numerous individuals who have contributed to the achievements of human history have been disproportionately non-heteronormative as represented by the father of computers, Alan Turing, indomitable author Oscar Wilde, Roman Emperor Hadrian, mercurial Isaac Newton, Walt Whitman, Leonardo DaVinci, Michelangelo Simoni, Pyotr Tchaikovsky, Little Richard, Virginia Woolf, Florence Nightingale, Marcel Proust, Freddy Mercury, Elton John, Tab Hunter, Billie Holiday, Allen Ginsburg, John Waters, Gore Vidal, Susan B. Anthony, civil rights giant Bayard Rustin, Tennessee Williams, Montgomery Clift, E.M. Forster, both Francis Bacons, George Washington Carver, Sally Ride, and Emily Dickinson, and that's not including people like Abraham Lincoln and Mahatma Ghandi who appear to also perhaps been queer. Otto Warburg, the Nobel prize winning scientist who discovered the Warburg Effect and whose work has been integral to the last hundred years of cellular biology was gay, with a loving partner of fifty-years, surviving even Nazi Germany though he was also Jewish. Not only is there nothing wrong with us, we are put here purposefully to help mankind find its better self, and if you are LGBTQI+ you are in very good company. Whether those around us accept the gift is not our responsibility, ours is only to show up for opportunity and do our best, and I would never have understood this nor my innate value as a human being which has nothing to do with why I am here, only that I am, if I had not practiced the personal inventory.

But don't press me for a conception of God. She-Ra is probably the closest description I could give you. I mean, why shouldn't the Master of the Universe be devastating in a white mini-skirt and gold armor, a magic sword in hand with hair piled high, sitting astride a rainbow-winged, speaking horse? To me that is a lot more impressive, and relatable, than an old white man sporting a long beard. It's certainly more like what I've come to know, and I very much prefer it.

CHAPTER 29

ACNE AND SKIN

I would say that as a teenager acne prevented me from getting many dates, but it's not true. Being a closeted gay boy did. While I harbored affections for a handful of my peers in secret (most of whom turned out *to also be gay* which would have dramatically altered my childhood narrative, had I known), I was content not to be involved in romance for the fear of being found out as gay, as well as being dishonest and hurting women (one girl attempted to date me and I went along for awhile, but ended it quickly when the guilt became too much). The acne, however, persisted long after I came out and was a constant source of mild anxiety, as it is for a great many people both young and old, across every race and religious affiliation. I would like to assure you that acne is not your problem, no matter how much you may think so. Acne might be the excuse for our self-doubt, anxiety, fears, and bad choices but it is our self-doubt, anxiety, fears, and bad choices that are the real problem, our failure to accept the conditions of mortality which sounds overly dramatized when talking about acne but it is still one of those things which we are not always in control. Overcoming the unpleasant emotional and social suffering surrounding the perception of acne requires self-searching, even as prescribed in the process of personal inventory, questioning what suffering means to us personally. When we can come to find the answer that life is trying to help us learn through adversity we then find relief from those things. Acne is just annoying.

As a teenager I was put on the drug Accutane, and while it saddled me with debilitating health problems it did not even lessen the amount of acne I continued to suffer. There are more treatments for acne than I can count, and how many of those permanently eradicate it? There are creams, washes, pastes, papers, peels, and prescriptions. For me and for many others the most effective treatments are antibiotics, but they only work while being used and can also come with a lot of serious side effects. That antibiotics are somewhat effective is a clue to the cause and solution for acne, but not in the way we are thinking. Yes, acne is caused by bacteria. We all know that. But then why do treatments which target this bacteria so often fail?

When I was twenty-six I did a cleanse that rid me completely of acne, but I'm not going to talk about it because it was dangerous, cleanses are bullshit, and turns out completely unnecessary. Other decisions I made around the time of the cleanse were also more important than the cleanse itself, such as attempting vegetarianism. Though vegetarianism is not the answer to acne either, in my particular vegetarianism where I also avoided wheat due to recently discovering its harmful effects on my digestion I inadvertently reduced exposure to iron, both from iron-fortification and heme iron found in meat which is iron bound to protein and very highly bioavailable. The cleanse also helped clear some excess iron out of my digestive system (this will happen naturally without a cleanse) while also supplementing extra salt which improves the immune system by providing extra chloride. My life up to this point included copious amounts of high-iron food from fortified wheat products and meat, strongly overloading my system with iron which then also strongly promotes all kinds of opportunistic microbes which use it to inactivate our immune system and find ingress into the human body.

The reason acne sets in during puberty and not before is that the iron content in the body, particularly the amount and how it is metabolized, is also mediated by the sex hormones. Estrogen in particular, which is a hormone of growth and helps bodies grow larger during puberty, causes cells to also accumulate iron. In both males and females estrogen levels rise at the onset of puberty and are never again as they were in childhood. It is supposed to be like this and the problem is not with the hormones but in how those hormones react to our inappropriate food sources and lifestyles, and because excess iron is caused by diet or supplements, acne thus begins in the gut.

For the same reason that milk is low in iron, to prevent excessive bacterial growth in the intestines, the body does not tend to excrete used or excess iron into the intestines, as it does for many other metabolic byproducts, to avoid feeding pathogenic bacteria (and viruses). Instead, the body mostly excretes iron through the skin, unless iron excess become so great that it also requires excretion in the gut, which is what promotes chronic gastrointestinal problems as discussed in the chapter on gut health. But this dermal excretory route is also why we tend to develop body odor along with acne when hitting puberty—the excreted iron on the skin allows more bacteria to begin growing there, and iron compounds produced by these bacteria are also smelly. Because the skin is naturally resistant to bacterial penetration, our internal health thus remains unaffected for much longer due to this evolutionary strategy. But because a full quarter of our biological iron is excreted through the skin (mainly by the sloughing of old skin), excess dietary iron is the root cause of acne.

Acne does not just occur on the face, although that is usually the source of our dislike since it muddies our appearance. The reason acne is typically so concentrated on the face is due to where the iron excreted originates. Iron seems to be excreted in the fastest direct route possible rather than circulating through the body, and while some organs like the liver and spleen will store iron the rest of the body does not readily release it back into the bloodstream once absorbed. In the case of the head, where large incidents of acne occurs, this iron comes from our most metabolically demanding organ—the brain, and since the brain is surrounded by skull, excreting iron would be extremely slow and difficult if it traveled through bone, so it instead it goes through the soft tissues of the oral and ocular cavity and out through the face, which is why acne tends to concentrate on the cheeks, temples, and forehead. When the diet contains an excess of iron than what is needed for health, this excess is excreted though the skin and thus promotes the growth of acne causing bacteria.

The worst dietary offenders for promoting acne are foods fortified with iron, excess meat consumption, and iron containing supplements. Iron fortification is nothing more than metal shavings, and can quickly contribute to iron overload and thence excessive iron burden on the body which can have worse effects than acne (yes there are such things). Adding additional iron from other food sources guarantees acne. The reason antibiotics help fix acne is because most antibiotics bind iron, preventing it from use by bacteria. So does aspirin which has long been used topically (salicylic acid) to prevent acne. But since problematic iron can be avoided in the diet, avoiding excess iron in the first place is the absolute best way to treat acne.

The two factors which regulate iron homeostasis most are vitamin A and vitamin D. Both of them, but more especially vitamin A, stimulate the release of iron from storage sites, such as the liver and spleen, into the bloodstream in turn by regulating the iron-regulating protein *hepcidin*. When I was experimenting with vitamin A supplementation it caused me to have a recurrence of acne, which I hadn't had in many years. This effect on iron metabolism is one of the reasons I strongly warn against using vitamin A in supplement form, as it can release enough iron that subsequent metabolic damage can result such as the increase in hair loss I experienced in the thinning parts of my scalp, since factors like zinc required to synthesize vitamin A from carotene would also be deficient meaning that the iron released by a supplement is not bound to protective proteins like heme or transferrin and instead circulates to react freely with other compounds and proteins. Vitamin A is a significant nutrient for the skin and, along with carotenoids, help protect the skin from sun damage and also promote skin renewal and regeneration, and deficiency of skin carotene can also result in and is the cause of many skin disorders like psoriasis and sensitivity to sunlight.

High microbial hydrogen sulfide production also strongly promotes acne because hydrogen sulfide binds and destroys heme which in turn forces the body to discard the resulting sulfur-iron complex and to absorb more dietary iron to replace it. This effect of hydrogen sulfide on the iron cycle in the body is the largest driver of iron excess and by extension acne (and other iron excretory routes like earwax). Most adults reach a point where they become populated by hydrogen sulfide producing microbes around the ages of thirty to forty, and find their skin to begin sloughing off at much increased rates. This is in fact why many spas offer skin scrubbing treatments, since many older people experience notable skin sloughing, but skin scrubbing is not really something that should be required for healthy skin and is in fact a symptom of microbial hydrogen sulfide production which increases the symptoms of aging due to interference with the immune system, increased iron metabolism, and increased oxidative and pathogenic stress which must be addressed by more frequent consumption of foods containing carotene as discussed in the chapter on vitamin D. Bad breath, foul smelling feces and flatulence, acne, skin sloughing, and excessive earwax production are all signs of hydrogen sulfide producing bacteria which must be addressed because without addressing the supply of iron which promotes and enables the pathogens which cause these problems it is impossible to suppress them no matter how many products or medicines are used. Since this condition also promotes other negative symptoms of aging, masking the problem with medicines or other treatments (for instance the use of mouthwash to mask oral malodor) will only deceive you into believing things are fine and will cause much more problems in later years. As excess hydrogens sulfide also impairs the immune system as discussed in the chapter on immunity this strategy will resolve skin problems through several different mechanisms.

The strategy for treating hydrogen sulfide producers is frequent intake of carotene, but carotene is also used in the skin to protect commensal skin microbes from irradiation by ultraviolet light which otherwise protect our skin from opportunistic and pathogenic microbes. In fact, the skin contains a layer of acidic, oily secretions which act as a barrier to ingress by opportunistic bacteria but you wash it off every day, sometimes two or three times, and without this protective layer our skin is exposed and vulnerable to acne causing microbes, drying, and our protective microbes die off which causes stress to the skin through reduced avail-ability of short chain fatty acids required for the skin to perform steroidogenesis that maintains hydration and endocrine function throughout the body. I made this realization around the time my acne disappeared and completely stopped washing my face with soaps, and except when experimenting with vitamin A I have not had acne in ten years. I have advised people of this but women especially often don't want to stop washing their face out of some misguided sense of cleanliness. The oil layer is much more antiseptic than our soap, and carotene in the skin is a highly effective barrier to ultraviolet damage, but a lot of people wear makeup to cover up poor skin quality which is caused by over-cleaning, drying, and killing of the commensal microbiome which would resolve itself if you just stopped using these fucking toxic chemicals on your living, breathing skin and ate carotene every day (but not so much that the skin turns orange).

As part of this natural defense barrier humans have a fatty acid called *sapienic acid* which is entirely unique in the animal kingdom, and it is excreted in the sebum from our sebaceous glands which occur in a high concentration on the facial skin precisely to protect against bacteria. The production of sapienic acid is inhibited by estrogen, though, and is another reason to maintain a diet that promotes a robust metabolic rate, as excess estrogen from depressed metabolisms promotes the uptake of additional iron, which is the reason why women can expe-rience cyclical cycles of acne development, and males who have acne whom are experiencing an increase rate testosterone aromatization such as those with slow metabolisms or those using steroids (which convert to estrogen due to stressful dieting and excessive exercise which lowers the metabolic rate). When estrogen is increased it inhibits the conversion of palmitic acid to sapienic, preventing the bactericidal properties of the skin. Excess iron can still establish acne even with this natural acidic barrier if enough is present, which is why it is important to avoid excess dietary iron in addition to leaving the acidic skin barrier intact and addressing microbial hydrogen sulfide.

Sulfur has traditionally been used as a remedy for acne precisely because of sulfur's strong affinity for iron, thus inhibiting the growth of bacteria on the skin (and elsewhere in the body), and the reason foods like garlic can make you smell bad is because its sulfur binds to excess iron which is then excreted through the skin in the same way as sulfide iron complexes and is a specific symptom of molyb-denum deficiency as discussed in the chapter on cardiovascular health and vitamin D required to change dietary sulfur into sulfate which is instead stored as glutathi-one. But for this same reason topical sulfur can be used to bind iron secreting from skin to help stop bacteria and other microbes which cause skin disorders like acne. To be clear, this is a temporary fix for acne and does not reverse the problem of iron excess and dysregulation which must be addressed through diet for long term resolution. Sublimed or powdered sulfur preparation in a good fat such as organic shea or cocoa butter or coconut oil can make topical treatment both pleasant and powerfully effective. Sulfur does pose a danger as even a little bit in the eyes can cause severe discomfort, and only about 1/8 tsp is needed in about 1/2 cup of oil to be effective. Daily use against acne and other skin conditions works rapidly. Pure sulfur does not have an odor—it only does when reacting with other compounds, so there is no need to worry about scent, but if you do smell a slight "rotten eggs" odor after applying it means sulfur is reacting with iron, though there shouldn't be enough to make an offensive amount of it, and never get sulfur near your eyes (if it does get in your eyes it just stings and isn't extremely harmful, and can be flushed out with water). Sulfur soap is excellent for this purpose—even though it removes the protective oil barrier, sulfur is so good at binding and removing the iron which is at the root of the bacterial growth that it can be very helpful in maintaining skin health, and using a topical application of shea butter or coconut oil can help replace the fats lost from using soap.

Skin issues also often also include injury such as burns, cuts, surgery, and scarring which can also all be treated with coconut oil too (not old scars, but to prevent scarring from fresh wounds). As related in my earlier stories about cutting off the tip of my finger with a mandolin when making potato gratin and healing my boyfriend's appendectomy incision with coconut oil and honey, coconut oil is high in lauric acid which converts to the master hormone pregnenolone in the body, and since the skin is a primary site of steroidogenesis application of coconut oil following any kind of skin injury can help to greatly increase healing. This is also achieved since coconut oil is a liquid medium and slightly antibiotic, so it helps to prevent skin from drying out which can also facilitate migration of stem cells to injuries to accomplish more complete healing (and it can help to keep the area covered fully such as with plastic wrap). Treatment of burns should especially be done in part with coconut oil since burns can often damage far beneath the surface skin layer, and keeping covered with coconut oil will help tissue to regenerate more fully than can be achieved otherwise.

Many skin conditions resemble acne but are in fact other types of infections. For years I experienced a strange condition where the hair follicles of my neck became infected if my facial hair grew out (opposite of most men who get infections if they shave). I tried many treatments for acne on this condition, but with no results. It turns out the infection was caused by demodex mites, which are an organism that commonly cohabitates with humans and feeds in hair follicles, which is why the infection worsened if I did not shave frequently, and was instead easily eradicated with the use of topical sulfur (a good sulfur soap should work nicely).

There are also an abundance of skin pathogens, such as dermatophyte fungi like Trichophyton which colonize skin and cause disorders as ringworm (it's fungi, not a worm), athletes foot, nail yellowing, jock rash, scaly skin, dandruff, etc., which feed on the keratin protein in skin and have traditionally been extremely difficult to eradicate, requiring weeks and even months of treatment with antifungal pharmaceuticals, which also do nothing to prevent reinfection and recolonization.

The elderly and those with compromised immune systems are highly vulnerable to dermatophyte infection, and any patches of skin and nails which are chronically scaly, red, yellow, peeling, or inflamed usually mean a chronic dermatophyte infection. Normally dermatophytes are easily eradicated from the deeper layers of skin by a competent immune system, so if infection is widespread, painful, and chronic this indicates severe failure of the immune system as discussed in that chapter and the need for increased daily intake of the halides chloride (dietary salt), iodine (a supplement), and cyanide (brassicas, yuca, bamboo shoots, etc.) in addition to resolving ammonia, hydrogen sulfide, and calcium dysregulation which impair the immune system. Other skin disorders like lupus, psoriasis, and eczema very likely also involve opportunistic dermatophytes, fungi, or parasites which penetrate deeper into the skin and which then elicit a more dramatic immune response which can and does appear as so-called "autoimmunity" conditions but which are in reality the uncontrolled oxidative cascade which occurs during dysregulated immune reactions due to immune problems like deficiency of vitamin E and vitamin C as discussed in the chapter on immunity, as there is in fact no such thing as autoimmunity as discussed in that chapter, and instead represents the presence of actual opportunistic pathogens living in those tissues.

In one square centimeter of skin there are also one billion microbes, and we are also normally protected from skin opportunists by our commensal skin microbiome, and any presentation of opportunistic skin microbes such as what cause these skin conditions is evidence of loss of protective skin microbes normally collected from the environment such as by interaction with other humans or healthy soils, plants, animals, etc., as is discussed in the chapter on diabetes. The protective acidic layer of the skin is a product of commensal microbes like Propionibacterium acnes producing short chain fatty acids from nutrients like proteins, sugars, and fats they receive from the skin itself, and behaviors like showering in fluoridated water, swimming in highly chlorinated water, engaging in low-carbohydrate diets, lacking dietary carotene, or exposure to sunlight while deficient in carotene (because it protects skin microbes from irradiation) all eradicate these commensal skin microbes which then predisposes us to colonization by opportunists. While it is true that the pH of the skin barrier is in the acidic range it is also not the pH which resolves fungal colonization such as during dermatophyte infection, so widely promoted treatments like application of vinegar, baking soda, lemon juice, etc., will do nothing to eradicate them but will irritate the skin and can promote pathogens due to their water and carbon content. Quite often the use of essential oils are recommended treatments too but you will remember from the chapter on oral health that essential oils strongly neutralize cellular polarity, which does damage microbes but also our own cells because our body also uses principles of polarity to run the nervous system and repel pathogens, and the use of essential oils likely promotes deeper penetration of fungal pathogens into the skin and peripheral neuropathy to cause more severe conditions and "autoimmunity" due to an impaired, chronic immune response, and can contribute to neurological problems if enough is used that it reaches the nervous system.

Sulfur is often an effective treatment for skin conditions, if the immune system is also restored and working, such as with sulfur soap or sulfur ointments, not only because the sulfur binds iron but also sulfites secreted by pathogens to dissolve disulfide protein bonds in skin, and I personally used a combination of sulfur powder and coconut oil daily for a few weeks to treat some toenail yellowing. There are, however, some dermatophytes which have evolved to colonize only the most outer layer of the skin (the stratum corneum) which helps them evade the immune system but cause chronic infection. Recurrent jock rash or jock itch is a primary symptom of chronic dermatophyte colonization and, contrary to accepted ideas of these conditions, is not a problem of hygiene but instead chronic persistence of these fungi in the outer layer of skin which evades normal clinical diagnosis. Especially in men this strongly affects sex hormone homeostasis, as these dermatophytes chronically interfere with testosterone by increasing aromatization through ammonia production and lower metabolic rate of the testicles through chronically decreased temperature of the testicles and scrotum, and symptoms of these dermatophytes are any chronic redness in skin, especially on exposure to sunlight, especially on the scrotal skin, perineum, anus, vulva, labia, inner thighs, buttocks, etc.

Medical professionals often also discuss hygiene and importance of keeping skin clean and dry for resolution of dermatophytoses like ring worm and jock rash, but these pathogens induce water seepage through the skin in order to provide the moisture they require, so hygiene strategies have very little to do with prevention, resolution, and treatment, and it technically should be possible to never shower and still not have jock rash which, if that is not the case (please do shower, though), is symptomatic of chronic colonization with dermatophytes which must be addressed. There are antifungal pharmaceutical treatments which can help resolve dermatophytoses, but these pathogens are highly adapted to persist in the environment through sporulation, and pharmaceuticals do not also protect against recolonization, and as discussed in previous chapters fungi like dermatophytes are inhibited instead by dietary *vitamin E* which prevents the formation of oxidized lipid products like oxylipin which otherwise derange metabolism and immune function by inhibiting chloride absorption, to enable colonization and cause such problems as type-two diabetes or chronic urogenital dysfunction. A healthy diet high in nuts and fruits and vegetables can contain plenty of vitamin E to keep us healthy, but sprouted nuts and grains are even higher in vitamin E, and leafy greens contain vitamin E too, and the vegetable purslane is extremely high in vitamin E, oxalate, and chloride since it also grows in high salt soil. But industrialized diets are typically low in vitamin E, and the saponification of fats in the gut by other opportunistic pathogens as discussed in the chapter on calcium also prevents absorption of requisite fat soluble nutrients like vitamin E, even when they are plentiful in the diet or supplemented. Any dermatophytosis likely reflects a deficiency of vitamin E and chloride both, and is then treated through the regular intake of salt with sources of vitamin E, such as sprouted, salted nuts, daily consumption of purslane, or the manual supplementation of salt in juice or sugar water with a little added supplement of natural vitamin E. One skin issue I never experienced after my recovery was dandruff, which is also caused by opportunistic fungi, which is probably due to the regular intake of dietary vitamin E, even when not using a supplement, and dandruff is probably a symptom of quite significant vitamin E deficiency which can be easily resolved through dietary or supplemental vitamin E.

Anyone in professions which risk close contact to a diverse population of other people such as the medical professions, dentistry, childcare, sex work, etc., should also preemptively protect themselves from dermatophyte colonization by always making sure they have vitamin C, vitamin E, and halides in the diet, daily, and once or twice a month making and consuming silicon ascorbate as described in the chapter on thyroid, and ceasing work if ever colonized by these microbes to avoid spreading them, until the infection is cleared up, and to avoid sexual intercourse with others if colonized by dermatophytes that affect the reproductive area, and to raise awareness of these pathogens in order to help limit their spread and impact on others.

As discussed in previous chapters, silicon in connective tissue, skin, and the basement membrane also acts as a mechanical barrier to ingress by opportunistic pathogens, since silicon polymerizes in alkaline pH, but deposition of silicon in connective tissue and skin requires vitamin C and halides as cofactors for synthesis, and after helping someone with years of recurrent eczema and migraine by using preparations of silicon as discussed in the chapter on migraine their eczema suddenly one day just completely disappeared. Fruit is high in silicon, vitamin C, and halides but is also especially helpful in combating acne as fructose is also involved in enzymes which regulate the desaturation of certain fatty acids which can otherwise cause metabolic decline of tissues like the skin, and fruit is also very high in cinnamic acids, especially those which have euphoric flavors like the Prunus family. But other high silicon foods like green beans and spinach as well as the use of silicon water made by boiling about 100 mg of silicon per liter of water or use of high silicon spring water can also be extremely useful not only for improving the health of skin (because silicon is mostly taken up in aquaporin channels which also take up water) but all other keratinous tissue like hair, nails, joints, and ligaments, and while I have not yet resolved them I suspect that the vertical lines in nails are probably also caused by dysregulation of silicon and first appear when we become colonized by alkalizing gut pathogens which disturb the normal digestion and integration of dietary silicon into tissues. Restoring silicon also restored the natural curl to my hair which, during the aging process, had become more dull and straightened. Potatoes for some inexplicable reason clear blackheads and impacted pore issues, so instead of digging at your skin just have some potatoes.

As we age skin can also start to appear dry and dull, and premature wrinkling and aging of the skin can be distressful for people who are not yet very aged. Catabolism of skin amino acids and fat because of undereating or problems with digestion induced by opportunistic microbes is the largest driver of this problem. For instance, proline is one of the most abundant amino acids in connective tissue, collagen, extracellular matrix, and many enzymatic pathways, but during glucose deficiency proline is catabolized as an efficient source of energy, destroying skin and connective tissue as the body struggles to keep itself alive during nutritional starvation. Remembering that a great deal of protein comes from a healthy gut microbiome, and our skin health is a direct reflection of the state of the gut and digestion which both provides nutrients for the skin and prevents skin catabolism by effectively breaking down food. As vitamin C is the primary requisite for the synthesis of collagen and renewal and regeneration of tissues, the impairment of vitamin C status by opportunistic, ammonia producing pathogens as discussed in earlier chapters prevents healthy protein synthesis, skin renewal, and impairs skin immunity. But this also not only a function of deficiency but also a regulatory one as skin metabolism changes during vitamin C deficiency to decrease blood flow since vitamin C is required for maintenance of enzymes that produce nitric oxide which increases blood flow to the skin (so that during times of vitamin C deficiency the body does not risk heat loss). As discussed in the chapters on erections and hormones, vitamin C is also the regulatory factor for hair distribution on the body, and deficiency whether dietary or pathogenic induces growth of our vestigial winter hair coat such as back hair, neck hair, and spreading of torso hair.

Of course, water is required by the skin to be hydrated and for the natural production of hydronium in sweat glands by commensal microbes. But most people think of skin hydration as being a primary function of water, which it absolutely is not, but instead is a function of the fat content of skin, which prevents evaporation of water and promotes local skin steroidogenesis. Many cosmetic formulations exploit this misunderstanding and even contain harmful chemicals which strongly stimulate the uptake of water into cells, causing damaging inflammation but which gives the skin a false appearance of fullness. Hyaluronic acid is a great example of this misunderstanding because hyaluronic acid is involved in the processes of cellular growth which is stimulated by water influx into cells, and exogenous hyaluronic acid and other harmful chemicals actually simulate thickening and stiffening of the skin and ironically accelerate aging through chronic inflammatory stress, since inflammation is the trigger for tissue proliferation, and commercial 'moisturizers' and cosmetics should be largely avoided, especially abrasives and chemical peels which tear off layers of skin as this triggers significant inflammation and can even induce fibrosis and scar tissue formation.

Fat also insulates skin and the body from heat loss which in turn facilitates higher cellular respiration of mammalian cells and thus an increase in CO_2 production, which is why those who retain more fat also so often have more youthful looking skin while those who are overly lean and chronically dieting with very low skin fat age more rapidly and present with more wrinkled and dull skin. Because most lotions and cosmetics try to achieve hydration through chemical interference of skin water management and stimulate inflammation, which is water influx into cells, this actually lowers cellular metabolism, CO_2 production, and promotes skin hypoxia. If you've ever noticed too after using a synthetic, commercial lotion it reemerges later during the day this is because it is made of harmful chemicals that are actually spit out by the skin. Good fats like coconut oil, olive oil, or shea butter can be very effective moisturizers for the skin because they are healthy, food-grade fats which the skin can actually absorb and metabolize, and don't reappear later because they are actually "eaten" by the skin as nutrition. The saturated fats in coconut oil, butter, and shea butter can even be used to effectively mitigate sunburn and block the itch of mosquito bites and other allergic skin reactions because such damage is caused primarily by oxidation of unstable polyunsaturated fats (which are also formed in the skin when skin temperature is too low due to dieting or metabolic disease).

As discussed in the chapter on hormones and pregnenolone the skin is also a primary site of steroidogenesis, and application of coconut oil (or other fat high in lauric acid) can actually stimulate the skin's production of pregnenolone which very strongly helps the skin manage electrolytes and water and even inhibit pathogens. This is especially useful for injury to the skin or underlying tissue, and especially for those suffering paralysis, as the local synthesis of pregnenolone will help reduce atrophy of the underlying tissue. Application of coconut oil to sites of herpes sores and cold sores (which are herpes viruses) as soon as activation is detected can often completely prevent them from erupting from the skin, because of the local production of steroids derived from topical lauric acid application.

Topical application of fats is not sufficient for the health of the skin, however, and this primarily comes from digestion of healthy fats which is instead strongly inhibited by saponification of dietary fats by opportunistic microbes as discussed in the chapters on calcium, parasitism, and hormones, since cholesterol is important for immunity, hormones, and thus also for skin, and the use of oxalates with dietary fats to prevent their saponification and resolution of calcium dysregulation and restoration of endogenous production of pregnenolone as discussed in the chapter on hormones can rapidly reverse many problems of skin aging through the increased production of cholesterol, steroids, and fat and cholesterol deposition in skin, without which skin health will only continue to deteriorate due to insufficient production of cholesterol and necessary dietary fats.

Sodium, you will remember from the chapter on cardiovascular disease, is also the primary tool which manages water in the body, and the skin is also a reservoir for sodium, which in turn promotes water retention in the skin while also preventing hypotonia (low electrolytes) otherwise caused by high water influx. Even sweat glands contain the epithelial sodium channels which reabsorb sodium from sweat to prevent its excessive loss from the skin during sweating (as well as the CFTR channel to reabsorb chloride). Because fructose is required for these channels to work properly, behaviors like dieting, starvation, and excess exercise rapidly deplete sodium and the body must then mobilize skin sodium which in turn diminishes the skin's ability to hold water and resist pathogenesis, and combined with increased catabolization of fats and amino acids from the skin during such stresses as dieting and illness promotes aging, dryness, thinning, and other characteristics of poor skin health. Raising skin sodium by reducing dietary and metabolic stress, resolving hyperammonemia and pathogenic ammonia producers, and regularly supplementing extra salt or sodium citrate or sodium acetate with sources of sugar will promote better skin hydration and restore a more glowing, hydrated, youthful quality and resolve problems of excessive sweating as discussed in the chapter on sleep. The effect of this strategy can begin to be seen in just a few days or weeks, and followed long term with other behaviors that improve digestion, hormones, and immunity can very effectively reverse much of the damage of metabolic stress on the skin. Iodine, probably through the promotion of thyroid hormone, can also strongly promote normal skin hydration and many people see an immediate increase in skin suppleness after restoring healthy levels of dietary iodine and thyroid function.

One exception to the usefulness of saturated fats in skin are the conditions chalazion or stye of the eyelids—Doctors do not know how to cure these conditions, usually resorting to cutting them out or other invasive procedure, as like many health problems they are completely misunderstood by medical science. As discussed in the chapter on hair loss the skin uses desaturase enzymes to desaturate fatty acids in the skin when the skin temperature drops significantly. If this was not the case the saturated fatty acids like lauric acid and palmitic acid solidify like butter in a refrigerator and are thence impossible for the body to move through cells and tissues, and styes and chalazion result from greatly reduced body temperature, cold skin, and deficiency of desaturase enzyme activity. Desaturase enzymes are zinc dependent, so zinc deficiency is the reason for low desaturase enzyme activity and a low-dose supplement can be taken to improve resolution. Pulse and body temperature as described in the chapter on self therapy can help elucidate the metabolic rate and it will be seen that the body temperature is consistently too low and must be raised in order to resolve these problems, while applying a very warm compress to the eye for as much time as is comfortable or spending time in a sauna will help soften the fats which are blocking the oil ducts. Maintaining an adequate body temperature and zinc repletion will thereafter prevent recurrence.

Lastly, vitamin E is also superbly protective against acne, as it both protects against iron accumulation and excess aromatization of testosterone to estrogen. As many vitamin E products are synthetic and even toxic, it is important to use an explicitly natural form of vitamin E such as from sprouted nuts and seeds or a natural supplement. I have found progesterone, which I discuss in another chapter, to also flush excess iron out of tissues and can temporarily cause an elevation in iron excretion and acne (no one under twenty should regularly use progesterone or thyroid or other medications, unless under a doctor's order, since children are so strongly affected by pharmaceutical intervention but also heal much more rapidly than adults). As long as the diet does not contain excess iron this effect should be short lived. Use of a sulfur soap occasionally to cleanse skin is very effective when paired with application of such topical fat, and in addition to not excessively washing skin antibiotic oils like coconut oil and shea butter can be used to topically moisturize as well as refatten skin and support the already antibacterial acidic layer. I think the skin condition vitiligo is [perfectly fine and doesn't need to be treated] a condition of fatty acid dysfunction in the skin, and application of these fats to the skin could also help.

Acne does not need to be suffered. Instead of simply avoiding the foods you might like which are high in iron replace them with better options. Your long term health will benefit too.

CHAPTER 30
LOVE AND HAPPINESS

"Nathan," said my new employer on a Thursday at lunch time. "It looks like we won't need you as long as we thought." My stomach suddenly jumped into my chest. I needed this money. I was only three weeks sober, deathly ill from cancer, and sleeping on a friend's couch. I had no money, except a little lent from my mom and dad. I had no car, no home, the few clothes which could fit into a duffle bag, and heartbroken over the demise of my relationship. It was my first non-remote job in a long time after having lived away from Los Angeles for three years. Thankfully I had marketable skills as a graphic artist and a long resume. But it was the only job I'd found after weeks of applications. In fact, it was the only response I'd gotten from any potential employer, and it was supposed to have gone for a whole month and would have supplied me with plenty of money to secure an apartment and lease a car. "Okay, for how long?" I asked. "Just till tomorrow," he said. My heart sank. I was glad to have enough money on the way to buy some food but it would not be enough to get an apartment or a car, never mind what to do for all the other things I needed money like health insurance for my cancer or to afford medication and supplements.

I hurried out of the office on my break before the tears came. I called my mother, that woman of all people who I knew would help me feel better, that woman who was not happy with my medical treatment when I broke my knee in ninth grade and didn't rest until she found me a good surgeon, who helped set up my first apartment, who asked about my first boyfriend when she realized I was in love, who came to visit me in Los Angeles a number of times and invited my once soon-to-be fiancé home to meet the family. Right before I'd gotten sober my parents had actually been volunteering at a Mormon A.A. group (A.A. is *not* supposed to be affiliated with religions though, and this is a highly misguided practice), and when I realized I was an alcoholic they stepped in to help with unconditional love and acceptance, not a hint of the condescension that I had expected and yet another in a long line of examples of God watching out for me, in spite of my best efforts. Initially alarmed by my sobbing she soon realized I was simply down in the dumps and encouraged me to remember it was okay, and things would work out. While talking with her I realized that taking some action to further my situation would make me feel better. After we hung up I called one of the large used car dealerships in Los Angeles and went through the approval process, even though I wouldn't have the money and had to believe another job would come, I could at least get an approval and set things in motion. The agent said he would email me once it went through, and I went back to work feeling a little better. But the hours passed and no email came. Soon I found myself more and more overwhelmed at my situation, and tears threatened to spill once more in front of my coworkers, drawing nearer the point where I might have to excuse myself. *Oh!* I thought suddenly, *the email is probably in the spam folder!* Excitedly I went searching for it. Sure enough there was an email that was not spam, though it wasn't from the car dealership.

'Hi Nathan,' it read, *'I don't know if you're getting my emails because our server has been acting up, but we love your reel and would like to you to come in on Monday if you're available.'* I was astonished. There was yet another email from the same person on Tuesday, also in my spam folder, and I would not have seen these if I had not been let go, called my mom, and resolved to apply for a car loan even though I couldn't afford it at the moment. I was safe once more, even if it was also temporary. In fact, when I went to that company on Monday it turned out they were only interviewing me, though it is unusual to interview freelance candidates since you can just not ask them back if they don't work out, and the person I met with was sour and unpleasant and they didn't end up hiring me. But already this serendipitous turn of events, like so many which have happened through the course of my life impressed upon me the realization that I was being taken care of, even when I couldn't see it and even when it seemed like I was alone. My life was not falling apart, but was being put back together when other things didn't work out. For the first time in thirty-four years I knew that things were always going to happen as they should, and that I needn't worry so much on the outcome. Funny enough, the employer who let me go did so because my work had, unknown to them, caught their project up so fast they were ahead of schedule. Without me they immediately fell behind again. They realized this and wasted no time hiring me back that following Thursday and kept me for an additional four weeks. I got a fat paycheck, secured the car lease, and moved into my own apartment. One day later after securing a new freelance job during which they offered me a full time position being paid a larger salary than I'd ever made in my life, I began to sob uncontrollably when driving home to my new apartment. I wondered why I was crying when things were so good. It dawned on me that I had never cried from happiness before. I was so happy I was crying.

I have had firsthand experience with the strains which money and resources bring to relationships, and indeed life itself. But many couples, parents, and even friends become entrenched in the stress of wants and needs, and even the most beautiful romances can be destroyed by conflicts which arise from financial and social insecurity. Though my own parents' fortunes rose and fell throughout the years and though they fought often about other things, their love was uniquely never burdened by financial stress, at least not openly, and they always seemed to have an appreciation for what they had even when that was very little, and most importantly when it was a lot. As I mentioned before, the opposite of depression is not happiness, but vitality, and when speaking of happiness here I am referring to that satisfaction in things which comes not from having but in appreciating, rather than the physiological state of depression which must be addressed through diet and overall physical wellness. Satisfaction is a more esoteric idea, and often people must go through much misery before they can know what real happiness is, and it always turns out to be different than we thought it would be.

The world is full of unhelpful, asinine advice on acceptance and fulfillment and people who preach about success but recognize value in nothing but money, and how much good does it actually do anyone? Many times while constructing this book and fighting the hatred it brought me when trying to free friends, family, and strangers from their diseases and trauma considered keeping everything in here to myself. Humanity is truly a pusillanimous sore on this beautiful planet, but I also knew that humanity would never get better unless someone could find solutions to the physical and mental illnesses which burden us. Indeed most awful people are just a result of parasitism and childhood trauma, and I eventually realized it was not my job to save people or determine the course of humanity but just to show up for opportunity and do my best, and perhaps my contributions might help future generations be better.

While perspective can greatly help improve the state of happiness, happiness is not a state of mind as is so commonly and derisively viewed. People with problems, real or imagined, being told by someone just to feel differently does not usually help or fix problems, and is in fact the opposite of what happiness embodies, which is not a mindset but a state of existence. So many therapy sessions spent with unhappy people being urged to just change their mindset, setting their intentions to be grateful, less quick to anger, or more forgiving toward themselves and their family continue to find themselves angry, upset, and unhappy because that advice is in fact nothing but an admonition to control life, which is the entire problem, and also entirely impossible to do. Changing mindset can be done but it never, ever comes from willpower and intention but from real behaviors and experiences. If your behavior is aimed to control that which you dislike or fear your mindset will never change. If instead your behaviors are opposite those of control, acceptance will take its place, which is achieved through behaviors like practicing inventory therapy (some people confuse healthy boundaries and control because our tools are limited to those born of trauma, where practicing inventory will clarify what is control and what is healthy boundary setting).

I was often struck by the thought of Wall Streeters jumping from buildings after the great stock crash of the Great Depression as if their fortunes could never be won back. What would a person feel to take such an extreme course of action over something like money that isn't even real? I myself tried to commit suicide over the rejection of my family and friends, does that mean these people regard money with the same devastating importance as people? Money is often regarded with derision too, as if it is dirty, or base, or beneath the dignity of a higher calling. The Dali Lama is quoted as shaming Western cultures for their consumerism, which is an absurd thing to say when you have your very own entourage (and later revealed himself to be a misogynist and probably a child abuser). While it is true that money cannot replace more important things like love and fellowship, money is always a representation of other ideals. To some money means food. To others it means clothes to wear. To others money means a job well done. Money can also be security or authority. Money has always existed because it is merely the form with which we exchange with one another. Money sometimes can even be a favor, where no actual bills or finical currency is exchanged but where the same intimate agreement is made and kept by those involved. Recognizing that money is simply a vehicle through which we interact with other humans helps to clarify what it does in our lives.

If happiness comes from connections to life and those around us then unhappiness comes when we become disconnected from that, and a great majority of people on this earth are in just such a state. The pursuit of money is merely one avenue by which people attempt to establish those connections when they lack the tools to do otherwise. Unable to reach out and say "will you be my friend," people get rich and flaunt their wealth so that others will be drawn to them. Unable to break the impassable walls of intimacy in a guarded relationship our focus drifts to things like money and finances which we use to control others, and then suddenly someone loses a job or gets cancer and can't work and the fraying tether of the relationship is fully severed. Or we find great success but still cannot draw near the person sleeping next to us. Men jumped from the towers of finance not because money has any real importance, but because their only connection to the people around them, a stupid and shallow control mechanism, was taken away and they had nothing left by which to achieve it.

Attaining happiness means to establish connections in life and the people in it without using control. This doesn't mean only reaching out to people, although that is important, but it means taking time to understand ourselves and why we do the things we do, why the things we have gone through needed to happen and how they affected us, and what we can do about moving forward in a way that looks out for our best interests without harming those of others, which on the surface may seem like selfish pursuits such as earning money, working out, or associating with exclusive people but these are only bandaids for deeper problems from which we suffer greatly. We only want money so that people will value us. We only want a good body so that people will desire us. We only want to be smart, or successful, or powerful, or even a nice person so that people will praise us.

But when we attract people with these qualities what they actually love is the thing which attracts them, not who we are, because it gives them a sense of control which in turn leaves both them and us dissatisfied since it is built on illusion and impermanence. Earning money is a replacement for self-worth, working out is a replacement for acceptance, and judging others is a replacement for intimacy and exposing ourselves to be hurt. As I increased in weight I withdrew from others, and then I saw my isolation as proof that weight was an impediment to love. In reality it was my fear of love and hurt, not my weight, which kept me from finding it. Instead of leaving his sorry ass and finding truer connections when the person I loved repeatedly cheated on and abused me and used my shortcomings as his excuse I stayed because I was afraid it was all I could get. But let me tell you my experience afterward showed me there is no shortage of men and women who will date and fall in love with someone for who they are rather than what they look like or how much money they earn, and countless others who need friends just as much as you, and that usually we just don't find them because we hide away out of fear, refusing to be the very thing we desire from others.

Sometimes we hold on to our unhappiness because we have deeply rooted trauma from our past that is difficult to let go of. This sounds a little esoteric, but take for instance that I was so miserable in love with a man who repeatedly lied and cheated and emotionally abused me yet was unable to gather the will to extract myself from the situation. There were perceptions of myself and life which gave me great fear that I would be abandoned, for various reasons, so I held onto that man as tightly as I could and in return tried to control him (which is also abuse). But oftentimes the only way that fear can be exorcised is by experiencing the very thing we are afraid of, in my sake getting fat, sick, and poor and being abandoned, and some part of me went and sabotaged my body, gaining weight and becoming so unhealthy that he would finally be forced to do what I could not—leave.

At the beginning of seventh grade I had only two friends. Already having moved many times throughout my young life a substantive accumulation of friendships had not been possible, and the raucous coalescence of children that occurs in middle school provided a new opportunity to expand my pool of friends, but also to drown in the choppy waters of social adversity. In the first half of the year I strived to find anyone who liked me. Dodging bullies who pulled supplies from my locker or made fun of my tumescent lower lip and lanky appearance, and abandoned by one of my two friends who was tempted away by promise of new pastures I finally began to find myself in the crosshairs of two eighth-grade girls and soon after regularly eating with a group of boys who inexplicably regarded me with some fraternity. But one day as winter break drew near I sat down at that table and stared at the faces of my new friends. An absence of feeling toward them alarmed me, it seemed that each was no more than a mound of soulless clay. I could not find any kind of emotion to remember them by. "I'm moving," I announced. Immediately each of their faces fell, a genuine look of surprise, and sorrow. It touched me that others cared, but I could not feel love for them. It had taken such effort, such vulnerability to find another place only to be ripped yet again from all my emotional links, and the void within me grew too great to evade.

We set out from Salt Lake City to a tiny town tucked into the corner of a great mountain range. "Oh, it's so pretty here!" my mother exclaimed as we pulled onto the small main road. "And look at that park!" Her joy was an overcorrection for what surely were feelings of guilt at yet again ripping their children from solid foundations, and though we went along with the script there was a heavy sinking feeling with the realization that life was never going to be for us the way it was for others. I cried the first day of school every year except sixth grade and my junior and senior years. I used to believe this happened because I was a wimpy, pigeon-toed, crybaby bedwetter and deeply ashamed of an inability to be tough. It wasn't until my late thirties I realized I cried because I had always alone, and grades six, eleven, and twelve were the only years of school I started bolstered by bonds of friendship. Not only was I alone at home, lost among the dregs of unbridled repro-duction and spiritually castrating religiosity, I was also required to navigate a sea of equally strange and unwelcoming peers and adults with no social tools at my disposal or friends to fall back on.

Which is why on my arrival to this small town when a friendly boy tried to insert himself into my life I failed to recognize that someone wanted me as a friend. He was gregarious, charming, the envy of everyone around him (including adults). He must have been flummoxed after spending so much effort inviting me to do things when I did not return the interest, perhaps even wondering if I liked him at all. I eventually fell in with a large group of mostly shallow and similarly indoctrinated friends, and a few of them did become dearly entangled in my own life in spite of my best efforts. But I have never been good at making friends. I know hundreds of people, and a thousand more recognize me for my conspicuous presence, but the key to their hearts eluded me in spite of a lifetime of trying. I am only now, at the age of thirty-seven, discovering what it means to be a friend, to draw close to people, which is admitting the need for them and not in going it alone. My self-destructive tendency to simply not notice when others were there for me came from a very real and debilitating dissociation caused from a childhood wrought with emotional, environmental, and nutritional challenges. But I mistook my readiness to protect myself from neediness and vulnerability as guarding against the appearance of ineptitude, of fear, or inadequacy. To appear strong means removing capacity for friendship, because friendship is based on our shared inability to survive alone. Those who make friends enthusiastically embrace our miserable reliance on each other, but it is not charity nor pity, simply the resolute understanding that a man is not whole unless he is accompanied by other men. We who cannot accomplish this have yet to see the solution in admitting a need for help, for some reason or another having gotten the impression that to do so meant the opposite of friendship.

In the middle of my ninth-grade year I realized one day when one of our friends did something funny that everyone around me was laughing, but I was not. Not out loud. It was a striking realization, that somewhere along the way and for an unknown amount of time I had lost my ability to laugh. Whenever something humorous occurred I would merely smile. Mortified, sad, and embarrassed, I set out to regain my laugh. Too nervous to do it during a spontaneous moment of levity I practiced laughing quietly at home in the mirror. Something that seemed to come naturally to others was for me a skill to be acquired. It sounded jarring and strange, but soon I began to feel more comfortable with the sound of my own laughter and gathered the courage to start sharing it quietly with friends at the right moments. Eventually I found the ability to laugh once again.

Although these things seem like they are only rooted in the mind they are actually also (and mostly) based in the endocrine system. Most of us have grown up with some kind of abusive or traumatic events and suffer to some degree or another from chronic imbalances in the endocrine system. Sometimes this can even simply be caused by some nutritional or environmental factor too. Lack of intimate parenting is pervasive among humanity because such derangements in the endocrine system permanently alter the character and ability of anyone to meet challenges which come later in life, and thus the cycle is perpetuated. Because the endocrine system is unseen we grasp at everything else to cope with the strain, but we fail because we are not working on the correct problem. My would be fiancé often bemoaned in a cyclical pattern his neglectful upbringing, descending into tirades of self pity in such a regular way that soon a connection with lapses in eating became obvious. I took it upon myself to feed him regularly, not just to care for the person I loved and to support his health but also his state of mind, and thus my own, as when he was fed he was a joy to be around and forgot the pain of his childhood. During my adult life, whenever my parents came to visit I experienced a marked improvement in some of the symptoms of my metabolic decline. Most notably the white tongue and leukoplakia which accompanied me for a decade. My parents had long ostracized me from the family for being gay, but also because of their own inability to connect to and to care for others our relationship was always lacking. When these improvements in my health occurred I always assumed it was due to an effect of something I had eaten, but the mind and body are sorely affected by social status and it is inextricably linked to our health prognosis as human animals. When the mind and body perceive isolation or social stress it automatically locks it down, slows the metabolic rate, and can contribute to long-term metabolic problems like weight gain, hair loss, and eventually cancer. The reason the body does this is because a state of isolation means the human animal must have more stores of nutrients and less rigorous use of them in order that they might better survive on their own. Obviously, we aren't really alone with the other millions of neighbors on this planet, but the psychological isolation created by dogma, prejudice, resentment, impatience, and self-righteousness both within families and throughout our society has the net effect of psychologically isolating people from others, thus triggering this metabolic survival mechanism which in turn lowers the long-term health of the individual, since high-metabolic functions like thyroid, thymus, and digestion go with it. This even, and especially, happens to the perpetrators and catalysts of these behaviors, the parents and leaders who demean, harass, and reject family, friends, and neighbors, because their own behavior causes them to be, in essence, isolated from human social intimacy and thus triggers metabolic stagnation within themselves, which can ironically further inflame and exacerbate their behavior from the discomfort and ill-feeling that such a state cultivates, lacking tools that would help them live more effectively are thusly burdened by constant stress, resentment, and disappointment. More severe states of unhappiness such as what accompany egregious behavior as murder, rape, war and violence, sexual abuse, racism, homophobia, etc., originate from a human animal's most basic survival instincts, triggered by ignorance and overwhelming fear of competition and death, those exhibiting such behavior sacrificed by their very biology to desperate acts of self-preservation at the cost of their own social welfare. The man I thought was the love of my life took all our furniture, money, and even my dogs as punishment for wasting his time, and along with the stress of losing my family, health, and difficulty making friendships I would have died if not for discovering these tools to heal my body, mind, and heart, let alone the kind of happiness and fulfillment I find every day, even when I have nothing.

To be truly happy there are only two fairly straightforward steps. The first is to properly care for the endocrine system. This is done by much of the points brought about in this book which include eating regularly to sustain blood sugar and protein levels, addressing physical ailments such as gut health, depression, hypothyroidism, etc., and maintaining a well running metabolic rate which can be measured by methods of pulse, temperature, finger color, and mood such as is outlined in the chapter on self therapy, and most importantly the regulation of the serotonergic center of the brain—the raphe nucleus—and its relationship to light as discussed in the chapter on depression. This takes care of the endocrine system and the balancing of the hormones to attain those which allow us to feel good regardless of what happens around us, which enables us to form bonds with others and repair the chronic pains of the past which originally upset the endocrinological balance. When I had that experience of realizing my life was going to be okay in spite of being let go it was in large part because I had already set out on a dietary and self-care path which was truly restoring the integrity of my endocrine system. This first and foremost allowed my brain chemistry to achieve the change in psyche which would not have happened otherwise, and indeed why I spent so many years suffocating within myself in spite of the same evidence occurring constantly.

The second step in achieving a happiness not dependent on external factors such as money, friends, success, love, health, etc., comes from the kind of enlightenment to our reality which is done through inventory therapy. Sometimes this can be achieved from other methods like mediation, prayer, mental health therapy, etc., but inventory is an easy, direct, and profoundly powerful way to accomplish the kind of perspective therapy through the subconscious which can help to remedy the past adulteration of our true selves which inhibit our connection to life and people. Human instinct is to control those things of which we are afraid, but control is the antagonist of happiness, and learning how to let go of control behaviors is the most effective course to achieving real happiness. Such a practice as inventory therapy which is outlined in the chapter on God and spirituality or my other book on childhood trauma and abuse, *The Perfect Child*, helps to illuminate those disconnections and thus enables their removal and creates space for recognizing exactly how our psyche can be damaged. The inventory therapy illuminates what skills we lack and what control behaviors and fears keep us down which in turn changes our behavior and we become empowered to teach ourselves those tools and life skills that have heretofore eluded us. Many people do not want to attempt such introspection because we most of all fear the confirmation of our insecurities, failures, and mistakes, but this resistance only serves to keep us willingly imprisoned in a cage where the door is in fact wide open and well we must do is walk through it. The writing of past traumas in the format of inventory is the open door, and all that needs be done is to sit down and write.

Like most I used to think that impediments to my happiness were based largely on external factors like my parents, a partner, or professional success (even if that just meant having a job), because such factors were so pervasive and profound in their effect upon my life and I went to great lengths to fight those which were standing in my way or exhaust myself trying to convince others that I was worth loving. More often than not this left me further defeated and falling into greater unhappiness, because the true source of happiness comes from an ability to establish bonds and connections with all parts of our life, even with coworkers and employers whom we might errantly regard as competition rather than compatriots. When we cannot find peace in our work, homes, or love life we must recognize how our internal hormonal state influences our ability to cope. I am always bothered when people say that relationships take work, as if the presence of someone who gives them sex and companionship requires an uncommon use of decency and empathy or employment of the most magnanimous of human qualities, passive-aggressively implying their own superiority and passing judgment on a person they are supposed to support and love unconditionally. Relationships are only difficult for those who are selfish and self-centered, and most difficult for those who lack empathy and self-awareness. Attraction is not love. Many people believe they must lie and scheme or employ other subterfuge in order to get laid, or get into or maintain a relationship. But women are just as horny as men are, and it is far more effective to be upfront and genuine with your intentions while accepting yourself as a human being with limitations, even if what you think you want is not within your power to obtain or somehow shameful, like getting someone into bed for only a night, which arises from attitudes toward your own self worth which were learned in childhood, which can be just as intimate and special as sex in a long term relationship when it is done with honesty and with respect for the other person. I am still friends with and have more intimate relationships with the boys I only used to fuck than those whom I dated or those who pretended to be my friend when really they wanted to get into my bed, because there was no dishonesty between us, and thus a deeper appreciation and admiration for each other, even if it only lasted an hour.

But we are not more powerful than our own biology, and often those who lack empathy and higher emotions are really just suffering from imbalances in the endocrine system caused by a life accumulation of stress both nutritional, social, and environmental. A perceived absence of money, love, or success does not cause unhappiness because we lack anything but the state of elevated stress hormones changes the thinking mind to more acutely recognize patterns of instability, that we may better navigate obstacles which potentially threaten our ability to survive. That is what stress hormones do—they enable us to better meet challenges that impede life. But especially in our high-stress, toxic societies this system is overactive and unhelpful, especially in our unnatural environment, which then causes inappropriate and heightened sensitivity to defects, deficits, and threats, and causes restlessness and discontent even when we have enough, or plenty, or too much, and the solution lies in discovering the proper way to care for oneself first which, while influenced by the psyche and benefits from practices like personal inventory, is primarily affected through the endocrine system. Then, reacting to that stress with ineffective life tools make our lives worse, not better.

One day in my youth during a heated row with my parents my mother exclaimed that family were the only ones who would be there for me, and not two years later they banned me from their home not because I was violent or abusive, or hateful or thieving or even rebellious, but because they didn't like who I was. It is true that parents believe such choices are from a place of love but it is not love for their child, only themselves, their reputations, security, power, and control. I am lucky, though, to have grown up in a less hateful and frightening time than other children like me, who are abused or killed by their parents, friends, and society.

Love is not harsh, it does not harm others even when it must correct. Love is simply the understanding that another person and myself are just as valuable in our respective conditions. If that valuation of another comes up short it is instead selfish, self-centered obsession. Even placing oneself subordinate to another is not love because voluntary subordination is a form of control, of devaluation to endear pity and thus manufacture attention from a target, and by ingenious scheming it devalues the other in seeking to force a response from them, which invalidates their autonomy as an equal and thus cheapens the response. Because love is the recognition of equality love is only reflected in action, in taking care of ourselves as much as we do others and of others as much as we do ourselves. When I was young and traumatized I did not recognize the mere presence of someone as a demonstration of love because I also did not (was not able) care for myself, but later when I learned that skill and finally recognized what love really looks like finally found it from others, because it was there all along and is everywhere in life and the world, but if we do not know what it is can be right under our nose and not even see it.

Much of my generation has learned hard corrections about the nature of love, empowered by the advent of mass interconnectedness in the age of the internet to affect real change within humanity. I love the film *Monsters INC* because the truth that love generates more for everyone, even those who seek personal gain, is a core reality of life. The reason that good always wins is not because good is inherently correct, although morally I believe it is, but that those who employ goodness recognize logical outcomes and those who employ divisiveness and subterfuge are intoxicated by errant and incorrect perceptions about reality and the course of cause and effect. The advent of historic conflicts such as the World Wars, the fall of Rome or the Soviet Union, the decline of the murderous and opportunist Catholic Church of past centuries are such courses of human activity which precipitate on assumptions of reality which actually differ from it. The United States right now is facing its own consequences of generations of exploitation and violence committed toward others and the epidemic of gun violence and political turmoil which is the natural result of past leaders acting on fear and hatred of others. Misunderstanding the boundaries of cause and effect the architects of anti-love think that gain lies through power and conflict, that security and wealth are the fruits of control and suppression, that adversaries are impediments to satisfaction no matter how many times history has proven this folly. The eventual outcomes of these kinds of world events, which finally restored the relative harmony and equanimity came not because good is inherently right but because good is based on logic, the unfearing recognition of facts as they are and not as self-serving interpretation. Operating on illogic, forces of antagonism always lose because they do not operate in reality, believing that things stay the same or that consequences do not exist, believing others to be different than is the case which then undermines their ability to act effectively as they are not in possession of reality.

On a less ridiculous and grandiose parallel our own capacity for enrichment, even for those in business, politics, and government, or as intimate as your marriage, or bond with a best friend, the achievement of success in any form as what comes to those who are the greatest, the wealthiest of men or the most content of hearts is found within the bounds of love, because love is founded on the recognition of equality in all things, the balance of nature, the price of give and take, the continual flux of life. To ignore that equality is to come up short, if not now, later, not only to lose profits of a material nature but also that which is immaterial, to have nothing even when you have everything, because the risks which were difficult to understand or inconvenient to acknowledge were laid by the wayside in deference of ego. To not love is outright stupid. Organic farmers, motivated by a love for their work, for food, integrity, the earth, or the quality of their product earn more from similar effort than the most industrious of agricultural conglomerates while greedy, commercial farmers in places like the Western United States who have gobbled up as much land and resources as possible now succumb to drought and economic ruin because they removed beavers from the land which would normally hold incredible amounts of water in their ponds and wetlands and act as firebreaks to stop raging wildfires. Despite having only two percent the population of the United States, Norway is now the second largest exporter of food in the whole world because their love of progress, of logic, and of human decency has led them to develop methods which are superior to those which only serve mammon. Medical products, supplements, and practices which respect the personal and not just the monetary value of their customers persist to accrue higher margins of profit because they acknowledge reality which thus enables them to persevere beyond the limitations of those which do not. The architects of the opioid crisis have now lost as much money as they ever made scheming to ruin the lives of countless people because they failed to consider the value of the lives they were taking, which mean more to their friends and family than any amount of money. Instead of recognizing the incompatibility of fossil fuels not only with the environment but also market forces, the feeble minds of a once influential industry find themselves up a creek, not because they are not intelligent nor capable but simply because they do not love their fellow man, and this impedes their ability to meet change with innovation because those who do not love do not see. Farmers who show no love for people and soil by using poison chemicals and ruining the natural water tables by clearcutting and destroying natural environments are finding that they themselves are victims in turn through others who lied about the safety of obviously unsafe chemicals, and with the microorganisms in their soil dead and water gone from the land are less able to generate healthy yields without increasingly expensive and contentious and still temporary solutions. To an astoundingly greater degree it profits any person from the poorest and lowest to the highest ranks of human society to first and foremost be motivated from love because it recognizes the boundaries of reality, the inconsequence of pride, the liability of stagnation, and the power of integrity.

I have been a vicim of my own lack of love. A greater force of self-interest ironically prevented me from getting what I wanted most, to be loved by friends and family and fulfilled in a good relationship. Instead of dating men with integrity I chose to date those who were broken and exhibited qualities which could be exploited. Of course, I did this because I had also been broken and my endocrinological systems were misaligned and I misunderstood my own value as a person, but nonetheless it failed to get me what I wanted and likewise it does for all those who act on self-interest, rather than love, regardless of context. Love must be given voluntarily and without expectation. But oftentimes there are psychological impairments to giving and receiving love in a healthy, unconditional manner. In families which are prone to abuse, whether physical or emotional, and most families have some degree of one or the other, there can then exist psychological divisions within each person according to their role and status within the family unit, which ultimately impair healthy bonding with others. This often takes the form of a child being abused in their childhood by parents who are incapable of containing the stress between them, then the child, traumatized by their experience, becomes unable to function as a whole person and takes their broken pieces with them into adulthood, unable to mend the fractured self nor function successfully as an adult. For some reason we expect or are expected to operate successfully even though we have never been given the skills to do so.

Reject connections built on superficial impermanence. Demand to be loved for who you are. Love others for who they are and not what they do or what they look like or how much money they have. Do not mistake your value to other humans originating from the physical body (and avoid those who value it only). Money can bring connection with others, but it is only a medium for something that is more profound and which can be had directly and without it. Besides, a person can be rich in things that are not money but which have real, immeasurable value in life such as good will, integrity, depth of spirit and intellect, contribution to the progress of man, and powers of creativity and talent which can have far more impact on the quality of life than mere material resources. For what good do riches a man without love? He may buy the whole world and have no one to fill it. You must contribute to your community rather than waiting for it to contribute to you. To partake in love we must participate and impart our value as a person, even if that value is merely our presence. If you think you live in a place that is devoid of love, friendship, and togetherness, it is only because you also withhold this from others. Get out and be among people, even if only to sit at a coffee shop or say hi to the person in line with you at the grocery store. Stop trying to control everyone and everything. Act from a place of love in all things. Work for love, community, and creation instead of profit and stuff. Recognize that everyone else, even the worst among us, is trying their best. Friendship is built through familiarity, so finding yourself in the same place repetitiously will naturally lead to an increase in community, no matter where you live. Love is something you must give first in order to receive it. And don't disparage anyone their mortality. Least of all yourself.

Travel With Me

Travel with me,
Across time, holding hands.
The place we left is no longer,
But we weren't going there anyway.

CHAPTER 31
AGING, GREYING, ARTHRITIS, ALZHEIMERS, ETC.

One day when I was seven, in the car with my mother and little sister we stopped at a red light. In the lane next to us was a nice elderly couple. At least, I assume they were nice people but my crazy little seven-year-old self had a different thought. "I hate them," I said out loud. "I hate them too," said my sister, following my lead. My mother turned around to look quizzically at us. "Why did you say that?" she said. "Because they're ugly," I replied. "Yeah, they're ugly," agreed my sister.

I'm not sure what formed this idea—that anyone less than the physical ideal was worth despising. Perhaps it was my mother's propensity to use comments about our appearance to shame us into always being happy. "You look so ugly when you talk like that," she would say when I was a brooding teenager, "I wish I could record you so you could see how ugly you are." Or perhaps it was because of every Disney movie I had ever seen, in which the antagonist is portrayed as physically undesirable. Even *Snow White*, where the evil queen is beautiful, does her misdeeds as an old crone. Obviously this is to pacify Snow White into believing she is harmless, but still, that a seven-year old could intuitively pick up this misguided perception of other people is confounding. My mother took the time to explain that hate was a word we use sparingly, and that it was not nice to judge people based on their outward appearance, but I didn't seem to grasp the lesson. In sixth grade my friends were rather rambunctious, and it was common to tease and cajole anyone who was different (that I was different of orientation not fully realized). It was all too common for us to make fun of a certain girl, who was large in figure. I have often thought of her over the years. She took our teasing in stride but we were pretty ruthless. I deeply regret how much pain I caused her, made worse by the fact that I did actually like her and had secretly wished we were real friends (that's the truth about bullies—we are insecure about our shared need of others).

By the time I was in seventh grade we had once again relocated, and I had to start over in the middle of a school year, by this point a fully developed dissociative personality to cope with inconsistent circumstances and frequent heartache. In spite of this and a strained effort to hide my ever-present fear of being found out as gay, I finally made one or two friends. One evening we attended an after school performance for the theater class, during which I thought to bond with my new friends by engaging in the same kind of disparaging antics I had with my old ones, so I leaned over and whispered, "She sucks doesn't she?" nodding to the girl who front and center was baring her soul in public. He looked at me, and smiled kindly, "that's my cousin." It was the last time I would ever openly mock someone for their vulnerabilities. That this boy continued to be my friend in spite of my reprehensible behavior, showing me the kind of love and acceptance I was not willing to show others made me want to never be like that again.

Thirty years later, having struggled with cancer and physical decline I now understand what it is to be rejected by the world because of mortality. Fear drives people to reject those in whom we see the manifestation of the limits of life, because nobody wants to be confronted by that reality, and evidence of mortality in others comes as a shock to those whom deny their own. Gay men often reject others with HIV even though we should be on the same side, because it represents everything harrowing about life. Straight men reject women who lose their physical appearance because to them it heralds their own oncoming decline. Women will openly mock and reject other women who possess less than they do, because a fear of want for means hits at the deepest fear of dying from lack of resources. We are all keenly aware of our mortality, though we probably don't think of it in those terms, and insecurities about our appearance, our talents, our status, or age paint starkly upsetting boundaries on what is possible in life, and rather than bravely face these realities it is mentally easier to draw attention to limitations in others. Though pointing out these limitations in others has the effect of drawing attention to those people, it is not why we do it—we do it to distract *ourselves* from what we prefer to ignore in ourselves, the fact that our life is also not really our own and that there is very little we actually control, certainly not mortality.

The most ominous marker of this ticking clock of our condition is the decline of the physical body, and seeing it in our parents, friends, partners, and strangers makes it impossible to ignore our own mortality, though we certainly try. Because of entropy, which is a law of the Universe without which we would not even exist, nothing is permanent. Death, heralded by the slow and persistent retreat from youth is unignorable, though some resort to insanity rather than face it. Divisive evangelism, destruction of families, rejection of bonds, pathologic cosmetic surgery, domestic violence, sociopathic focus on money, God, sex, and even wellness fixation are all attempts to put makeup on the face of death. Countless generations have come and gone, and the wisest in every single one have all come to only one conclusion—the only true cure for the fear of death is the acceptance of it. No matter your belief or lack thereof in the supernatural, the truth is none of us actually know what happens after we die. Maybe we do go to heaven, or maybe we are reincarnated to gather more life experience for our soul, or maybe we all simply return to the consciousness which populates all life, but no matter what happens it will be as it is intended, and we can rest easy at night knowing we have made amends for the wrongs we have caused and that whatever happens after death is exactly which is meant to happen, and in all likelihood is just as wonderful as our small chance at life.

Similarly, the way to handle aging, as I understand it, is to work with the conditions of mortality, not to fight them. Nothing in my work or natural process-es is stronger than destructive forces. This is what entropy is, and the reason that our very existence is possible. If it weren't for entropy, and destruction, nothing in our universe would be here. Other things, like stars, must be destroyed for life to develop. To restore aging is to work with the natural ways of biological chemistry as much as is possible, while also avoiding those things which interfere with the biological process, without a concern for preventing the inevitable. Trying instead to force reality and biology to do our will always results in the opposite results we desire, because we are not the ones who control reality.

Being in my early forties there is much I do not know about aging, and I can't imagine I will live to a very old age considering the enormous health stress I've endured, but many of my own conditions were those of premature aging and it has also provided insight into the aging process. Aging is essentially a problem of normal production of energy (ATP) which is no longer efficient or effective and results in an increase in oxidative stress during energy production primarily due to pathogens which colonize the adult human body, and reversing colonization by pathogens and maintaining a diet and behaviors which reduce stress and support the immune system as discussed in earlier chapters helps to arrest or possibly reverse the aging process. But those driven by fear do things like try to eradicate pathogens, which is not the same as supporting the immune system and, like the mass fluoridation of water intended to fight cavities but which also poisons the immune system, instead also kills off our commensal microbes on which we are wholly dependent for B vitamins, short chain fatty acids, and a constant supply of healthful amino acids. While there is nothing wrong with wanting to be healthy, for many the desire to conquer aging is simply a control mechanism for coping with the fear of death, and even if it were possible to live for thousands of years it would never resolve this fear, which is instead a product of childhood trauma that can only ever be resolved through practices like inventory therapy and effective resolution of childhood trauma.

One issue is that aging people often receive artificial replacements for deteri-orating joints or failing organs, because the pain of aging is often unbearable. But artificial body parts are not as wonderful as they seem and in fact can contribute to further rapid deterioration of the human body because our tissues do not ignore foreign implants, even if they are manufactured to a high quality, and one of the mechanisms by which life organizes itself is to communicate with its environment, meaning that when foreign material that is not supposed to be in tissue is detected the body actively produces enzymes to dissolve and detoxify those foreign bodies. An artificial knee, for instance, is slowly but actively dissolved by the body, which not only keeps our healing metabolic pathways around the implant chronically turned on (which is inflammation) but then also actively spreads foreign materi-al like the metals of which it is made throughout the entire body. Large artificial implants start a countdown to death which cannot be reversed since such proce-dures usually also remove living tissue which has been thrown in the trash, and of the many persons I know who have received artificial joint replacement all have shown obvious and remarkable metabolic decline afterward. Taking out body parts is not something which can be easily restored (organ transplant is probably a good idea for those missing their thyroids, parathyroid, etc), and since aging is consid-ered a source of revenue by the medical industry joint replacement and other reception of artificial body parts which cannot self-heal the way our own body does should always be the very, very last consideration in acceptance of the end of life, not its extension.

Very often joint mobility and chronic pain can be resolved rapidly by simply applying topical coconut oil to the skin, which results in local increase in steroid production, as well as a weak aqueous solution of topical *magnesium chloride* as discussed in the chapter on calcium. Also discussed in that chapter is that all pain is mediated by calcium, and joints become stiff also due to calcification, so efforts to restore normal metabolism of calcium not only assists the body in reversing calcification of soft tissue to relieve pain and restore mobility but also to help resolve colonization by opportunistic microbes at the root of disease and aging which used calcium to buffer themselves from the immune system. Similarly, many problems of aging like incontinence, insomnia, fatigue, etc., are primarily rooted in the chronic loss of electrolytes caused by microbes which produce ammonia and dysregulate ATPase pathways as discussed in earlier chapters. The chapter on immunity discusses how failure of the esophageal sphincter muscle due to chloride loss during hypochlorhydria results in acid reflux, but there are other sphincter muscles in the body such as for the bladder and the rectum, so incontinence in aging people is similarly caused by simple deficiency of chloride for the same reasons which prevent those sphincter muscles from working properly.

Common problems of aging also include *osteoporosis* and thinning bones, which ironically also presents with increased calcification of soft tissue as discussed in the chapter on calcium. But what most people do not know is that bone is mostly cartilage, and this gives bones more resilience against breaks and fractures since more brittle things break more easily. Cartilage throughout the body calcifies and stiffens, and arthritis is primarily caused by opportunistic pathogens which long ago accessed the bloodstream and are distributed through-out the body, consuming connective tissue for its amino acids (like glycine and arginine), and becoming inflamed due to chronic but ineffective immune activity. Silicon is one of the primary factors in collagen, which is why collagen has similar physical properties to silicon kitchen implements, being both bendy and stiff and resistant to breaking, so impairment of silicon absorption by ammonia produc-ers and other factors which disturb digestion and the commensal microbiome as discussed in the chapters on cancer, parasitism, and immunity, causes the body to increasingly leach silicon from bones and connective tissue as it tries to maintain mitochondrial silicon to support normal production of energy, and without the resilient properties of silicon, bones become more brittle and joints and other connective tissue more stiff, easily inured, and slower to regenerate. This problem is also compounded by the fact that vitamin C is required to synthesize collagen, and since vitamin C uptake is also silicon dependent as discussed in the chapter on immunity, restoration of silicon absorption with vitamin C by consuming foods high in both silicon and vitamin C, such as lots of fruit, or preparing silicon ascorbate as discussed in the chapter on immunity after meditating resolution of ammonia excess can help bones to regenerate and entirely prevent osteoporo-sis. Sudden repletion with silicon does seem to make old injuries more prone to re-injury, however, as newly available silicon stimulates bone remodeling and new remineralization, so care should be taken when attempting this to protect old inju-ries from pressure and stress, and taking excess silicon ascorbate in desperation to get well can excessively oxidize glutathione to cause significant oxidative stress, patience is key and using only as directed.

Vitamin C deficiency also directly promotes *atherosclerosis* which is the condition that often causes problems like heart attack, stroke, and contributes to thrombosis. This is caused by oxidized forms of cholesterol which build up in the bloodstream to create blockages, but it also affects the body as a whole because cholesterol is required to produce hormones and vitamin D as discussed in the chapter on hormones. Animals which produce their own vitamin C (which primates such as ourselves do not) are shown to be highly resistant to atherosclerosis, and this occurs because copper dysregulation and excessive free circulating copper oxidizes cholesterol, causing it to stick together. Normally vitamin C circulating in the blood scavenges this copper, and studies show that both the reduced and oxidized forms of vitamin C form a complex with copper to liberate cholesterol from its atherosclerotic effect, so cardiovascular problems associated with age can also be reversed by restoring vitamin C through the simultaneous combination with silicon as directed (without using excess which can and will overly oxidize our glutathione).

I found my first grey hair at the age of twenty-one and, like all of my health problems, it was a disheartening development far before its time, not because there is anything wrong with having grey hair but because it was yet another unwelcome omen to portend the end of my already unfulfilled youth, and sure enough my hair readily increased in greyness across the span of my twenties, and when my once thick mat of hair also began fleeing my scalp the combination of hair loss and leaching tint added to my fatigued appearance and served to make me appear approaching fifty rather than my early thirties. I never did put color in my hair, thinking that doing so accentuates a person's age rather than defy it, so I bore my grey hair and enjoyed all the exclamations of "daddy" which came with it. Just as with hair loss and many other health issues the cause of grey hair has many theories, assumptions, and mistruths as there are products and books to sell. Some of them are based in some truth but not exactly the way or reasons which are commonly discussed. Early greying is often a symptom of cystic fibrosis, which is why it happened in my early twenties, but children as young as seven with severe cystic fibrosis will also present with greying hair because the pathway at issue in the condition of cystic fibrosis (as discussed in the chapter on immunity) causes excess release of chloride which then increases the production of hypochlorous acid (which is chlorine bleach) while also causing chloride deficiency.

Melanin pigment in skin and hair is made by copper dependent *tyrosinase* enzymes, but free calcium caused by calcium dysregulation which impairs immunity and promotes tissue calcification also destabilizes copper status, as copper is released from its chaperone proteins by environmental pH, not enzymes as usually occurs with other chaperones, in order to intoxicate pathogens and make them easier to eradicate but then, over time and chronic colonization, more and more disrupts copper status. Simply taking a copper supplement as do most delusional people trying to control mortality mostly causes copper poisoning, because the problem isn't copper but its regulation by complex factors like the production of hydrogen sulfide by microbes, dysregulation of calcium, and disruptions in environmental pH. In fact, because copper metabolism requires functioning biology free of pathogenic interruption, markers of aging and illness we see reflected in our appearance such as the greying of hair and mottling of skin is functionally a reflection of copper status. Vitamin C is also shown in studies to promote copper retention, which it likely does through forming the complex which also protects cholesterol from copper-mediated oxidation. Other studies show that the enzyme which produces the active form of testosterone, dihydrotestosterone, which gives men their most male characteristics is inhibited by free copper, so features of youth and gender are very likely also themselves functions of vitamin C repletion, which is also required for so many other fundamental pathways like collagen, immunity, respiration, etc.

One day at a spa about two years into my recovery I ran into an old acquaintance. I hadn't seen him for almost four years and the last time was not even at the trough of my physical deterioration. He is a specimen of a young man with flawless skin, wavy, deep colored hair, a well formed physique and lean, taught waist. I couldn't help but admire his beauty, especially since he was standing completely naked in the giant hot tub next to me. We got to talking and I mentioned the development of my cancer and subsequent return to physical health. "It's so weird how much younger you look," he said. It was true that I had regrown hair, had a reduction in greying and an improvement in the quality of my skin as well as some restoration of a physique, but I still had a long way to go and would again experience aging as I studied infectious oral pathogens and the function of the immune system in later years. As my aging improves I continue to find restoration of hair, which is now grown almost back to the hairline of my teenage years, as well as skin which gets less fatigued by the day and muscles which are large and easy to maintain. None of this is brought about by products, procedures, discipline, or dieting. The body cannot be restored by cutting, lasers, pharmacological intervention, self-will, or deprivation. The youthful quality of appearance—or rather, *healthy* quality of appearance is determined solely by the proper function of metabolic pathways which maintain the structural integrity of cells, organs, and systems. It is why even wealthy people and celebrities with their limitless resources fail to retain youth, even looking ghoulish as they carve up their bodies and pad it with plastic and silicon, as there is absolutely no artificial way to preserve that which is living.

Many centenarians cite chocolate as a reason for their longevity, but chocolate is just a good source of dietary oxalate, stable saturated fats, citrulline, and copper that are also available from other foods and resources. Chocolate is also a fermented microbial product, made by allowing cocoa to ferment in large containers for several days before distribution and further refining, and so it also contains B vitamins and short chain fatty acids which not only support our health but also that of our commensal microbiome the same way that high prebiotic sources like coffee and tea also support our microbiome. Other fats like butter, coconut oil, and olive oil also contain good, stable fats which directly support metabolic stability (if bile is working properly). Because the skin is a major site of steroidogenesis applying a little coconut oil, cocoa butter, or shea butter to the skin can help it produce its own local pregnenolone to boost skin quality and youthfulness in support of other healthy dietary and behavioral factors required to reverse pathogenic colonization, calcification, etc.

At one former place of employment I noticed that many of the young, new hires who started their employment bright-eyed and cheery would in just six months begin showing sagging eyes, acne, weight gain, and emotional frustration, depression, and anxiety. Casual observers might attribute it to the stress of the job, but honestly it wasn't that bad and these people were so young that such stress should not take that kind of toll on the appearance nor physical and emotional health. At this same place there were video editors who sat in dimly lit rooms all day long, employed by the same people and who worked even longer hours but whom did not display this same accelerated decline in their appearance. These editors proactively turned off the offensive *fluorescent lights* in their bays and instead installed several dim incandescent lamps. The areas where everyone else worked was brightly lit by very strong fluorescent lights. Unfortunately I did not notice this trend until after I also suffered a reversal in my hard-won return to some youthfulness, but which brings me to the final important factor in the aging process—which is light. We get so much free energy from the sun, if you're very perceptive you may have noticed that you or people around you have marked declines in youthfulness immediately at the end of and after wintertime. Oppositely, summertime is an active promoter of health and wellness because of the composition and availability of sunlight. Obviously this requires exposure to such light in the first place in order to benefit, but light is not all good in general. The blue side of the wavelengths of light such as occurs in artificial fluorescent lighting and wintertime stimulate ATP *consumption*, not production, and it is the red and warmer wavelengths in light which stimulate ATP production. It is not that blue light is bad, only that in excess or in isolation it stimulates too much energy consumption, and during too much blue light exposure the body uses up ATP without a coordinate production of ATP from complimentary red light, such as occurs in natural sunlight, and this imbalance contributes to an acceleration in aging since ATP provides our cells with energy and without sufficient energy our bodies cannot resist stress.

The reason fluorescent lights are installed in workplaces, aside from being less expensive than incandescent light, is precisely because the cold spectrum of light was found in studies to stimulate alertness and biological activity. This was thought to encourage productivity and reduce sleepiness, to force workers to work faster and be more productive and so entire businesses and industries installed these lights as an authoritarian, dystopian way to manipulate workers. But the reality is these lights deplete workers of energy, and quite rapidly too, as well as preventing the normal function of vitamin D by simulating the wintertime composition of sunlight, as it does not also provide for ATP replenishment. Sunlight has by percentage more red light, especially during the summertime, because the gasses in our atmosphere scatter a lot of the blue end of the spectrum (which is why the sky is blue), lowering the effective amount which reaches our skin and increasing that of red, especially in the morning and evening hours. But UV light has a higher frequency than the warm spectrum so it penetrates the atmosphere whereas the wavelengths toward the red spectrum bounce off it when not direct. It is important to have exposure to only healthy sources of light, to prevent premature aging and even reverse it, but also to prevent fatigue and exhaustion during the workday, and businesses would do well by their employees and promote stability and productivity by replacing lights with those that have a color temperature of 3000k or less.

Because aging is essentially a deficiency of ATP and a collection of impairments to production of energy, reversing any potential inhibition of energy production such as from microbial ammonia, hydrogen sulfide, deficiency of sunlight, vitamin C deficiency, and immune dysfunction since pathogens are primary inhibitors of energy production can help slow or arrest the aging process. Several times helping women in their fifties through changing their diets, eating behaviors, and self care skills as described in this book found their menstrual cycles restored (which was more likely in that age group since they had not long lost it), as it has been so common for women to enter menopause too early due to harmful ideas about dieting, food, and self worth that most women experience menopause far too early, and even simple dietary practices like starting each day with sugar, sunlight, and vitamin C or blocking avidin's binding of biotin by using vinegar in eggs and salads since this increases production of glutamine can easily accomplish health benefits that slow the aging process and even reverse some symptoms of aging.

Writing this book and making the discoveries I have naturally led me to contemplate a world in which people live far longer than has heretofore been possible. While this is an exciting prospect for the individual it also brings complications of overpopulation and dystopian futures of resource depletion, conflict, and systemic corruption. This is not so likely a scenario as might seem, however, which is mostly an entertainment from popular media since it assumes that all humans will have the ability, access, and more importantly a desire to adopt the practices and principles of this book. That to become a long-lived human requires resolution of stress and trauma which underlie and motivate participation in corruption, conflict, and antisocial behavior it is far more likely that a future of long-lived humans is more peaceable and cooperative than dystopian. This is in fact already the case as seen in cities such as Los Angles, New York, Tokyo, Kinshasa, etc., whose populations alone exceed the historic entirety of living humans at many points in our past but whom live in unprecedented peace and harmony because humans are, in fact, naturally cooperative, empathetic, kind, and helpful. When humans are stressed, uneducated, oppressed, and lacking in resources it shortens lifespan and increases conflict and reproduction rates, while peace and prosperity lengthens lifespan and decreases conflict and reproduction rates. Given these truths there is no real danger of catastrophic overpopulation even in a world where people live decades longer than is typical. Because corruption and crime are driven by trauma that must be resolved to live longer, longer age simply means more time to provide for oneself and contribute to society, especially when supported by policies and institutions, and if systems of universal education and basic guaranteed income are implemented to support the autonomy of citizens and stability of markets it will naturally inhibit corruption and the self-interested in favor of cooperative competition, and the problems of overpopulation will never actualize due to the liabilities of self-interest and denial of reality and the positive sides of human nature that naturally regulate itself.

Almost two years after my cancer diagnosis my health improved to the point of being nearly better than it was in my late twenties. I looked younger and felt better than I had in many years, and finally had enough energy to go dancing with my friends one night at one of my favorite clubs. We danced for hours, on two floors packed with people. I was sweaty and gross but I couldn't remember the last time I had danced like this or that had much fun. While taking a breather I sat down on a bench with a Coke and took in sights that made me feel a little out of place, considering my age, but which filled me with the joy of being alive. An overly intoxicated girl was helped to the bathroom by her only slightly less intoxicated friends. A guy bought two women drinks at a nearby bar. A crowd of college students danced apart from the main room near a large speaker under a closed circuit television playing music videos.

Suddenly a beautiful boy stepped toward me from the crowd. "Hi," he said. I looked behind me, certain I was not the target of his gesture because he was at least fifteen years younger, but there was no one else around. "Hi?" I replied. He smiled, and it gave me pause, his fresh face and bright, beautiful blue eyes which stood out starkly against his dark skin was the kind of beauty that will make me start to laugh because it's so overwhelmingly wonderful to see. I was sure he was going to ask if I knew where the bathroom was. "Want to dance?" he said, a hint of nervousness in his voice. This had to be a mistake."I need to take a break," I said, a little confused by what was happening, pointing at my sweaty tank top. His face fell for the briefest instant. I smiled. "Want to sit with me?" I said. He smiled again and sat down, and suddenly I noticed his hands shaking ever so slightly, unsure of what position to be in. He really was hitting on me, and I couldn't believe it. I'd gone out with one or two handsome guys over the last two years, but nobody as beautiful as this had ever looked at me even when I was younger, let alone approached me on purpose.

"I'm Alfred," he said.

"Hi, I'm Nathan."

We talked for a little while. He was twenty-one and an architecture student, a Los Angeles native and possessed of all the innocent love that such newly minted adults bring straight from childhood. I wanted to draw out that moment into eternity, to spend forever like this with someone who didn't know what pain life could bring. He was charming and sweet, and a little brazen (obviously). He asked me about myself and before long my energy returned and we went to the dance floor. He was so nervous he danced stiff and rigid. I placed my hands around his waist and led him into a gentle, fluid sway to the music, showing him how to relax and dance close with an object of desire, not dissimilar from that boy who taught me to kiss all those years ago. It was easy because I desired him too. After a few minutes he caught on and our bodies pressed together in a smooth and passionate rhythm amongst a sea of throbbing, young, sweaty life as the music penetrated our very beings. He looked into my eyes, unafraid and happy, and I kissed him. He kissed me back, and we became those people locked at the lips on the dance floor for what must have been an hour or more. *I am way too old to be doing this*, I thought. But I didn't care. He felt amazing in my arms, his soft lips against mine. I felt alive again.

He gave me his number, but I didn't call because I would have immediately fallen in love with him, and I still had health issues to deal with and work to do which would have destroyed a budding romance, especially with someone so young. I might not be giving him enough credit—he could have been a golden-hearted boy who would love me until I lay down in my grave. I'd like to believe he was. It was written all over his face. More likely our ages and issues would have been too disparate to really work. I was also afraid I could not survive another heartbreak, should he see me in bright daylight no longer through beer-goggles and decide he had made a mistake. So instead I cherish that night, a moment when I came back to life because of someone brave enough to approach a stranger.

The years since my recovery have been nothing if not a rebirth, and while there is not yet a happy ending to my story I suppose there is a happy ending to this book, since my depression has been gone now for nearly a decade, no longer suffering under the stress of sleepless nights and physical illness, without the requirement for medical support and for the first time in my life I am happy alone, finding the absence of anyone or anything in my life strangely and paradoxically holding a thrill of greatest promise, as if I were a teenager once again and had my whole life ahead of me. In a way I do, no longer restrained by the chains of the past both psychological and physical the way forward will be something new, with richer depths and deeper, truer love. My achievements uncovering the mysteries to health issues which have plagued humanity has given me a chance to age backward, to recapture a bit of my lost youth and a new birth at life. Maybe there is a second chance to it better this time. If only I had known how much people love each other. If only I could go back to kindergarten and start over. There is so much I wish I could do differently. But then, this book would not exist.

For more information on health, wellness, and living in harmony with the human condition, recipes which fit within the dietary guidelines proposed throughout this book, and to stay up to date on my latest work please visit fuckportioncontrol.com. *The Perfect Child* is my book on psychology which explores the trauma and abuse of childhood and how to be a better parent through self-care and resolution of unresolved trauma, and *Under A Libra God* explores scientific justifications for spirituality.

A special thank you also to all the many people who have supported my work over the years and made this research and writing possible, without your financial and moral support my work would not have been possible.

www.ingramcontent.com/pod-product-compliance
Lightning Source LLC
Chambersburg PA
CBHW060018030426
42334CB00019B/2082